PRINCIPLES and BIOMECHANICS of ALIGNER TREATMENT

PRINCIPLES and BIOMECHANICS of ALIGNER TREATMENT

Ravindra Nanda, BDS, MDS, PhD
Professor Emeritus
Department of Orthodontics
University of Connecticut Health Center
Farmington, Connecticut, USA

Tommaso Castroflorio, DDS, PhD, Ortho. Spec.
Department of Surgical Sciences, Postgraduate School of Orthodontics
Dental School, University of Torino
Torino, Italy

Francesco Garino, MD, Ortho. Spec.
Private Practice
Torino, Italy

Kenji Ojima, DDS, MDSc
Private Practice
Tokyo, Japan

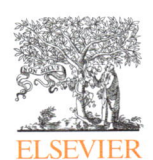

ELSEVIER

Elsevier
3251 Riverport Lane
St. Louis, Missouri 63043

PRINCIPLES AND BIOMECHANICS OF ALIGNER TREATMENT, FIRST EDITION

ISBN: 9780323683821

Copyright © 2022 by Elsevier, Inc. All rights reserved.

No part of this publication may be reproduced or transmitted in any form or by any means, electronic or mechanical, including photocopying, recording, or any information storage and retrieval system, without permission in writing from the publisher. Details on how to seek permission, further information about the Publisher's permissions policies and our arrangements with organizations such as the Copyright Clearance Center and the Copyright Licensing Agency, can be found at our website: www.elsevier.com/permissions.

This book and the individual contributions contained in it are protected under copyright by the Publisher (other than as may be noted herein).

Notices

Practitioners and researchers must always rely on their own experience and knowledge in evaluating and using any information, methods, compounds or experiments described herein. Because of rapid advances in the medical sciences, in particular, independent verification of diagnoses and drug dosages should be made. To the fullest extent of the law, no responsibility is assumed by Elsevier, authors, editors or contributors for any injury and/or damage to persons or property as a matter of products liability, negligence or otherwise, or from any use or operation of any methods, products, instructions, or ideas contained in the material herein.

ISBN: 9780323683821

Content Strategist: Joslyn Dumas
Content Development Manager: Ellen Wurm-Cutter
Content Development Specialist: Rebecca Corradetti
Publishing Services Manager: Shereen Jameel
Project Manager: Nadhiya Sekar
Design Direction: Patrick Ferguson

Printed in India

Last digit is the print number: 9 8 7 6 5 4 3

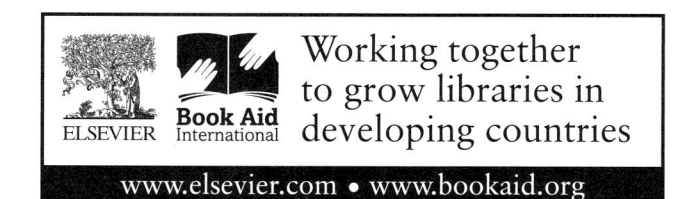

To Catherine, for her love, support, inspiration, and encouragement.
RN

To Katia, for showing me what love is and for keeping my feet on the ground. To Alessandro, Matilda, and Sveva, because you made the world a brighter place. To my friends, Francesco and Kenji, for your passion, enthusiasm, commitment, and support: you are always an example to follow. To Ravi, for your trust and friendship, for your guidance and leadership: you have translated a vision into reality. It was a wonderful journey with you; thanks for your time and for sharing your experience.
TC

I would like to dedicate this book to all my family with a special thought to my dad, mentor and a visionary, who shared with me a passion in aligner orthodontics for 20 years.
FG

My thanks to Francesco and Tommaso for sharing their friendship with me over so many years. The time I spent writing this book with Ravi was amazing, like a dream for me. I am truly grateful to my family for all of their support.
KO

Contributors

Masoud Amirkhani, PhD
Institute for Experimental Physics
Ulm University
Ulm, Germany

Sean K. Carlson, DMD, MS
Associate Professor
Department of Orthodontics
School of Dentistry, University of the Pacific
San Francisco, California, USA

Tommaso Castroflorio, DDS, PhD, Ortho. Spec.
Researcher and Aggregate Professor
Department of Surgical Sciences, Postgraduate School of Orthodontics
Dental School, University of Torino
Torino, Italy
Orthodontics Unit
San Giovanni Battista Hospital
Torino, Italy

Chisato Dan, DDS
Private Practice
Smile Innovation Orthodontics
Tokyo, Japan

Iacopo Cioffi, DDS, PhD
Associate Professor
Division of Graduate Orthodontics and Centre for Multimodal Sensorimotor and Pain Research
Faculty of Dentistry
University of Toronto
Toronto, Ontario, Canada

David Couchat, DDS, Ortho. Spec.
Private Practice
Cabinet d'Orthodontie du dr. Couchat
Marseille, France

Fayez Elkholy, DDS
Senior Physician
Department of Orthodontics
Ulm University
Ulm, Germany

Francesco Garino, MD Ortho. Spec.
Private Practice
Studio Associato dott.ri Garino
Torino, Italy

Aldo Giancotti, DDS MS
Researcher and Aggregate Professor
Department of Clinical Sciences and Translational Medicine
University of Rome "Tor Vergata"
Rome, Italy

Juan Pablo Gomez Arango, DDS, MSc
Associate Professor
Orthodontics Program
Universidad Autonoma de Manziales
Manziales, Colombia

Mario Greco, DDS, PhD
Visiting Professor
University of L'Aquila
L'Aquila, Italy
Visiting Professor
University of Ferrara
Ferrara, Italy

Luis Huanca, DDS, MS, PhD
Research Associate
Department of Orthodontics
University of Geneva
Geneva, Switzerland

Josef Kučera, MUDr., PhD
Assistant Professor
Department of Orthodontics
Clinic of Dental Medicine
First Medical Faculty
Charles University
Prague, Czech Republic
Lecturer
Department of Orthodontics
Clinic of Dental Medicine
Palacký University
Olomouc, Czech Republic

Bernd G. Lapatki, DDS, PhD
Department Head and Chair
Department of Orthodontics
Ulm University
Ulm, Germany

Luca Lombardo, DDS, Ortho. Spec.
Chairman and Professor
Postgraduate School of Orthodontics
University of Ferrara
Ferrara, Italy

Tiantong Lou, DMD, MSc
Division of Gradual Orthodontics and Centre for Multimodal Sensorimotor and Pain Research
Faculty of Dentistry
University of Toronto
Toronto, Ontario, Canada

Kamy Malekian, DDS, MSc
Private Practice
Clinica Bio
Madrid, Spain

Gianluca Mampieri, DDS, MS, PhD
Researcher and Aggregate Professor
Department of Clinical Sciences and Translational Medicine
University of Rome "Tor Vergata"
Rome, Italy

Edoardo Mantovani, DDS, Ortho. Spec.
Research Associate
Department of Surgical Sciences, Postgraduate School in Orthodontics
Dental School, University of Torino
Torino, Italy

Ivo Marek, MUDr., PhD
Assistant Professor
Department of Orthodontics
Clinic of Dental Medicine
Palacký University
Oloumouc, Czech Republic
Consultant
Department of Orthodontics
Clinic of Dental Medicine
First Medical Faculty
Charles University
Prague, Czech Republic

Ravindra Nanda, BDS, MDS, PhD
Professor Emeritus
Division of Orthodontics
Department of Craniofacial Sciences
University of Connecticut School of Dental Medicine
Farmington, Connecticut, USA

Kenji Ojima, DDS, MDSc
Private Practice
Smile Innovation Orthodontics
Tokyo, Japan

Simone Parrini, DDS, Ortho. Spec.
Research Associate
Department of Surgical Sciences, Postgraduate School in Orthodontics
Dental School, University of Torino
Torino, Italy

Serena Ravera, DDS, PhD, Ortho. Spec.
Research Associate
Department of Surgical Sciences, Postgraduate School in Orthodontics
Dental School, University of Torino
Torino, Italy

Gabriele Rossini, DDS, PhD, Ortho. Spec.
Research Associate
Department of Surgical Sciences, Postgraduate School in Orthodontics
Dental School, University of Torino
Torino, Italy

Waddah Sabouni, DDS, Ortho. Spec.
Private Practice
Cabinet d'Orthodontie du dr. Sabouni
Bandol Rivage
Sanary-sur-Mer, France

Silva Schmidt, DDS
Department of Orthodontics
Ulm University
Ulm, Germany

Jörg Schwarze, DDS, PhD, Ortho. Spec.
Private Practice
Kieferorthopädische Praxis Dr. Jörg Schwarze
Cologne, Germany

Giuseppe Siciliani, MD, DDS
Chairman and Professor
School of Dentistry
University of Ferrara
Ferrara, Italy

Ali Tassi, BSc, DDS, MCID (Ortho)
Assistant Dean and Chair
Division of Graduate Orthodontics
Schulich School of Medicine and Dentistry
The University of Western Ontario
London, Ontario, Canada

Johnny Tran, DMD, MCID
Division of Graduate Orthodontics
Schulich School of Medicine and Dentistry
The University of Western Ontario
London, Ontario, Canada

Flavio Uribe, DDS, MDentSc
UConn Orthodontics Alumni/Nanda Orthodontics Endowed Chair
Program Director and Chair
Division of Orthodontics
Department of Craniofacial Sciences
University of Connecticut
School of Dental Medicine
Farmington, Connecticut, USA

Benedict Wilmes, DDS, MSc, PhD
Professor
Department of Orthodontics
University of Düsseldorf
Düsseldorf, Germany

Foreword

Aligners represent the new frontier in the art and science of orthodontics. This new frontier offers new opportunities and challenges, but also requires the need for additional knowledge. A rethinking of biomechanics and force delivery concepts is needed along with the role of materials used for aligners. There is a need for combining established concepts with new tools and technologies which aligner treatment requires.

When considering new methodologies, orthodontists should always remember that technology is a tool and not the goal. Diagnosis, treatment plan, and biomechanics are always the key elements of successful treatment, regardless of the treatment methodology. Aligner orthodontics is quite different than traditional methods with brackets and wires. Force delivery with aligners is through plastic materials. Thus, the knowledge of the aligner materials, physical properties, attachment design, and the sequentialization protocol is crucial for treatment of malocclusions. It is also imperative to understand limitations of aligner treatment and how to overcome them with the use of miniscrews and auxiliaries.

Aligner treatment requires new knowledge; the number of clinical and scientific reports about all the different aspects of aligner orthodontics is increasing year by year. This book represents an up-to-date summary of the available research in the field as well as a clinical atlas of treated patients based on the current evidence. We have made an attempt to provide benchmark for clinicians, researchers, and residents who want to improve their skills in aligner orthodontics.

We would like to express our great appreciation to all the friends and colleagues who have contributed to this book. It was a pleasure to work with all these talented orthodontists.

We would like to say thank you to the Elsevier team for their support, patience, and guidance during the challenging Covid pandemic.

Ravindra Nanda
Tommaso Castroflorio
Francesco Garino
Kenji Ojima

Contents

1 *Diagnosis and Treatment Planning in the Three-Dimensional Era* 1
TOMMASO CASTROFLORIO, SEAN K. CARLSON, and FRANCESCO GARINO

2 *Current Biomechanical Rationale Concerning Composite Attachments in Aligner Orthodontics* 13
JUAN PABLO GOMEZ ARANGO

3 *Clear Aligners: Material Structures and Properties* 30
MASOUD AMIRKHANI, FAYEZ ELKHOLY, and BERND G. LAPATKI

4 *Influence of Intraoral Factors on Optical and Mechanical Aligner Material Properties* 35
FAYEZ ELKHOLY, SILVA SCHMIDT, MASOUD AMIRKHANI, and BERND G. LAPATKI

5 *Theoretical and Practical Considerations in Planning an Orthodontic Treatment with Clear Aligners* 42
TOMMASO CASTROFLORIO, GABRIELE ROSSINI, SIMONE PARRINI

6 *Class I Malocclusion* 51
MARIO GRECO

7 *Aligner Treatment in Class II Malocclusion Patients* 66
TOMMASO CASTROFLORIO, WADDAH SABOUNI, SERENA RAVERA, and FRANCESCO GARINO

8 *Aligners in Extraction Cases* 83
KENJI OJIMA, CHISATO DAN, and RAVINDRA NANDA

9 *Open-Bite Treatment with Aligners* 95
ALDO GIANCOTTI and GIANLUCA MAMPIERI

10 *Deep Bite* 109
LUIS HUANCA, SIMONE PARRINI, FRANCESCO GARINO, and TOMMASO CASTROFLORIO

11 *Interceptive Orthodontics with Aligners* 121
TOMMASO CASTROFLORIO, SERENA RAVERA, and FRANCESCO GARINO

12 *The Hybrid Approach in Class II Malocclusions Treatment* 137
FRANCESCO GARINO, TOMMASO CASTROFLORIO, and SIMONE PARRINI

13 *Aligners and Impacted Canines* 149
EDOARDO MANTOVANI, DAVID COUCHAT, TOMMASO CASTROFLORIO

14 *Aligner Orthodontics in Prerestorative Patients* 168
KENJI OJIMA, CHISATO DAN, and TOMMASO CASTROFLORIO

15 *Noncompliance Upper Molar Distalization and Aligner Treatment for Correction of Class II Malocclusions* 190
BENEDICT WILMES and JÖRG SCHWARZE

16 *Clear Aligner Orthodontic Treatment of Patients with Periodontitis* 202
TOMMASO CASTROFLORIO, EDOARDO MANTOVANI, and KAMY MALEKIAN

17 *Surgery First with Aligner Therapy* 235
FLAVIO URIBE and RAVINDRA NANDA

18 *Pain During Orthodontic Treatment: Biologic Mechanisms and Clinical Management* 252
TIANTONG LOU, JOHNNY TRAN, ALI TASSI, and IACOPO CIOFFI

19 *Retention and Stability Following Aligner Therapy* 259
JOSEF KUČERA and IVO MAREK

20 *Overcoming the Limitations of Aligner Orthodontics: A Hybrid Approach* 275
LUCA LOMBARDO and GIUSEPPE SICILIANI

Index 290

1 Diagnosis and Treatment Planning in the Three-Dimensional Era

TOMMASO CASTROFLORIO, SEAN K. CARLSON, and FRANCESCO GARINO

Introduction

Orthodontics and dentofacial orthopedics is a specialty area of dentistry concerned with the supervision, guidance, and correction of the growing or mature dentofacial structures, including those conditions that require movement of teeth or correction of malrelationships and malformations of their related structures and the adjustment of relationships between and among teeth and facial bones by the application of forces and/or the stimulation and redirection of functional forces within the craniofacial complex.[1]

To accurately diagnose a malocclusion, orthodontics has adopted the problem-based approach originally developed in medicine. Every factor that potentially contributes to the etiology and that may contribute to the abnormality or influence treatment should be evaluated. Information is gathered through a medical and dental history, clinical examination, and records that include models, photographs, and radiographic imaging. A problem list is generated from the analysis of the database that contains a network of interrelated factors. The diagnosis is established after a continuous feedback between the problem recognition and the database (Fig. 1.1). Ultimately, the diagnosis should provide some insight into the etiology of the malocclusion.[2]

Orthodontics diagnosis and treatment planning are deeply changing in the last decades, moving from two-dimensional (2D) hard tissue analysis and plaster cast review toward soft tissue harmony and proportions analyses with the support of three-dimensional (3D) technology. A detailed clinical examination remains the key of a good diagnosis, where many aspects of the treatment plan reveal themselves as a function of the systematic evaluation of the functional and aesthetic presentation of the patient.[3]

The introduction of a whole range of digital data acquisition devices (cone-beam computed tomography [CBCT], intraoral and desktop scanner [IOS and DS], and face scanner [FS]), planning software (computer-assisted design and computer-assisted manufacturing [CAD/CAM] software), new aesthetic materials, and powerful fabrication machines (milling machines, 3D printers) is changing the orthodontic profession (Fig. 1.2).

As a result, clinical practice is shifting to virtual-based workflows.[4] Today it is common to perform virtual treatment planning and to translate the plans into treatment execution with digitally driven appliance manufacture and placement using various CAD/CAM techniques from printed models, indirect bonding trays, and custom-made brackets to robotically bend wires or aligners. Furthermore, it is becoming possible to remotely monitor treatment and to control it.[5]

The introduction of aligners in the orthodontics field led the digital evolution in orthodontics. The two nouns *evolution* and *revolution* both refer to a change; however, there is a distinctive difference between the change implied by these two words. Evolution refers to a slow and gradual change, whereas revolution refers to a sudden, dramatic, and complete change. What has been claimed as the "digital revolution" in orthodontics should be claimed as the "digital evolution" in orthodontics. Orthodontics and biomechanics have always had the same definitions, and we as clinicians should remember that technology is an instrument, not the goal. This differentiates orthodontists from marketing people.

The diagnosis and problem list is the framework that dictates the treatment objectives for the patient. Once formulated, the treatment plan is designed to address those objectives.[2] In aligner orthodontics, CAD software displays treatment animations, helping the clinician to visualize the appearance of teeth and face that is desired as treatment outcome; however, those animations should be deconstructed by the orthodontist frame by frame or stage by stage, to define how to address the treatment goal from mechanics to sequence. Only an accurate control of every single stage of the virtual treatment plan can produce reliable results. As usual, it is the orthodontist rather than the technique itself that is responsible for the treatment outcome.

Contemporary records should facilitate functional and aesthetic 3D evaluation of the patient.

Intraoral Scans and Digital Models

IOSs are quickly replacing traditional impressions and plaster models. These scanners generally contain a source of risk for inaccuracy because multiple single 3D images are assembled to complete a model. Recent studies, however, have shown that the trueness and precision of IOSs of commercially available scanning systems are excellent for orthodontic applications.[6] Digital models are as reliable as traditional plaster models, with high accuracy, reliability, and reproducibility (Fig. 1.3).

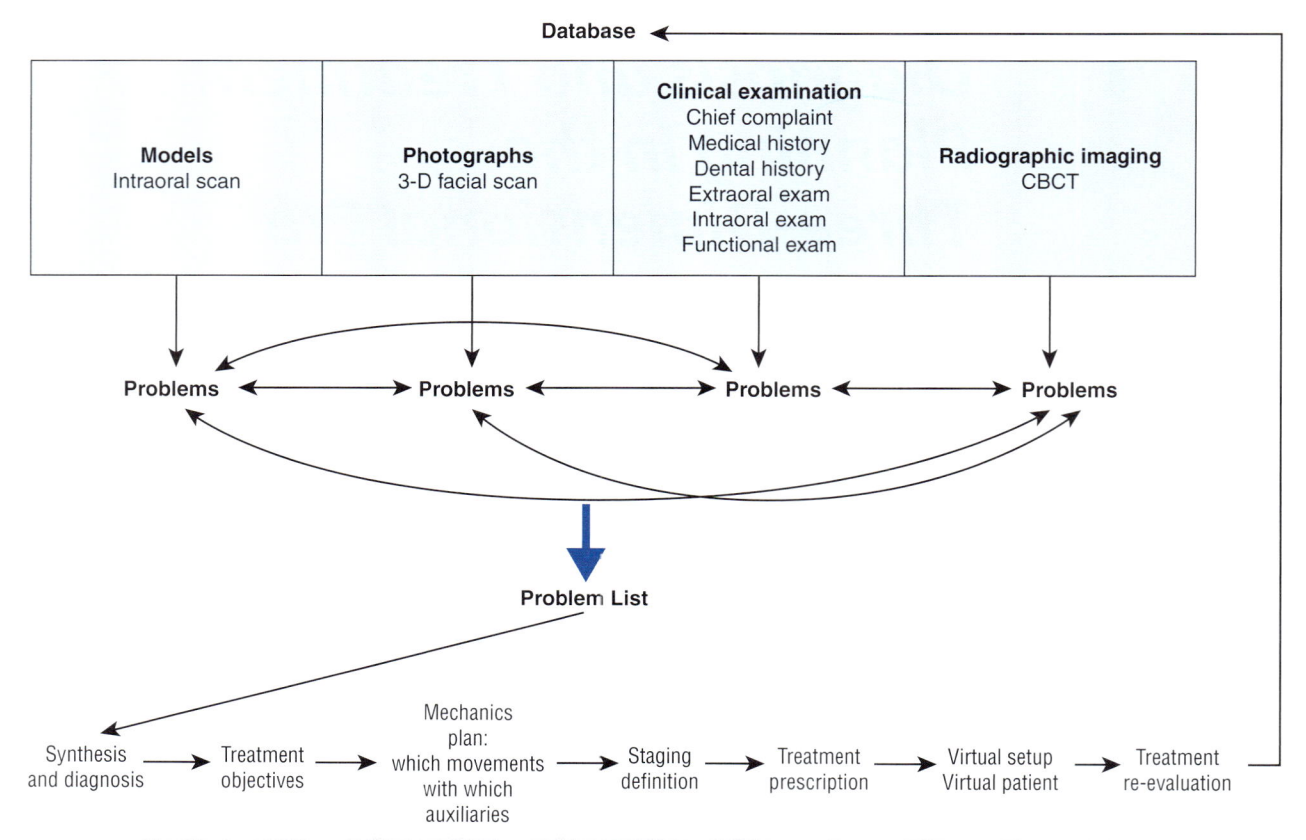

2   Principles and Biomechanics of Aligner Treatment

```
                              Database ←─────────────────────────────┐
                                                                      │
┌──────────────┬──────────────┬──────────────────┬──────────────────┐ │
│              │              │ Clinical examination                │ │
│              │              │   Chief complaint                   │ │
│   Models     │ Photographs  │   Medical history │ Radiographic    │ │
│ Intraoral scan│ 3-D facial scan│ Dental history │   imaging       │ │
│              │              │   Extraoral exam  │     CBCT        │ │
│              │              │   Intraoral exam  │                 │ │
│              │              │   Functional exam │                 │ │
└──────┬───────┴──────┬───────┴─────────┬────────┴────────┬─────────┘ │
       ↓              ↓                 ↓                 ↓           │
   Problems ←──→  Problems  ←──→    Problems  ←──→    Problems        │
                                                                      │
                              ↓                                       │
                         Problem List                                 │
                              ↓                                       │
                                                                      │
                         Mechanics                                    │
                           plan:                                      │
  Synthesis  → Treatment → which movements → Staging   → Treatment → Virtual setup → Treatment ──┘
and diagnosis  objectives  with which        definition  prescription Virtual patient re-evaluation
                           auxiliaries
```

Fig. 1.1 Steps in diagnosis and treatment planning in the digital orthodontics era. (Modified from Uribe FA, Chandhoke TK, Nanda R. Individualized orthodontic diagnosis. In: Nanda R, ed. *Esthetics and Biomechanics in Orthodontics.* 2nd ed. St Louis, MO: Elsevier Saunders; 2015:1-32.)

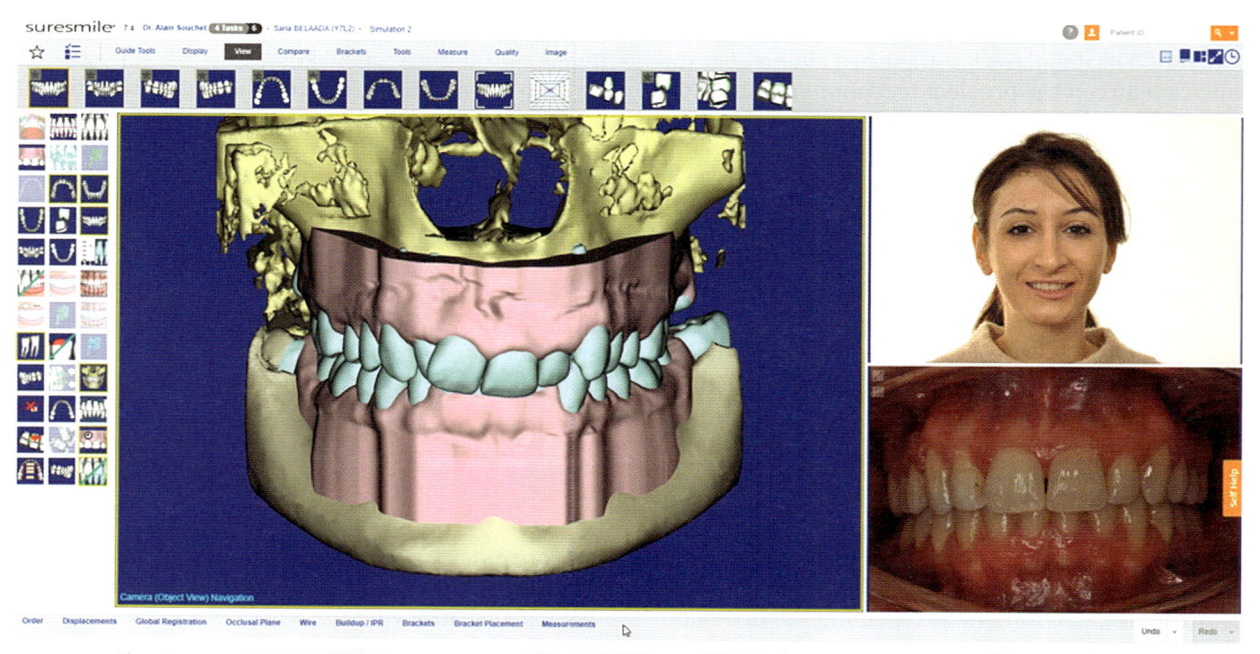

Fig. 1.2 Integration of cone-beam computed tomography data, facial three-dimensional scan, digital models from intraoral scans, and virtual orthodontic setup. Courtesy of dr. Alain Souchet, Mulhouse, France.

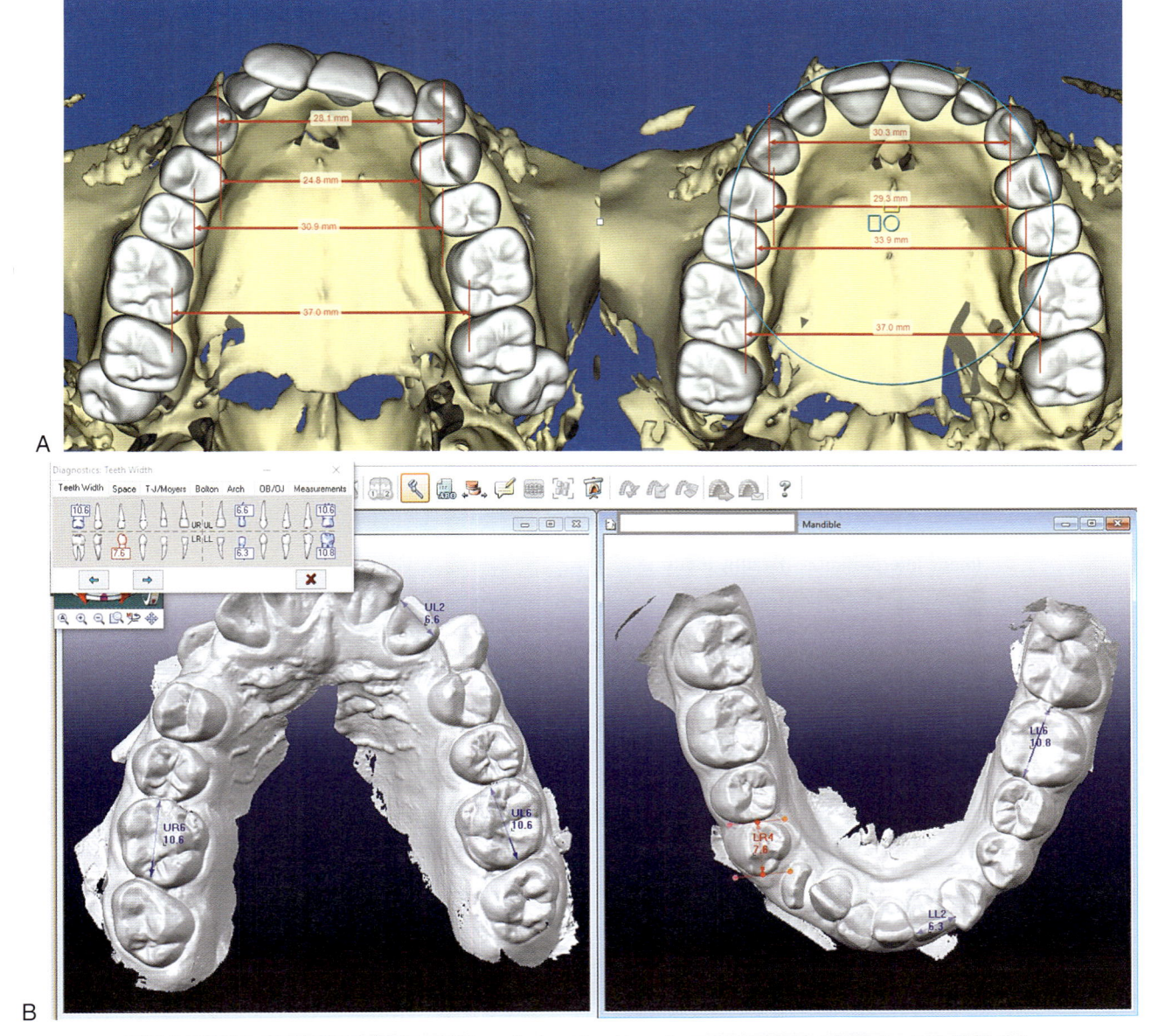

Fig. 1.3 (A) Digital models and measurements obtained from cone-beam computed tomography data. (B) Digital models and measurements obtained from intraoral scans.

Furthermore, the models can also be used in various orthodontic software platforms to allow the orthodontist to perform virtual treatment plans and explore various treatment plans within minutes as opposed to expensive and time-consuming diagnostic setups and waxups. Performing digital setups not only allows the clinician to explore a number of treatment options in a simple manner but also facilitates better communication with other dental professionals, especially in cases that require combined orthodontic and restorative treatments. The virtual treatment planning also allows for better communication with patients and allows them to visualize the treatment outcome and understand the treatment process.[5]

Further advantages of virtual models of the dental arches are related to study model analysis, which is an essential step in orthodontic diagnostics and treatment planning. Compared to measurements on physical casts using a measuring loop and/or caliper, digital measurements on virtual models usually result in the same therapeutic decisions as evaluations performed the traditional way.[7] Furthermore, with their advantages in terms of cost, time, and space required, digital models could be considered the new gold standard in current practice.[6]

Digital impressions have proven to reduce remakes and returns, as well as increase overall efficiency. The patient also benefits by being provided a far more positive experience. Current development of novel scanner technologies (e.g., based on multipoint chromatic confocal imaging and dual wavelength digital holography) will further improve the accuracy and clinical practicability of IOS.[7]

Recently near infrared (NIR) technology has been integrated in IOS. The NIR is the region of the electromagnetic spectrum between 0.7 and 2 μm (Fig. 1.4). The interaction of specific light wavelengths with the hard tissue of the

4 Principles and Biomechanics of Aligner Treatment

NIRI - A reflective concept of light and its mechanism of action

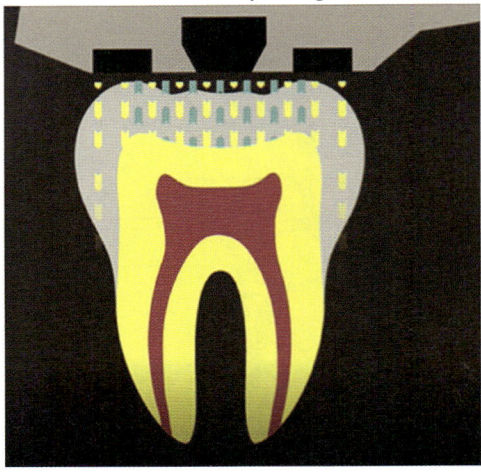

The iTero Element 5D intraoral scanner uses light of 850nm that penetrates into the tooth structure to produce a NIRI image

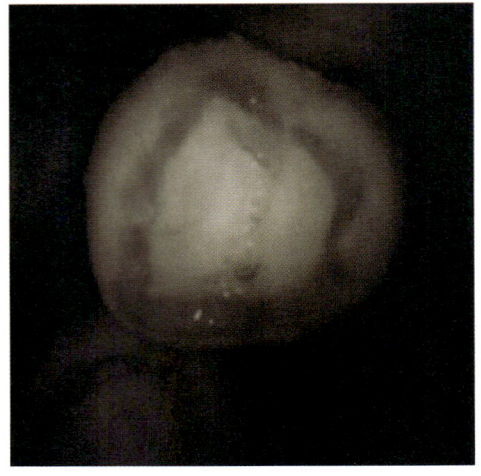

NIRI image of a healthy tooth

Image interpretation - Healthy tooth

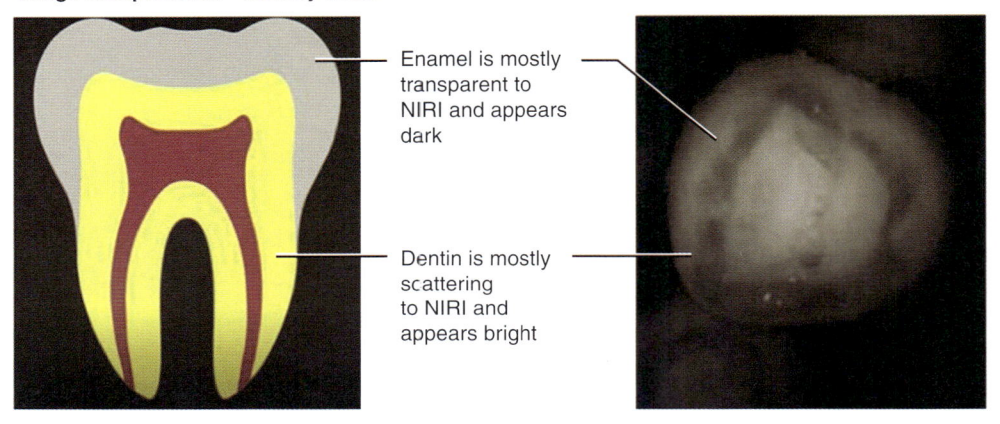

- Enamel is mostly transparent to NIRI and appears dark
- Dentin is mostly scattering to NIRI and appears bright

Image interpretation - Tooth with caries

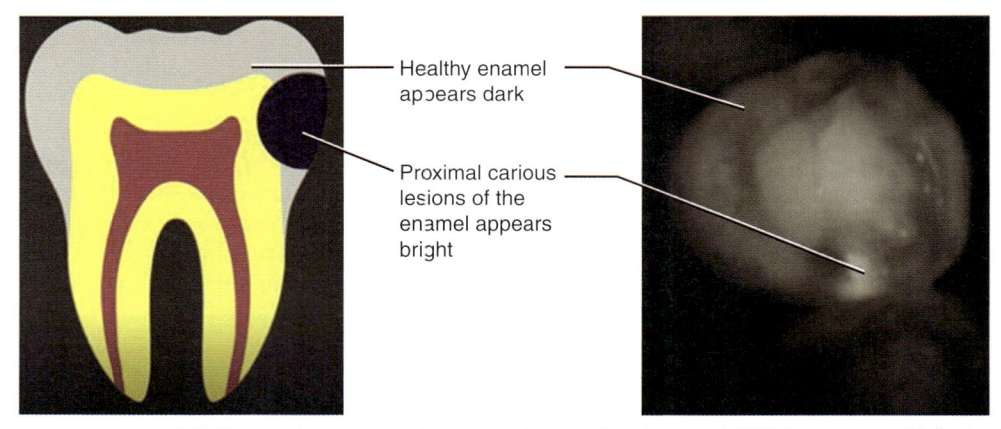

- Healthy enamel appears dark
- Proximal carious lesions of the enamel appears bright

A

Fig. 1.4 New generation of intraoral scanners with integrated near infrared (NIR) technology. (A) Itero Element 5D (Align Technology, San José, CA, USA) decays detection scheme.

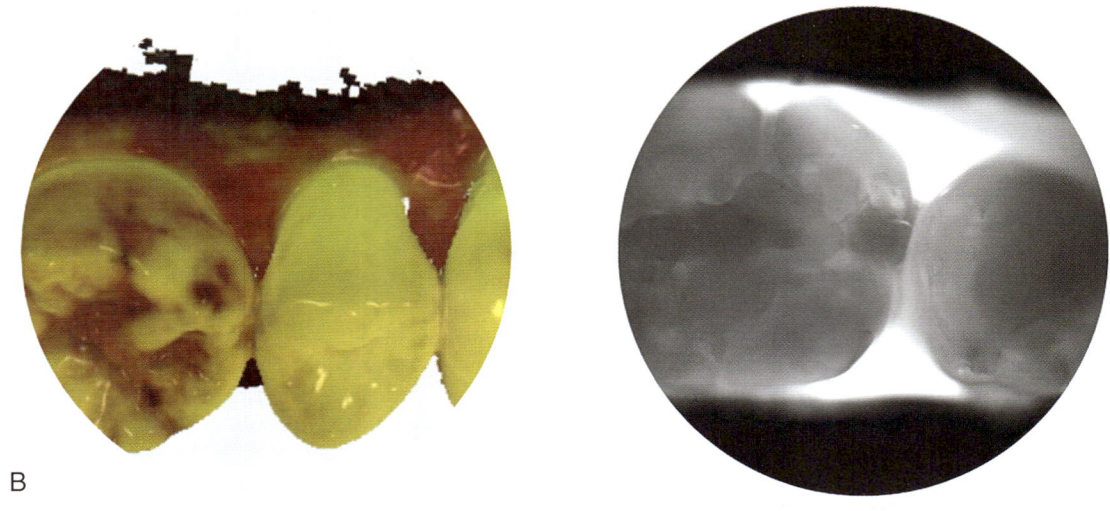

Fig. 1.4, cont'd (B) 3Shape Trios 4 (3Shape A/S, Copenhagen, Denmark) fluorescent technology for surface decay detection *(left)* and NIR technology for interproximal decay detection *(right)*.

tooth provides additional data of its structure. Enamel is transparent to NIR due to the reduced scattering coefficient of light, allowing it to pass through its entire thickness and present as a dark area, whereas the dentin appears bright due to the scattering effect of light caused by the orientation of the dentinal tubules. Any interferences/pathologic lesions/areas of demineralization appear as bright areas in a NIR image due to the increased scattering within the region. Therefore IOS provides information regarding possible decays without any x-ray exposure.[8]

Through the use of digital impression making, it has been determined that laboratory products also become more consistent and require less chair time at insertion.[9]

3D Imaging

CONE-BEAM COMPUTED TOMOGRAPHY

3D imaging has evolved greatly in the last two decades and has found applications in orthodontics as well as in oral and maxillofacial surgery. In 3D medical imaging, a set of anatomic data is collected using diagnostic imaging equipment, processed by a computer and then displayed on a 2D monitor to give the illusion of depth. Depth perception causes the image to appear in 3D.[10] Over the last 15 years, CBCT imaging has emerged as an important supplemental radiographic technique for orthodontic diagnosis and treatment planning, especially in situations that require an understanding of the complex anatomic relationships and surrounding structures of the maxillofacial skeleton. From the introduction of the cephalostat, Broadbent stressed the need for a perfect matching of the lateral and posteroanterior x-rays to obtain a perfect 3D reproduction of the skull.[11] CBCT imaging provides unique features and advantages to enhance orthodontic practice over conventional extraoral radiographic imaging.[12] Lateral cephalometrics provides information on the sagittal and vertical aspects of the malocclusion with little contribution about unilateral or transversal discrepancies. The latter seem to be related to urbanization and industrialization becoming more frequent in the last decades.[13-15] Therefore, the need for a diagnostic tool providing information on the 3D aspects of the dentoskeletal malocclusion is increasing. While the clinical applications span from evaluation of anatomy to pathology of most structures in the maxillofacial area, the key advantage of CBCT is its high-resolution images at a relatively lower radiation dose.[16]

Exposing patients to x-rays implies the existence of a clinical justification and that all the principles and procedures required to minimize patient exposure are considered. The ALARA concept should always be kept in mind: ALARA is an acronym used in radiation safety for <u>a</u>s <u>l</u>ow <u>a</u>s <u>r</u>easonably <u>a</u>chievable. This concept is supported by professional organizations as well as by government institutions.[17,18] Recognizing that diagnostic imaging is the single greatest source of exposure to ionizing radiation for the US population that is controllable, the National Commission on Radiation Protection and Measurements has introduced a modification of the ALARA concept.[19] ALADA represents <u>a</u>s <u>l</u>ow <u>a</u>s <u>d</u>iagnostically <u>a</u>cceptable. Implementation of this concept will require evidence-based judgments of the level of image quality required for specific diagnostic tasks as well as exposures and doses associated with this level of quality. Little research is currently available in this area.

For 2D imaging modalities used in orthodontics, the radiation dose for panoramic imaging varies between 4 and 10 μSv, while a cephalometric exam range is between 3 and 5 μSv. A full mouth series ranges from 12 to 58 μSv based on the type of collimation used.[16] While 2D and 3D radiation doses are often compared for reference, they cannot truly be compared because the acquisition physics and the associated risks are completely different and cannot be equated. The actual risk for low-dose radiographic procedures such as maxillofacial radiography, including CBCT, is difficult to assess and is based on conservative assumptions as there are no data to establish the occurrence of cancer following exposure at these levels. However, it is generally accepted that any increase in dose, no matter how small, results in an incremental increase in risk.[20] Therefore there is no safe limit or safety zone for radiation exposure in orthodontic diagnostic imaging.[12] A recent meta-analysis about the effective dose of dental CBCT stated that the mean adult effective doses grouped by field of view (FOV) size were 212 μSv (large), 177 μSv (medium), and 84 μSv (small). Mean child doses were 175 μSv (combined large and medium) and 103 μSv (small). Large differences were seen between different CBCT units.[19]

The American Dental Association Council on Scientific Affairs (CSA) proposed a set of principles for consideration in the selection of CBCT imaging for individual patient care. According to the guidelines, clinicians should perform radiographic imaging, including CBCT, only after professional justification that the potential clinical benefits will outweigh the risks associated with exposure to ionizing radiation. However, CBCT may supplement or replace conventional dental x-rays when the conventional images will not adequately capture the needed information.[17]

Recently, a number of manufacturers have introduced CBCT units capable of providing medium or even full FOV CBCT acquisition using low-dose protocols. By adjustments to rotation arc, mA, kVp, or the number of basis images or a combination thereof, CBCT imaging can be performed at effective doses comparable with conventional panoramic examinations (range, 14–24 μSv).[21] This is accompanied by significant reductions in image quality; however, viewer software can be helpful in improving the clinical experience with low-quality images. Even at this level, child doses have been reported to be, on average, 36% greater than adult doses.[21] The use of low-dose protocols may be adequate for low-level diagnostic tasks such as root angulations.

BENEFITS OF CBCT FOR ORTHODONTIC ASSESSMENT

The benefits of CBCT for orthodontic assessment include accuracy of image geometry. CBCT offers the distinct advantage of 1:1 geometry, which allows accurate measurements of objects and dimensions. The accuracy and reliability of measurements from CBCT images have been demonstrated, allowing precise assessment of unerupted tooth sizes, bony dimensions in all three planes of space, and even soft tissue anthropometric measurements—things that are all important in orthodontic diagnosis and treatment planning.[22-24]

The accurate localization of ectopic, impacted, and supernumerary teeth is vital to the development of a patient-specific treatment plan with the best chance of success. CBCT has been demonstrated to be superior for localization and space estimation of unerupted maxillary canines compared with conventional imaging methods.[25,26] One study indicated that the increased precision in the localization of the canines and the improved estimation of the space conditions in the arch obtained with CBCT resulted in a difference in diagnosis and treatment planning toward a more clinically orientated approach.[25] CBCT imaging was proven to be significantly better than the panoramic radiograph in determining root resorption associated with canine impaction.[27,28] One study supported improved root resorption detection rates of 63% with the use of CBCT when compared with 2D imaging.[28] When used for diagnosis, CBCT has been shown to alter and improve the treatment recommendations for orthodontic patients with impacted or supernumerary teeth.[29,30]

Based on the findings of a recent review[30] and in accordance with the DIMITRA (Dentomaxillofacial Paediatric Imaging: An Investigation Towards Low Dose Radiation Induced Risks) project,[31] CBCT can be considered also in children for diagnosis and treatment planning of impacted teeth and root resorption (Fig. 1.5).

Maxillary transverse deficiency may be one of the most pervasive skeletal problems in the craniofacial region. Its many manifestations are encountered daily by the orthodontist.[32]

Although many analyses of the lateral cephalometric headfilm have been developed for use in orthodontic and orthognathic treatment planning, the posteroanterior cephalogram has been largely ignored. The diagnosis of transverse discrepancy is quite challenging in the daily practice because of several methodologic limitations of the proposed methods.[33]

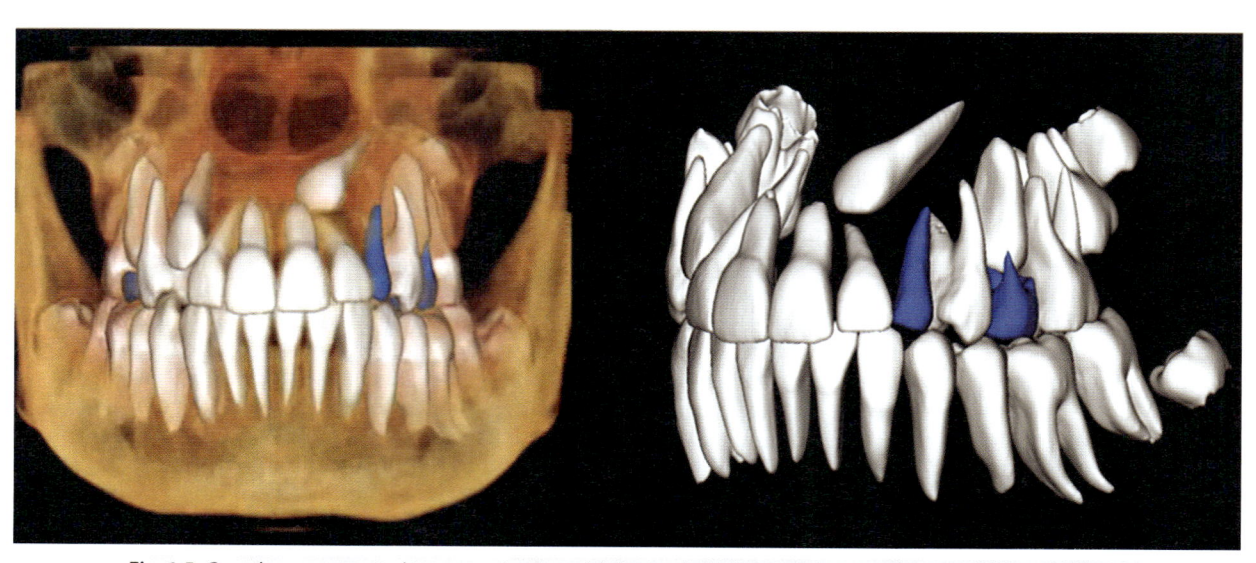

Fig. 1.5 Cone-beam computed tomography data elaboration for enhancing diagnosis and treatment planning.

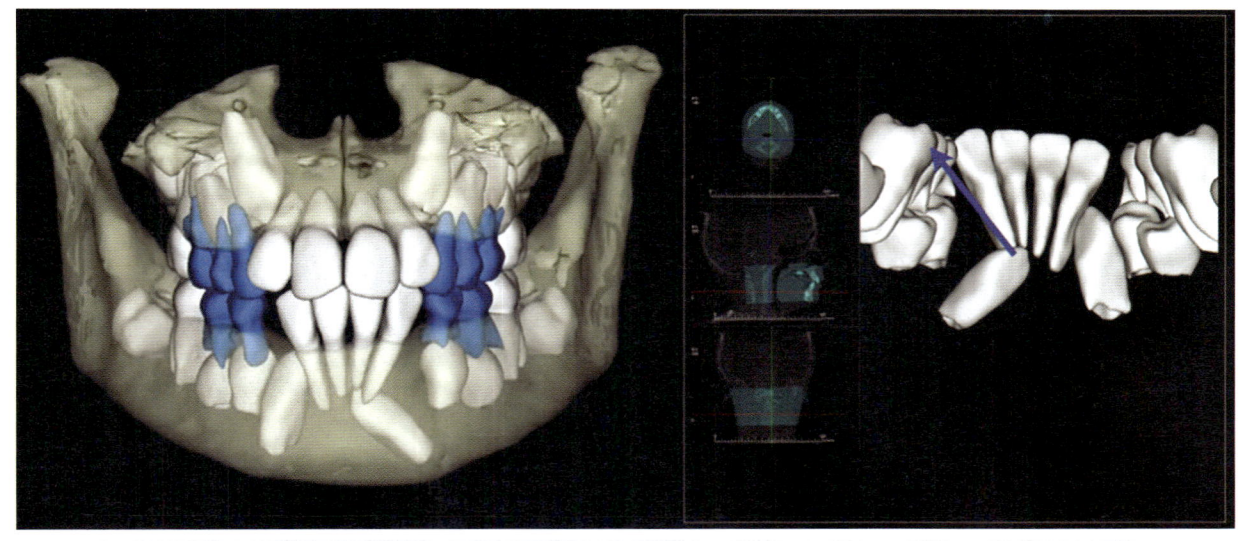

Fig. 1.6 Case of impacted lower canine in which the cone-beam computed tomography data are helpful in defining the right mechanics.

The maxillary and mandibular skeletal widths at different tooth level, buccolingual inclination of each tooth, and root positions in the alveolar bone can be determined and evaluated from the CBCT (Fig. 1.6). With this information, the clinician can make a proper diagnosis and treatment plan for the patient.

The temporomandibular joint (TMJ) can be assessed for pathology more accurately with CBCT images than with conventional radiographs. The CBCT volume for orthodontic assessment will generally include the TMJ and therefore is available for routine review. Several retrospective analyses of CBCT volumes indicate 15% to 18% of incidental findings are related to TMJ (Fig. 1.7), which is significant enough for further follow-up or referral.[34]

CBCT data can also be used to obtain the volumetric rendering of the upper airways. Studies of the upper airway based on CBCT scans are considered to be reliable in defining the border between soft tissues and void spaces (i.e., air), thus providing important information about the morphology (i.e., cross-sectional area and volume) of the pharyngeal airway[35] (Fig. 1.8). However, despite the potentials offered by the technique in this field and the potential role of orthodontists as sentinel physicians for sleep breathing disorders, limited, poor quality, and low evidence level literature is available on the effect of head posture and tongue position on upper airway dimensions and morphology in 3D imaging. Natural head position at CBCT acquisition is the suggested standardized posture.[36] However, for repeatable measures of upper airway volumes it may clinically be difficult to obtain. Indications and methods related to tongue position and breathing during data acquisition are still lacking. Furthermore, a recent study focusing on the reliability of airway measurements stated that the oropharyngeal airway volume was the only parameter found to have generalized excellent intra-examiner and inter-examiner reliability.[37]

In orthognathic surgery, Digital Imaging and Communications in Medicine (DICOM) data from CBCT can be used to fabricate physical stereolithographic models or to generate virtual 3D models. The 3D reconstructions are extremely useful in the diagnosing and treatment planning of facial asymmetry cases. They can also be used to generate substitute grafts when warranted. CBCT can be useful as a valuable planning tool from initial evaluation to the surgical procedure and then the correction of the dental component in the surgery-first orthognathic approach.[16]

In addition, databases may be interfaced with the anatomic models to provide characteristics of the displayed tissues to reproduce tissue reactions to development, treatment, and function. The systematic summarization of the results presented in the literature suggests that computer-aided planning is accurate for orthognathic surgery of the maxilla and mandible, and with respect to the benefits to the patient and surgical procedure it is estimated that computer-aided planning facilitates the analysis of surgical outcomes and provides greater accuracy[38] (Fig. 1.9).

A recent systematic review[39] was conducted to evaluate whether CBCT imaging can be used to assess dentoalveolar relationships critical to determining risk assessment and help determine and improve periodontal treatment needs in patients undergoing orthodontic therapy. The conclusion was that pretreatment orthodontic CBCT imaging can assist clinicians in selecting preventive or interceptive periodontal corticotomy and augmentation surgical requirements, especially for treatment approaches involving buccal tooth movement at the anterior mandible or maxillary premolars to prevent deleterious alveolar bone changes. This assumption seems more suitable for skeletally mature patients presenting with a thin periodontal phenotype prior to orthodontic treatment (Fig. 1.10).

3D FACIAL RECONSTRUCTION TECHNIQUES

The accurate acquisition of 3D face appearance characteristics is important to plan orthognathic surgery, and excellent work is based on an exact 3D face modeling. A precise approach to 3D digital face profile acquiring, which is applied to simulate and design an optimal plan for face surgery by modern technologies such as CAD, is required.

Three types of 3D face modeling methods are currently used to extract human face profiles: CT technology,[40,41]

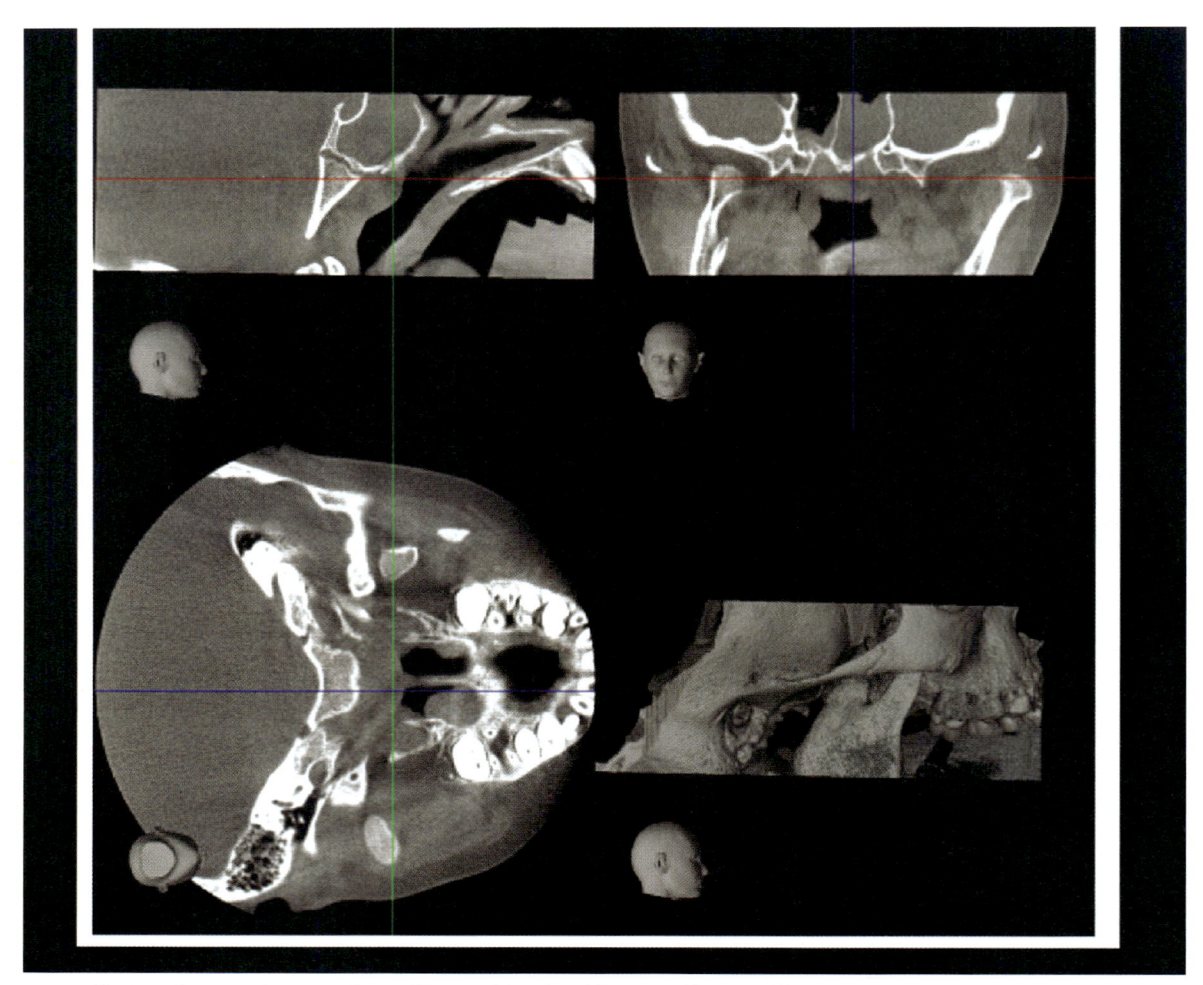

8 | Principles and Biomechanics of Aligner Treatment

Fig. 1.7 Occasional report of misunderstood right condyle neck fracture results in a 9-year-old child being prescribed cone-beam computed tomography for orthodontic reasons.

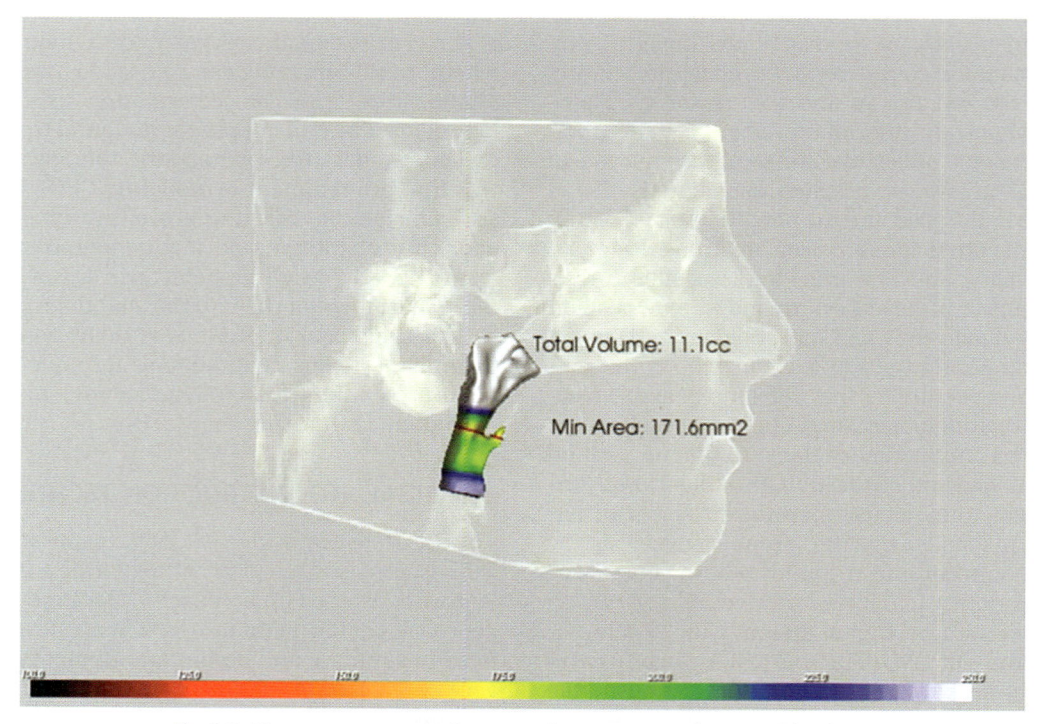

Fig. 1.8 Airway measurements from cone-beam computed tomography data.

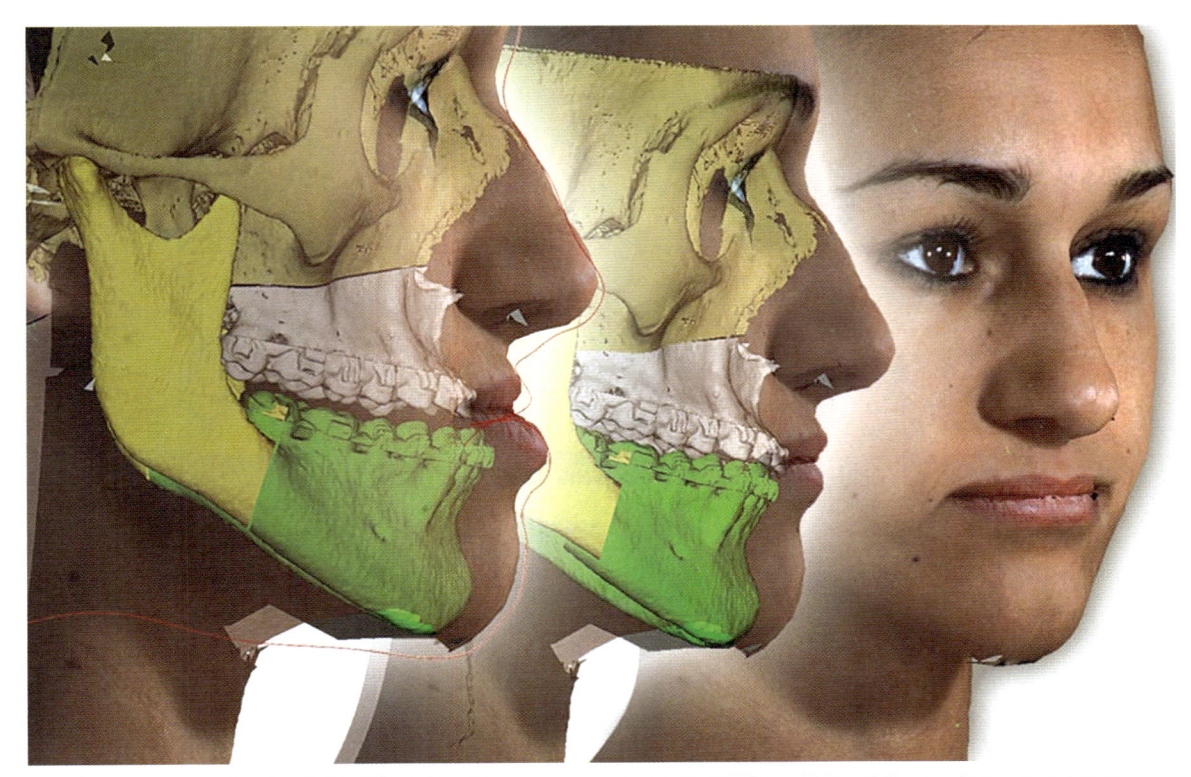

Fig. 1.9 Example of cone-beam computed tomography data integration in a surgery three-dimensional planning software. (Dolphin Imaging, Chatsworth, CA, USA.)

the passive optical 3D sensing technique,[42] and the active optical 3D sensing technique.[43] The 3D reconstruction method based on CT technology is sensitive to the skeleton and can be conveniently utilized for craniofacial plastics, as well as the oral and maxillofacial correction of abnormalities.[44] Soft tissue data extraction, or segmentation, can be created using a dedicated software. For orthodontic purposes, the image should be recorded with eyes open and with the patient smiling. The smiling image will permit the use of dental landmarks to superimpose the digital models on the 3D face reconstruction for treatment planning purposes. Novel technologies aiming at acquiring facial surface are available. Stereophotogrammetry and laser scanning allow operators to quickly record facial anatomy and to perform a wider set of measurements[45] not exposing patients to radiation (Fig. 1.11). Stereophotogrammetry still represents the gold standard with respect to laser scanning at least for orthodontic applications since it is characterized by good precision and reproducibility, with random errors generally less than 1 mm.[45] With this method, 3D images are acquired by combining photographs captured from various angles with synchronous digital cameras, with the main advantage of reducing possible motion artifacts. The main limitation at this stage is represented by the high cost of the instrumentation.

According to Sarver and Jacobson[46] and Sarver and Ackerman,[47] it may be inappropriate to place everyone in the same esthetic framework and even more problematic to attempt this based solely on hard tissue relationships since the soft tissues often fail to respond predictably to hard tissue changes. Integrating CBCT data, facial 3D reconstruction, and digital models with specific simulation software will provide useful indications in relation to orthodontic treatment results and the eventual need of interdisciplinary intervention.

VIRTUAL SETUP

Several software programs are available on the market to create virtual setups able to produce the sequence of physical models on which thermoforming plastic foils are used to create aligners.

Setup accuracy is improved when virtual teeth segmentation is applied on digital models obtained by IOS or digitization of plaster casts, reducing the loss of tooth structure observed during the cutting process of the plaster in conventional plaster and wax setups.

The segmentation process starts with marking mesial and distal points on each tooth or simply indicating the center of the crown on the occlusal view of the arches, depending on the software used. Then the software generally identifies the gingival margin. Teeth segmentation and the tooth-tooth-gingiva segmentation are executed semiautomatically, but the operator can always correct the automatic process. Once teeth are segmented they are separated from the gingiva, and a mean virtual root (shape and length are derived from proprietary databases) is applied. Recently, virtual setup software programs are starting to use real root morphologies derived from patient CBCT data when available. Tooth segmentation from CBCT images in those cases is a fundamental step. Recent engineering innovations made the process simple and timesaving with respect to the past.[48]

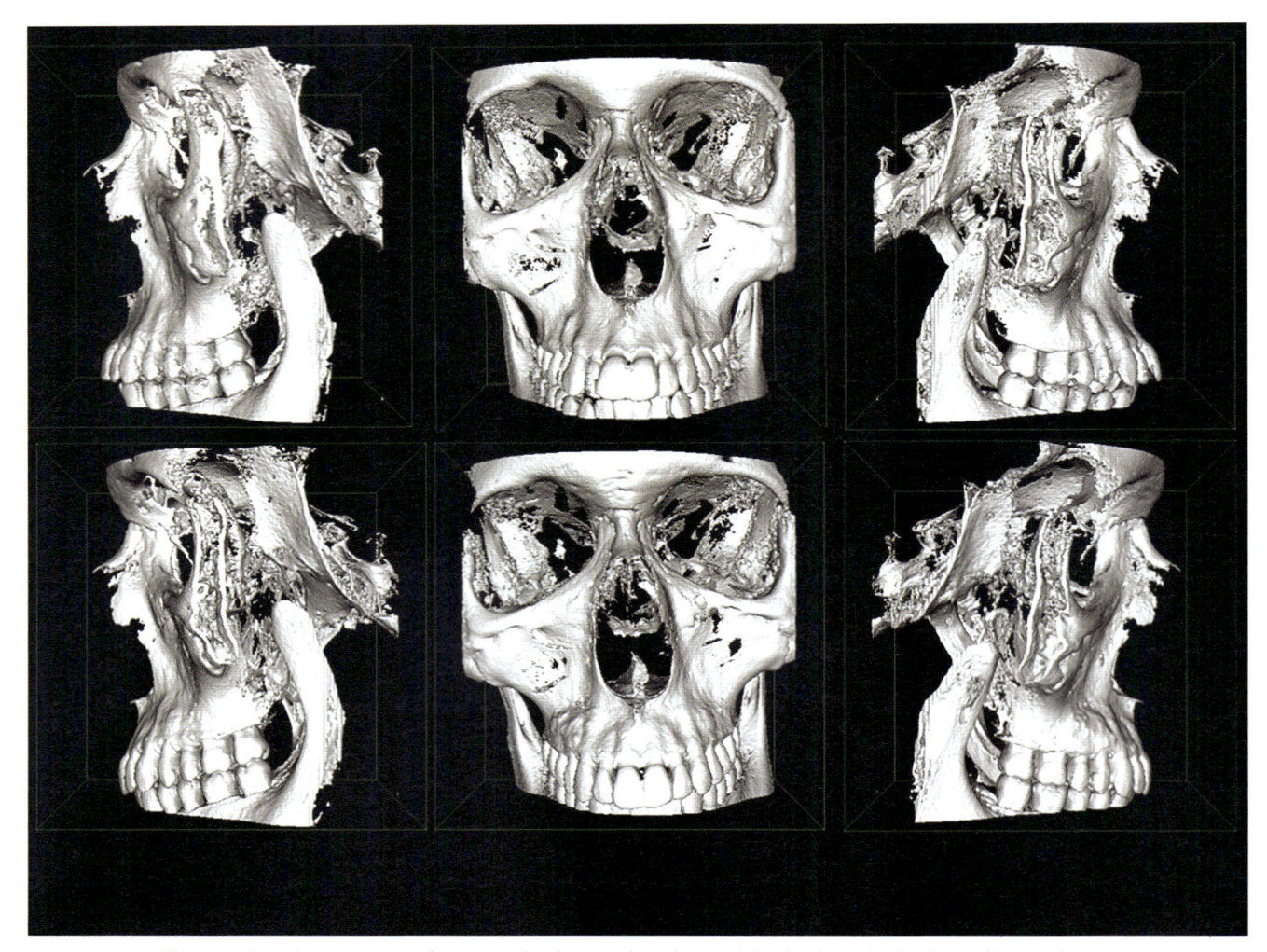

Fig. 1.10 Cone-beam computed tomography data used to plan an orthodontic expansion in a subject with poor periodontal support *(upper)*. Orthodontic expansion, corticotomies, and bone grafts were planned to obtain an excellent final result without bone dehiscence *(lower)*.

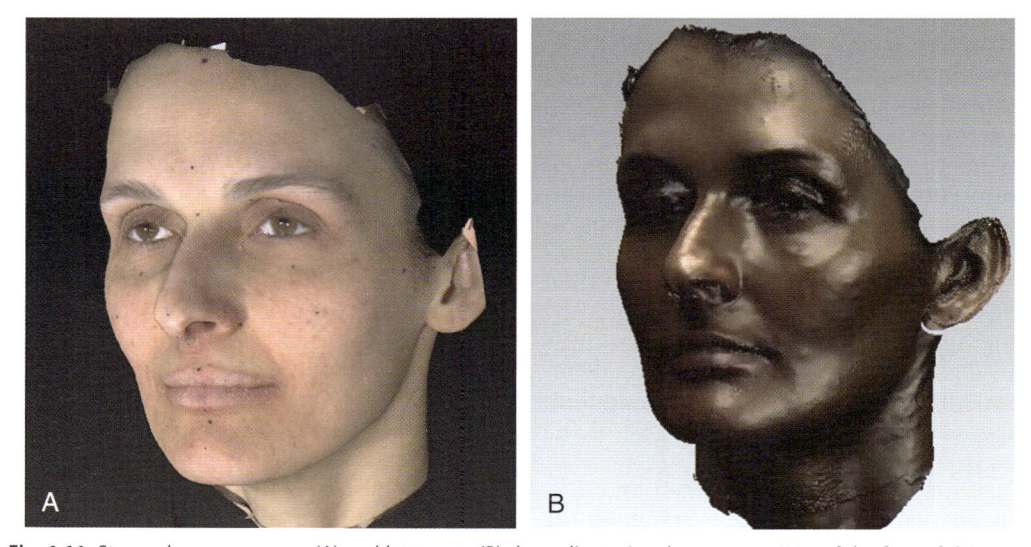

Fig. 1.11 Stereophotogrammetry (A) and laser scan (B) three-dimensional reconstructions of the face of the same patient. (From Gibelli D, Pucciarelli V, Poppa P, et al. Three-dimensional facial anatomy evaluation: reliability of laser scanner consecutive scans procedure in comparison with stereophotogrammetry. *J Craniomaxillofac Surg.* 2018;46: 1807-1813.)

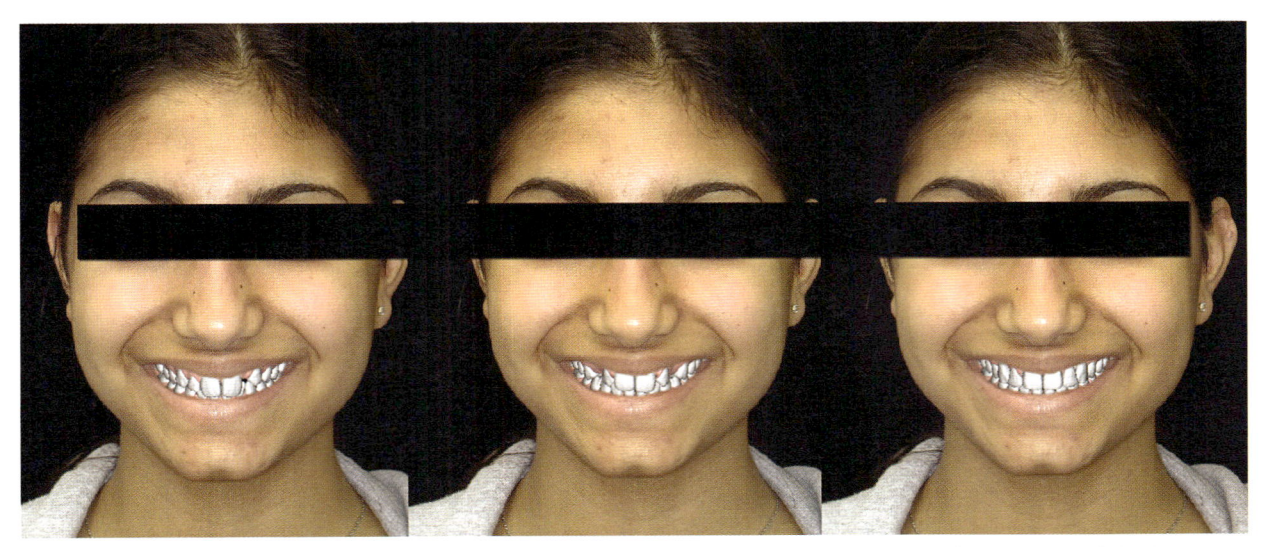

Fig. 1.12 Superimposition of the virtual setup on the smile picture of a patient with unilateral agenesis, visualizing from left to right the initial situation, the postorthodontic situation, and the final smile with restorative simulation.

Once the teeth have been segmented and the interproximal contacts defined, the arch form is adjusted using software tools that can create an individual arch form. Digital arch templates are also available, while several software programs consider the WALA (an acronym for Will Andrews and Larry Andrews) ridge.

The occlusal plane as well as the original vertical plane are used as reference.[49] Each tooth can be moved in the space since the required final position has been achieved. It is important to mention that tooth movements on computers are unlimited. Tooth alignment and leveling can be planned on the computer screen, but this result may not be realistic for that specific patient. Obviously, tooth movement has its biologic limitations. On the basis of the used system the virtual setup could be prepared by a trained dental technician or by a software expert; however, every setup should be based on biologic principles and on a biomechanics background making the orthodontist the initial designer and the final reviewer of every setup.

As progress in digital imaging techniques accelerates and tools to plan medical treatments improve, the use of virtual setups in orthodontics before and during treatment will become the mainstream in orthodontics (Fig. 1.12).

3D DATA INTEGRATION

The creation of a virtual copy of each patient is dependent upon the integration of 3D media files and the possibility of their fusion into a unique and replicable model. CBCT data can be used as a platform onto which other inputs can be fused with acceptable clinical accuracy. These data sources include light-based surface data such as photographic facial images and high-resolution surface models of the dentition produced by direct scans intraorally or indirectly by scanning impressions or study models. The integration of hard and soft tissues can provide a greater understanding of the interrelationship of the dentition and soft tissues to the underlying osseous frame.[12] Individual 3D models of tooth are needed for the computer-aided orthodontic treatment planning and simulation. With the novel 3D superimposition techniques, clinicians are able to simulate the outcome of both the osseous structures and the soft tissue posttreatment.

The 3D data integration makes the diagnostic process and the treatment planning more accurate and complete, provides an effective communication tool and a method for patients to visualize the simulated outcomes, instills motivation, and encourages compliance to achieve the desired treatment outcome (Fig. 1.13).[16]

What technology is providing to orthodontists is amazing; however, what is still missing is the fourth dimension (i.e., the dynamic movements of the mandible and the surrounding tissues integrated in the virtual model). Idealistically, the capture of digital data for virtual modeling should happen in a one-step, single-device approach to improve accuracy. Future research will fill this gap and will realize the dream of the real virtual patient.

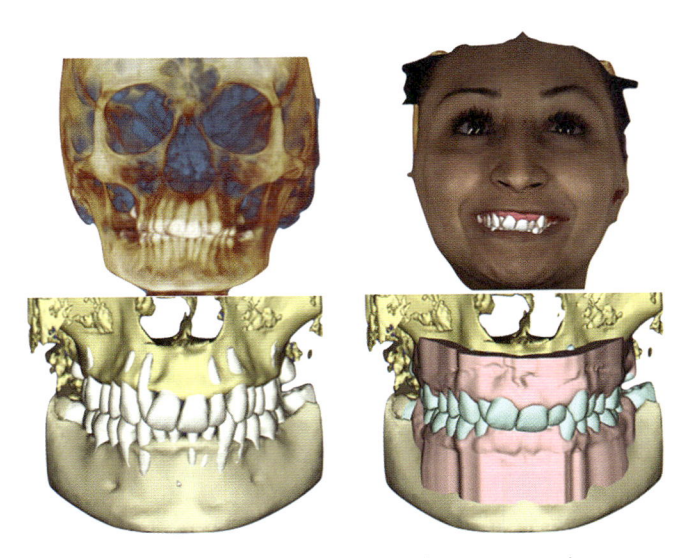

Fig. 1.13 The virtual patient in which cone-beam computed tomography data, facial three-dimensional reconstruction, and virtual setup obtained after teeth segmentation are superimposed. Courtesy of dr. Alain Souchet, Mulhouse, France.

References

1. American Association of Orthodontists. Clinical practice guidelines for orthodontics and dentofacial orthopedics. AAO; 2017. https://www.aaoinfo.org/d/apps/get-file?fid=12939
2. Uribe FA, Chandhoke TK, Nanda R. Individualized orthodontic diagnosis. In: Nanda R. ed. *Esthetics and Biomechanics in Orthodontics*. 2nd ed. St Louis, MO: Elsevier Saunders; 2015:1-32.
3. Sarver D, Yanoski M. Special considerations in diagnosis and treatment planning. In: Graber LW, Vanarsdall RL, Vig KWL, eds. *Orthodontics. Current Principles and Techniques*. 5th ed. Philadelphia, PA: Mosby; 2012:59-98.
4. Mangano C, Luongo F, Migliario M, et al. Combining intraoral scans, cone beam computed tomography and face scans: the virtual patient. *J Craniofac Surg*. 2018;29:2241-2246.
5. Tarraf NA, Daredeliler AM. Present and the future of digital orthodontics. *Semin Orthod*. 2018;24:376-385.
6. Rossini G, Parrini S, Castroflorio T, et al. Diagnostic accuracy and measurement sensitivity of digital models for orthodontic purposes: a systematic review. *Am J Orthod Dentofacial Orthop*. 2016;149:161-170.
7. Claus D, Radeke J, Zint M, et al. Generation of 3D digital models of the dental arches using optical scanning techniques. *Semin Orthod*. 2018;24:416-429.
8. Kühnisch J, Söchtig F, Pitchika V, et al. In vivo validation of near-infrared light transillumination for interproximal dentin caries detection. *Clin Oral Investig*. 2016;20:821-829.
9. Nayar S, Mahadevan R. A paradigm shift in the concept for making dental impressions. *J Pharm Bioallied Sci*. 2015;7(1):S213-S215.
10. Hajeer MY, Millett DT, Ayoub AF, et al. Applications of 3D imaging in orthodontics: part I. *J Orthod*. 2004;3:62-70.
11. Broadbent BS. A new x-ray technique and its application to orthodontia. *Angle Orthod*. 1931;1:45-66.
12. Scarfe WC, Azevedo B, Toghyani S, et al. Cone beam computed tomographic imaging in orthodontics. *Aust Dent J*. 2017;62(1):S33-S50.
13. Corruccini RS, Flander LB, Kaul SS. Mouth breathing, occlusion, and modernization in a north Indian population. An epidemiologic study. *Angle Orthod*. 1985;55:190-196.
14. Camporesi M, Marinelli A, Baroni G, et al. Dental arch dimensions and tooth wear in two samples of children in the 1950s and 1990s. *Br Dent J*. 2009;207:e24.
15. Lindsten R, Ogaard B, Larsson E. Transversal dental arch dimensions in 9-year-old children born in the 1960s and the 1980s. *Am J Orthod Dentofacial Orthop*. 2001;120:576-584.
16. Tadinada A, Schneider S, Yadav S. Role of cone beam computed tomography in contemporary orthodontics. *Sem Orthod*. 2018;24:407-415.
17. American Dental Association Council on Scientific Affairs. The use of cone-beam tomography in dentistry. An advisory statement from the American Dental Association Council on Scientific Affairs. *J Am Dent Assoc*. 2012;143:899-902.
18. Horner K. SEDENTEXCT guideline development [panel]. In: *Cone Beam CT for Dental and Maxillofacial Radiology (Evidence Based Guidelines) (Radiation Protection Series)*. Luxembourg: European Commission: Directorate-General for Energy; 2012:154.
19. Ludlow JB, Timothy R, Walker C, et al. Effective dose of dental CBCT—a meta-analysis of published data and additional data for nine CBCT units. *Dentomaxillofac Radiol*. 2015;44(1):20140197.
20. Valentin J. The 2007 recommendations of the International Commission on Radiological Protection. Publication 93. *Ann ICRP*. 2007;37:1-332.
21. Ludlow JB, Walker C. Assessment of phantom dosimetry and image quality of i-CAT FLX cone-beam computed tomography. *Am J Orthod Dentofacial Orthop*. 2013;144:802-817.
22. Berco M, Rigali Jr PH, Miner RM, et al. Accuracy and reliability of linear cephalometric measurements from cone-beam computed tomography scans of a dry human skull. *Am J Orthod Dentofacial Orthop*. 2009;136:17.e1-e9.
23. Fourie Z, Damstra J, Gerrits PO, et al. Accuracy and repeatability of anthropometric facial measurements using cone beam computed tomography. *Cleft Palate Craniofac J*. 2011;48:623-630.
24. Lagravère MO, Carey J, Toogood RW, et al. Three-dimensional accuracy of measurements made with software on cone-beam computed tomography images. *Am J Orthod Dentofacial Orthop*. 2008;134:112-116.
25. Botticelli S, Verna C, Cattaneo PM, et al. Two-versus three-dimensional imaging in subjects with unerupted maxillary canines. *Eur J Orthod*. 2011;33:344-349.
26. Hodges RJ, Atchison KA, White SC. Impact of cone-beam computed tomography on orthodontic diagnosis and treatment planning. *Am J Orthod Dentofacial Orthop*. 2013;143:665-674.
27. Ngo CTT, Fishman LS, Rossouw PE, et al. Correlation between panoramic radiography and cone-beam computed tomography in assessing maxillary impacted canines. *Angle Orthod*. 2018;88:384-389.
28. Jawad Z, Carmichael F, Houghton N, et al. A review of cone beam computed tomography for the diagnosis of root resorption associated with impacted canines, introducing an innovative root resorption scale. *Oral Surg Oral Med Oral Pathol Oral Radiol*. 2016;122:765-771.
29. Haney E, Gansky SA, Lee JS, et al. Comparative analysis of traditional radiographs and cone-beam computed tomography volumetric images in the diagnosis and treatment planning of maxillary impacted canines. *Am J Orthod Dentofacial Orthop*. 2010;137:590-597.
30. De Grauwe A, Ayaz I, Shujaat S, et al. CBCT in orthodontics: a systematic review on justification of CBCT in a paediatric population prior to orthodontic treatment. *Eur J Orthod*. 2019;41:381-389. doi:10.1093/ejo/cjy066.
31. Oenning AC, Jacobs R, Pauwels R, et al. Cone-beam CT in paediatric dentistry: DIMITRA project position statement. *Pediatr Radiol*. 2018;48:308-316.
32. McNamara JA. Maxillary transverse deficiency. *Am J Orthod Dentofacial Orthop*. 2000;117:567-570.
33. Miner RM, Al Qabandi S, Rigali PH, et al. Cone-beam computed tomography transverse analysis. Part I: normative data. *Am J Orthod Dentofacial Orthop*. 2012;142:300-307.
34. Larson BE. Cone-beam computed tomography is the imaging technique of choice for comprehensive orthodontic assessment. *Northwest Dent*. 2014;93:17-20.
35. Shokri A, Miresmaeili A, Ahmadi A, et al. Comparison of pharyngeal airway volume in different skeletal facial patterns using cone beam computed tomography. *J Clin Exp Dent*. 2018;10:e1017-e1028.
36. Gurani SF, Di Carlo G, Cattaneo PM, et al. Effect of head and tongue posture on the pharyngeal airway dimensions and morphology in three-dimensional imaging: a systematic review. *J Oral Maxillofac Res*. 2016;7(1):e1.
37. Zimmerman JN, Vora SR, Pliska BT. Reliability of upper airway assessment using CBCT. *Eur J Orthod*. 2019;41:101-108.
38. Haas Jr OL, Becker OE, de Oliveira RB. Computer-aided planning in orthognathic surgery-systematic review. *Int J Oral Maxillofac Surg*. 2014;S0901-5027(14):00430-00435.
39. Mandelaris GA, Neiva R, Chambrone L. Cone-beam computed tomography and interdisciplinary dentofacial therapy: an American Academy of Periodontology best evidence review focusing on risk assessment of the dentoalveolar bone changes influenced by tooth movement. *J Periodontol*. 2017;88:960-977.
40. Schmelzeisen R, Schramm A. Computer-assisted reconstruction of the facial skeleton. *Arch Facial Plast Surg*. 2003;5:437.
41. Bell RB. Computer planning and intraoperative navigation in craniomaxillofacial surgery. *Oral Maxillofac Surg Clin North Am*. 2010;22:135-156.
42. Hirshmüller H, Innocent PR, Garibaldi J. Real-time correlation-based stereo vision with reduced border errors. *Int J Comput Vis*. 2002;47:229-246.
43. You Y, Shen Y, Zhang G, et al. Real-time and high-resolution 3D face measurement via a smart active optical sensor. *Sensors (Basel)*. 2017;17:e734.
44. Troulis MJ, Everett P, Seldin EB, et al. Development of a three-dimensional treatment planning system based on computed tomographic data. *Int J Oral Maxillofac Surg*. 2002;31:349-357.
45. Gibelli D, Pucciarelli V, Poppa P, et al. Three-dimensional facial anatomy evaluation: reliability of laser scanner consecutive scans procedure in comparison with stereophotogrammetry. *J Craniomaxillofac Surg*. 2018;46:1807-1813.
46. Sarver DM, Jacobson RS. The aesthetic dentofacial analysis. *Clin Plast Surg*. 2007;34:369-394.
47. Sarver DM, Ackerman MB. Dynamic smile visualization and quantification: part 2. Smile analysis and treatment strategies. *Am J Orthod Dentofacial Orthop*. 2003;124:116-127.
48. Xia Z, Gan Y, Chang L, et al. Individual tooth segmentation from CT images scanned with contacts of maxillary and mandible teeth. *Comput Methods Programs Biomed*. 2017;138:1-12.
49. Camardella LT, Rothier EK, Vilella OV, et al. Virtual setup: application in orthodontic practice. *J Orofac Orthop*. 2016;77:409-416.

2 Current Biomechanical Rationale Concerning Composite Attachments in Aligner Orthodontics

JUAN PABLO GOMEZ ARANGO

Introduction

The orthodontic technique that we now call "aligner orthodontics" has evolved considerably over the last 20 years. Improvements in behavior of aligner plastics, treatment planning software, and three-dimensional (3D) printing have served one basic but fundamental intention: to mitigate the biomechanical limitations inherent to aligner-based tooth movement. Another significant development designed to overcome the aforementioned biomechanical shortcomings of aligner systems has been the continuous improvement of biomechanically complementary composite attachments. Attachments were conceived to produce supplementary force vectors that, when applied to teeth by the aligner material, transform the resultant system, allowing complex tooth movements. The application of one of the initial geometric configurations was initially presented by the clinical team from Align Technology Inc., as basic 1 x 3 mm rectangular structures, bonded to the lower incisor buccal surface, in an attempt at controlling undesired tipping during space closure after incisor extraction (Fig. 2.1A).[1] As the incisors adjacent to the extraction space begin to incline mesially, the rigid, fixed structure of the attachment collides with aligner plastic, producing force couples that counteract the initial moment, reducing undesired tipping (see Fig. 2.1B).

Orthodontic tooth movement with conventional bracket techniques can deliver sophisticated force systems due to the manner in which the rigid ligature-archwire-bracket scheme "grasps" the malaligned tooth. This particular arrangement allows broad control of magnitude and direction of applied force vectors, and, consequentially, of tooth movement (Fig. 2.2).

It is important to keep in mind that attachments work, not as *active* agents that produce forces, but by passively "getting in the way" of plastic as it elastically deforms due to lack of coincidence between tooth position and aligner material ("mismatch"), establishing the force vector that subsequently affects the tooth (Fig. 2.3).

Biomaterials used for attachment fabrication must assure that requirements in adhesion, wear resistance, and esthetics are fulfilled. A recent study[2] suggests that contemporary microfilled resin composites provide sufficient wear resistance to deliver a stable attachment shape during treatment, assuring its functionality. Mantovani et al.[3] also concluded that the use of bulk-filled resins for attachment fabrication improved dimensional stability when compared to low-viscosity resins, which experience higher polymerization shrinkage. The use of translucent composites generally provides sufficient esthetic acceptance and stain resistance as long as an adequate bonding technique is executed, in which voids (bubbles) in attachment surface and excessive residue (flash) left on tooth surface[4] are avoided.

Several considerations come into play when determining the optimal attachment design for a specific clinical objective: geometry, location, and size.

Geometry (Active Surface Orientation)

At the time of aligner insertion, orthodontic forces will be produced in response to the particular complex pattern of mismatches between plastic and tooth structure. This pattern of mismatch–plastic deformation–orthodontic force is critical for attachment design during digital simulation to produce specific areas (active surfaces) that will contact aligner plastic with predetermined force magnitudes, producing the desired force vectors and consequent tooth movements. Not all the surface area of attachments will be in direct contact with the aligner. The active or functional surfaces can and should be determined with thoughtful biomechanical intentionality, in accordance with clinical objectives (Fig. 2.4A). While the magnitude of the force produced is determined by the amount of mismatch (along with the characteristics of aligner material), the direction of the force will depend on the orientation of the active surface. The principles of mechanics state that the direction of the normal component of the contact force (the vector that in this case acts upon the active surface of the attachment) will always be perpendicular to that surface (see Fig. 2.4B). Identifying the direction of these complementary force vectors is essential for treatment planning, especially when more than one force acts simultaneously. In these cases, the resultant forces must be properly recognized to deliver predictable tooth movements (see Fig. 2.4C).

14 Principles and Biomechanics of Aligner Treatment

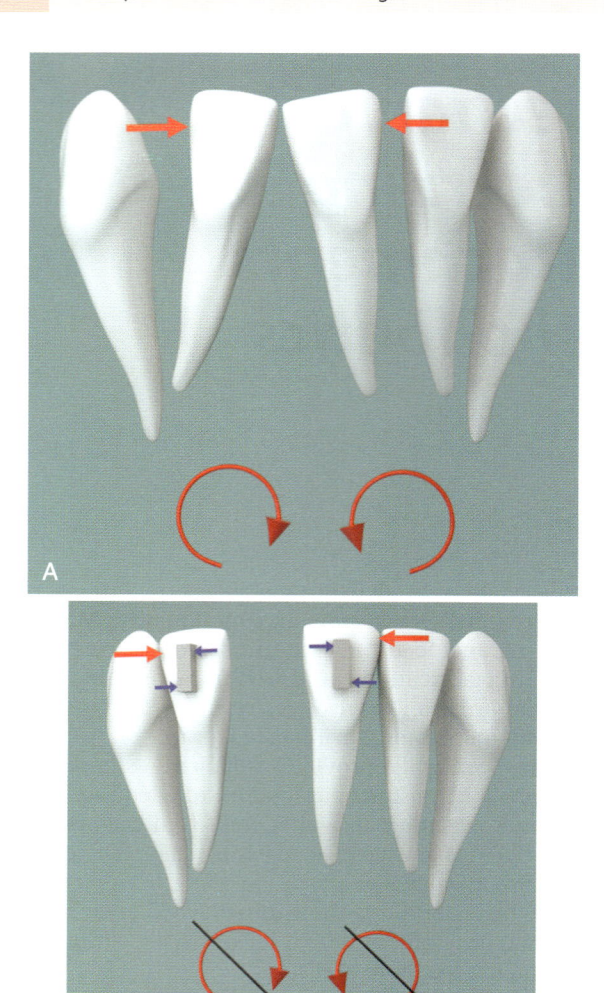

Fig. 2.1 (A) Mesial tipping moments *(red curved arrows)* produced by aligner forces *(red arrows)* occurring during space closure. Antitipping moments *(blue curved arrows)* produced by forces *(blue arrows)* acting at rectangular vertical attachments (B). Opposing moments are canceled out, promoting bodily movement.

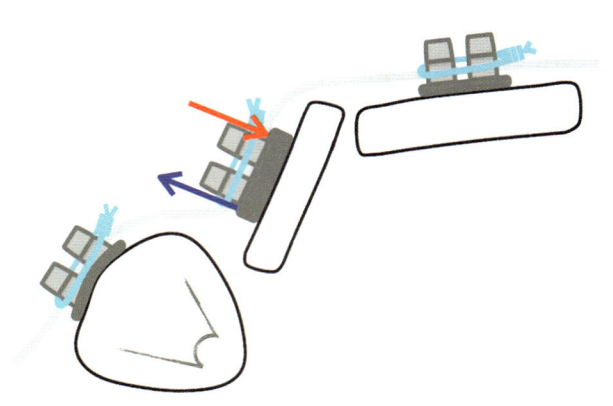

Fig. 2.2 The typical force couple generated during bracket-based alignment of rotated tooth with a fully engaged 0.014 NiTi archwire consists of two force vectors: one that pushes against the posterior wall of the slot *(red arrow)* and a second that pulls away from the same wall *(blue arrow)*.

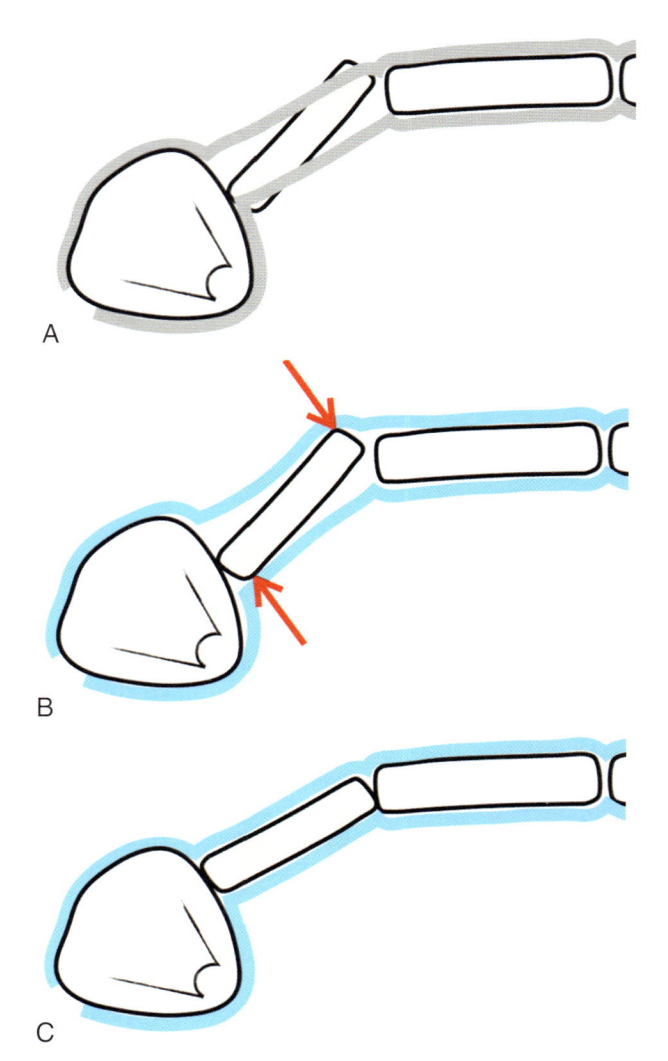

Fig. 2.3 (A) Aligner-tooth mismatch. (B) Elastic aligner deformation and activation of forces upon aligner insertion. (C) Tooth alignment after aligner sequence.

Location

Based on the premise that the magnitude of a moment is proportional to the perpendicular distance between the line of action and the center of resistance, to fully understand the effect of aligner-based orthodontic forces being applied in any particular moment, it is essential to establish this distance in the three planes of space. Once this correlation has been clearly established and quantified, there will be a much clearer picture of the effectiveness of expected rotational moments as well as the possibility of anticipating undesired occurrences such as buccolingual and mesiodistal tipping and intrusion. In a case in which mesiolingual rotation of the tooth is required, localization of attachment A will produce a strong mesial tipping moment and a weak mesiolingual rotational moment (Fig. 2.5A). In this specific clinical situation, a better alternative would be with attachment location B, in which modification in distance from line of action to center of resistance would reduce tipping

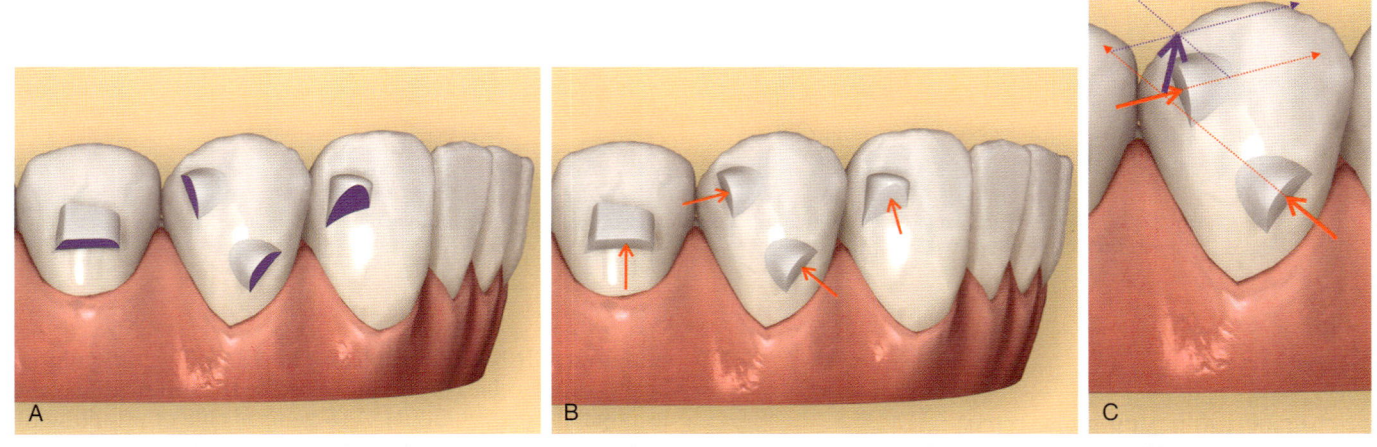

Fig. 2.4 (A) Active surfaces of attachments. (B) Direction of forces acting at active surfaces. (C) Resultant force affecting the first premolar will produce extrusion and clockwise, second-order rotation.

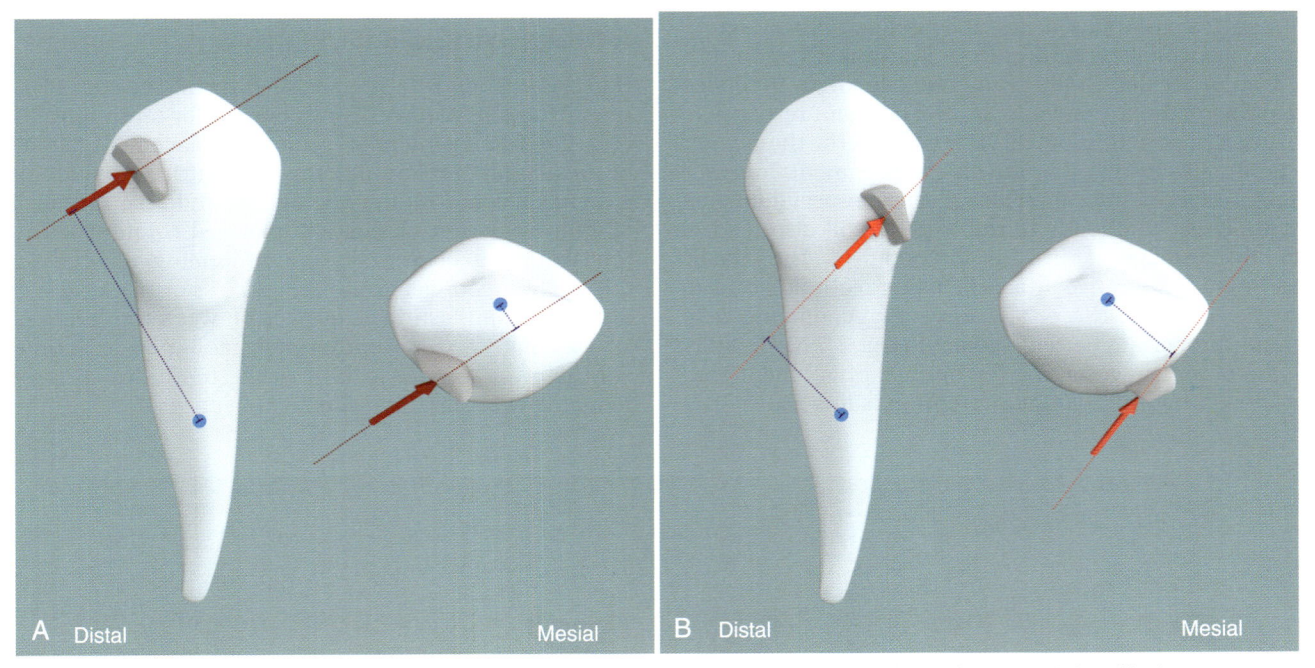

Fig. 2.5 (A) Due to the distance between the center of resistance *(blue dot)* and the line of action *(red dotted line)*, large mesial tipping and negligible mesiolingual rotational moments should be expected. (B) A more mesial and apical attachment location will result in reduced mesial tipping and increased mesiolingual rotational moments, increasing clinical efficacy.

tendency as well as increase mesiolingual rotational capacity (see Fig. 2.5B).

Another example of the influence of attachment localization is observed during transverse arch expansion, when buccal tipping of posterior segments is detrimental to treatment objectives. A recent unpublished finite element analysis (FEA) study[5] of the mechanical effects of the bonding position of rectangular horizontal attachments found that the resultant tipping moment acting on the molars was greater when located on the lingual surface of the first upper molars versus the labial surface (Fig. 2.6).

Size

Attachment size is important because of its mechanical and esthetic implications. Small configurations are desirable because they are less noticeable; however, as size diminishes, so does the ability to produce predictable forces due to reduced active surface area. On the other hand, larger attachment designs are desirable because of their increased biomechanical capabilities, but they result in increased aligner retention (with subsequent patient discomfort) and negative esthetic perception, especially with high-profile configurations in anterior teeth.

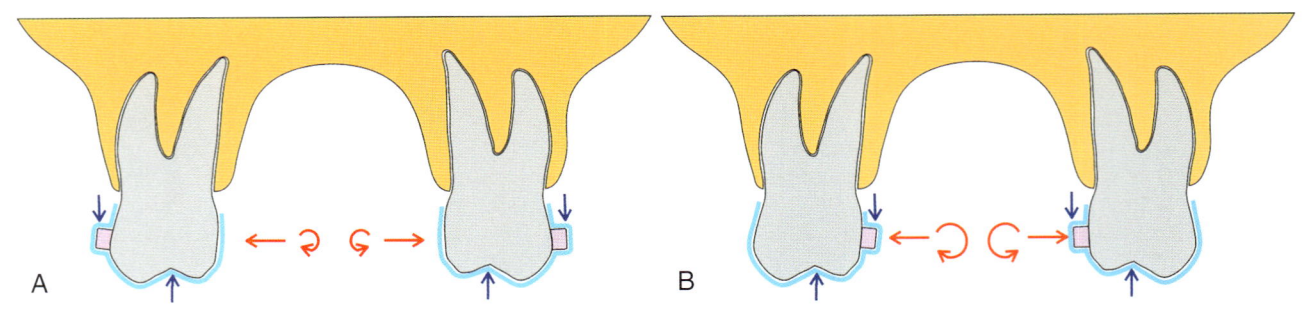

Fig. 2.6 During expansion, labial attachment location (A) produced smaller net buccal molar tipping moments than lingually bonded attachments (B).

Functions

PROVIDING ALIGNER RETENTION

For aligner-based orthodontic forces to affect teeth as conceived in digital simulation, the aligner must be stably seated after insertion and remain so for the duration of treatment. Occasionally, deficient adaptation of the aligner may occur, usually resulting from faulty fabrication, but may also occur due to the many reactive forces produced once properly fitted. For example, as a frequent response to intrusive forces acting on the posterior teeth, the aligner will tend to be dislodged in the anterior segment, and vice versa. The use of intermaxillary elastics, especially when they are engaged directly to the aligner, will also tend to vertically dislodge it in the direction of the elastic force. Bonding retentive attachments on teeth adjacent to those receptors of the elastic force is recommended to maintain proper aligner engagement (Fig. 2.7A). A study by Jones et al.[6] suggests that the optimal attachment configuration, when high aligner retention is imperative, is a nongingivally beveled (such as a horizontal rectangular or occlusally beveled) design, as close to the gingival margin as possible (see Fig. 2.7B). As a general rule of attachment design, occlusal beveling will facilitate aligner insertion due to the inclined plane configuration as well as increase force (and discomfort) required for aligner removal.

AVOIDING ALIGNER "SLIPPING"

Especially when rotating rounded teeth, the sum of a series of tangential forces is responsible for tooth movement (Fig. 2.8A), causing inconvenient displacement (slipping) of the aligner in relation to the tooth surface, reducing the system's efficacy and predictability, and resulting in lack of full expression of digitally planned rotation with the tooth lagging behind the corresponding aligner stage. Clinically, incomplete rotation and loss of tracking will be observed, manifesting as a space between tooth and plastic (see Fig. 2.8B). Appropriately designed attachments can help the aligner lock in to the tooth crown, greatly reducing this undesired slipping effect.

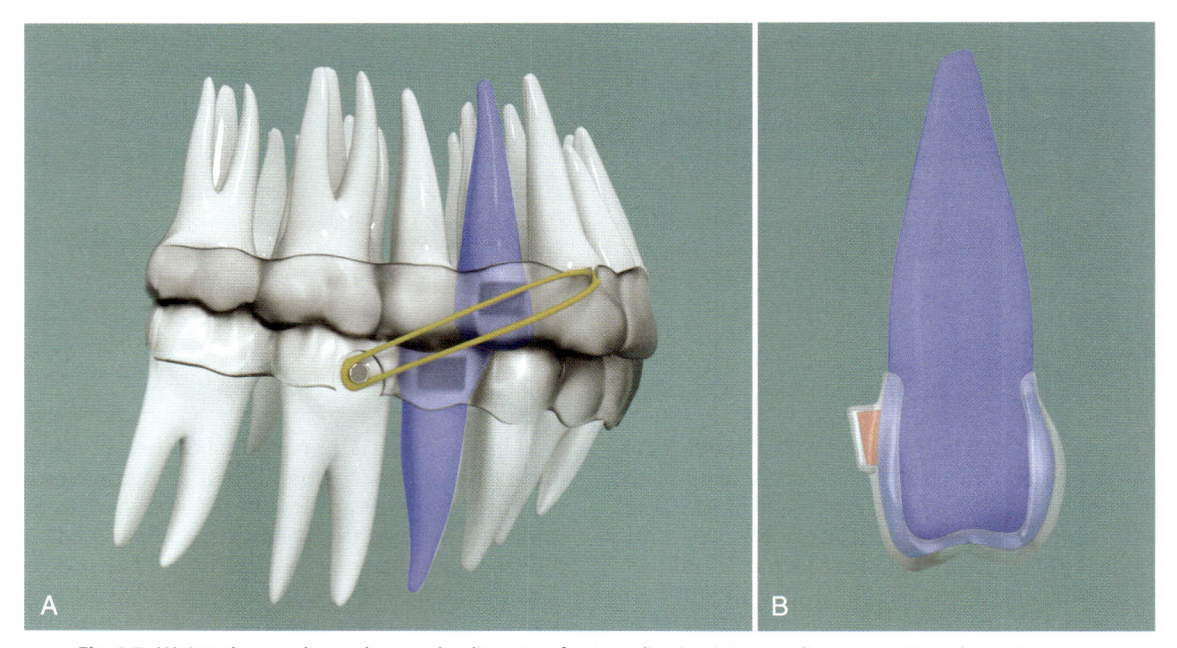

Fig. 2.7 (A) Attachments located on teeth adjacent to force application increase aligner retention when using intermaxillary elastics. (B) Attachment position close to the gingival margin and occlusally beveled geometry is ideal for aligner retention.

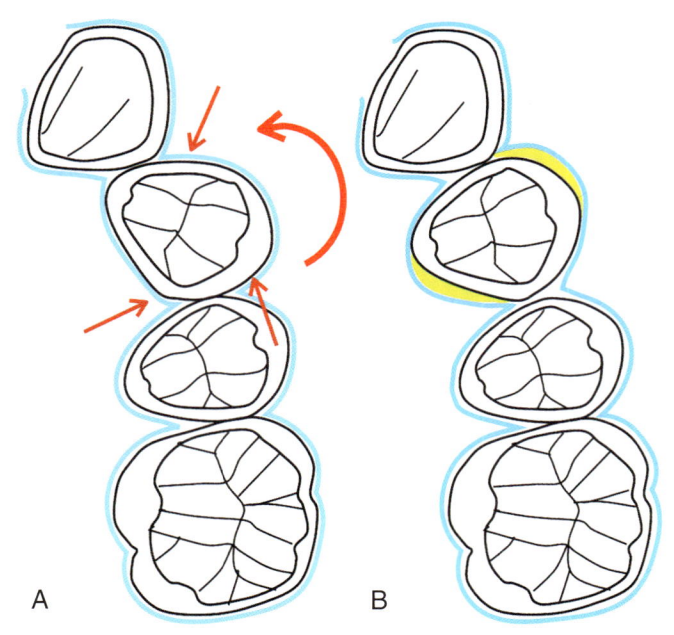

Fig. 2.8 (A) Multiple tangential forces *(red arrows)* acting during aligner-based, bicuspid rotation. (B) Due to slipping effect, incomplete expression of expected rotation with space between tooth and aligner *(in yellow)* will be observed.

DELIVERING PREDETERMINED FORCE VECTORS

The fundamental purpose of composite attachments in aligner orthodontics is to produce specific, complementary force vectors required for predictable tooth movement, which are not possible with the sole use of aligners thermoformed with existing materials (Fig. 2.9A).

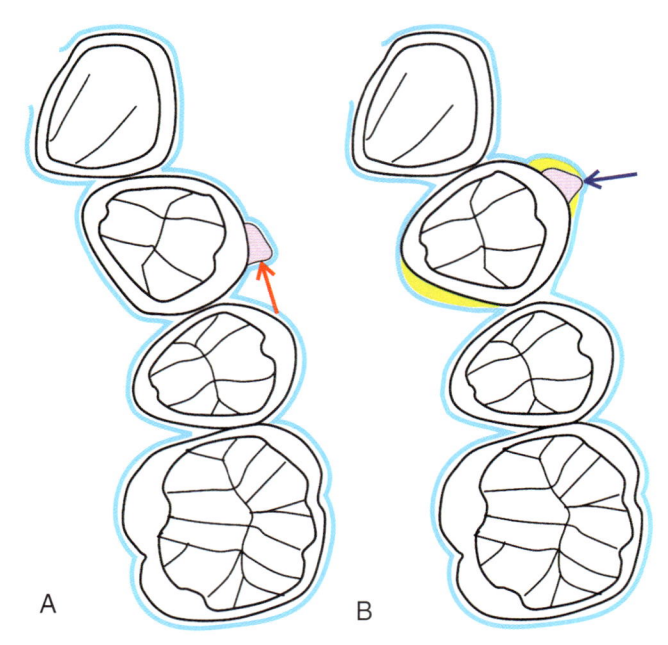

Fig. 2.9 (A) Properly designed attachments produce complementary force vectors required for predictable tooth movement. (B) Polymer stress relaxation and creep, along with incomplete rotation and unintended force *(blue arrow)*, may occur during sequence of aligner-based, tooth rotation stages.

Unfortunately, to harness the full clinical potential of bonded attachments, current polymers have yet to resolve limitations associated with their viscoelastic and hygroscopic nature. Once inserted, the initial force produced by the aligner after it is elastically deformed is not constant and will decline with time. This time-dependent reduction of force under constant deformation is called stress relaxation.[7,8] Not infrequently, due to unwarranted localized stress (caused by excessive mismatch), lack of compliance, or shortcomings inherent to the polymer, the aligner is not able to accommodate the attachment. When forces exerted upon the aligner exceed its capability to adjust to the new position, unintended forces will appear, the tooth will lag behind, and control will be lost (see Fig. 2.9B). Fig. 2.9 illustrates how this phenomenon is responsible for the incomplete expression of the expected tooth movement, where only 35 of the 45 degrees of predicted rotation were achieved after completion of the entire sequence of stages. In this case, after the aligner is removed, plastic deformation of the aligner material is evident. This time-dependent plastic deformation under constant force is called creep and is attributed to reorganization of polymer chains.[9] It is important to underline that this permanent deformation, so detrimental to clinical performance of plastic aligners, is not caused by a violation of the materials' elastic limit but is due to a time-dependent, mechanochemical phenomenon of a different nature.

This inherent flaw of aligner plastics is the major cause behind the inconsistent force levels and plastic deformation that result in one of the most dreaded occurrences for orthodontists practicing aligner orthodontics, now commonly referred to as loss of tracking. Fig. 2.10 illustrates an example of the clinical manifestations of this complex reality in which mesiolingual rotation and extrusion of a first upper left bicuspid were incorporated in the digital treatment plan but did not fully occur. The lack of coincidence between the attachment and its corresponding recess in the aligner is unambiguous evidence of loss of tracking, a contingency that in many cases must be resolved by obtaining updated digital dental models from which a new treatment sequence must be designed.

Basic Attachment Configurations in Current Aligner Orthodontics

The evolution of attachments, derived from a better understanding of the effect of geometry, location, and size of the composite structure, has resulted in a diverse array of configurations with well-defined biomechanical objectives.

VERTICAL CONTROL

The tendency of conventional fixed orthodontics to increase vertical dimension, especially in open-bite patients with increased anterior facial height, has been studied.[10] Aligner-based treatment has proven to be an effective alternative for open-bite correction[11-13] with encouraging results.[13] Successful treatment often includes the sum of complementary clinical strategies such as the combined effect of counterclockwise mandibular rotation, posterior intrusion, and anterior extrusion.[14]

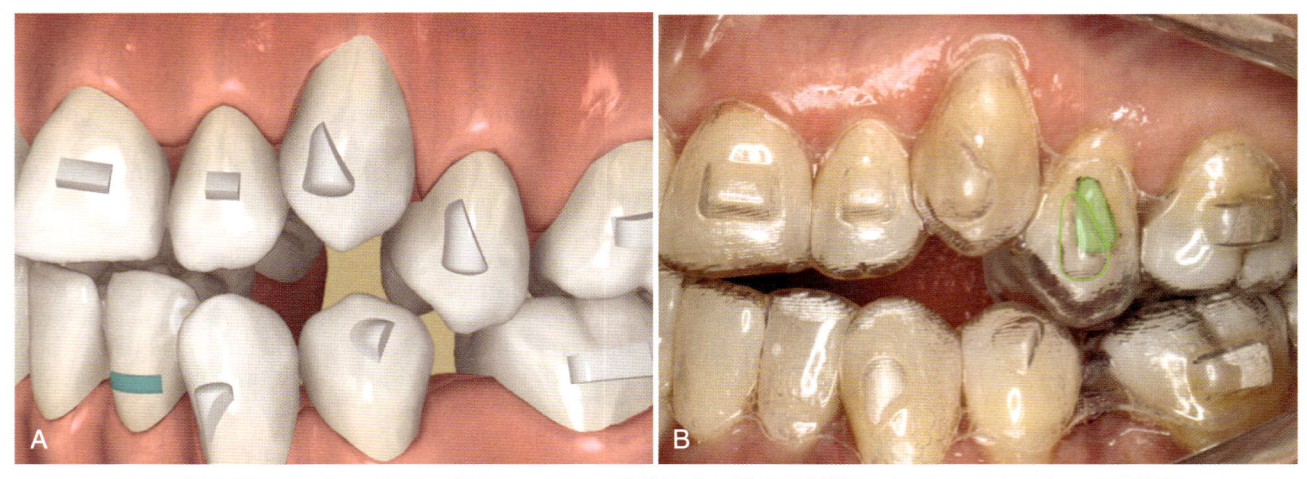

Fig. 2.10 (A) Image from ClinCheck treatment plan. (B) Loss of tracking with incomplete expression of rotation and extrusion of left upper bicuspid. Lack of coincidence between attachment *(green shaded area)* and its corresponding recess in the aligner *(green outline)* is observed.

ANTERIOR EXTRUSION

Correction of open bite based solely on anterior extrusion is to be viewed with caution because of possible negative effects such as root resorption, periodontal deterioration, instability, and unfavorable esthetics.[15,16] Along with these clinical restrictions, aligner extrusion poses mechanical limitations in anterior teeth in which buccal and lingual crown surfaces converge towards the incisal edge (Fig. 2.11A), facilitating aligner dislodgement and rendering this type of tooth movement virtually impossible (see Fig. 2.11B) without the use of supplementary composite attachments. A gingivally oriented, inclined plane configuration (Fig. 2.12) provides a force system that improves predictability of this type of movement. The importance of attachment design can be illustrated with a graphic simplification of a complex interaction of vectors. The resultant force acting on the

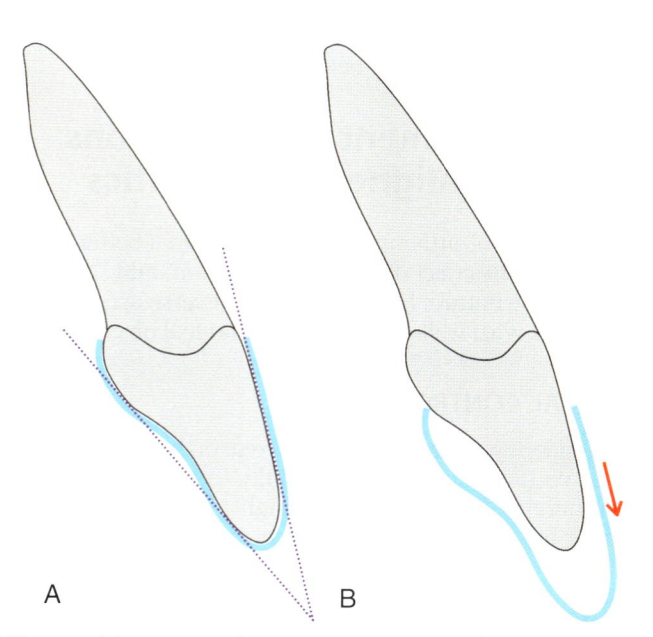

Fig. 2.11 (A) Converging buccal and lingual crown surfaces. (B) Undesired aligner dislodgment during extrusive movement.

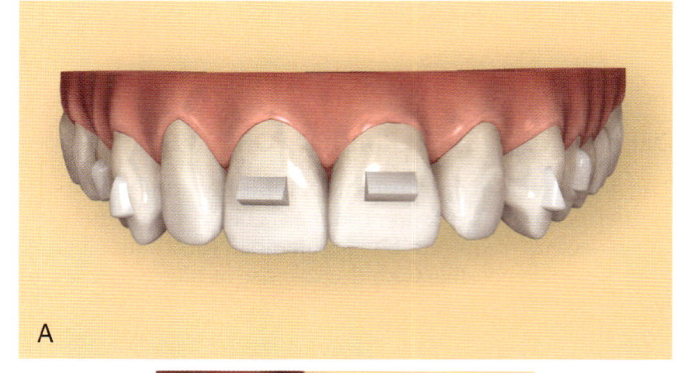

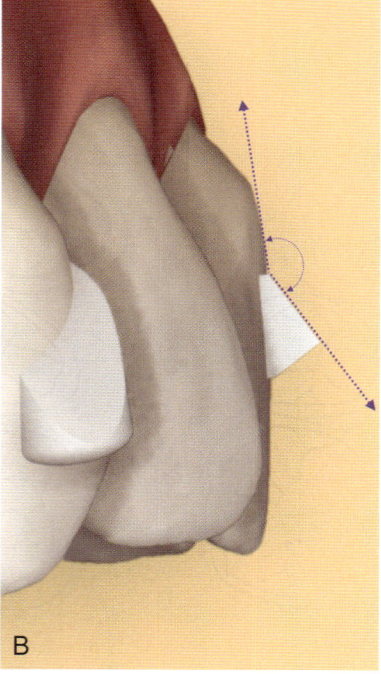

Fig. 2.12 (A) Optimized Extrusion Attachments (Align Technology, Santa Clara, CA) on central incisors. (B) Gingivally oriented inclined plane with optimal active surface angulation.

2 • Current Biomechanical Rationale Concerning Composite Attachments in Aligner Orthodontics

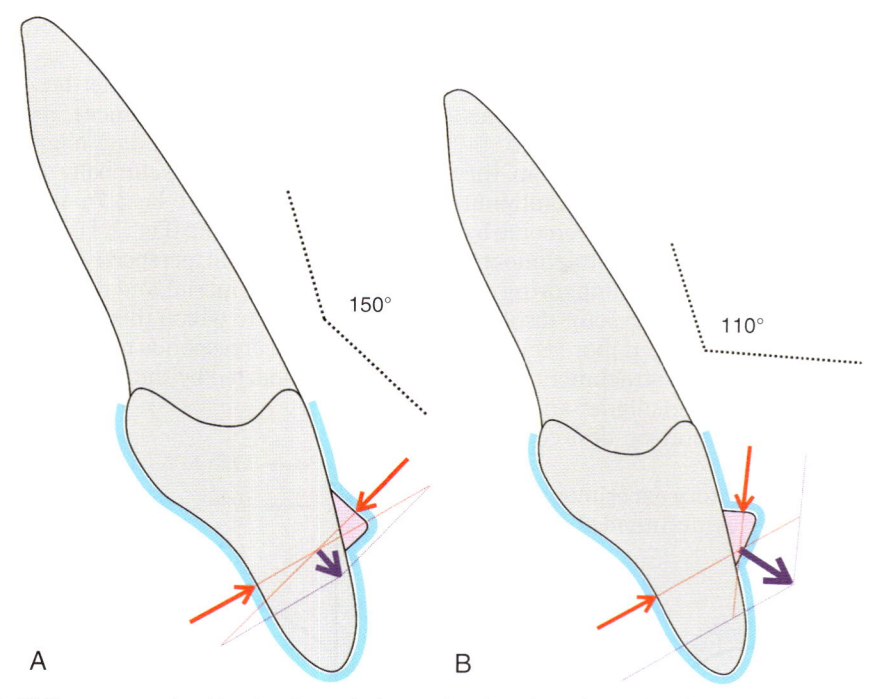

Fig. 2.13 (A) Forces transmitted by the aligner (red arrows) and resultant forces (purple arrows) acting on the tooth. (B) A reduction of the angle between active attachment surface and buccal tooth surface produces stronger resultant extrusive forces.

incisor is derived from the two red arrows that represent buccal and lingual forces present during aligner-based extrusion (Fig. 2.13A). Reducing the angle formed by the active surface of the attachment and the buccal surface of the tooth will result in a stronger resultant force (see Fig. 2.13B). Clinicians must be wary of excessive reduction of this angle, which along with excessive force may produce difficulty of aligner-attachment engagement with the ensuing localized plastic deformation.

POSTERIOR INTRUSION

Recent studies suggest that the presence of interocclusal plastic during aligner treatment[17,18] may produce a bite-block effect that potentiates bite closure and posterior intrusion capabilities. This improves treatment outlook, especially in cases in which anterior extrusion is not desirable and intrusion of posterior teeth, with the consequent mandibular rotation, are to be considered as part of the strategy for bite closure. As mentioned previously, intrusive forces acting in the posterior region will tend to dislodge the aligner in the occlusal direction. Even with light posterior intrusive forces, an opposite, reactive force should be expected in the anterior arch that will tend to vertically dislodge the aligner (Fig. 2.14). Gingivally positioned rectangular horizontal or occlusally attachments beveled towards the incisal edge should provide the necessary aligner stability for optimal treatment progress.

FIRST-ORDER CONTROL

Rotation

Rotation of teeth with rounded anatomies such as bicuspids and molars is another movement particularly difficult[19] to accomplish with plastic aligners without the help

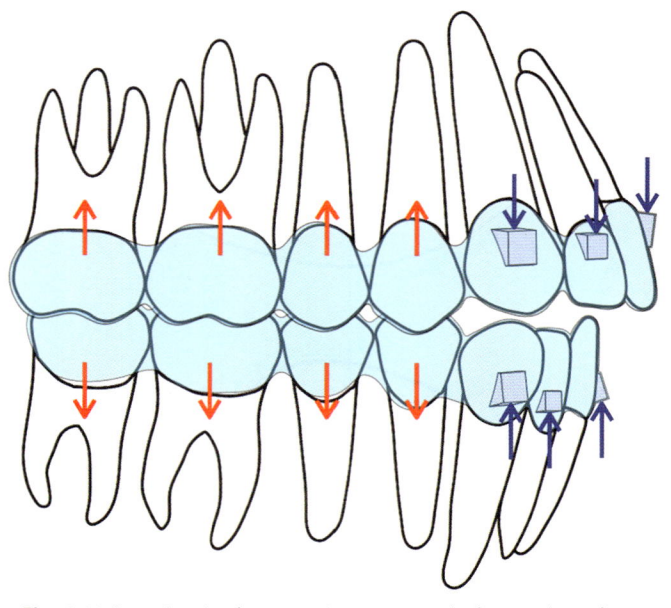

Fig. 2.14 Intrusion in the posterior segment (red arrows) produces reactive forces that will tend to dislodge the aligner anteriorly (blue arrows). Adequate attachment selection on anterior teeth will counteract this undesired occurrence.

of specialized attachments, which improve biomechanical capabilities.

The limitations associated with rounded crown morphologies are due to some extent to three particular realities:

- As mentioned previously, in rounded crown configurations, the tangential nature of the forces produced during aligner-based tooth rotation, along with very

low coefficient of friction between the two surfaces, facilitates a slipping effect between the aligner and tooth.
- The line of action of the normal force vectors resultant from tangential forces delivered during rotation of rounded crowns crosses at a short distance from the center of resistance, resulting in weaker rotational moments (Fig. 2.15A). These difficulties are overcome by means of specifically designed composite attachments, with properly oriented active surfaces, reconfiguring resultant force vectors with increased intervector distance (see Fig. 2.15B) and resulting in stronger, more effective rotational moments. Additionally, the attachment structure blocks the slipping effect between aligner and tooth surface, allowing a fuller expression of desired tooth movement.
- Another effect observed in laboratory experimentation[20] as well as in clinical practice is unintended intrusion during rotational tooth movement. In another study using finite element analysis,[21] researchers demonstrated that during aligner-based rotation of an upper canine without attachment, not only did the tooth lag behind the corresponding aligner stage almost by 30%, but it also displayed clinically significant intrusive forces that were found to be 3.71 times greater without than with attachments (Fig. 2.16). The same numeric model, from an incisal perspective, revealed distinct pressure areas on the mesial and distal slopes of the incisal ridge (Fig. 2.17), to which this undesirable effect can be attributed and corresponds to the normal components of the forces imparted by the aligner. Due to the orientation of

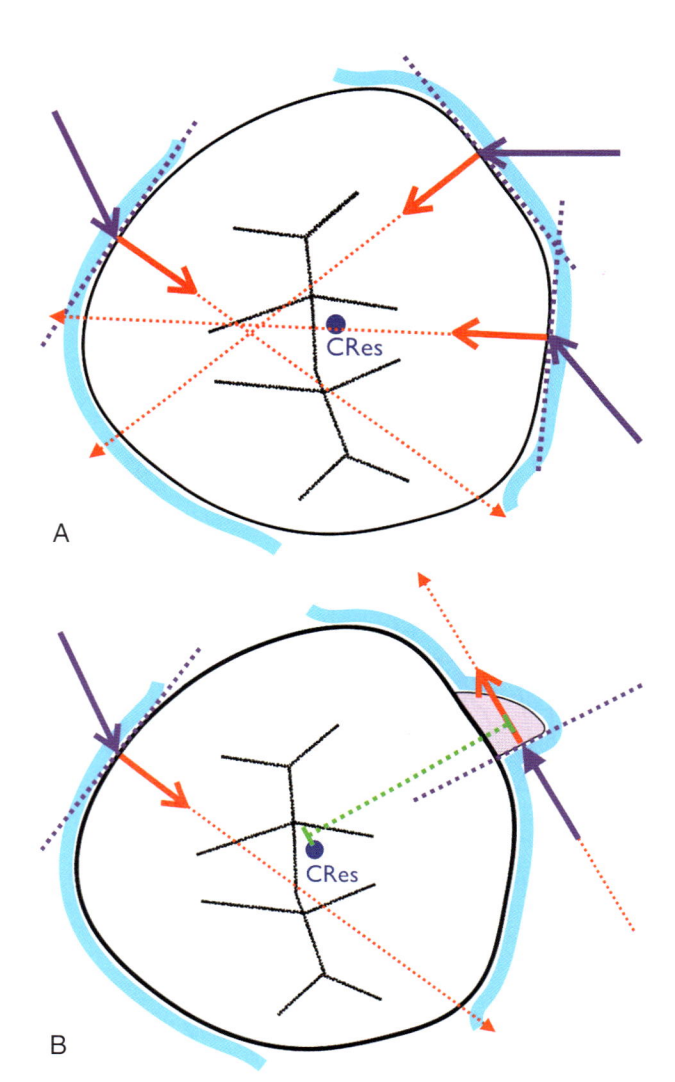

Fig. 2.15 (A) Rotational forces produced by the aligner *(purple arrows)* are transmitted to the tooth as normal force components *(red arrows)*, which are perpendicular to tooth surface tangents *(purple dotted lines)*. (B) Incorporation of bonded attachment increases the magnitude and efficacy of rotational moment by increasing the perpendicular distance *(green dotted line)* between the line of action *(red dotted line)* and the center of resistance *(CRes)*.

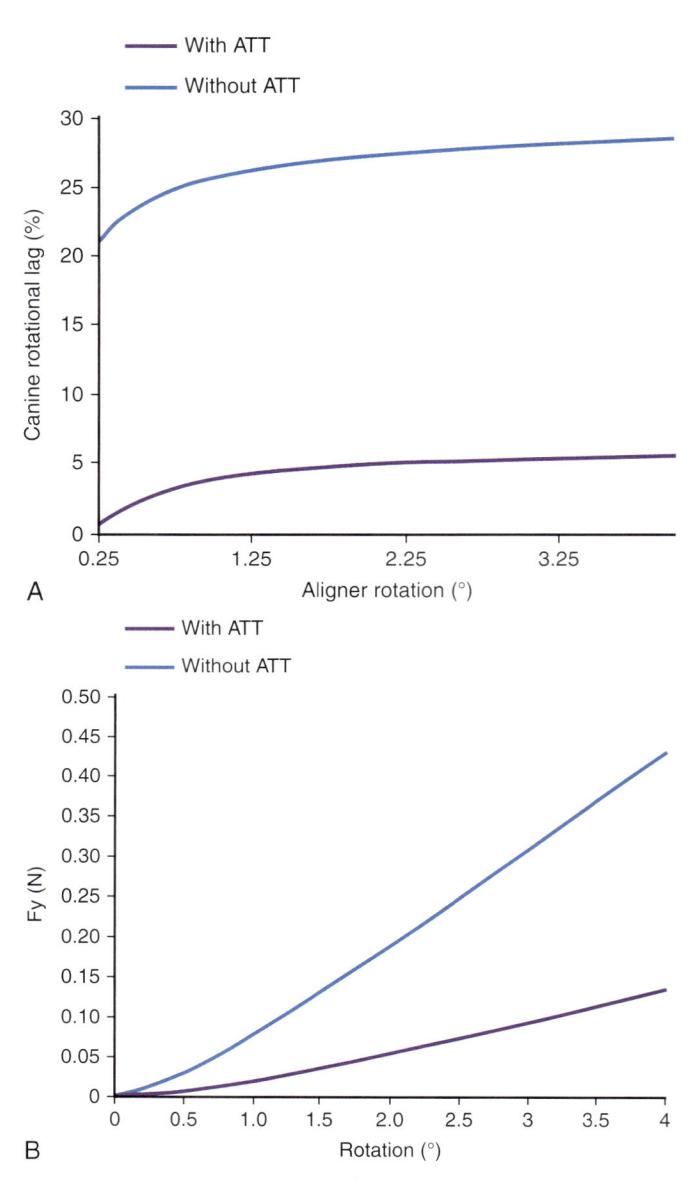

Fig. 2.16 (A) Without attachment, the tooth lagged behind the aligner almost by 30%. With attachment incorporation, this lag dropped to 5%. (B) Intrusive forces observed at the periodontal ligament without attachments was 0.078 N for every degree of rotation, while with attachments the load was reduced to 0.021 N for every degree. *ATT*, Attachment. (Adapted from Gómez JP, Peña FM, Valencia E, et al. Effect of composite attachment on initial force system generated during canine rotation with plastic aligners: a three dimensional finite elements analysis. *J Align Orthod.* 2018;2[1]:31-36.)

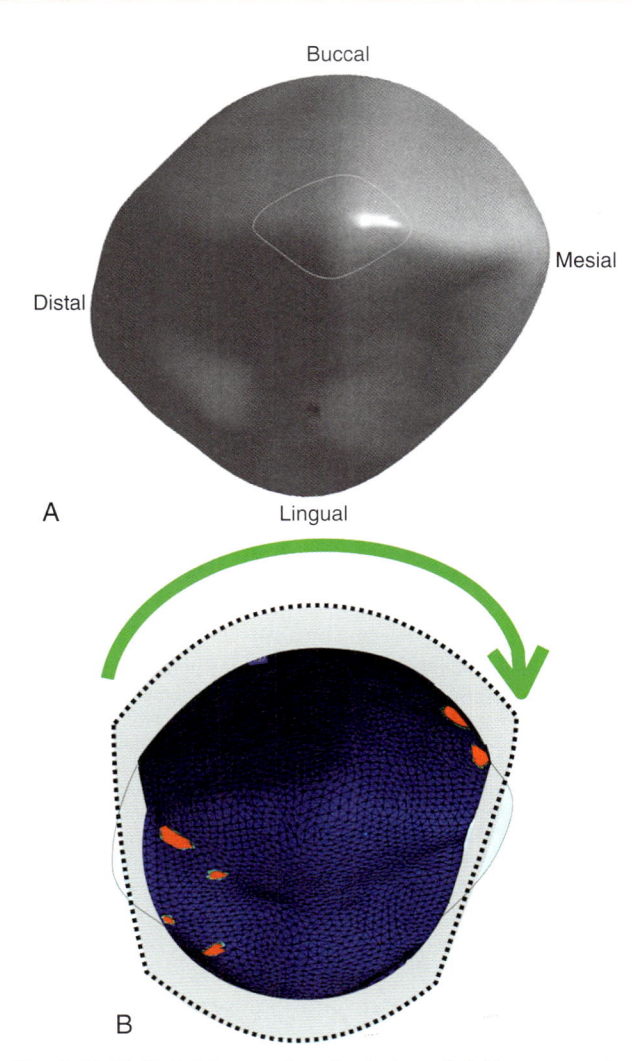

2 • Current Biomechanical Rationale Concerning Composite Attachments in Aligner Orthodontics   21

Fig. 2.17 (A) Digital image of occlusal view of right upper canine. Occlusal view of finite element method simulation of upper right canine during mesiolingual rotation. (B) Distinctly intrusive pressure areas (red) on mesiolabial and distolingual aspects of the tooth crown appear upon aligner insertion. The dotted line represents the aligner's profile. (Adapted from Gómez JP, Peña FM, Valencia E, et al. Effect of composite attachment on initial force system generated during canine rotation with plastic aligners: a three dimensional finite elements analysis. J Align Orthod. 2018;2[1]:31-36.)

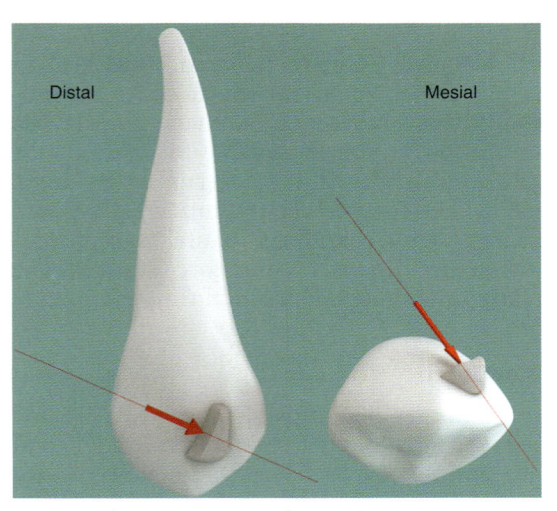

Fig. 2.18 Optimized Rotation Attachment (Align Technology, Santa Clara, CA) with active surface oriented to provide a compensatory extrusive force.

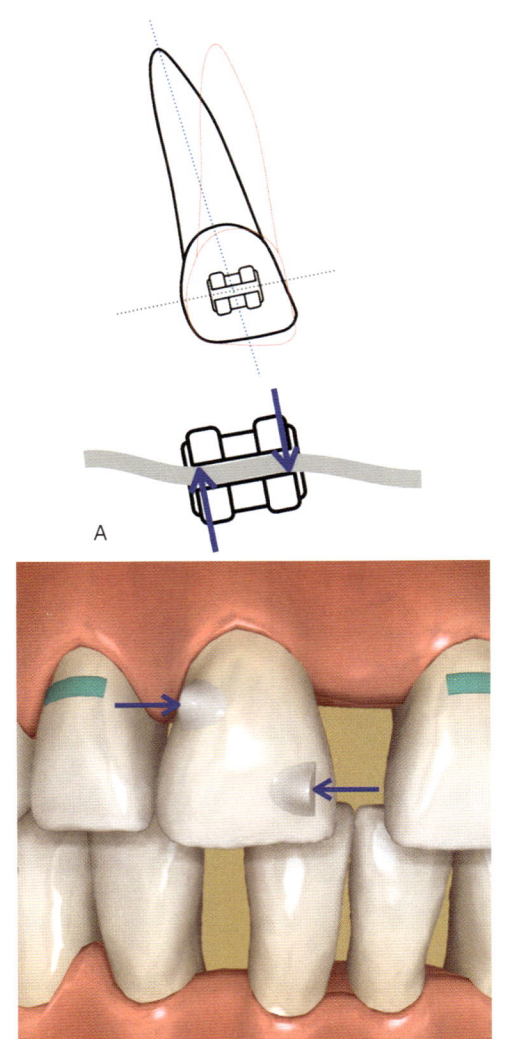

Fig. 2.19 (A) Force couple produced during bracket-based correction of excessive mesial tip. (B) Equivalent force couple produced at Optimized Root Control Attachments (Align Technology, Santa Clara, CA) during aligner-based tipping.

the surface area, these forces are clearly intrusive. This undesirable intrusive effect can be reduced with appropriate attachment design, orienting the active surface at an angle in which the normal component of the force transmitted by the aligner will express an extrusive tendency (Fig. 2.18).

SECOND-ORDER CONTROL

Tipping movements are easily achieved with bracket-based biomechanics (Fig. 2.19A). On the other hand, aligners lack control of mesiodistal root position due to the system's inability to produce the required force couples, explaining why modification of anterior teeth angulation is so challenging. To improve second-order capabilities, aligner-based systems rely on specialized attachments that generate equivalent force couples (see Fig. 2.19B).

Anterior Teeth

Successful closure of extraction spaces with aligners is also particularly difficult without excessive tipping in the direction of tooth movement. Numeric models[22] describing tooth displacement (Fig. 2.20) and periodontal ligament (PDL) strain (Fig. 2.21) patterns during distal tooth movement have shown that Optimized Root Control Attachments (Align Technology, Santa Clara, CA), when bonded to upper cuspids, produce force systems capable of controlling undesired inclination during extraction space closure.

Posterior Teeth

In the posterior segment, tipping movements are not easily obtained with aligner-based mechanics without combining fixed auxiliaries (such as buccal tubes, power arms, etc.), and these tooth movements, although possible, require sophisticated treatment planning, clinical expertise, and patient cooperation. Additionally, as with most complex force systems, specialized attachments must be designed to enhance the biomechanical capabilities of the aligner. The goal of this configuration of composite attachments is to produce a force couple (and its corresponding moment) that will incline the tooth in the desired direction (Fig. 2.22A). Alternatively, the rectangular, horizontal attachment can be replaced with two shorter attachments, with variable distance separating them according to the clinician's plan (see Fig. 2.22B). It is important to remember that the magnitude of the moment will depend on the amount of activation (and corresponding mismatch) prescribed in the digital treatment plan. On the other hand, the magnitude of the individual force vectors acting at the

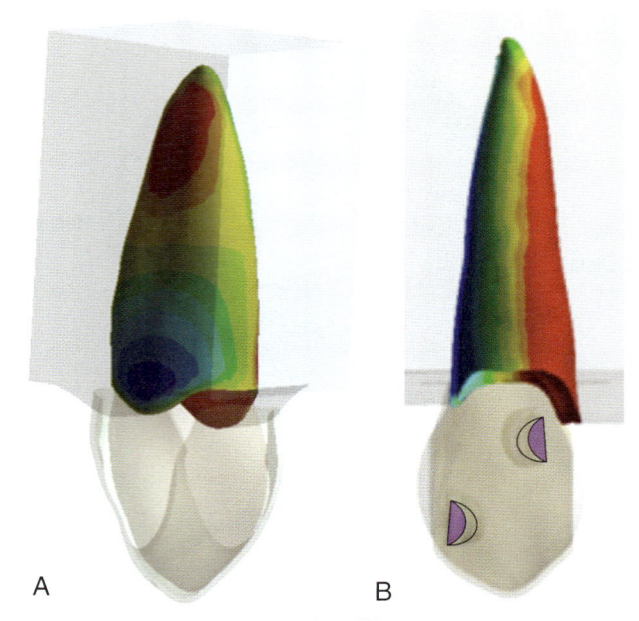

Fig. 2.21 Periodontal ligament strain patterns during aligner-based distalization of upper right canine. (A) Without attachments, distocervical pressure *(in blue)* and distoapical tension *(in red)* areas were observed, typical of uncontrolled distal tipping. (B) With attachments, uniform pressure along the distal root surface *(in blue)* and uniform tension *(in red)* along the medial surface, typical of distal bodily movement, were observed. (Adapted from Gomez JP, Peña FM, Martínez V, et al. Initial force systems during bodily tooth movement with plastic aligners and composite attachments: a three-dimensional finite element analysis. *Angle Orthod.* 2015;85[3]:454-460.)

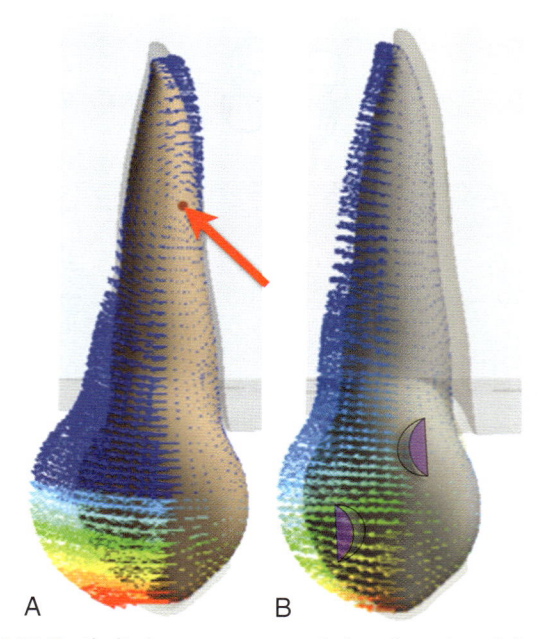

Fig. 2.20 Tooth displacement patterns during aligner-based distalization of upper right canine. (A) Without attachments, distinct uncontrolled distal tipping was observed, with center of rotation between apical and middle thirds of the root *(red arrow)*. (B) With attachments, the canine expressed distal bodily movement. (Adapted from Gomez JP, Peña FM, Mart√≠nez V, et al. Initial force systems during bodily tooth movement with plastic aligners and composite attachments: a three-dimensional finite element analysis. *Angle Orthod.* 2015;85[3]:454-460.)

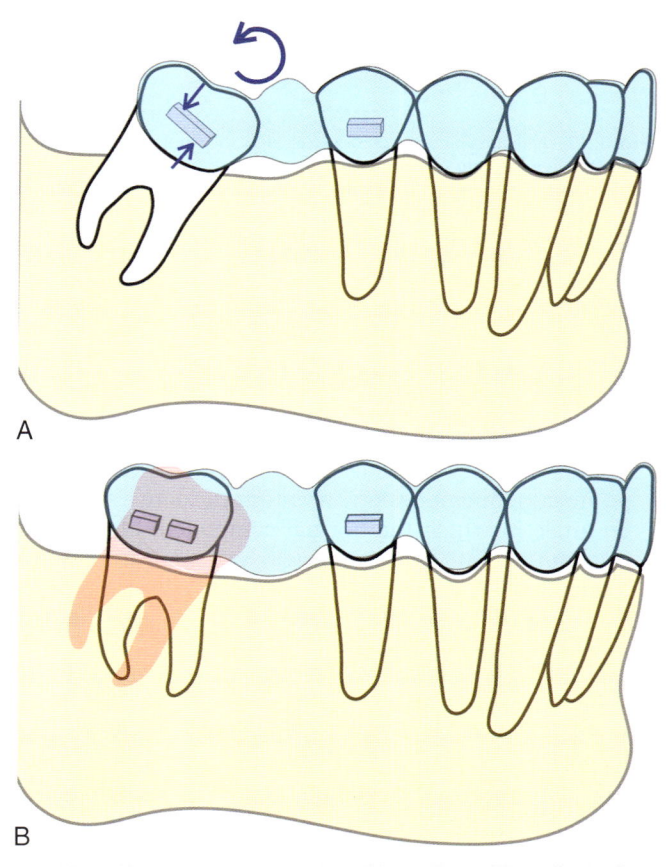

Fig. 2.22 (A) Uprighting moment produced at single rectangular horizontal attachment. (B) Alternative twin attachment configuration.

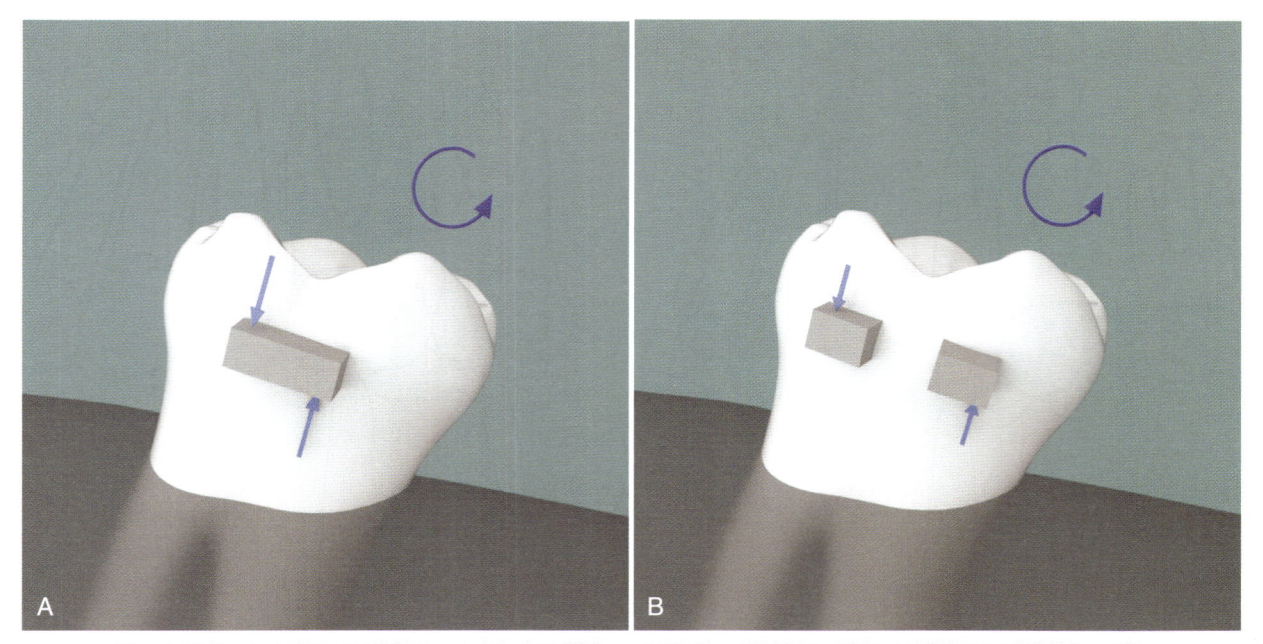

2 • Current Biomechanical Rationale Concerning Composite Attachments in Aligner Orthodontics   23

Fig. 2.23 Producing equivalent moments *(curved arrows)*, an increase in intervector distance proportionately reduces force magnitude *(blue arrows)* acting at attachment surface. Two degrees of distal tipping with a 4-mm rectangular attachment (A) will produce higher forces on the aligner than with a two-attachment configuration that significantly separates the force vectors (B) of the acting couple.

aligner-attachment contact will depend on the distance between these two vectors. As the distance between the vectors decreases, the forces produced at the active surfaces of the attachments to produce an equal uprighting moment will increase (Fig. 2.23). This is an extremely important detail, considering aligner polymers' high susceptibility to creep-related plastic deformation, which requires the use of the lowest forces possible.

Differential Moments

An effective strategy for controlling anchorage during extraction space closure is anterior and posterior moment to force ratio manipulation in favor of the segment that requires anchorage.[23] As shown in Fig. 2.24A, a reciprocal moment to force ratio between anterior (alpha) and posterior (beta) segments will result in group B space closure, in which both segments will meet at the middle of the extraction space resulting in class II malocclusion (see Fig. 2.24B). To obtain class I occlusion, posterior anchorage must be reinforced. Bonding rectangular horizontal attachments on the buccal surface of posterior teeth (Fig. 2.25A) will result in clockwise moments that will resist mesialization of posterior teeth, resulting in group A space closure and the desired class I occlusal outcome (see Fig. 2.25B).

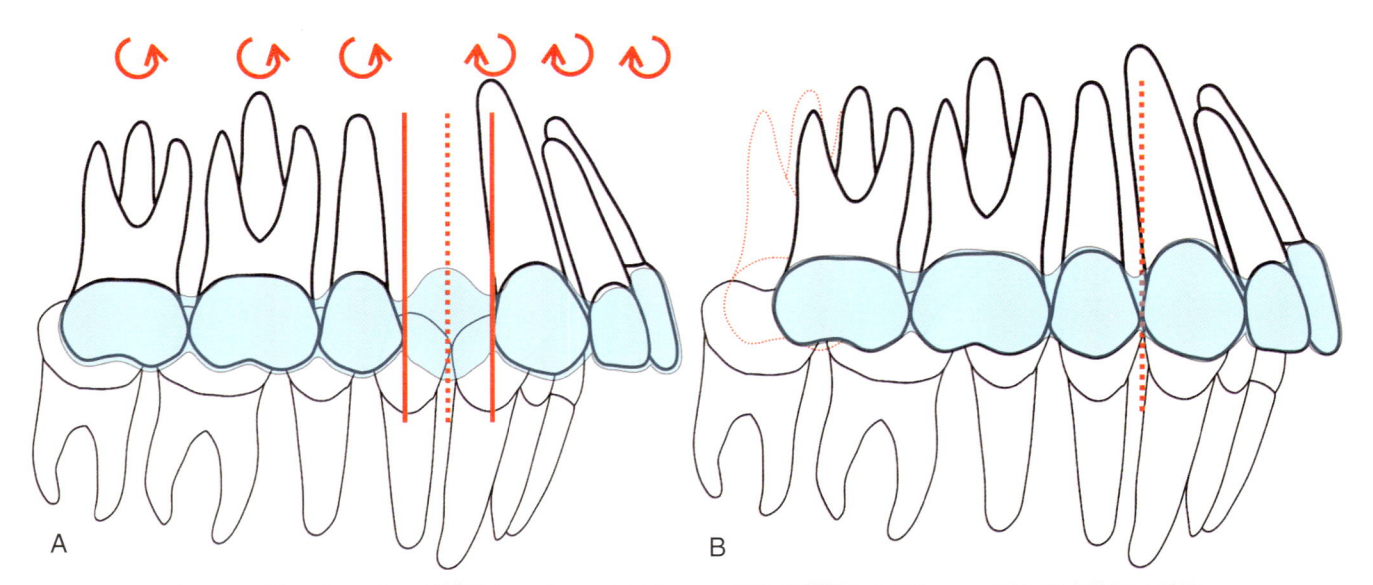

Fig. 2.24 Class II case in which reciprocal moments between anterior and posterior segments during extraction space closure (A) will result in 50% anchorage loss and class II occlusion (B).

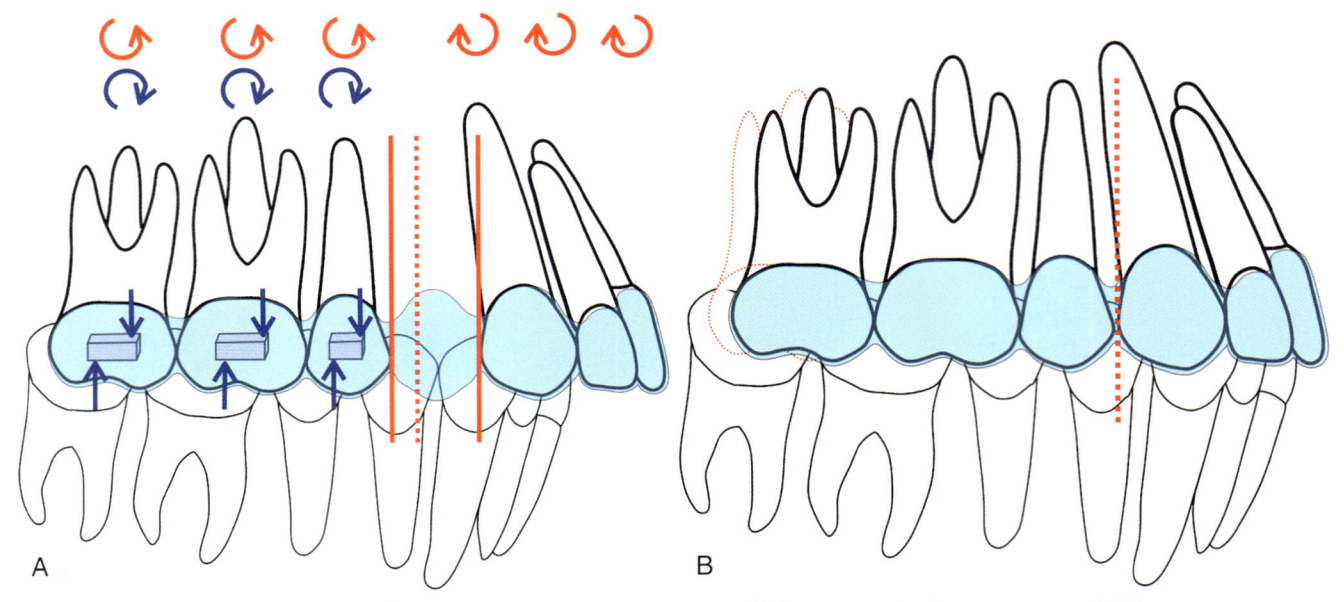

Fig. 2.25 Clockwise moments *(blue curved arrows)* produced by attachments bonded to posterior teeth (A) will counteract posterior anchorage loss, reducing it to 25%, resulting in class I occlusion (B).

THIRD-ORDER CONTROL

Anterior Torque

Torque modification of anterior teeth with conventional brackets is easily achieved by means of preactivation of the rectangular archwire, producing a complex, high-force couple when fully engaged in the rectangular slot (Fig. 2.26A). Accomplishing the same type of movement with plastic aligners demands an equivalent couple, derived from horizontal, parallel, and opposing forces applied on buccal and lingual surfaces (see Fig. 2.26B). Because of the relatively ample distance between the couple vectors, force magnitudes required for third-order control are significantly lower than those required in equivalent bracket-based force systems.

Posterior Torque

Correction of transverse deficiencies by expansion of the dental arch continues to be a challenging clinical objective with current aligner-based techniques.[24] This has led to a widespread tendency of clinicians to overcorrect expansive movements in 3D treatment planning.[25] The main reasons for lack of efficacy and predictability in the transverse plane are excess buccal tipping and insufficient force levels.

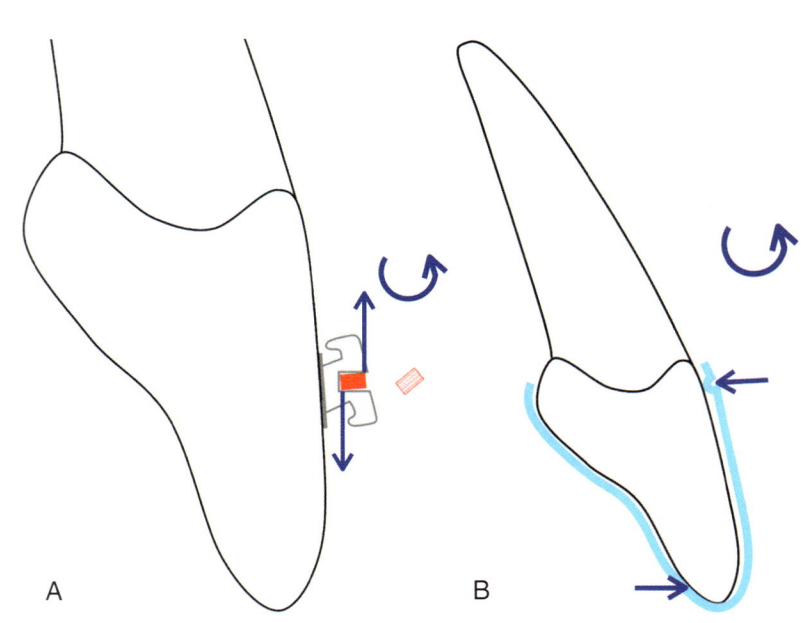

Fig. 2.26 (A) By preactivating (red shaded) and subsequently inserting (red) the archwire, a force couple *(blue arrows)* and its corresponding counterclockwise moment *(blue curved arrow)* will be produced. (B) The same positive torque can be achieved with aligners by producing an equivalent couple, with lower forces and increased intervector distance.

Excess Buccal Tipping

Because forces act at a distance from the molar's center of resistance (Fig. 2.27A), buccal tipping must always be expected when expansive forces are applied, especially when aligner-based forces are used.[26] With negligible friction (and consequent pervasive sliding effect) between plastic and tooth crown, and relatively low stiffness as uncontrolled tipping occurs during expansion, the aligner will tend to flare, losing control as dissociation between tooth and plastic occurs (see Fig. 2.27B).

The use of attachments (horizontal rectangular or occlusally beveled) bonded to the buccal surface of posterior teeth helps improve third-order control by counteracting the undesired tipping moment as a result of a couple with opposite forces acting at the occlusal surface and at the gingival aspect of the attachment (Fig. 2.28).

Insufficient Force Levels

Due to their horseshoe-shaped geometry, orthodontic aligners deliver expansive forces in a particular manner in which an anteroposterior decreasing force gradient will be observed (Fig. 2.29). Because of this distinct mode of force transmission, researchers have found that efficacy (planned vs. final increase in arch width) of upper arch expansion dropped from 70% at first premolars to 29% at the second molar.[24,25] Increasing force levels during arch expansion by using thicker or lower elastic modulus polymers for aligner fabrication would improve this shortcoming, but not without the inconvenient increase in force levels of all other tooth movements programmed during the expansive stages. An alternative solution is the use of intermaxillary elastics, especially in cases with reduced anterior facial height, in which buccolingual tipping and

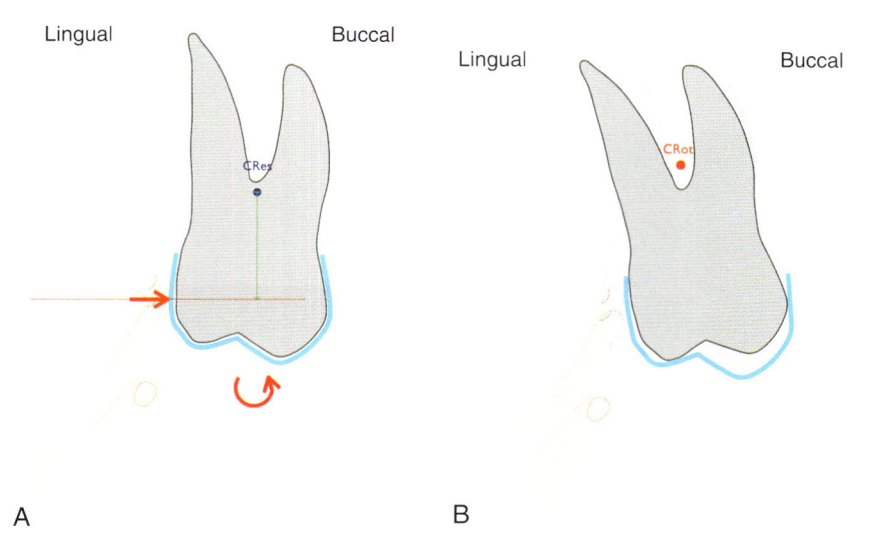

Fig. 2.27 (A) Aligner-based expansive force *(red arrow)* applied at a distance from the center of resistance *(CRes)* will produce counterclockwise moment *(red curved arrow)*. (B) Without preventive measures, buccal tipping with center of rotation *(CRot)* above the furcation will occur, followed by aligner deformation and loss of control.

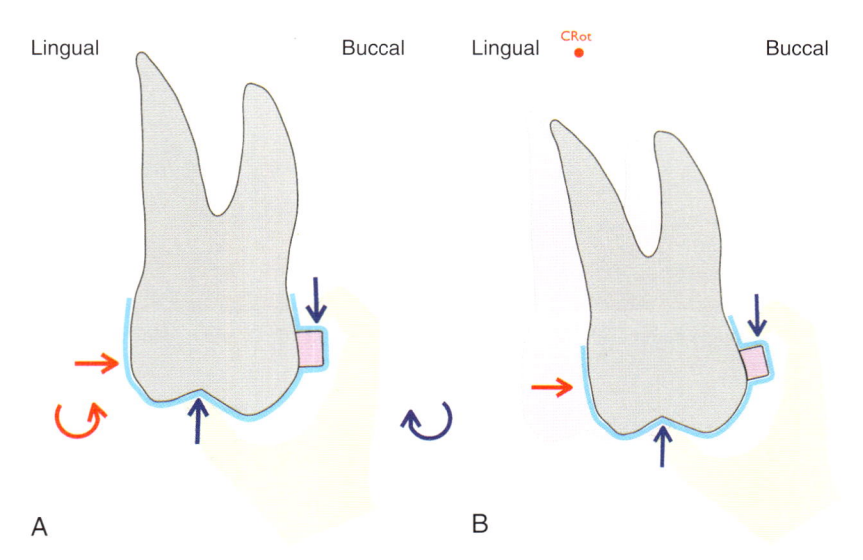

Fig. 2.28 (A) Opposing forces *(blue arrows)* acting at the occlusal surface and gingival aspect of a rectangular horizontal buccal attachment will provide a clockwise moment *(blue curved arrow)* that reduces buccal tipping, with apical migration of the center of rotation *(CRot)* (B).

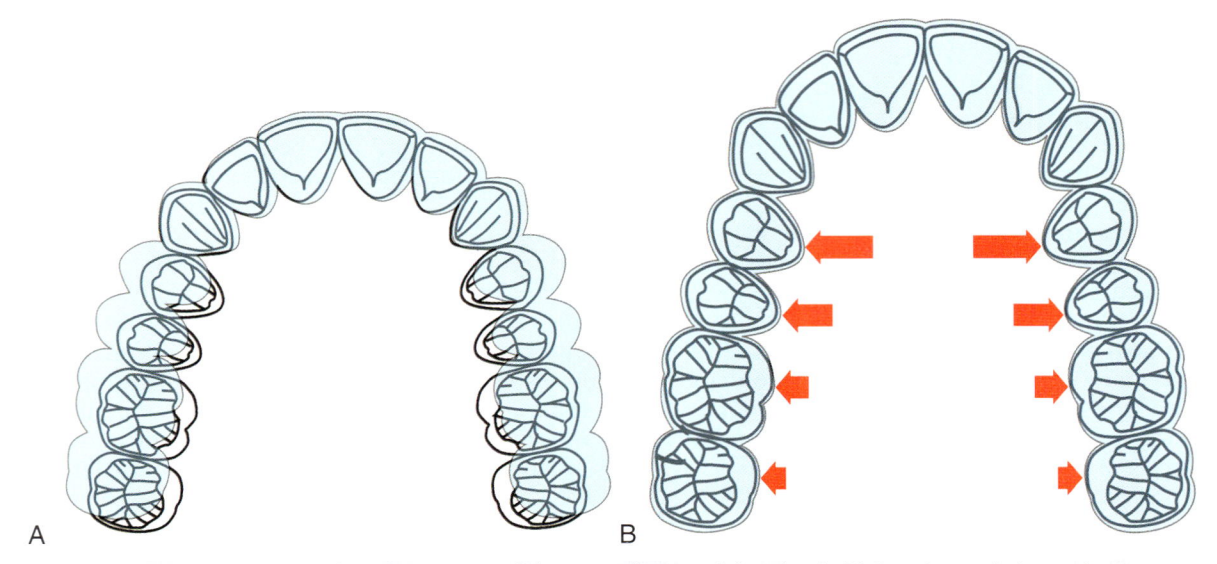

Fig. 2.29 (A) Programmed expansive mismatch between aligner and dental arch. (B) Once inserted, the resultant expansive forces will have a distally decreasing magnitude gradient.

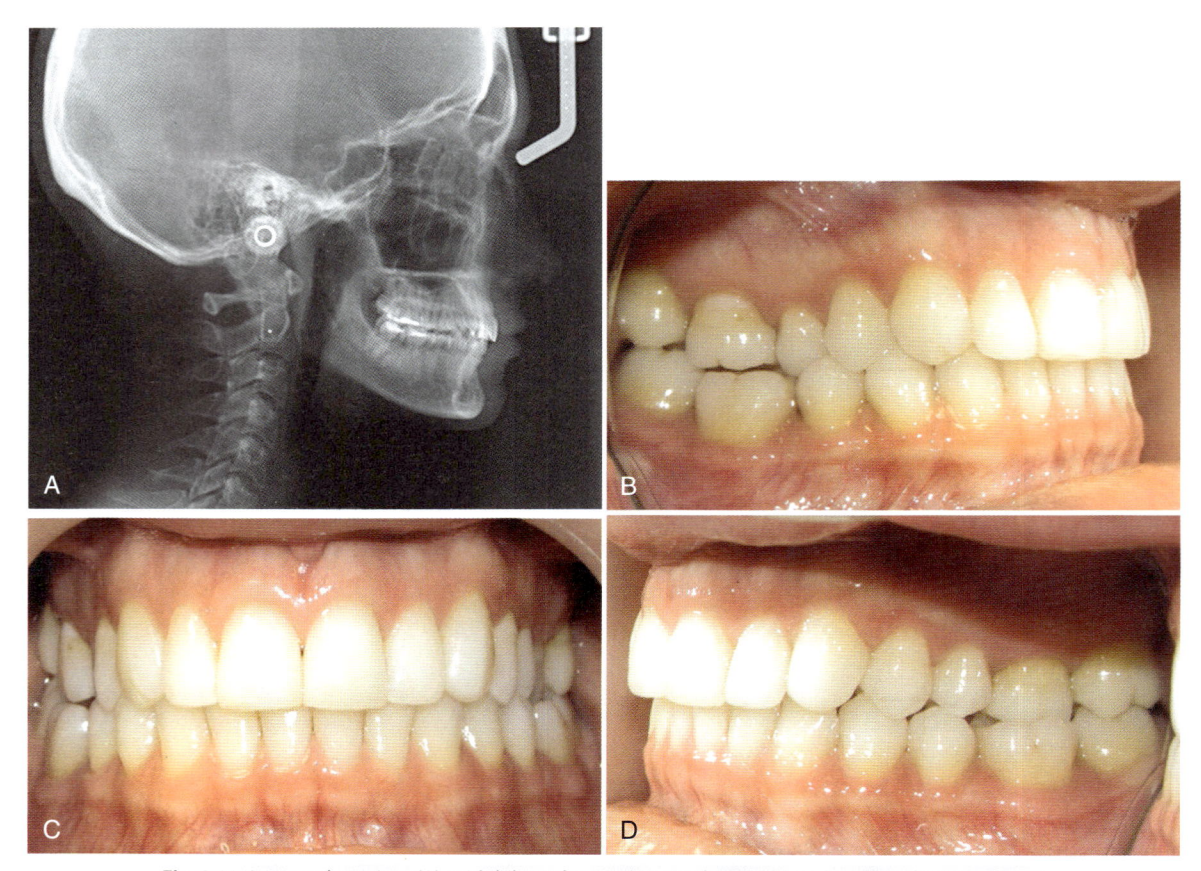

Fig. 2.30 Low angle patient (A), with bilateral posterior crossbite (B, D) and midline discrepancy (C).

extrusion of posterior segments are acceptable (Fig. 2.30). Elastic forces originated from buttons bonded to palatal upper and buccal lower aspects of molars (Fig. 2.31) will produce a force vector with vertical and horizontal components of clinically relevant magnitudes that must be considered during treatment planning. In the example in Fig. 2.32, a 100-gmf vector produced by a crossed intermaxillary elastic will be transmitted to the system as 90 gmf of horizontal and 40 gmf of vertical force. As mentioned previously, horizontal rectangular attachments are effective in mitigating undesired tipping by counteracting excessive rotational moments (Fig. 2.33). By controlling vertical and transverse force levels, as well as desired and undesired tipping moments, predictable aligner-based treatment of different types of transverse discrepancies is possible (Fig. 2.34).

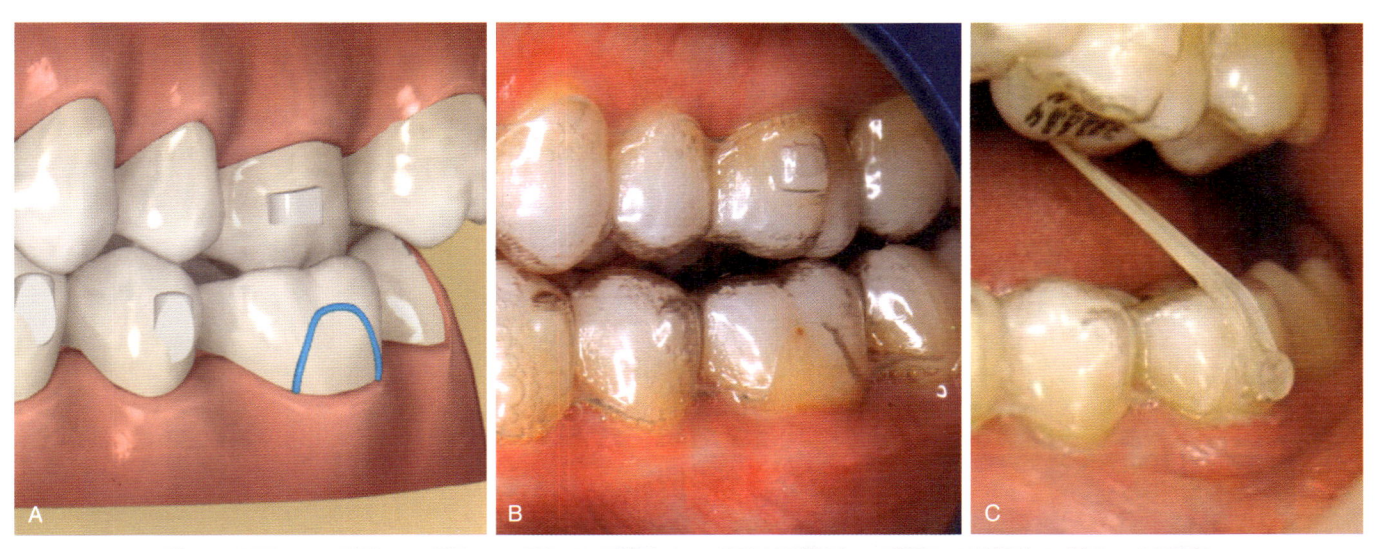

2 • Current Biomechanical Rationale Concerning Composite Attachments in Aligner Orthodontics   27

Fig. 2.31 (A) Initial ClinCheck stage. (B) Aligners inserted, prior to bonding of upper palatal and lower buccal buttons. (C) Crossbite elastic.

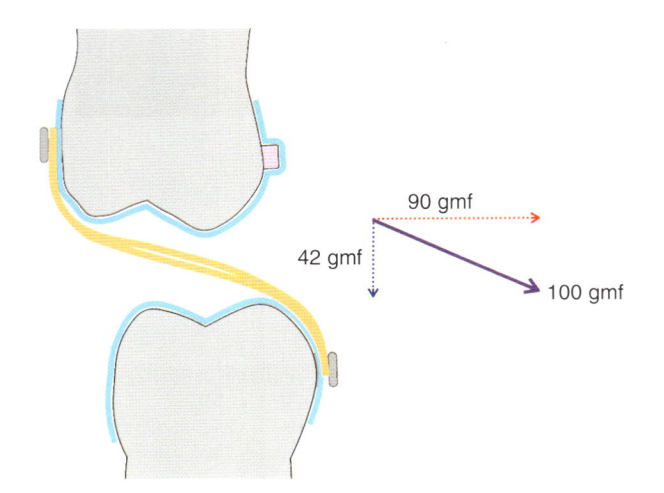

Fig. 2.32 A 100-gmf intermaxillary elastic force will produce a 90-gmf effective transverse force, expanding the upper arch and compressing the lower arch. Additionally, 42 gmf of extrusive force will equally influence upper and lower arches.

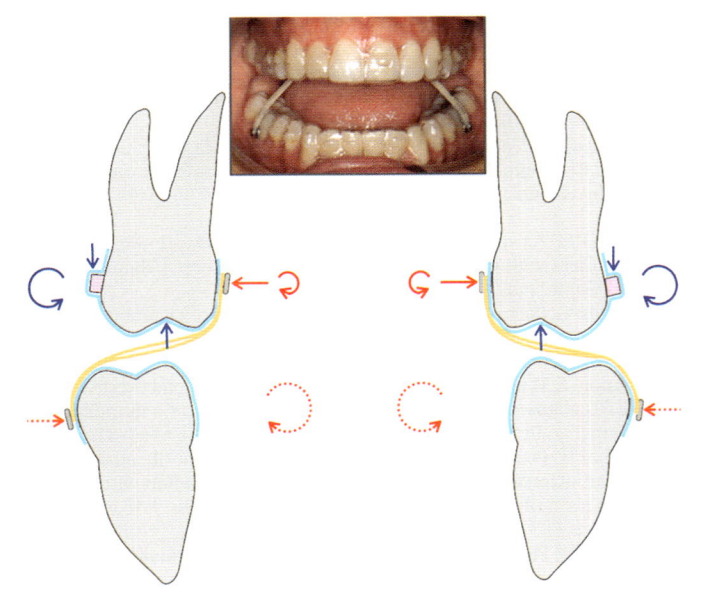

Fig. 2.33 In the upper arch, the moments provided by upper buccal attachments *(blue curved arrows)* will counteract moments *(red curved arrows)* produced by elastic expansive forces *(red arrows)*, reducing undesired upper tipping. In the lower arch, unopposed lingual elastic forces *(dotted red arrows)* will result in expected lingual tipping *(dotted red curved arrows)*.

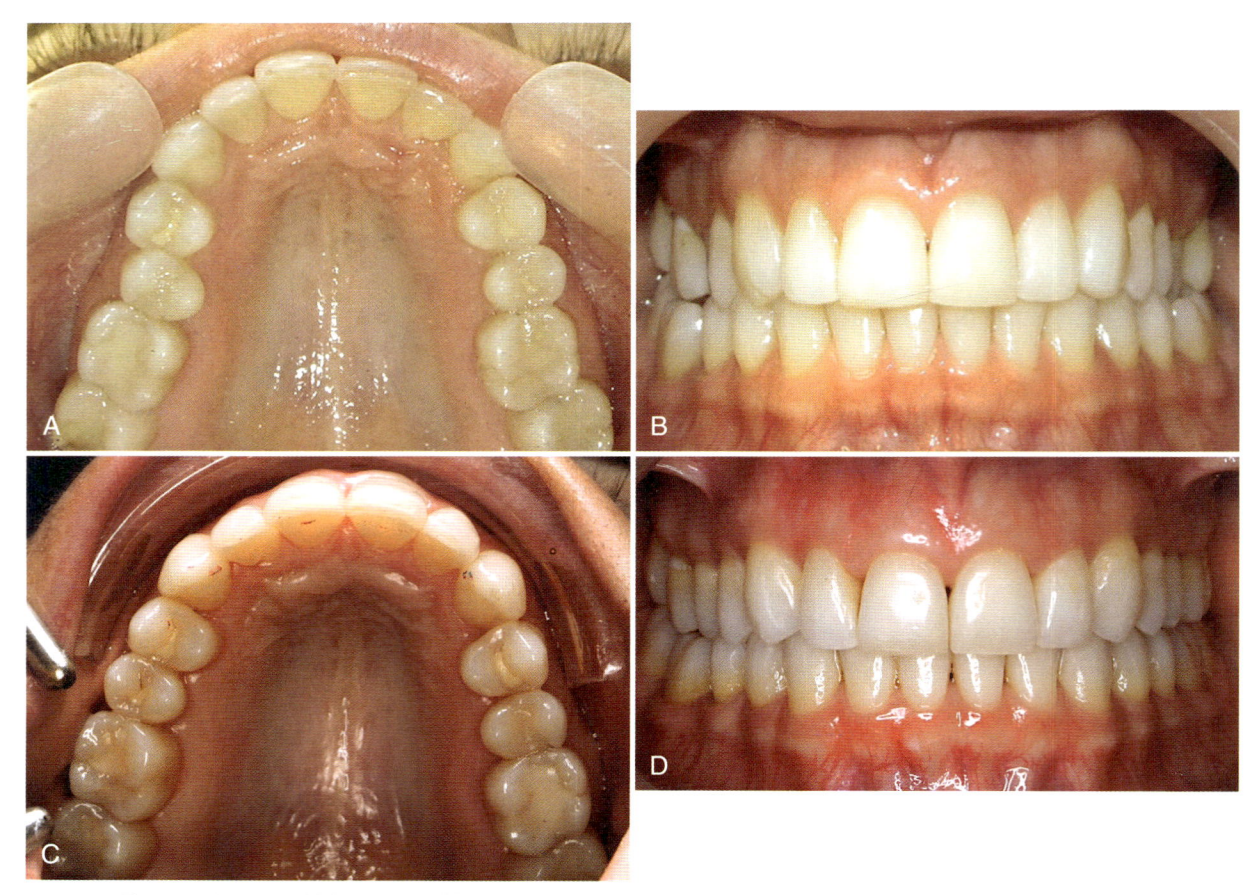

Fig. 2.34 (A, B) Initial bilateral crossbite and midline discrepancy. (C, D) Aligner-based correction with complementary use of intermaxillary elastics.

References

1. Miller RJ, Duong TT, Derakhshan M. Lower incisor extraction treatment with the Invisalign system. *J Clin Orthod.* 2002;36:95-102.
2. Barreda GJ, Dzierewianko EA, Muñoz KA, et al. Surface wear of resin composites used for Invisalign® attachments. *Acta Odontol Latinoam.* 2017;30(2):90-95.
3. Mantovani E, Castroflorio E, Rossini G, et al. Scanning electron microscopy analysis of aligner fitting on anchorage attachments. *J Orofac Orthop.* 2019 Mar;80(2):79-87.
4. Feinberg KB, Souccar NM, Kau CH, et al. Translucency, stain resistance, and hardness of composites used for Invisalign attachments. *J Clin Orthod.* 2016;50(3):170-176.
5. Aristizabal JS, García JI, Peña FM. Valoracion del efecto biomecánico en el ligamento periodontal durante la expansión en el arco maxilar, de canino a molar, usando alineadores termo-formados con aditamentos biomecánicos complementarios, mediante métodos computacionales (MSc thesis). Cali, Colombia: Universidad del Valle;2019
6. Jones M, Mah J, O'Toole B. Retention of thermoformed aligners with attachments of various shapes and positions. *J Clin Orthod.* 2009;43(2):113-117.
7. Lombardo L, Martines E, Mazzanti V, et al. Stress relaxation properties of four orthodontic aligner materials: a 24-hour in vitro study. *Angle Orthod.* 2017;87(1):11-18.
8. Fang D, Zhang N, Chen H, et al. Dynamic stress relaxation of orthodontic thermoplastic materials in a simulated oral environment. *Dent Mat J.* 2013;32(6):946-951.
9. Alexandropoulos A, Al Jabbari YS, Zinelis S, et al. Chemical and mechanical characteristics of contemporary thermoplastic orthodontic materials. *Aust Orthod J.* 2015;31(2):165-170.
10. Moshiri S, Ara√∫jo EA, McCray JF, et al. Cephalometric evaluation of adult anterior open bite non-extraction treatment with Invisalign. *Dental Press J Orthod.* 2017;22(5):30-38.
11. Guarneri MP, Oliverio T, Silvestre I, et al. Open bite treatment using clear aligners. *Angle Orthod.* 2013;83(5):913-919.
12. Giancotti A, Garino F, Mampieri G. Use of clear aligners in open bite cases: an unexpected treatment option. *J Orthod.* 2017;44(2):114–125.
13. Kau CH, Feinberg KB, Christou T. Effectiveness of clear aligners in treating patients with anterior open bite: a retrospective analysis. *J Clin Orthod.* 2017;51(8):454-460.
14. Garnett BS, Mahood K, Nguyen M, et al. Cephalometric comparison of adult anterior open bite treatment using clear aligners and fixed appliances. *Angle Orthod.* 2018 Jan;89(1):3-9.
15. Sherwood KH, Burch JG, Thompson WJ. Closing anterior open bites by intruding molars with titanium miniplate anchorage. *Am J Orthod Dentofacial Orthop.* 2002;122(6):593-600.
16. Proffit WR. *Contemporary Orthodontics.* Toronto: Elsevier; 2013.
17. Boyd RL. Complex orthodontic treatment using a new protocol for the Invisalign appliance. *J Clin Orthod.* 2007:41(9):525-547; quiz 523.
18. Klein BM. A cephalometric study of adult mild class II nonextraction treatment with the Invisalign system [master's thesis]. Saint Louis, MO: Saint Louis University; 2013.
19. Rossini G, Parrini S, Castroflorio T, et al. Efficacy of clear aligners in controlling orthodontic tooth movement: a systematic review. *Angle Orthod.* 2015;85(5):881-889.
20. Elkholy F, Mikhaiel B, Schmidt F, et al. Mechanical load exerted by PET-G aligners during mesial and distal derotation of a mandibular canine: an in vitro study. *J Orofac Orthop.* 2017;78(5):361-370.
21. Gómez JP, Peña FM, Valencia E, et al. Effect of composite attachment on initial force system generated during canine rotation with plastic aligners: a three dimensional finite elements analysis. *J Align Orthod.* 2018;2(1):31-36.
22. Gomez JP, Peña FM, Martínez V, et al. Initial force systems during bodily tooth movement with plastic aligners and composite

attachments: a three-dimensional finite element analysis. *Angle Orthod.* 2015;85(3):454-460.
23. Nanda R. *Biomechanics and Esthetic Strategies in Clinical Orthodontics.* St. Louis, MO: Elsevier; 2005.
24. Solano-Mendoza B, Sonnemberg B, Solano-Reina E, et al. How effective is the Invisalign® system in expansion movement with Ex30' aligners? *Clin Oral Investig.* 2017;21(5):1475-1484.
25. Houle JP, Piedade L, Todescan Jr R, et al. The predictability of transverse changes with Invisalign. *Angle Orthod.* 2017; 87(1):19-24.
26. Zhao X, Wang HH, Yang YM, et al. Maxillary expansion efficiency with clear aligner and its possible influencing factors. *Zhonghua Kou Qiang Yi Xue Za Zhi.* 2017;52(9):543-548.

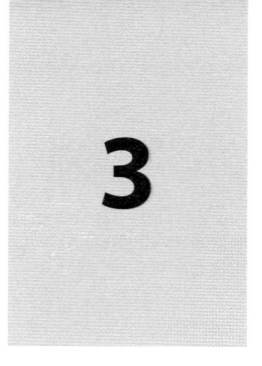

3 Clear Aligners: Material Structures and Properties

MASOUD AMIRKHANI, FAYEZ ELKHOLY, and BERND G. LAPATKI

Introduction

The continued improvement of medical treatment demands easy to use, cheaper, and more durable products without compromising the treatment outcome itself. Due to inherent properties and availability, polymeric materials show high potential for medical applications. Polymeric materials are lightweight, easy to manufacture, cheap, and versatile. These properties allow them to be used in diverse medical applications such as implants, prostheses, and orthodontic appliances. As of any material used for medical applications (and intraoral applications in particular), the polymer must be biocompatible and must not induce adverse reactions.[1,2] The restrictions and the standard in choosing a polymer depend on the type of application.

In orthodontic applications, polymers are exposed to the intraoral environment, which comprises several different substances including water, electrolytes, enzymes, bacteria, among other components.[3] Additionally, consuming different food and drink changes the acidity and ion concentration and may temporarily introduce organic solvent (e.g., alcohol) to the polymer environment. This means that the polymer must be resistant to chemical corrosion. Principally, corrosion causes a particle release, which—depending on the size and form of particles—might influence the mechanical properties of the polymer as well.

Another important aspect is the thermal properties of the polymer. Although the intraoral temperature remains relatively constant (near 37°C), a polymer could be subjected to varying temperature during intraoral application. This means that the intraoral temperature might change from a subzero range (e.g. while eating ice cream) to values as high as 60°C (e.g., while drinking tea). Such temperature variations lead to expansion or contraction of the material, which might have an influence on the interaction between the polymer and the teeth. Thus, a polymer must be able to tolerate temperature alteration without a pronounced volume and mechanical performance change.

The mechanical stability of the polymer also plays an important role in orthodontic applications. For instance, a polymer used for aligners must withstand high occlusal forces; otherwise, fractures or deformation might occur.[4] A change in the mechanical properties of the polymer during the intraoral application period could also lead to unwanted changes of the mechanical loads applied to the teeth. Even for a chemically stable material (i.e., a material showing no corrosion), the mechanical properties of the polymer can still vary over time due to aging and creep.[5-7]

There are two types of aging: physical and chemical aging.[5,6] Both chemical and physical aging render the polymer brittle and stiffer, thus a lower strain may be generated during the application.

This chapter will focus on the basic properties of polymers typically used for aligners. It will also include an explanation of the chemical structure and thermal properties of these polymers. As the effectiveness of a polymer for dental use depends on thermal, chemical, and mechanical stability, these issues also will be discussed briefly. Finally, future perspectives of polymers used for aligners are described.

Polymer Molecular Structure and Thermal Properties

Polymers are very long and entangled molecules with nonconventional thermal and mechanical behavior. In this section, the structure of a polymer and its thermal behavior will be described. This comprises the specification of glass transition, aspects of aging, and the stability of the polymer in the intraoral milieu.

WHAT IS A POLYMER?

The word *polymer* is derived originally from the Greek words *poly* ("many") and *méros* ("units"). This indicates that polymers consist of many repeating units connected to each another through chemical bonding. Normally, if a substance contains just a few molecules, an addition or removal of only a few atoms would change the material properties significantly. For example, if one would add just CH_2 to heptane (C_7H_{16}), then the boiling point of the resulting molecule (C_8H_{18}) increases by 27°C. With polymers, in contrast, the number of repeating units could be changed by one or more units without any noticeable change in the polymer properties.

Typically, a polymer chain is made of several thousand repeating units with a length of several micrometers and a diameter just around 1 nm. The polymer chain is usually flexible, twisted, and intertwined. The molecular weight and chemical structure of the polymer determine most of its properties. In contrast to small molecules having a specific size and molecular weight (expressed in g/mol or kg/mol), a polymer bulk contains polymer chains with many different sizes and molecular weights. Hence the molecular weight of the polymer reflects an average of many different polymer chains.

Fig. 3.1 Chemical structure of polyethylene terephthalate glycol material (PET-G).

Fig. 3.2 Chemical structure of polyurethane material (PU).

Based on their thermal behavior, the three different classes of polymers are thermoplastic, elastomer, and thermoset.[8] Clear aligners belong to the thermoplastic group. Thermoplastic polymers melt and flow upon heating above a certain temperature. Two widely used polymers for aligners are polyethylene terephthalate glycol (PET-G) and thermoplastic polyurethane (TPU).[9-11] The latter is a special thermoplastic form of polyurethane which melts by heating, facilitating the thermoforming process. Both of these thermoplastic materials are transparent in the visible light spectrum, are impact-resistant, and highly ductile. Just these properties in particular make them very suitable for use as aligner material.

PET-G is a copolymer that constitutes two repeating units (Fig. 3.1): polyethylene terephthalate and glycol. The addition of glycol prevents the crystallization of the PET upon heating. This makes PET-G less brittle and more resistant to mechanical stress. PET-G is a versatile polymer used in many other applications such as protective cover (e.g., smart card), electronic devices, food containers, and medical instruments. One can thermoform, print, drill, bend, polish, and cut PET-G easily without noticeable impact on its stability and physical properties. As PET-G can be easily thermoformed and also recycled, it is also the material of choice for three-dimensional printing.

The building block of polyurethane is urethane (Fig. 3.2). PU is available in both soft and rigid form, making it ideal for automotive interiors, packaging, coating, flexible foam, and construction. PU is impact resistant, is a good electrical isolator, bonds well with other material, and is chemically stable in the presence of water and oil. The versatility of PU is due to the fact that one can link urethane molecules using different chemicals in very different structures. This allows tailoring the hardness of PU to the specific application. In general, PU is biocompatible, but to make it applicable as aligners, PU is usually combined with other material.

GLASS TRANSITION-THE MACROMOLECULAR BASIS OF VISCOELASTICITY

Depending on the temperature, most materials exist in a solid, liquid, or gas state. Each of these states could be precisely described by thermodynamics laws. However, the investigation of polymers revealed that most of them do not follow these basic material states. Instead, they show fluid or solidlike, time-dependent characteristics.[12]

More specifically, if a polymer is observed in a short time scale, it behaves like a solid material. If the experiment, however, is performed during a longer time period, polymers may flow and show a liquidlike behavior.

This phenomenon is to be exemplified on the basis of the behavior of a simple liquid (ethanol), which normally crystallizes. Let us assume that the liquid is cooled below its melting point. Fig. 3.3 illustrates the change of the specific volume of the material versus its temperature. The specific volume, defined as volume divided by mass, is the reverse of the density. During cooling, the specific volume of the liquid decreases continually as long as it is still in the liquid phase. There exists, however, a point (the freezing point) at which the specific volume will decrease drastically and form a crystalline solid. Such volume discontinuity is related to the reduction of specific volume due to the crystallization. Below the freezing point, the specific volume remains almost constant even though the cooling process is continued. The freezing or melting point is a material property and does not depend on the cooling rate or method of the measurement. It also has a clear thermodynamic definition without any room for interpretation.

Under certain conditions, small molecules and many types of polymers, however, do not follow the mentioned

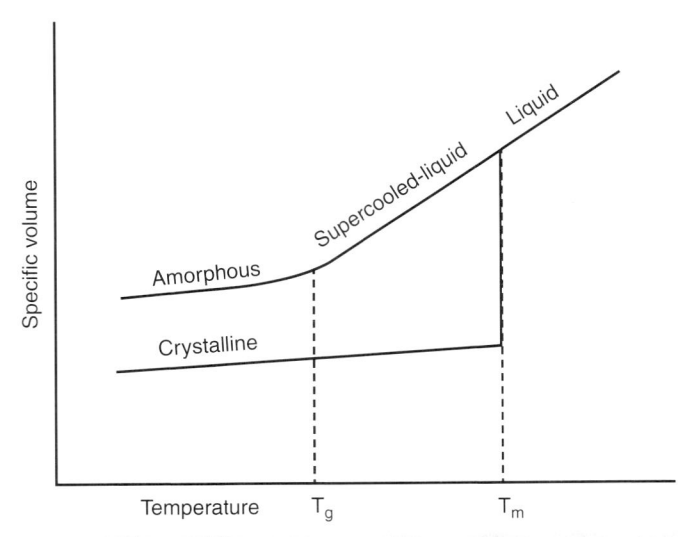

Fig. 3.3 Specific volume versus temperature. T_m represents the melting temperature and T_g the glass transition temperature.

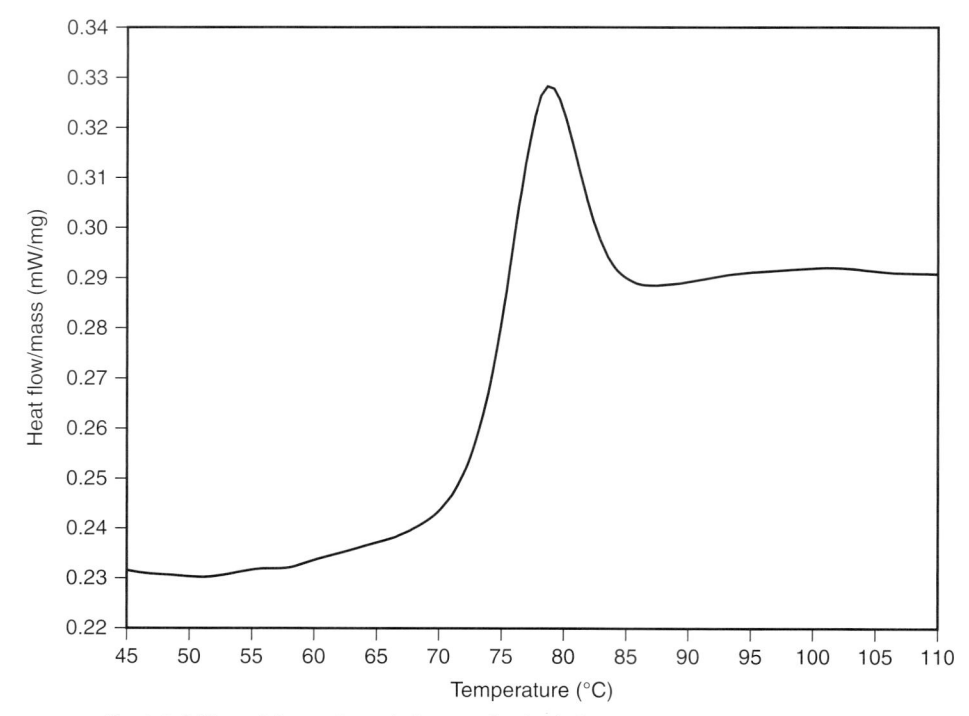

Fig. 3.4 Differential scanning calorimetry of polyethylene terephthalate glycol (PET-G).

scenario but demonstrate another behavior. This is even applicable to simple liquids such as ethanol (small molecules). If a very pure ethanol is stored in a bowl with no corner and in a refrigerator without vibration, it can be cooled to below freezing temperature without freezing. Hence there exists a temperature range below the melting point (called the supercooled region) in which the substance remains liquid.[13] If the cooling process is continued, a temperature range will be reached at which the supercooled liquid transforms into a glassy state called the glass transition temperature (T_g). In this solidlike form, the substance has very different properties than the crystalline state. Glassy material is an amorphous material, which does not have a long-range order. The structure of material in the glassy form is therefore more similar to a liquid than to a crystalline structure. Except for only a few examples, solid polymeric materials mainly exist in such an amorphous state. This is primarily related to the fact that the polymer's long chain is entangled with other chains. Hence it is usually difficult for the polymer chains to orientate and build an ordered crystalline structure.

It has to be noted that simple polymers may actually show crystallization if the cooling rate is low enough so that the polymer chains are allowed to find their minimum state of energy (i.e., their equilibrium). However, for many polymers with entangled chains, movements of polymer chains are hindered too much, making it physically impossible to reach the crystalline state.[14] The usual state of polymers is, consequently, solidlike with an amorphous structure. Nevertheless, the polymer chains retain their tendency to orient and to achieve an equilibrium state. This tendency is the source of the specific behavior of (amorphous) polymers, which is plastic and elastic-like, and might alter between these characteristics throughout time.

These aspects explain why the glass transition temperature plays an important role in defining a polymer's properties, though it must be mentioned that the glass transition temperature is an ill-defined transition. The latter means that different measurement techniques may lead to different T_g values. Differential scanning calorimetry (DSC) is a widely accepted technique for determination of the T_g value. Fig. 3.4 shows results of DSC measurements for PET-G. Usually the middle of this range (i.e., 75°C for PET-G) is taken as the determined T_g value.

From an application-oriented view, any thermoforming must occur above the T_g temperature. The exemplified DSC curve further indicates that, if PET-G is heated above 60°C, its mechanical properties will change drastically. More specifically, around a temperature of 60°C, PET-G will start to get softer and deform easier. Intraorally, this temperature is usually not exceeded for a sufficiently long time, so PET-G stays mechanically stable during dental applications.

Physical and Chemical Aging of Aligner Polymers

In the fabrication process, aligners go through thermoforming. During subsequent clinical application, they are in contact with saliva, food, drinks, among other chemicals. Consequently, as the orthodontist requires a reliable appliance, sufficient material stability is needed under varying conditions. The stability of the aligner is measured by its aging (i.e., the change of its properties over time). Polymer aging has several sources. With respect to intraoral application of polymers, two aspects of aging should be considered in particular: physical and chemical aging.[5,6]

PHYSICAL AGING OF POLYMERS

Physical aging of polymers principally occurs, as mentioned earlier, in an amorphous (i.e., nonequilibrium) form. Every system with the nonequilibrium state tends to decrease its energy to thus approach its equilibrium state. If enough mobility is obtained, the chains may rearrange themselves to their lowest energy state, which might be compared to crystallization. This in turn will lead to a decrease of the specific volume, a decrease of the enthalpy, an increase of the hardness and brittleness, and changes to other properties.[15] This effect particularly changes the mechanical properties of the polymer. Accordingly, physical aging can be defined as the relaxation of a polymer toward a more stable energy state. If the usage of a polymer occurs far below its T_g temperature, the polymer chains will not have enough kinetic energy to move and rearrange. Hence, by choosing an aligner with a T_g value much higher than the intraoral temperature, physical aging might be largely avoided. It is important to note in this context that a polymer's T_g value may also change due to environmental influences.

Physical aging of polymers can be influenced by exposure to water and many other kinds of molecules in the intraoral medium. As mentioned, the specific volume of an amorphous polymer is high in comparison to a crystalline polymer. This means there exists a lot of free volume in the amorphous polymer below the T_g temperature. Consequently, for prolonged exposure of such a polymer to water, water molecules could diffuse into the material alongside other molecules. The latter is one of the reasons for discoloration of aligners. It is important to note that the absorption of these molecules may also change the properties of the polymer. A typical change is called the plasticizing effect.[16] To explain further, consider using spaghetti as an example. Provided that a bowl contains spaghetti without sauce, the noodles cannot move as easily because they stick together. However, by adding a sauce to the bowl, the spaghetti noodles separate, which enables them to slip along each other. In polymers, the plasticizing effect follows almost the same logic: the small, embedded molecules are placed between the polymer chains to increase the mobility of the chains. The plasticizing effect will reduce the glass transition, and therefore the polymer will be more affected by physical aging.

From a clinical perspective, physical aging can affect an aligner in two ways. Initially, the polymer will become softer due to the plasticizing effect. As a result, force magnitudes applied to the individual teeth are reduced. In the long run, however, due to the effect of classical physical aging, aligner polymers become harder (which will increase the applied forces) and more brittle (increasing the risk of breakage).

CHEMICAL AGING OF POLYMERS

As introduced, aligners may also suffer from chemical aging, which is the result of a chemical interaction between a polymer and its medium. At present, none of the available aligner materials is inert, which means that these materials do react with certain chemicals included in saliva, drink, or food. Chemical aging can affect a polymer via different mechanisms. For example, water molecules can break the polymer chains and shorten them (hydrolysis), or a similar reaction can occur due to the interaction between the oxygen and polymer (oxidation). A polymer suffering from chemical aging is more likely to develop cracks and induce notch effects.

Note, too, the time dependency of the mechanical properties of an aligner might be related to creep (which will be explained in the next chapter). Creep is different from aging phenomenon. It occurs due to application of mechanical stress to the material, whereas aging is the result of a polymer's nonequilibrium state or medium, which occurs without any external stress application. Both phenomena are similar to each other, but they are related to quite different mechanisms and should therefore not be confused.

Conclusions and Outlook

The two aligner materials mainly used (i.e., TPU and PET-G) have a distinct chemical structure leading to different responses to thermoforming, exposure to the intraoral milieu, and mechanical stress. Hence it is of great importance not to generalize the characteristics determined for one aligner material (even one brand). Methodologic conditions for material tests must be as realistic as possible. For example, the mechanical properties of aligner materials differ greatly before and after thermoforming. Thus a realistic test should include the thermoformed material specimen or aligners. Furthermore, stress measurements should be performed in a simulated intraoral medium. Also, the production process (the method of molding, cooling, etc.) affects polymer structure, which in turn might alter the performance of aligner materials. To obtain valid comparisons between tested materials and to achieve reliable treatment results, test procedures and clinical application protocols should be standardized. Only then will the full potential of clear aligners be revealed. Aligner manufacturers or dental suppliers should inform users (i.e., orthodontists) about any changes in the chemical composition and production process. Nevertheless, it is often rather difficult to obtain such information.

References

1. Williams DF. On the mechanisms of biocompatibility. *Biomaterials*. 2008;29:2941-2953.
2. Pires F, Ferreira Q, Rodrigues CAV, et al. Neural stem cell differentiation by electrical stimulation using a cross-linked PEDOT substrate: expanding the use of biocompatible conjugated conductive polymers for neural tissue engineering. *Biochim Biophys Acta*. 2015;1850:1158–1168.
3. Humphrey SP, Williamson RT. A review of saliva: normal composition, flow, and function. *J Prosthet Dent*. 2001;85:162–169.
4. Hidaka O, Iwasaki M, Saito M, et al. Influence of clenching intensity on bite force balance, occlusal contact area, and average bite pressure. *J Dent Res*. 1999;78:1336-1344.
5. Hodge IM. Physical aging in polymer glasses. *Science*. 1995;267:1945–1947.
6. Crissman JM, McKenna GB. Physical and chemical aging in PMMA and their effects on creep and creep rupture behavior. *J Polym Sci B Polym Phys*. 1990;28:1463-1473.
7. Riggleman RA, Schweizer KS, Pablo JJd. Nonlinear creep in a polymer glass. *Macromolecules*. 2008;41:4969-4677.
8. Bower DI. *An Introduction to Polymer Physics*. Cambridge: Cambridge University Press; 2002.

9. Lombardo L, Martines E, Mazzanti V, et al. Stress relaxation properties of four orthodontic aligner materials: a 24-hour in vitro study. *Angle Orthod.* 2017;87:11-18.
10. Mancini G, Carinci F, Zollino I, et al. Simplicity and reliability of Invisalign® system. *Eur J Inflamm.* 2011;9:13-52.
11. Alexandropoulos A, Al Jabbari YS, Zinelis S, et al. Chemical and mechanical characteristics of contemporary thermoplastic orthodontic materials. *Aust Orthod J.* 2015;31:165-170.
12. Aleksandrov AP, Lazurkin YS. A study of polymers. I. Highly elastic deformation of polymers. *Rubber Chem Technol.* 1940;13:886-898.
13. Gedde UW. *Polymer Physics.* Dordrecht: Springer Netherlands; 1999.
14. Doi M, Edwards SF. *The Theory of Polymer Dynamics.* Oxford: Clarendon Press; 1986.
15. Struik LCE. *Physical Aging in Amorphous Polymers and Other Materials.* Elsevier Science; 1977.
16. Amirkhani M, Gorini G, Leporini D. Second harmonic generation studies of intrinsic and extrinsic relaxation dynamics in poly(methyl methacrylate). *J Non Cryst Solids.* 2009;355:1707-1712.

4 Influence of Intraoral Factors on Optical and Mechanical Aligner Material Properties

FAYEZ ELKHOLY, SILVA SCHMIDT, MASOUD AMIRKHANI, and BERND G. LAPATKI

Introduction

The triad of success of orthodontic therapy comprises patient compliance, biomechanical knowledge, and, for the therapy with aligners, sufficient understanding of the thermoplastic material used. Chapter 3 addressed the basic chemical and mechanical properties of commonly used aligner materials. This chapter will focus on the influence of different intraoral factors on the mechanical and optical properties of aligner materials.

To achieve an efficient orthodontic tooth movement, single aligners are usually worn for a period of 7 to 10 days and approximately 22 hours per day.[1] During their period of use, aligners are subjected to a prolonged exposure to different factors that are influencing their properties. They can be subdivided into two main categories. On the one hand, there are factors inducing optical material changes, either in the form of discoloration or increased opacity; such effects are related to the presence of salivary enzymes, plaque, and food and beverage coloring.[2-5] On the other hand, there are factors affecting the mechanical properties of aligners, including the periodic loading and unloading of the material during its clinical handling, combined with uneven local stress and strain distribution. It must be noted, too, that excessive occlusal forces (e.g., during involuntary clenching or grinding) and intraoral temperature fluctuations may influence an aligner's properties.[6,7] As this appliance, however, is to be removed during food or liquid intake and worn for only a relatively short period, the clinical relevance of the latter two factors may not be overemphasized.

The following sections will discuss the mechanisms of how intraoral factors influence optical and mechanical aligner properties and describe the clinical implications. Particular attention will be given to describing the material-specific characteristics of the two aligner materials mainly used (i.e., thermoplastic polyurethane [TPU] and polyethylene terephthalate glycol [PET-G]). TPU is used, for instance, in the Invisalign system (Align Technology, Santa Clara, CA, United States) or F22 Aligner (Sweden & Martina, Due Carrare, Padova, Italy), whereas PET-G is used in the Clear Aligner system (Duran, Scheu Dental GmbH, Iserlohn, Germany) and the Essix system (Essix A+, Dentsply Raintree Essix, Sarasota, FL, United States).[8]

Water Absorption

Aligners are constantly subjected to saliva, which consists of 99% water. Hence it is crucial to understand the mechanism and effects of water absorption as well as the influence of water absorption on the mechanical material properties. As stated in Chapter 3, amorphous polymers such as TPU and PET-G possess relatively low molecular density, which provides free volume for water intake. A previous study comparing these two materials showed that TPU shows higher water absorption characterized by a weight increase of 1.45% after a 1-week water storage than PET-G showing only a 0.84% increase.[9] Besides this weight effect, penetration of thermoplastic materials by water molecules also leads to modification of their internal structure. As explained in Chapter 3, this will result in plasticization because links between polymer chains are weakened or even destroyed, which reduces the internal cohesion and increases the molecular mobility.[10] The resulting loss of elasticity might explain the appearance of internal cracks observed in aligners after clinical usage.[6] It is interesting to note in this context that own studies on PET-G material characteristics using three-point bending of thermoformed rectangular specimens revealed that the sole water storage without subjecting the material to any mechanical loads has only a minor impact on the mechanical material characteristics (Fig. 4.1). In contrast, if PET-G is subjected to both water and a continuous mechanical load, the effect on the mechanical properties is much more pronounced, as indicated by the reduction of the bending forces of up to 43% (see Fig. 4.1).

Principally, water absorption could also induce dimensional changes of the aligners, known as hygroscopic expansion. In theory, this factor—besides other factors such as the initial play between the aligner and the setup model[11-13]—might affect the fit of the aligners and, consequently, might also induce an alteration of the forces applied to the individual teeth.[9,14] A previous study on water adsorption of thermoplastic materials, however, did not find significant and plausible correlations between the rate of water absorption and the amount of hygroscopic expansion.[9] For instance, TPU showed a lower hygroscopic expansion, although it showed the highest water absorption rates.

Bending forces for PETG specimens

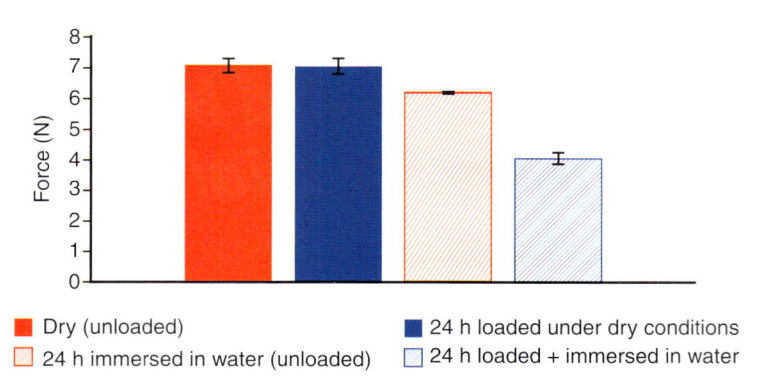

Fig. 4.1 Bending forces depending on the (dry or wet) storage conditions and the unloaded or loaded condition. Note 0.75-mm polyethylene terephthalate glycol *(PET-G)* specimens were investigated in a three-point bending setting with a span length of 8 mm at a deflection of 0.1 mm. The specimens were either only thermoformed and then underwent only one short deflection with simultaneous force, stored for 24 hours in water without loading, loaded continuously for 24 hours without water immersion, or loaded continuously for 24 hours with water immersion. The error bars represent the standard deviation for the different measurements.

Optical Changes

One of the main reasons for the popularity of aligners with patients lies in the invisibility or (better) the transparency of this appliance.[15-17] These characteristics should be maintained throughout the treatment period because a discolored or opaque aligner (Fig. 4.2) might jeopardize the patient's motivation and compliance.

Aligner discoloration is primarily related to superficial absorption or penetration of pigmentations in food and beverages. Coffee (i.e., the highest chromogenic agent), black tea, and red wine play a prominent role.[2,3,18] It is noticeable in this context that the rate and extent of discoloration is material-specific.[2] It seems that TPU-based aligners might exhibit faster discoloration rates than PET-G aligners. A possible explanation for this difference is the higher water absorption capability of TPU facilitating the accumulation of the pigments.[9] In addition, the higher surface roughness of TPU might also facilitate the adhesion of pigments on the polymer film's surface.[4]

Aligners might also lose translucency by the development of internal microcracks, formation of calcific integuments, or the accumulation of plaque on the aligner surface.[5-7,19] Obviously, the two latter changes do not have a significant impact on the treatment success due to the short application period of each single aligner of maximally 2 weeks. Moreover, the loss of translucency can be minimized by maintaining good aligner hygiene through regular brushing with neutral soap and the use of denture-cleaning effervescent tablets containing sodium bicarbonate or sodium sulfate.[5]

Short-Term Mechanical Loading of Aligner Materials

SINGLE SHORT-TERM LOADINGS

For viscoelastic materials, it is known that during very short loading periods the elastic component dominates. This thesis was also confirmed by (unpublished) investigation of PET-G specimens by our group, consisting of two short loading-measuring cycles with a duration of only ca. 0.1 second each and a 2-minute break in between. The comparison of the

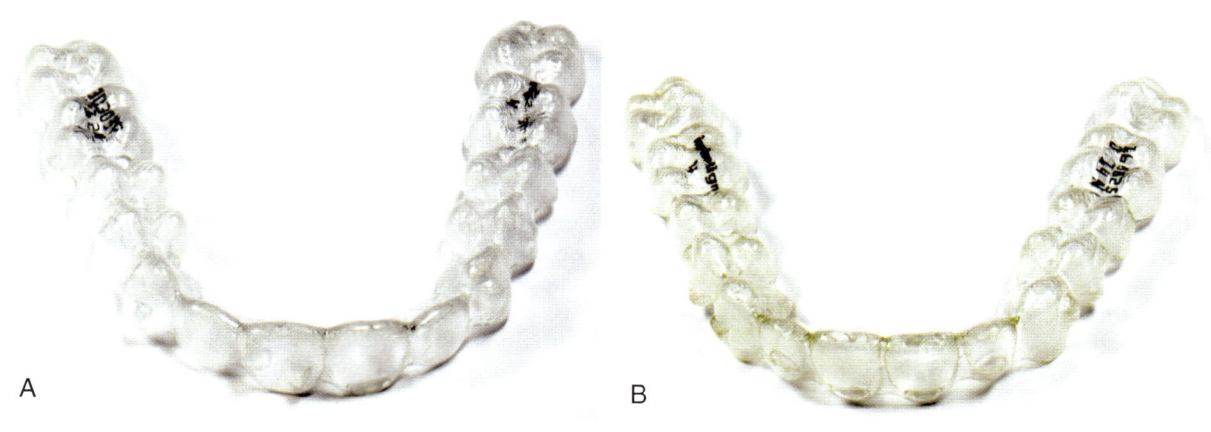

Fig. 4.2 Invisalign aligners. (A) Prior to first intraoral application. (B) After a 1-week wearing period.

Force measured at short-term deflection

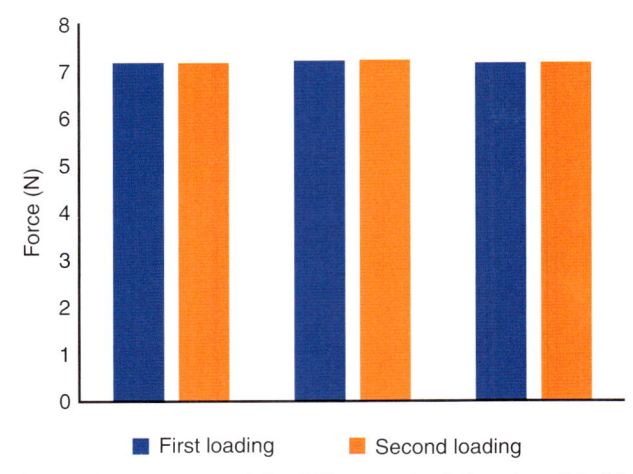

Fig. 4.3 Forces measured for 0.75-mm polyethylene terephthalate glycol (PET-G) specimens in a three-point bending setup with a span length of 8 mm. The central support was deflected by 0.1 mm. Two short loading-measuring cycles with 0.1-second duration, separated by a 2-minute recovery break, were performed.

forces obtained by the first and second measurements did not show a significant difference (Fig. 4.3).

MULTIPLE SHORT-TERM LOADING CYCLES

During clinical application, aligners are removed multiple times for food and liquid intake as well as during the regular oral hygiene procedures. To simulate or exemplify such scenarios, our group conducted an in vitro study, including cyclic loading of 0.75-mm-thick PETG specimens using a three-point bending setup. Each of the 12 cycles consisted of a 5-minute loading interval, followed by a nearly unloaded interval of 10 minutes during which the deflection was reduced to a level at which the remaining force was just above 0 N (to maintain contact between the force-measuring device and the specimen). As revealed by Fig. 4.4, the PET-G specimen showed a continuous stress relaxation behavior during the 5-minute loading periods with a force reduction of ca. 2% average over the 12 loading-unloading cycles. It was also observed that during the 10-minute (quasi unloaded) period, a slight average increase of the deflection forces by ca. 0.5% occurred. Such force increase indicates a slight recovery of the PET-G material (see Fig. 4.4). In some studies, such recovery is described as "relaxation"; the latter expression, however, should not be mistaken for "stress relaxation," which describes a completely opposite phenomenon.

It is noteworthy that a similar material behavior was found in another in vitro study in which PET-G-aligners were repeatedly removed from a test model.[20] This previous study observed a clear decrease of aligner force delivery in the course of the 50 aligner seating-removal procedures. Moreover, the force reduction showed a nearly linear relation with the frequency of the cycles, with force values dropping down to 50% of the initial forces after 50 cycles (Fig. 4.5).[20] Further work is required to systematically examine this aspect for other materials than PET-G.

OCCLUSAL FORCES

In addition to the specific loading of aligners related to repeated intraoral seating and removal, aligners are also potentially exposed to relatively high mechanical loads occurring during occlusal contacting. Such bite forces are particularly relevant in patients showing clenching or grinding where they may reach force values up to 35 N per single molar.[21]

Although TPU possesses higher abrasion resistance than PET-G, available studies indicate that both materials showed delamination and abrasion as well as an increased Vickers hardness, particularly in the posterior region of the dental arch.[6,7,14,19,22,23] The latter was observed after a 2-week wear period and was traced back to the changes in the crystalline structure of the polymer under cold work.[7] Nevertheless, the clinical impact of these changes appears unproblematic for two reasons: First, those teeth mainly affected by the altered material behavior (i.e., the buccal teeth) are moved to a minor extent during aligner therapy; second, the wearing period of an aligner ranging between 1 and 2 weeks seems too short for the mechanical destruction of an aligner by contact forces.

Long-Term Loading

Aligner materials such as TPU and PET-G show a viscoelastic behavior. Hence they show both elastic and viscous characteristics when undergoing loading, resulting in a time-dependent deformation. During very short loading periods, the elastic component dominates. The time-dependent viscous component, in contrast, reveals primarily during prolonged loading.[24] The viscoelastic behavior can be mathematically described as standard linear solid models (Fig. 4.6). Such models consist of springs and dashpots representing the elastic and viscous material components, respectively.

Experimental description of the mechanical behavior of a viscoelastic material is possible by two variables: creep or stress relaxation. It is important to clarify the difference between these two parameters (Fig. 4.7). Creep describes the phenomenon of increasing mechanical strain over time in case of a constantly applied stress or force, respectively. Since the mechanical load (stress) is maintained at a constant level, creep experiments induce a continuous deformation (strain) (see Fig. 4.7A) until a maximum strain is reached. Stress relaxation, in contrast, describes the gradual stress decrease over time under a constant strain and deformation, respectively (see Fig. 4.7B). As a result, the force level drops continually until a certain equilibrium state is reached at a reduced stress level.[25,26]

To ensure a better understanding of the viscoelastic properties of polymers, it is important to consider the specific test method applied. Creep is usually examined either by tensile measurements or by instrumental indentation tests.[8,27,28] Tensile measurements are usually performed by loading the specimens at a certain force level, which is then maintained for a certain period. The rate of elongation of the specimen describes the creep rate of the tested material. Instrumental indentation is more common and usually quantitatively evaluated by calculating the percentage difference between

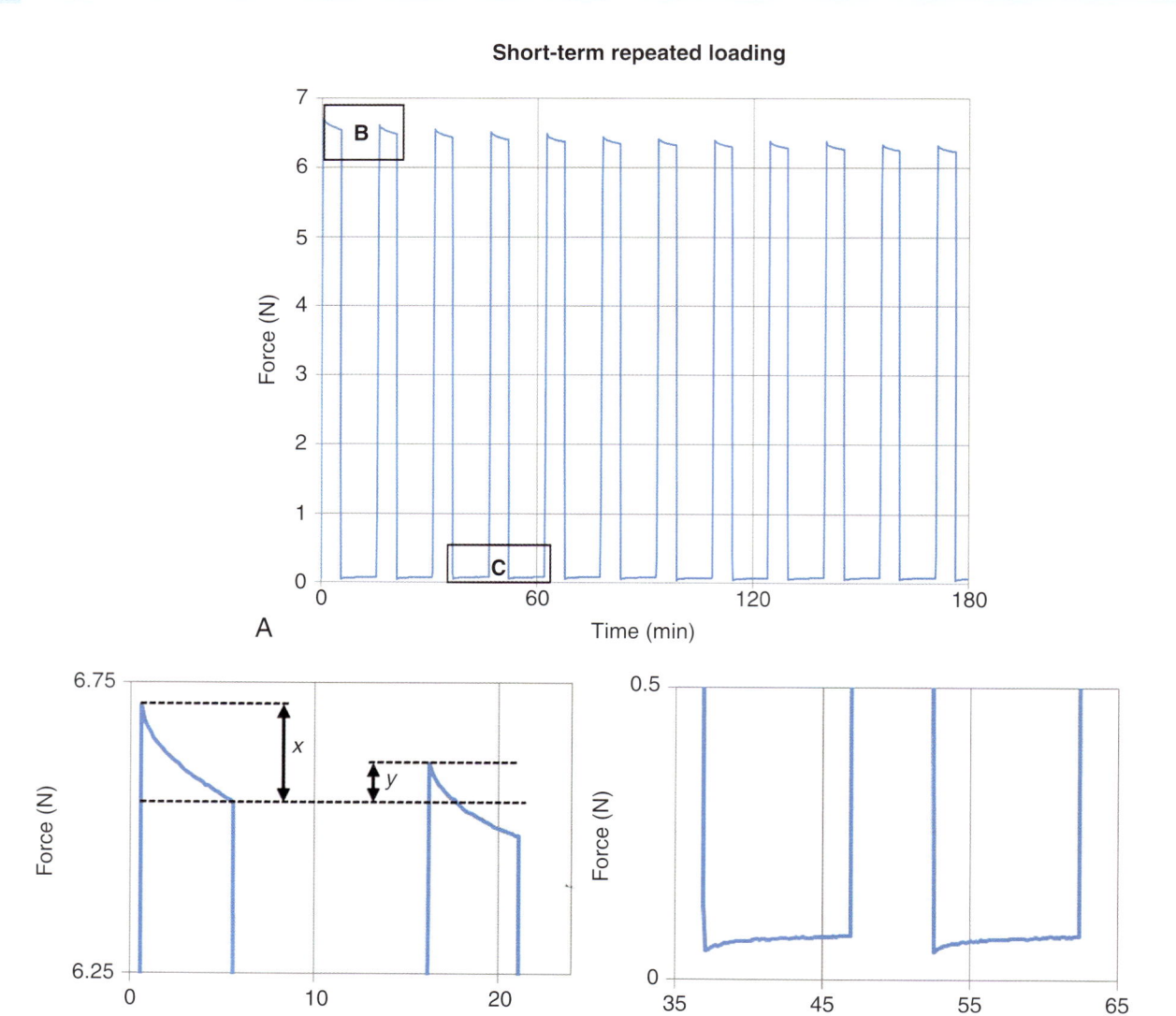

Fig. 4.4 (A) Forces measured during multiple 5-minute loading and 5-minute loading cycles for a 0.5-mm polyethylene terephthalate glycol (PET-G) specimen in a three-point bending setup with a span length of 8 mm and a deflection of 0.2 mm. (B) Enlargement of a data segment *(see top of A)* showing the gradual force decrease during the 5-minute loading time. (C) Enlargement of a data segment *(see bottom of A)* showing the slight force increase during the 10-minute minimal load time at the corresponding deflections.

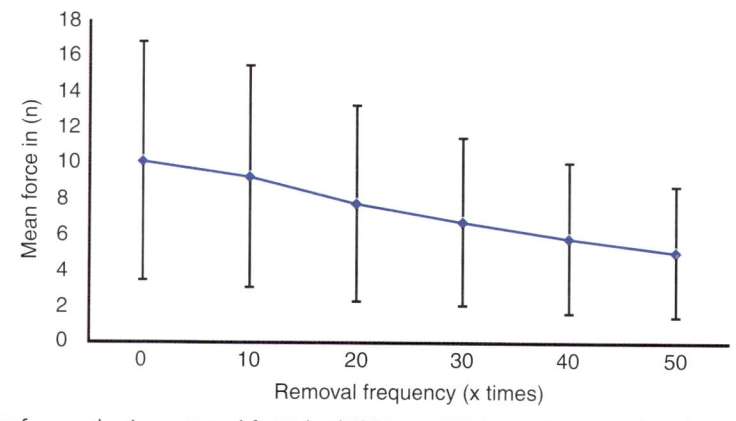

Fig. 4.5 Average force reduction reported for polyethylene terephthalate glycol (PET-G) aligners in the course of 50 aligner seating-removal procedures based on the data published by Skaik et al.[20] The error bars indicate the standard deviation.

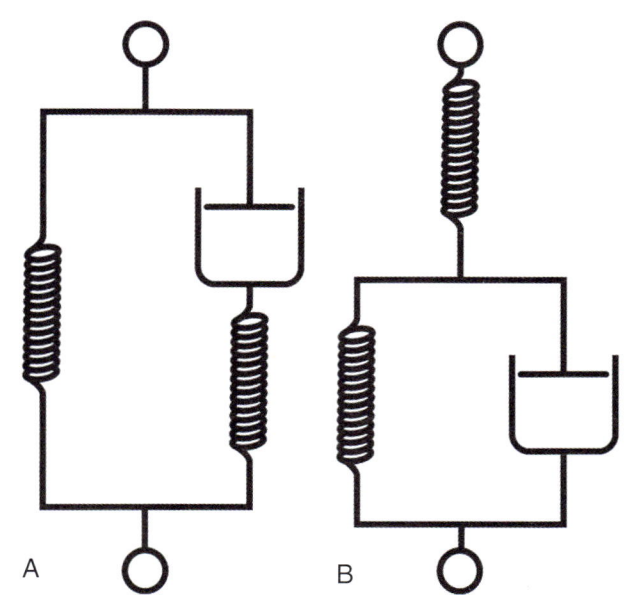

Fig. 4.6 Schematic modeling of viscoelastic material behavior using a standard linear solid model. (A) Maxwell representation of a standard linear solid model. (B) Kelvin representation of a standard linear solid model. Such models combine springs and dashpots in a certain arrangement to describe the overall behavior of a system under different loading conditions. Springs represent the elastic component of a viscoelastic material, whereas dashpots represent the viscous component.[30] Due to combination of such elements, an applied stress varies with the time-dependent change of the strain.

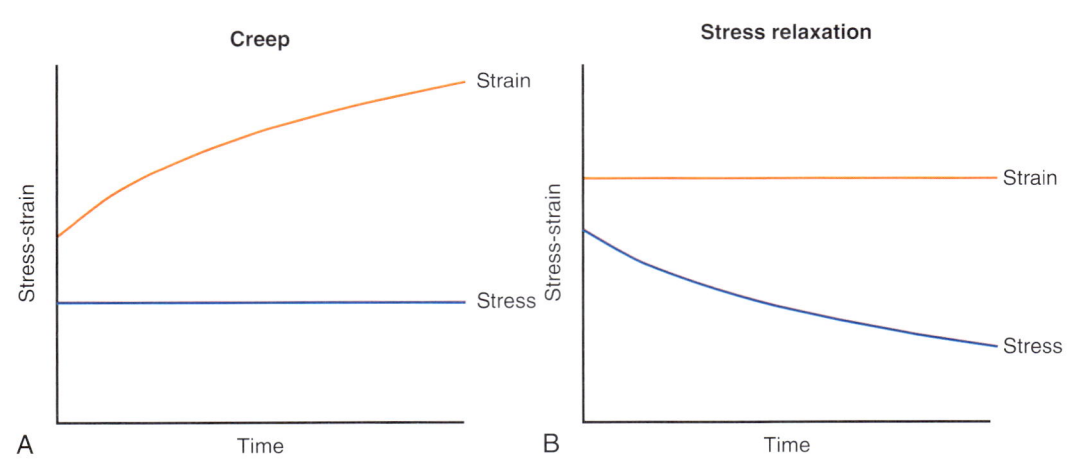

Fig. 4.7 Two fundamentally different experiments and parameters, respectively, describing the time-dependent behavior of a viscoelastic aligner material. (A) The creep phenomenon is observed if the load (and stress level, respectively) is kept constant over time. (B) The stress relaxation behavior is characterized by loading the material under constant strain and deflection, respectively.

the initial and final indentation depth during the constant force application period. Hence it is determined how deep the material has been penetrated over the designated period.[27] Stress relaxation, on the other hand, can be tested either by three-point bending or in tensile experimental setups.[25,29] A common feature of both setups is the constant deflection (strain) of the specimen for a defined period during which the time-dependency of the stress is registered. The difference between the initial and residual values over time defines the stress relaxation rate.

Aligner materials with lower creep resistance tend to a faster strain (deformation) under constant mechanical stress. When transferred to the clinical situation, such behavior would reduce the mechanical load applied to the teeth because the relative discrepancy between the actual tooth position and its position in the aligner would diminish. A previous study investigated the creep behavior of the different thermoplastic raw films used in the Invisalign (Align Technology, Santa Clara, CA, USA), Clear Aligner (Scheu Dental GmbH, Iserlohn, Germany), and Essix A+ (Dentsply Raintree Essix, Sarasota, FL, USA) systems by means of indentation creep experiments.[8] The indentation creep behavior was characterized by the percentage increase of the indentation depth within an interval of 2 minutes in with the specimens were subjected to a constant indentation force.[8,27] Results of this study revealed more pronounced creep for modified TPU, which is the material of Invisalign aligners (3.7%) compared to the corresponding percentage for PET-G (2.7%). Another study observed that the creep of TPU was even more pronounced after aging, with an increased indentation depth of 4%.[27]

Previous research determining the stress relaxation behavior of commercial aligner materials revealed that most materials show a relatively high stress relaxation rate in the first 8 hours of loading, followed by a nearly steady plateau.[25,26] The stated stress decay, however, showed a material-dependent pattern with the highest stress relaxation for PET-G with 44% of the initial stress values, followed by the stress relaxation of TPU with 40.5%.[25] After the 24-hour loading period, a similar material-dependent pattern was observed with residual stresses of 45.5% and 38% of the initial values for the TPU and the PET-G materials, respectively.[25] Similar stress relaxation patterns were found by our group investigating PET-G specimens (Clear Aligner, Scheu Dental GmbH, Iserlohn, Germany) during a 1-week constant deflection period with water immersion of the specimens. Our results also indicated relatively rapid stress relaxation during the first day, followed by a slower stress reduction. At the end of the longer 1-week loading period, stress values approximated a residual stress value of only 17% of the initial stress (Fig. 4.8).

Clinical Loading Patterns of Aligner Materials

As mentioned, aligner materials possess elastic elements, which are of utmost importance for maintaining a certain force level on the teeth. If their load-deflection behavior would be purely elastic, and the strain would be kept within the elastic range, then the force and moment components applied to the teeth would be directly proportional to the discrepancy between the actual tooth position and the programmed tooth position in the aligner. Furthermore, the stiffness of the aligner material would describe the slope of this interrelation. As pointed out earlier, in case the load is maintained for a longer time, these materials also show a viscous behavior that can be quantified, for instance, by stress relaxation experiments. It is important to note that both the amount and the rate of deformation of thermoplastic materials depend on the loading time scheme and the stress magnitude, and both are affected by collateral factors such as the temperature and material-specific water absorption properties. Another important characteristic of thermoplastic aligner materials is observed in cases where the load is removed. Under this condition, thermoplastic materials may show a certain rebound effect. Obviously such a phenomenon might be of practical importance; as during clinical therapy, aligners are usually removed periodically (e.g., for food intake).

To investigate this characteristic, recent research in our lab aimed at the examination of the influence of repeated 18-hour loading/6-hour unloading cycles on the force application of PET-G aligner materials over a total period of 1 week. An example of a measurement curve is presented in Fig. 4.9. Similar to the experiments with constant strain, the results indicated a relatively high force decay in the first few hours to a level less than 40% of the initial

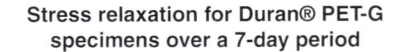

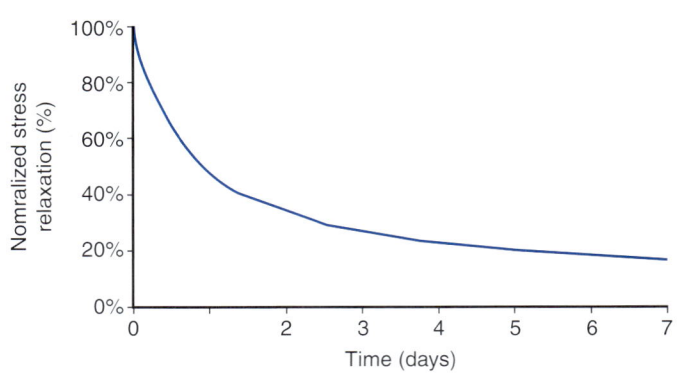

Fig. 4.8 Normalized stress relaxation for polyethylene terephthalate glycol (PET-G) materials loaded for 1 week in a three-point bending setup with a constant deflection of the specimen leading to a constant strain.

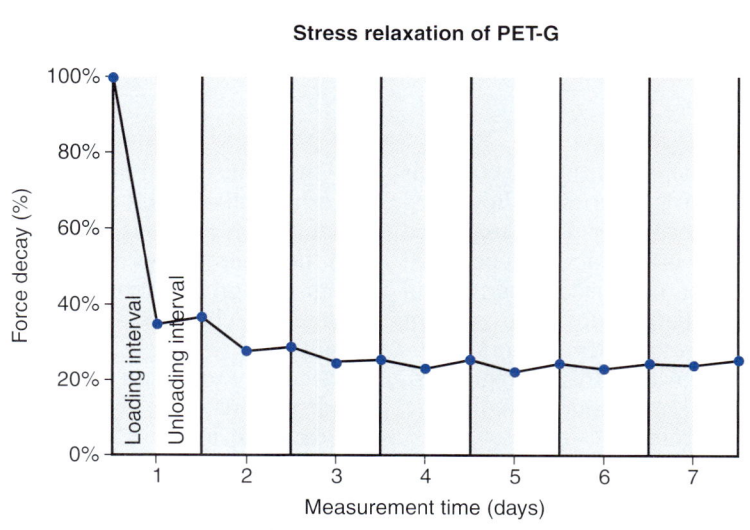

Fig. 4.9 Decay of the forces measured after the loading and unloading periods during the 1-week observation time.

force indicating a clear stress relaxation. After the 6-hour periods without loading, only slight force increases were observed. Even though after the second and following loading periods stress relaxation could be observed, the latter was much less pronounced than that occurring in the first loading period. Based on these findings, we concluded that the stress relaxation behavior of PET-G, which is related to repeated loading and unloading intervals (with similar lengths as those typically occurring during clinical therapy), tends to stabilize at a level between 20% and 25% of the initial stress.

References

1. Boyd RL, Miller RJ, Vlaskalic V. The Invisalign system in adult orthodontics: mild crowding and space closure cases. *J Clin Orthod*. 2000;34:203-212.
2. Liu CL, Sun WT, Liao W, et al. Colour stabilities of three types of orthodontic clear aligners exposed to staining agents. *Int J Oral Sci*. 2016;8:246-253.
3. Zafeiriadis AA, Karamouzos A, Athanasiou AE, et al. In vitro spectrophotometric evaluation of Vivera clear thermoplastic retainer discolouration. *Aust Orthod J*. 2014;30:192-200.
4. Fernandes ABN, Ruellas ACO, Araújo MVA, et al. Assessment of exogenous pigmentation in colourless elastic ligatures. *J Orthod*. 2014;41:147-151.
5. Levrini L, Novara F, Margherini S, et al. Scanning electron microscopy analysis of the growth of dental plaque on the surfaces of removable orthodontic aligners after the use of different cleaning methods. *Clin Cosmet Investig Dent*. 2015;7:125-131.
6. Eliades T, Bourauel C. Intraoral aging of orthodontic materials: the picture we miss and its clinical relevance. *Am J Orthod Dentofacial Orthop*. 2005;127:403-412.
7. Schuster S, Eliades G, Zinelis S, et al. Structural conformation and leaching from in vitro aged and retrieved Invisalign appliances. *Am J Orthod Dentofacial Orthop*. 2004;126:725-728.
8. Alexandropoulos A, Al Jabbari YS, Zinelis S, et al. Chemical and mechanical characteristics of contemporary thermoplastic orthodontic materials. *Aust Orthod J*. 2015;31:165-170.
9. Ryokawa H, Miyazaki Y, Fujishima A, et al. The mechanical properties of dental thermoplastic materials in a simulated intraoral environment. *Orthod Waves*. 2006;65:64-72.
10. Boubakri A, Elleuch K, Guermazi N, et al. Investigations on hygrothermal aging of thermoplastic polyurethane material. *Mater Des*. 2009;30:3958-3965.
11. Elkholy F, Panchaphongsaphak T, Kilic F, et al. Forces and moments delivered by PET-G aligners to an upper central incisor for labial and palatal translation. *J Orofac Orthop*. 2015;76:460-475.
12. Elkholy F, Schmidt F, Jäger R, et al. Forces and moments applied during derotation of a maxillary central incisor with thinner aligners: an in-vitro study. *Am J Orthod Dentofacial Orthop*. 2017;151:407-415.
13. Elkholy F, Mikhaiel B, Schmidt F, et al. Mechanical load exerted by PET-G aligners during mesial and distal derotation of a mandibular canine an in vitro study. *J Orofac Orthop*. 2017;78:361-370.
14. Zhang N, Bai Y, Ding X, et al. Preparation and characterization of thermoplastic materials for invisible orthodontics. *Dent Mater J*. 2011;30:954-959.
15. Jeremiah HG, Bister D, Newton JT. Social perceptions of adults wearing orthodontic appliances: a cross-sectional study. *Eur J Orthod*. 2010;33:476-482.
16. Rosvall MD, Fields HW, Ziuchkovski J, et al. Attractiveness, acceptability, and value of orthodontic appliances. *Am J Orthod Dentofacial Orthop*. 2009;135:276, e1-12; discussion 276-277.
17. Shalish M, Cooper-Kazaz R, Ivgi I, et al. Adult patients' adjustability to orthodontic appliances. Part I: a comparison between Labial, Lingual, and Invisalign™. *Eur J Orthod*. 2012;34:724-730.
18. Schott TC, Göz G. Color fading of the blue compliance indicator encapsulated in removable clear Invisalign Teen® aligners. *Angle Orthod*. 2011;81:185-191.
19. Gracco A, Mazzoli A, Favoni O, et al. Short-term chemical and physical changes in invisalign appliances. *Aust Orthod J*. 2009;25:34-40.
20. Skaik A, Wei XL, Abusamak I, et al. Effects of time and clear aligner removal frequency on the force delivered by different polyethylene terephthalate glycol-modified materials determined with thin-film pressure sensors. *Am J Orthod Dentofacial Orthop*. 2019;155:98-107.
21. Hattori Y, Satoh C, Kunieda T, et al. Bite forces and their resultants during forceful intercuspal clenching in humans. *J Biomech*. 2009;42:1533-1538.
22. Pejaković V, Jisa R, Franek F. Abrasion resistance of selected commercially available polymer materials. *Finn J Tribol*. 2015;33:21-27.
23. Poomali S, Suresha B, Lee JH. Mechanical and three-body abrasive wear behaviour of PMMA/TPU blends. *Mat Sci Eng A-Struct*. 2008;492:486-490.
24. Rust W. *Nichtlineare Finite-Elemente-Berechnungen*: Kontakt, Geometrie, Material. 2nd ed. Wiesbaden: Vieweg+Teubner Verlag / Springer Fachmedien Wiesbaden GmbH Wiesbaden; 2011.
25. Lombardo L, Martines E, Mazzanti V, et al. Stress relaxation properties of four orthodontic aligner materials: a 24-hour in vitro study. *Angle Orthod*. 2017;87:11-18.
26. Li X, Ren C, Wang Z, et al. Changes in force associated with the amount of aligner activation and lingual bodily movement of the maxillary central incisor. *Korean J Orthod*. 2016;46:65-72.
27. Bradley GT, Teske L, Eliades G, et al. Do the mechanical and chemical properties of Invisalign TM appliances change after use? A retrieval analysis. *Eur J Orthod*. 2016;38:27-31.
28. Condo' R, Pazzini L, Cerroni L, et al. Mechanical properties of "two generations" of teeth aligners: change analysis during oral permanence. *Dent Mater J*. 2018;37:835-842.
29. Fang D, Zhang N, Chen H, et al. Dynamic stress relaxation of orthodontic thermoplastic materials in a simulated oral environment. *Dent Mater J*. 2013;32:946-951.
30. Roylance D. *Engineering Viscoelasticity*. Cambridge, MA: Massachusetts Institute of Technology; 2001:02139.

5 Theoretical and Practical Considerations in Planning an Orthodontic Treatment with Clear Aligners

TOMMASO CASTROFLORIO, GABRIELE ROSSINI, and SIMONE PARRINI

Introduction

After the Stone Age, the Iron Age, and the Bronze Age, are we switching to the Polymer Age? This question is legitimate when examining the increase of plastic materials production during the last half-century.

In the last decades, plastics have permeated industrial technology. Plastic materials have replaced many materials used in the past, and they have made possible industrial and medical applications that would not have been possible with older technologies. The key to the widespread dissemination of these materials is their incredible versatility.[1]

Furthermore, we are living in the personalized medicine era. Personalized medicine represents the natural evolution of health care. When medicine is informed solely by clinical practice guidelines, the patient is not treated as an individual but as a member of a group. Personalized or precision medicine characterizes unique biologic characteristics of the individual to tailor diagnostics and therapeutics to a specific patient. Personalized medicine uses additional information about the individual derived from knowing the patient as a person.[2]

Orthodontists have always been educated in collecting and analyzing patients' individual characteristics to perform a diagnosis and define a personalized treatment plan. In this view, orthodontics will be the pioneer in guiding dentistry into the personalized medicine process. What is still missing is the integration of biologic markers into the diagnostic process and treatment planning, but researchers are going to fill the gap.[3-5]

In the last century, orthodontics was mostly a matter of metals and predefined prescriptions. In the last decades, the introduction of clear aligners moved the attention toward thermoplastic materials and their possible applications and personalized prescriptions. In clear aligner therapy (CAT), every aligner is built for a specific stage of orthodontic tooth movement (OTM) of a specific patient. Aligners are comfortable, less visible, and more aesthetically pleasant compared with buccal fixed appliances; they can be removed for eating and oral hygiene procedures, reducing the occurrence of emergencies. Despite those advantages making clear aligner increasingly requested by patients in our beauty-conscious society, there was always a great debate involving efficacy and efficiency of this appliance in controlling OTM. For instance, questions have been raised regarding the extent to which aligners can control extrusion, rotation, bodily movement, and torque.

As stated by Proffit in 2013, effectiveness, efficiency, and predictability are the three things orthodontists need to know about the treatment they are providing.[6] A recent review[7] stated that CAT can control complex movements as maxillary molars bodily distalization and extraction spaces close and that the buccolingual inclination of incisors is well controlled in mild to moderate malocclusions. Furthermore, in a recent research paper, Grünheid et al.[8] analyzed the differences between predicted and achieved tooth positions and found statistically significant differences for all teeth except maxillary lateral incisors, canines, and first premolars. In general, anterior teeth were positioned more occlusally than predicted, rotation of rounded teeth was incomplete, and movement of posterior teeth in all dimensions was not fully achieved. However, except for excessive posttreatment of buccal crown torque of maxillary second molars, these differences were not large enough to be clinically relevant.

Therefore, with respect to what was possible a few years ago when the recommendation was to treat only simple malocclusions with aligners, the growing base of common knowledge regarding the control of OTM made it possible to use this technique even in more complex cases with good results when compared to conventional fixed orthodontics. Those results were made possible thanks to orthodontists who started to consider the virtual setup not only to visualize moving teeth but as an instrument to design the proper biomechanics, starting to transfer well-known concepts in this field.

As stated by Burstone[9] during a *JCO* interview:

The nice thing about scientific biomechanics is that it is not dependent on any given appliance or technique. No matter what appliance you use, it allows you to use it better with more predictable results. Today, we have much too much commercialism in orthodontics; a healthy dose of science in understanding appliances and how they work is a good antidote. It is interesting to note that many of the new appliances that are suggested are nothing more than reinventions of old appliances.

Theoretical and Practical Considerations in CAT

Based on these assumptions and on clinical and laboratory research,[10-13] the biomechanics of clear aligners could be described as a sequence of crown tipping and root uprighting. The first part of movement occurs in the occlusal part of the tooth because the aligner envelopes the entire tooth crown, while the interactions between aligner and attachments determine root movement. Therefore, when designing a virtual treatment plan, we must always remember which is the interaction surface between the aligner and the tooth, which is the effect of the force application at the crown level, and which is the anchorage unit required to avoid undesired movements.

The analysis of a virtual treatment plan using dedicated software should be based on the following steps:

1. Analysis of the final position
2. Analysis of the movements occurring at each stage for each tooth

ANALYSIS OF THE FINAL POSITION

According to Sarver et al.[14,15] it may be inappropriate to place everyone in the same esthetic framework and even more problematic to attempt this based solely on hard tissue relationships since the soft tissues often fail to respond predictably to hard tissue changes. Nevertheless, it is accepted that esthetic considerations are paramount in planning appropriate treatment but that rigid rules cannot be applied to this process. In view of our inability to apply rules defining optimal esthetics, the use of scientific methods to plan the most esthetic treatment may therefore be complicated. Nevertheless, it is clear that laypeople can identify various factors affecting smile esthetics. Thus clinicians can expect their patients to be more attentive to some dental esthetic factors than they are to others.[16]

A recent review was conducted to define the minimum level of esthetic harmony that can be approved as pleasurable by an external observer.[17] The indications provided in Fig. 5.1 represent the threshold of acceptance of smile esthetics provided by laypeople that should be considered when analyzing the final position of front teeth.

Regarding the final position of upper maxillary molars, it is recommendable to refer to the position indicated by Ricketts in 1974 in which the line connecting the distobuccal and the mesiolingual cusps of the upper first molar is passing through the cusp of the opposite canine at the end of treatment.[18] This final position is based on precise anatomic landmarks and can prevent misunderstandings between the prescribing clinician and the technician transferring the information in the virtual treatment plan.

Furthermore, when defining the final position, the clinician should always consider the buccal and the frontal limits of the arches, considering bone and periodontal support and the cephalometric information. Those indications are very important to avoid excessive expansion and/or proclination movements that can result in severe periodontal iatrogenic effects.[19,20]

ANALYSIS OF THE MOVEMENTS OCCURRING AT EACH STAGE FOR EACH TOOTH

The analysis of movements occurring in every stage should consider three different aspects:

1. Aligner auxiliaries
2. Anchorage management and movement sequentialization
3. OTM staging

Aligner Auxiliaries

Since the introduction of orthodontic aligners in early 2000s, several auxiliaries have been adopted from manufacturing companies and from clinicians to prevent anchorage loss and maximize treatment efficiency.

The most commonly adopted auxiliaries could be classified as follows:

- Attachments and pressure areas
- Intraoral elastics
- Interproximal enamel reduction (IPR)
- Temporary anchorage devices (TADs)

Attachments and Pressure Areas.
Using aligners without attachments is something like orthodontics but not orthodontics. Attachments are useful to guide teeth in a determined direction but are also useful in providing anchorage control depending on the type of

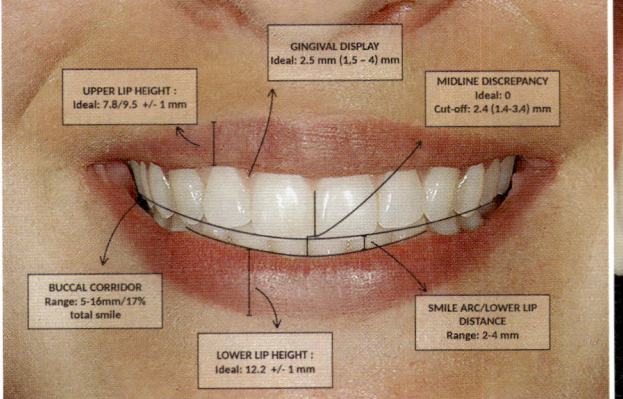

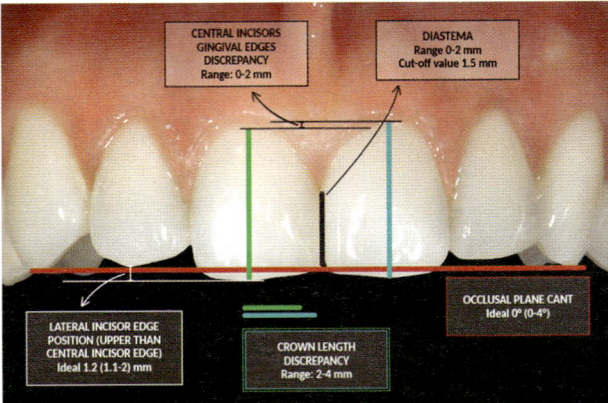

Fig. 5.1 Thresholds of acceptance of smile esthetics from laypeople point of view.

planned orthodontic movement. The use of attachments is crucial to achieve effective treatments. Ravera et al.[21] and Garino et al.[22] demonstrated the importance of using attachments to improve the root control of distalizing molars in class II treatments. In an in vitro study, Simon et al. demonstrated that load transfer from aligners to teeth without the use of attachment is possible only to a limited extent.[11]

Attachments are divided into two categories:

1. Conventional attachments (rectangular, beveled, or ellipsoid)
2. Optimized attachments

Conventional attachments (Figs. 5.2, 5.3, and 5.4) can be positioned by the clinician on every tooth (compatibly with tooth dimension) and can be oriented in any direction. Rectangular attachments are usually placed to increase anchorage in posterior teeth or to reinforce the retention of the aligner.

Optimized attachments (Fig. 5.5) are positioned by technicians, and the orthodontist is not able to modify their position, dimension, and orientation. This kind of attachment was introduced to generate a dedicated couple of force during rotations, especially in canines and premolars.

The "play" of aligners on teeth and attachments is another key factor in producing desired outcomes, which is strictly related to attachment application. An in vitro study by Dasy et al.[23] demonstrated that attachment shape affects retention: Rectangular attachments are more retentive than ellipsoid ones. Two in vitro studies demonstrated that aligners produced by different companies (Invisalign, Align Technology, San José, CA, USA; CA Clear Aligner, Scheu-Dental, Iserlohn, Germany; F22 Aligner, Sweden & Martina, Due Carrare, Italy) showed excellent fitting on teeth and attachments.[24,25] F22 aligners seem to have the best values in terms of fitting on attachments: the values range from 1 to 178 μm. The Invisalign fitting ranges from 5 to 212 μm. The measured values for CA Clear Aligner analysis range from 7 to 298 μm. Dasy et al. demonstrated that edgeless aligners generated significantly lower forces than those with a wider edge. The increased force might be due to the enhanced stiffness caused by material shape. Consequently, the enhanced stiffness may reduce the fitting of the aligner on the attachments. This could be the reason why CA aligners showed the worst results in terms of fitting. However, despite the statistical significance, measured differences might not be clinically relevant. Therefore the play of aligners on teeth and attachments is minimal, resulting in a precise transfer of the mechanical properties of the thermoplastic material to teeth.

From a biomechanical point of view, only a few studies in existing literature have analyzed the interaction between aligners and attachments. An efficient method for studying aligner mechanics is the finite element method (FEM). Applications of FEM on aligner studies will be presented in the next parts of this chapter. Except for the Yokoi et al. study,[26] reported FEM results will refer to the initial instance of

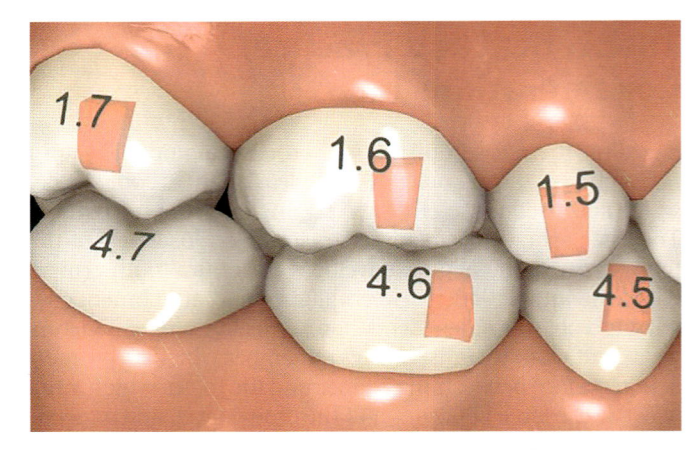

Fig. 5.4 Rectangular attachments on posterior teeth in Align Technology ClinCheck software.

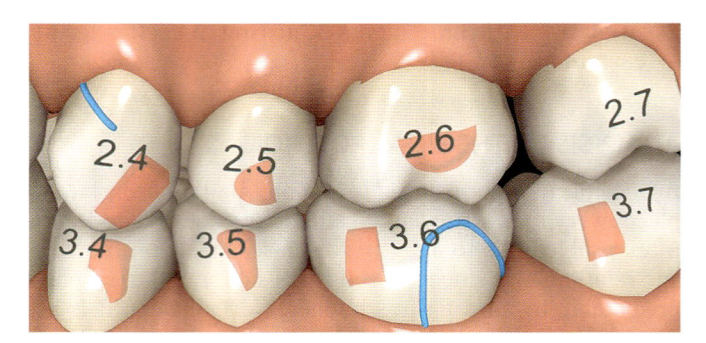

Fig. 5.5 Optimized and conventional attachments in Align Technology ClinCheck software.

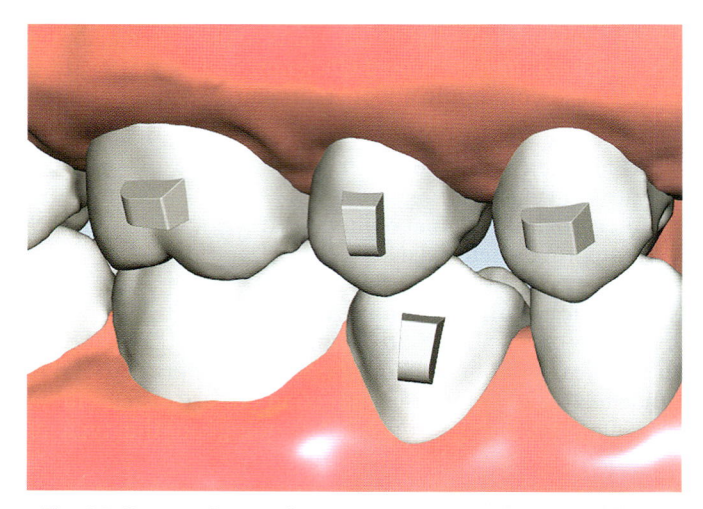

Fig. 5.2 Rectangular attachments on posterior teeth in CA Digital software.

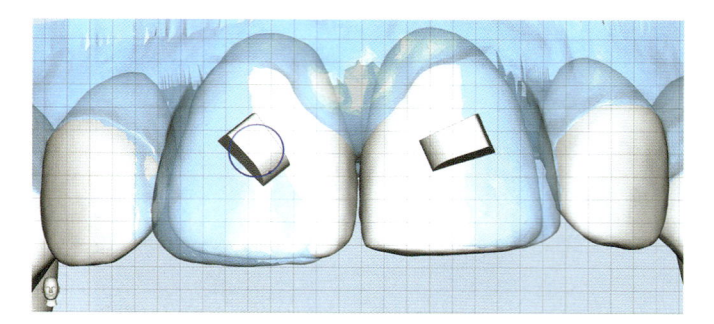

Fig. 5.3 Rectangular attachments on anterior teeth in CA Digital software.

aligner wearing; thus these results should be considered in terms of initial force systems and displacements, not taking into account such precise measurements of the amount of movement expressed by the aligner on teeth.

Using FEM, Gomez et al. investigated a theoretical 0.15-mm displacement of an isolated upper canine with and without a composite attachment.[27] The attachment considered for this analysis was inspired by the "optimized attachments" adopted by Align Technology to increase root control during distalization. The authors observed uncontrolled distal crown tipping without the attachment and a displacement similar to bodily movement with the attachment. Thus the authors highlighted the difficulty to obtain a controlled movement in CAT using only aligners and suggested the use of composite attachments to increase root control.

The biomechanical explanation of attachments usefulness in controlling tooth movement could be related to the role of braces in fixed orthodontics. While in fixed appliance orthodontics the moment is developed in the bracket itself by the engagement of the wire, in CAT it is developed by the interaction of aligner and auxiliaries.[28] The aligner without attachments tends to move away from the teeth in its gingival edge. In such eventuality, all force is concentrated only in the occlusal part, and no couple of force could be generated. When recurring to attachments, the interaction between the displacement applied to the aligner and the attachment generates the adequate forces and moments to obtain a more controlled movement.

Yokoi et al. in 2019 published a paper that demonstrated these concepts using FEM to compare upper incisor diastema closure without attachments and with optimized ones. As reported by authors, the initial displacement corresponded to uncontrolled crown tipping for both the simulations; however, after hundreds of iterations that simulated the bone remodeling process, the simulation without attachments resulted in uncontrolled tipping, while bodily movement was observed in the simulation with optimized attachments.[26]

Regarding pressure areas, the kind of movements in which they are adopted depends on the aligner manufacturer. Usually, pressure areas are adopted to improve efficiency in crown tipping, rotations, and root torquing. Barone et al. in their FEM study from 2016 reported that pressure areas are the most effective auxiliaries in lower incisors tipping, even more than rectangular attachments.[12]

A study by Castroflorio et al. regarding control of root movement demonstrated the efficacy of pressure areas to improve this type of movement.[29] The force couple generated by an aligner torquing a tooth consists of a force near the gingival margin and a resulting force produced by movement of the tooth against the opposite inner surface of the appliance near the incisal edge.[30] Since the gingival edge of the aligner is elastic, it is difficult to control the forces applied in this region without an altered geometry.[27]

Intraoral Elastics.
Regarding intraoral elastics, three main variables could influence the right choice for the planned treatment:

1. Force/length
2. Application point
3. Application surface

Figs. 5.6 through 5.11 refer to upper molar distalization, which will be thoroughly analyzed in the following chapters, and present the effects of elastics on teeth and aligners while changing application point. The same elastic (0.25 in., 8 oz) was applied so that the force/length variable would not affect the analyzed ones. The difference in aligner deformation and teeth initial displacement during second upper molar distalization could be observed.

In the previously cited study, Gomez et al. observed an intrusive effect on the canine due to an unexpected deformation of the aligner during distalization.[26] A loose fitting between aligner and tooth would achieve inadequate contact with the gingival optimized attachment and thus fail to produce a correct couple of force. This eventuality could be avoided by class II elastic that assists during distalization movement providing anchorage with the sagittal component of elastic force and preventing intrusion thanks to its vertical component.

Interproximal Reduction.
Since first described by Ballard in 1944, IPR has been a procedure dedicated to mild-to-moderate crowning cases.[31] However, in the last years, the digitalization of treatment planning increased the adoption of this technique to obtain

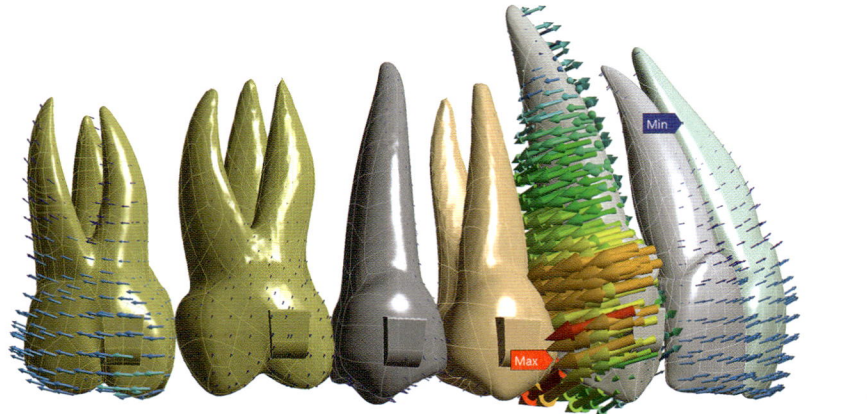

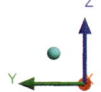

Fig. 5.6 Initial tooth displacement of second molar distalization with class II elastics applied directly on upper canine *(sagittal view)*.

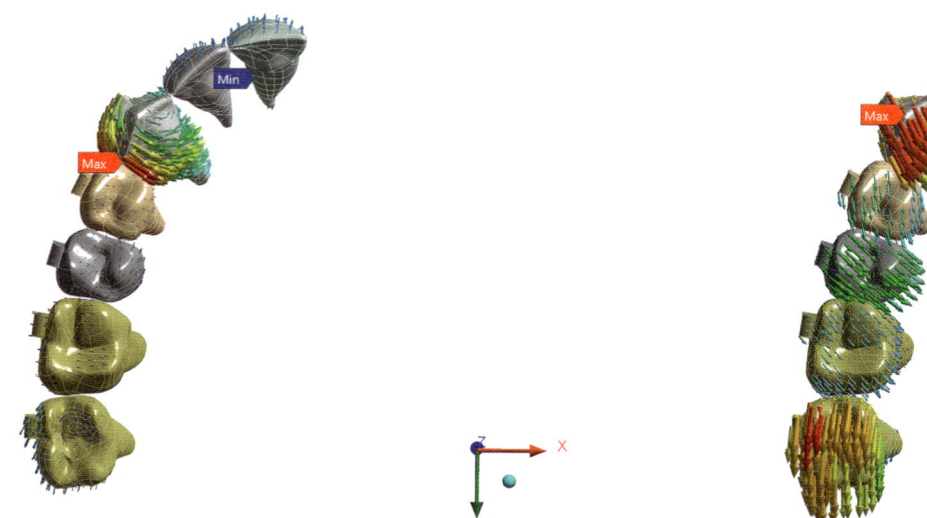

Fig. 5.7 Initial tooth displacement of second molar distalization with class II elastics applied directly on upper canine *(occlusal view)*.

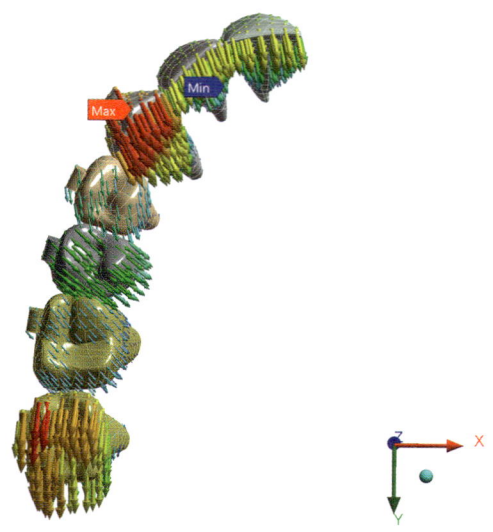

Fig. 5.9 Initial tooth displacement of second molar distalization with class II elastics applied on aligner at upper canine level *(occlusal view)*.

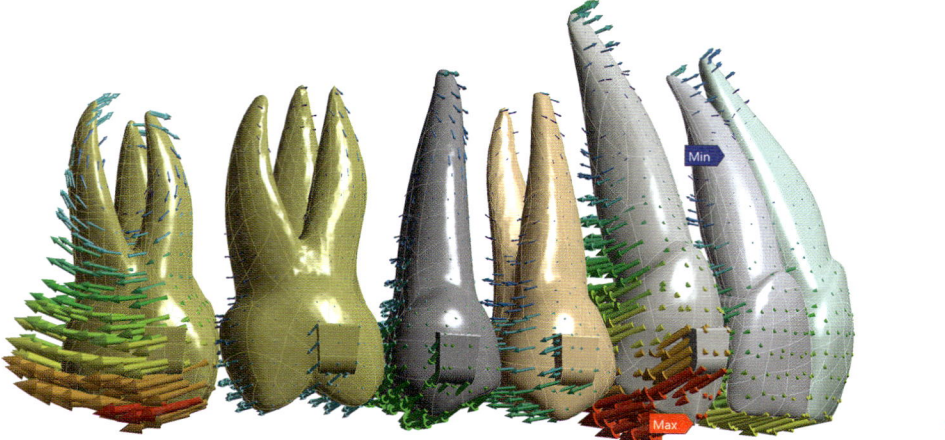

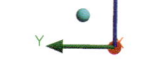

Fig. 5.8 Initial tooth displacement of second molar distalization with class II elastics applied on aligner at upper canine level *(sagittal view)*.

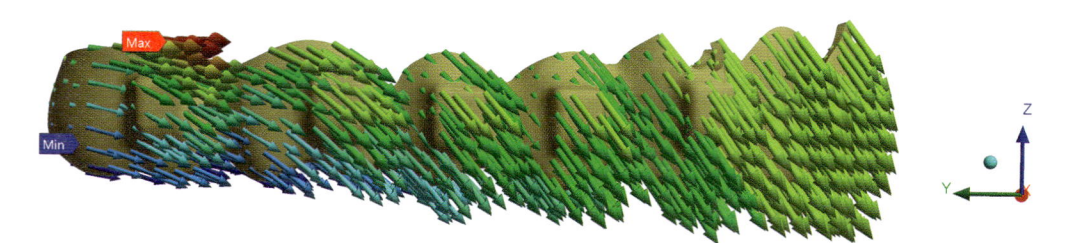

Fig. 5.10 Initial aligner displacement of second molar distalization with class II elastics applied directly on upper canine.

space during orthodontic treatment, also improving its accuracy and precision. During CAT digital planning, the IPR amount is calculated based on digitally performed dental index scores (Bolton index, Little index, space analysis, etc.), and the timing of IPR is programmed to obtain the best interproximal surface access and to avoid premature tooth surface collisions. As demonstrated by several authors, IPR is a safe procedure for tooth health, which does not increase the risks of interproximal cavities and tooth demineralization.[32,33] Regarding IPR maximum amount, in 2015 Sarig et al. analyzed 109 extracted intact anterior and posterior teeth from both maxilla and mandible.[34] The authors reported that the existing guidelines of 0.5-mm max IPR for each interproximal space could be confirmed for anterior region, while in the posterior region it could be increased to 1 mm.

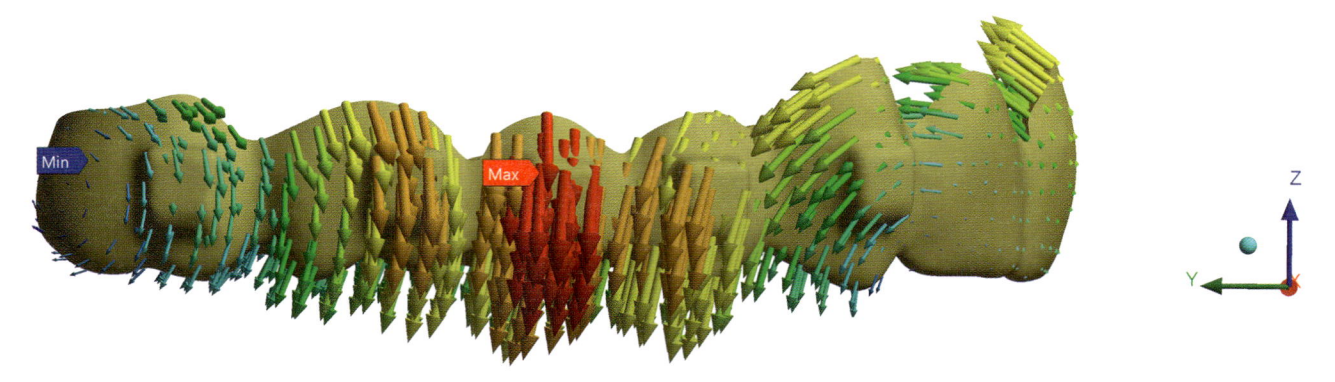

Fig. 5.11 Initial aligner displacement of second molar distalization with class II elastics applied on aligner at upper canine level.

Temporary Anchorage Devices.

Aligner treatment with TADs is thoroughly analyzed in Chapter 15.

Anchorage Management and Movements Sequentialization

Anchorage management represents the key for a successful orthodontic treatment. In fixed orthodontic treatment, auxiliaries such as lacebacks, tiebacks, and elastics are adopted to reinforce anchorage when needed, principally during the working phase of treatment. Despite the widespread use of aligner orthodontics, no biomechanical studies are present to date to verify the efficiency of aligners alone in maintaining anchorage.

In aligner orthodontics, as well as in conventional orthodontics, anchorage loss could result in inefficacy of programmed movements or in undesired movements of anchorage unit. A paper by Cortona et al. reported the effects of anchorage loss on a contralateral premolar during rotation of a lower premolar without attachments.[35]

Anchorage in aligner orthodontics depends on two key factors: sequentialization of movements and aligner deformation.

Sequentialization in aligner orthodontics is intended as the order in which teeth are moved during the treatment. Movement sequentialization allows a proper anchorage control, reducing the risk of undesired displacements. Multiple movements at the same time should be avoided unless we are referring to small amounts of movement on several teeth, as in such cases when we are aligning and leveling the arches in mild class I malocclusions, for example. Multiple complex movements as well as lingual root torque movement associated with rotation and extrusion or intrusion movements of an upper incisor, as an example, should be always avoided. In cases when multiple movements have been planned on a specific tooth, the best option is to split movements based on their complexity. Therefore, torque movement should be performed a second time, at least once rotational and tipping movements have been completed. More detailed sequentialization protocols will be analyzed in dedicated chapters. Among sequentialization resides also the concept of "differential forces and moments." This concept is the result of the biomechanical design of a force system, which by the way of its application can distribute the reciprocal forces and moments over significantly different root areas with the objective of eliciting a differential response.[36] Several studies demonstrated the efficiency of this method in preserving anchorage and anterior torque during space closure after a premolar extraction.[37,38] In aligner orthodontics, these concepts have been introduced by Align Technology with the so-called G6 protocol for first premolar extraction.[39] Differential moments are produced with a combination of optimized attachments and aligner activation; however, no detailed force systems are publicly available and to date no trials have been conducted to measure the outcomes of this clinical protocol.

Aligner deformation is intended as the response of the whole aligner to the stress caused by fitting it on teeth. During aligner wearing, a push and pull force system involves not only the teeth for which movements are planned but also adjacent teeth and the aligner itself. Fig. 5.12 shows the tooth displacement during upper second molar distalization in an efficient force configuration; note that while 0.2 mm of movement was planned for tooth 1.7, 0.1 mm is efficiently applied on the tooth, while the other amount results in mesial displacement of the aligner. Another example of anchorage loss due to aligner deformation is reported in Fig. 5.13, in which mesial displacement of molars is highlighted during sequential distalization of premolars. First and second molars, in this simulation, were set as an anchorage unit. However, without proper auxiliaries to increase anchorage and manage aligner deformation, even a good movement sequentialization could be not adequate.

OTM Staging

In aligner orthodontics, staging is intended as the amount of programmed movement per tooth in each aligner. Staging amount is determined by each aligner company based on internal research, thus default staging settings may differ between one another. Regarding scientific literature, evidence-based data about staging are very poor. Simon et al., in their 2014 in vitro study, tested different amounts of staging for premolar rotation.[10] The accuracy for this movement was halved when a rotation greater than 1.5 degrees per aligner was planned (<1.5 degrees: 41.8 +/− 0.3%; >1.5 degrees: 23.2 +/− 0.2%). The importance of staging for tooth rotation could be highlighted in the paper by Cortona et al.[36] A simulation, including an ideal dental arch with element 4.5 rotated 30 degrees mesially, was tested with different staging and attachment configurations for premolar distal rotation. Staging of 1.2 and 3 degrees of rotation per

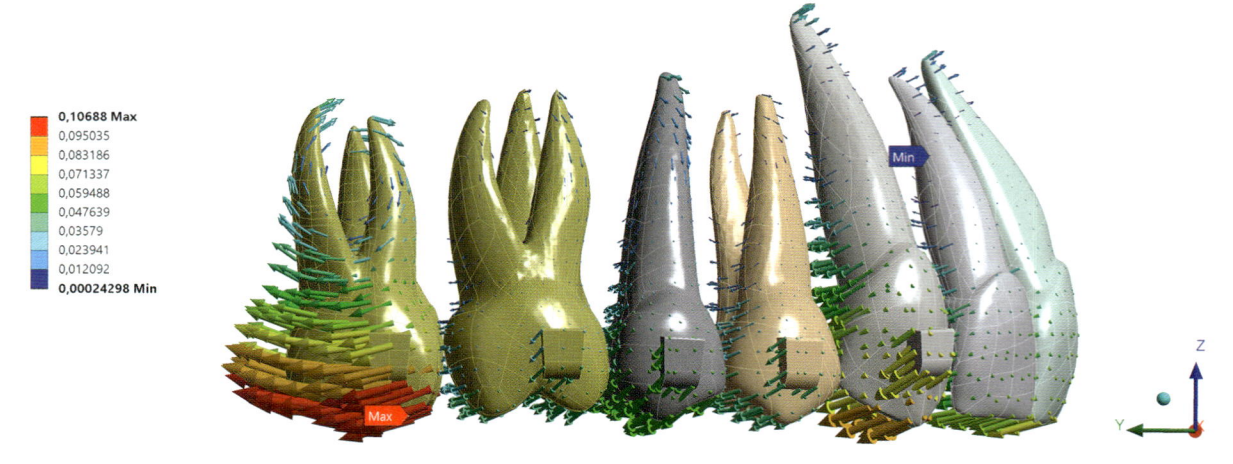

Fig. 5.12 Initial tooth displacement of second molar distalization with class II elastics applied on aligner at first premolar level. Initial displacement amount is shown in the attached legend.

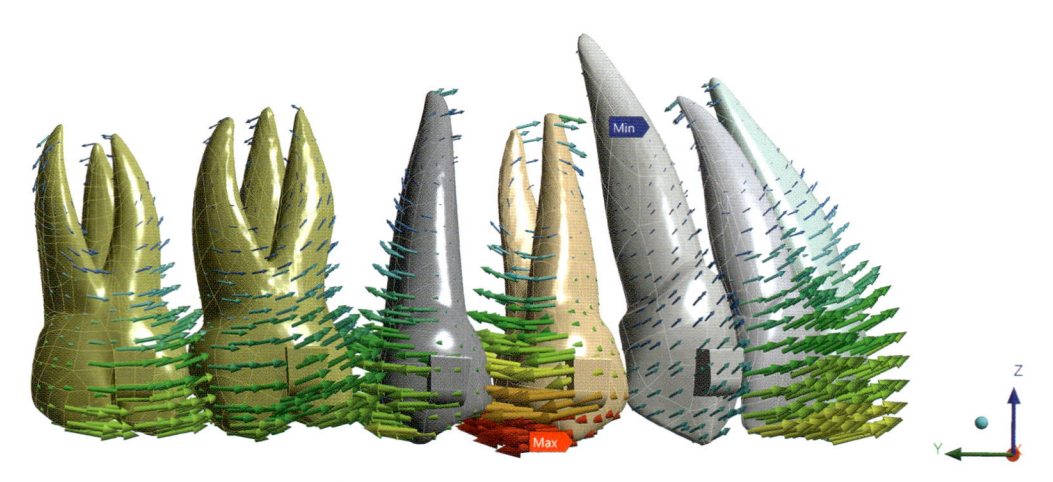

Fig. 5.13 Initial tooth displacement of first molar and second premolar distalization without class II elastics. The mesial shift of posterior teeth is clinically relevant.

aligner was compared and the difference in periodontal ligament (PDL) pressure on tooth 4.5 between the different amount of staging with rectangular attachments from tooth 4.4 to 4.6 was reported. Planned rotation of 1.2 degrees produced 22.5 mmHg of pressure on periodontal ligament, while 3 degrees of planned rotation obtained pressure of 412.53 mmHg. Thus the model with attachments from 4.4 to 4.6 and 1.2 degrees of activation was the most reliable and efficient configuration for lower premolar rotation.

Evidence-based data regarding staging for other movements may be derived from in vitro and clinical studies, but there is a lack of dedicated trials. Table 5.1 reports the suggested amount of movement per aligner based on scientific literature and clinical expertise of the authors.

Table 5.1 Suggested Amount of Movement per Aligner

Rotation[10,11,36]	<1.5°
Intrusion/Extrusion[40]	0.2 mm
Linear Movement[10,11,21,22]	0.2 mm
Root Torque[10,11,30]	1°

Biologic Considerations in Aligner Orthodontics

As stated at the beginning of this chapter, personalized medicine applied to orthodontics is based not only on dedicated mechanics but also on the knowledge of each patient's biology.

The application of an orthodontic force produces a tissue reaction resulting from the perturbation generated by the orthodontic appliance and the modeling and remodeling of the alveolar bone.[41] Kuncio et al. suggested that teeth moved with aligners did not undergo the typical stages of movement, as described by Krishnan and Davidovitch, because of the intermittent forces applied by the aligners.[42] However, light, continuous forces seem to be perceived as intermittent forces by the periodontium due to its viscoelastic nature, and orthodontic intermittent forces can produce OTM with less cell damage in the periodontium.[43] Castroflorio et al., in analyzing the biologic response to the application of aligners distalizing a maxillary molar in a single tooth movement design study, showed that the force delivery produces an increased concentration of bone modeling and remodeling mediators at both pressure sites (interleukin 1 beta [IL-1β], receptor activator of nuclear factor kappa-B ligand [RANKL]) and tension sites (transforming growth factor beta [TGFβ], osteopontin [OPN]). In other words, aligners seem to be capable of inducing the same biologic responses described for other appliances at least in the very early stages of orthodontic treatment.[44]

Patient Compliance

Despite all biologic and biomechanical aspects, the success of an orthodontic treatment strictly depends on patient compliance. Compliance with removable orthodontic aligners is fundamental for the efficiency and success of CAT in the short and long term.

A 2017 systematic review built on previous primary research confirmed suboptimal levels of compliance with a variety of removable orthodontic adjuncts, alluding to actual wear durations of 5.7 hours per day less than recommended.[45]

The influence of treatment progress appeared to be significant to motivate compliance, although it could be argued that facial and occlusal improvement is most likely in more compliant patients anyway. Notwithstanding this, demonstrable change was frequently reported as a facilitator of appliance wear. As such, the importance of encouragement and positive reinforcement by clinicians and family members in encouraging appliance wear is clear.[46]

Pilot studies in the field have demonstrated that known monitoring increases patient compliance.[47,48] The use of an app was effective in increasing patient compliance in a fixed-appliance population.[49] Customized reminders may help to promote enhanced levels of compliance with aligners thanks to teleorthodontics. Teleorthodontics is a broad term that encompasses remote provision of orthodontic care, advice, or treatment through the medium of information technology. Teleorthodontics platforms using artificial intelligence to remotely monitor patient adherence to the prescribed wearing time are available (e.g., Dental Monitoring, Paris, France) and have been demonstrated to be effective in enhancing patient compliance.[50]

CAT Fundamentals Recap

Considering all the premises, aligner orthodontics is a mature orthodontic technique requiring orthodontists to manage it properly. Some limitations in the appliance system remain, but they in no way suggest unsatisfactory treatment results. Diagnosis and treatment plans still remain the responsibility of clinicians and cannot yet be overcome by artificial intelligence.

It is clear that treatment progress is not as easy and predictable as dictated by computer animation. Therefore, giving priority to technology instead of orthodontics is dangerous. The knowledge of biomechanics is crucial to properly manage clear aligner therapy. Moreover, like any other orthodontic technique, auxiliaries are mandatory to perform an efficient and predictable orthodontic treatment.

References

1. Seymour RB. Polymers are everywhere. *J Chem Educ.* 1988;65(4):327.
2. Ziegelstein RC. Personomics: the missing link in the evolution from precision medicine to personalized medicine. *J Pers Med.* 2017;7(4):11. doi:10.3390/jpm7040011.
3. Han Y, Jia L, Zheng Y, et al. Salivary exosomes: emerging roles in systemic disease. *Int J Biol Sci.* 2018;14(6):633-643. doi:10.7150/ijbs.25018.
4. de Aguiar MC, Perinetti G, Capelli Jr J. The gingival crevicular fluid as a source of biomarkers to enhance efficiency of orthodontic and functional treatment of growing patients. *Biomed Res Int.* 2017;2017:3257235.
5. Yashin D, Dalci O, Almuzian M, et al. Markers in blood and saliva for prediction of orthodontically induced inflammatory root resorption: a retrospective case controlled-study. *Prog Orthod.* 2017;18(1):27.
6. Proffit W, Fields H. *Contemporary Orthodontics.* 5th ed. St. Louis: Mosby; 2013.
7. Rossini G, Parrini S, Deregibus A, et al. Controlling orthodontic tooth movement with clear aligners: an updated systematic review regarding efficacy and efficiency. *J Aligner Orthod.* 2017;1(1):7-20.
8. Grünheid T, Loh C, Larson BE. How accurate is Invisalign in nonextraction cases? Are predicted tooth positions achieved? *Angle Orthod.* 2017;87(6):809-815.
9. Burstone CJ. Charles J. Burstone, MS. Part 2: biomechanics. Interview by Dr. Nanda. *J Clin Orthod.* 2007;41(3):139-147.
10. Simon M, Keilig L, Schwarze J, et al. Treatment outcome and efficacy of an aligner technique—regarding incisor torque, premolar derotation and molar distalization. *BMC Oral Health.* 2014;14:68. doi:10.1186/1472-6831-14-68.
11. Simon M, Keilig L, Schwarze J, et al. Forces and moments generated by removable thermoplastic aligners: incisor torque, premolar derotation, and molar distalization. *Am J Orthod Dentofacial Orthop.* 2014;145(6):728-736.
12. Barone S, Paoli A, Razionale AV, et al. Computational design and engineering of polymeric orthodontic aligners. *Int J Numer Method Biomed Eng.* 2017;33(8):e2839.
13. Hennessy J, Garvey T, Al-Awadhi EA. A randomized clinical trial comparing mandibular incisor proclination produced by fixed labial appliances and clear aligners. *Angle Orthod.* 2016;86(5):706-712.
14. Hayes RJ, Sarver DM, Jacobson A. The quantification of soft tissue cervicomental changes after mandibular advancement surgery. *Am J Orthod Dentofacial Orthop.* 1994;105(4):383-391.
15. Sarver DM, Ackerman JL. Orthodontics about face: the re-emergence of the esthetic paradigm. *Am J Orthod Dentofacial Orthop.* 2000;117(5):575-576.
16. Flores-Mir C, Silva E, Barriga MI, et al. Lay person's perception of smile aesthetics in dental and facial views. *J Orthod.* 2004;31(3):204-209.
17. Parrini S, Rossini G, Castroflorio T, et al. Laypeople's perceptions of frontal smile esthetics: a systematic review. *Am J Orthod Dentofacial Orthop.* 2016;150(5):740-750.
18. McNamara Jr JA, Brudon WL. *Orthodontic and Orthopedic Treatment in the Mixed Dentition.* Ann Arbor: Needham Press; 1993.
19. Rafiuddin S, Yg PK, Biswas S, et al. Iatrogenic damage to the periodontium caused by orthodontic treatment procedures: an overview. *Open Dent J.* 2015;9:228-234.
20. Jati AS, Furquim LZ, Consolaro A. Gingival recession: its causes and types, and the importance of orthodontic treatment. *Dental Press J Orthod.* 2016;21(3):18-29.
21. Ravera S, Castroflorio T, Garino F, et al. Maxillary molar distalization with aligners in adult patients: a multicenter retrospective study. *Prog Orthod.* 2016;17:12. doi:10.1186/s40510-016-0126-0.
22. Garino F, Castroflorio T, Daher S, et al. Effectiveness of composite attachments in controlling upper-molar movement with aligners. *J Clin Orthod.* 2016;50(6):341-347.
23. Dasy H, Dasy A, Asatrian G, et al. Effects of variable attachment shapes and aligner material on aligner retention. *Angle Orthod.* 2015;85(6):934-940. doi:10.2319/091014-637.1.
24. Mantovani E, Castroflorio E, Rossini G, et al. Scanning electron microscopy evaluation of aligner fit on teeth. *Angle Orthod.* 2018;88(5):596-601. doi:10.2319/120417-827.1.
25. Mantovani E, Castroflorio E, Rossini G, et al. Scanning electron microscopy analysis of aligner fitting on anchorage attachments. *J Orofac Orthop.* 2019;80(2):79-87. doi:10.1007/s00056-018-00167-1.

26. Yokoi Y, Arai A, Kawamura J, et al. Effects of attachment of plastic aligner in closing of diastema of maxillary dentition by finite element method. J Healthc Eng. 2019;2019:1075097.
27. Gomez JP1, Peña FM, Martínez V, et al. Initial force systems during bodily tooth movement with plastic aligners and composite attachments: a three-dimensional finite element analysis. Angle Orthod. 2015;85(3):454-460.
28. Brezniak N. The clear plastic appliance: a biomechanical point of view. Angle Orthod. 2008;78(2):381-382.
29. Castroflorio T, Garino F, Lazzaro A, et al. Upper-incisor root control with Invisalign appliances. J Clin Orthod. 2013;47:346-351.
30. Grünheid T, Gaalaas S, Hamdan H, et al. Effect of clear aligner therapy on the buccolingual inclination of mandibular canines and the intercanine distance. Angle Orthod. 2016;86(1):10-16.
31. Ballard ML. Asymmetry in tooth size, a factor in the etiology, diagnosis, and treatment of malocclusion. Angle Orthod. 1944;14:67-69.
32. Koretsi V, Chatzigianni A, Sidiropoulou S. Enamel roughness and incidence of caries after interproximal enamel reduction: a systematic review. Orthod Craniofac Res. 2014;17:1-13.
33. Zachrisson BU, Nyøygaard L, Mobarakc K. Dental health assessed more than 10 years after interproximal enamel reduction of mandibular anterior teeth. Am J Orthod Dentofacial Orthop. 2007;131:162-169.
34. Sarig R, Vardimon AD, Sussan C, et al. Pattern of maxillary and mandibular proximal enamel thickness at the contact area of the permanent dentition from first molar to first molar. Am J Orthod Dentofacial Orthop. 2015;147:435-444
35. Cortona A, Rossini G, Parrini S, et al. Clear aligner orthodontic therapy of rotated mandibular conical teeth: a finite element study. Angle Orthod. 2019 Submitted for publication (minor revision).
36. Nanda R. Dr. Ravindra Nanda on orthodontic mechanics. Interview by Robert G Keim. J Clin Orthod. 2010;44(5):293-302.
37. Kuhlberg AJ, Priebe D. Testing force systems and biomechanics—measured tooth movements from differential moment closing loops. Angle Orthod. 2003;73:270-280.
38. Davoody AR, Posada L, Utreja A, et al. A prospective comparative study between differential moments and miniscrews in anchorage control. Eur J Orthod. 2013;35(5):568-576.
39. Jie RKPLK. Treating bimaxillary protrusion and crowding with the invisalign G6 first premolar extraction solution and invisalign aligners. APOS Trends Orthod. 2018;8:219-224.
40. Liu Y, Hu W. Force changes associated with different intrusion strategies for deep-bite correction by clear aligners. Angle Orthod. 2018;88(6):771-778.
41. Krishnan V, Davidovitch Z. Biological Mechanisms of Tooth Movement. 2nd ed. Hoboken, NJ: Wiley-Blackwell; 2015.
42. Kuncio D, Maganzini A, Shelton C, et al. Invisalign and traditional orthodontic treatment postretention outcomes compared using the American Board of Orthodontics objective grading system. Angle Orthod. 2007;77(5):864-869.
43. Cattaneo PM, Dalstra M, Melsen B. Strains in periodontal ligament and alveolar bone associated with orthodontic tooth movement analyzed by finite element. Orthod Craniofac Res. 2009;12(2):120-128.
44. Castroflorio T, Gamerro EF, Caviglia GP, et al. Biochemical markers of bone metabolism during early orthodontic tooth movement with aligners. Angle Orthod. 2017;87(1):74-81.
45. Al-Moghrabi D, Salazar FC, Pandis N, et al. Compliance with removable orthodontic appliances and adjuncts: a systematic review and meta-analysis. Am J Orthod Dentofacial Orthop. 2017;152(1):17-32.
46. El-Huni A, Colonio Salazar FB, Sharma PK, et al. Understanding factors influencing compliance with removable functional appliances: a qualitative study. Am J Orthod Dentofacial Orthop. 2019;155(2):173-181.
47. Pauls A, Nienkemper M, Panayotidis A, et al. Effects of wear time recording on the patient's compliance. Angle Orthod. 2013;83(6):1002-1008.
48. Arreghini A, Trigila S, Lombardo L, et al. Objective assessment of compliance with intra- and extraoral removable appliances. Angle Orthod. 2017;87(1):88-95.
49. Li X, Xu ZR, Tang N, et al. Effect of intervention using a messaging app on compliance and duration of treatment in orthodontic patients. Clin Oral Investig. 2016;20(8):1849-1859.
50. Hansa I, Semaan JS, Vaid NR, et al. Remote monitoring and "tele-orthodontics": concept, scope and applications. Semin Orthod. 2018;24(4):470-481.

6 Class I Malocclusion

MARIO GRECO

Introduction

Class I malocclusions represent one of the most common conditions in the daily clinical practice and one of the most elective conditions to be treated with aligners, since the primary patients' concern is often represented by crowded anterior teeth, especially in the mandibular arch.[1]

Working with clear aligners challenges the paradigm on which we, as orthodontists, based the traditional fixed mechanics approach. Working with aligners means that we need to plan everything in advance and not on a monthly basis, defining final teeth position from the beginning and spending more time in treatment plan design and staging than at the chairside.[2-3]

Diagnostic Reference

When dealing with class I malocclusion, the first step to consider is the definition of the biologic limits of the arches. We should identify anterior, frontal, and vertical limits. All the limits represent both a morphologic limit (torque posterior and anterior) strictly connected to bone and teeth pattern of movement and an esthetic indication to define exactly the ideal teeth positioning in relationship to lips and face.

More specifically, during treatment plan in class I malocclusion a very schematic approach could be focused on the observation and respect of the following key points:

- Esthetic key points: face midline, smile arc, intraarch symmetry
- Occlusal key points: Bolton analysis, overjet, incisors inclination

Substantially the esthetic indicators represent the limits in which teeth need to be moved on the horizontal plane (arch symmetry, face midline) and on the vertical plane (smile arc); the occlusal indicators are useful to define the proper Overjet needed to ensure anterior clearance and avoiding premature anterior contacts (causing posterior open bite) in relationship to dental size and anterior limit of dentition.

Treatment Plan

The development of proper treatment plan in class I malocclusion starts from the definition of correct staging of movement to create a reliable digital setup and to reach a predictable result with high superimposition between the real and the digital settings.[4] The ideal approach in terms of treatment staging should be based on curve of Spee leveling, incisor control, arch development, rotation control, attachment choice, and interproximal reduction (IPR).

CURVE OF SPEE LEVELING

To avoid anterior premature contacts, to create the proper cuspids and molars intercuspations, and to allow lower incisor leveling and correct anterior relationship related to guidance function, flattening of the curve of Spee is required. Moreover, the assessment of the amount of leveling will give information about the space needed for curve flattening.[5]

INCISOR CONTROL

Having in mind the precise angular inclination of lower incisors according to the cephalometric references and using the superimposition tool (and/or the movement table tool), together with the grid tool of digital setup software, is possible to determine the amount of proclination or retroclination required to properly locate the lower incisors on the sagittal plane.[6]

ARCH DEVELOPMENT

In terms of treatment approach, expansion represents a very common solution to treat crowding and transverse discrepancy. Buccal tipping movement is more predictable than bodily movement when planning arch expansion with aligners. This should be kept in mind when defining the buccolingual inclination of canine premolars and molars respecting the periodontal condition.[7]

ROTATION CONTROL

Rotation of small teeth or round teeth such as premolars could be considered a difficult movement to achieve because of the reduced tooth surface on which the force can be applied. Complex rotations should be managed by first creating the mesial and distal spaces required to rotate teeth and then choosing the proper attachment.[8]

ATTACHMENT CHOICE

Attachments represent a useful tool to increase the surface on which orthodontic forces could be applied (Fig. 6.1). See previous chapters for more details.[9]

INTERPROXIMAL REDUCTION

One common procedure in aligner technique is represented by the IPR, which ideally should be limited to 0.3 mm per interproximal point to avoid too wide enamel reduction. The management of IPR is fundamental not only for fixing crowding problems and finding more space but also to control the

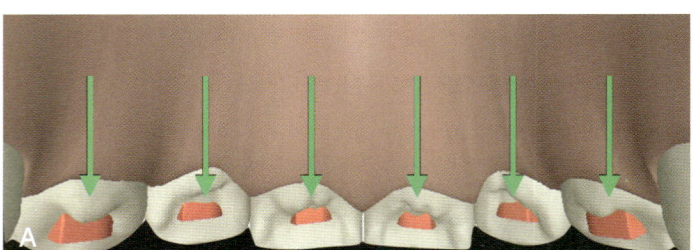

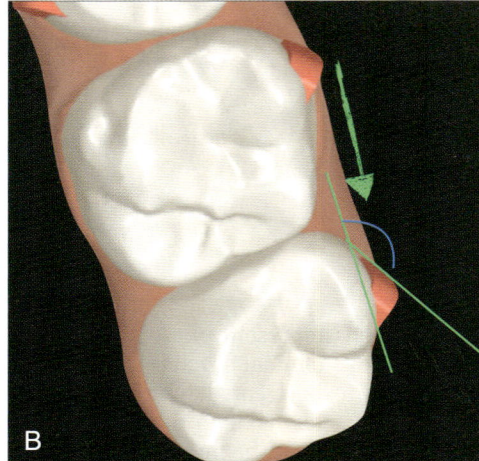

Fig. 6.1 Biomechanical design of conventional attachments for extrusion (A) and distal rotation (B)

incisor inclination (i.e., creating space with IPR could represent a reliable system to upright upper or lower incisors), to compensate Bolton discrepancy by reducing teeth excess, and to create symmetric dimension between left and right sides.[10]

Class I Conditions

Class I malocclusions can be divided into different categories following the principal condition that affects specifically one or more dimensions of the space (transverse or vertical) or which creates a determinate discrepancy. For this reason they will be discussed separately.

DENTOALVEOLAR DISCREPANCY

The most common condition is represented by crowding in the upper or lower arch or both. The clear aligner treatment (CAT) of crowding is highly predictable when approached with the proper staging such as expansion, small proclination, reduced IPR, and torque correction. Normally, being able to avoid extractions means that treatment options available are related to expansion (2 mm per quadrant) and IPR (0.3 mm maximum per interproximal space). The severity of crowding, particularly in the lower jaw, significantly affects the possibility of avoiding extraction treatment. Conditions in which it is reasonable to treat without extraction are as follows:

- Light crowding, with normal amount of IPR (0.1/0.2 mm)
- Mild to moderate crowding, with combination of expansion without changing intercanine width and maximum rate of 0.3 mm of IPR per interproximal space
- Moderately severe crowding, combining the 0.3-mm IPR per interproximal space with torque correction of lower premolars to create a positive torque up to a maximum of -3 degrees of buccal torque inclination

This means that when the crowding is lower than 4 mm per quadrant, the possibility to combine expansion and IPR could represent a reliable solution to recreate ideal alignment, but some options during the digital setup planning need to be controlled to avoid collateral effects, as follows:

- Avoid excessive proclination of lower incisors by means of using the superimposition tool and the grid tool of the software and by favoring transverse expansion and consequently a more uprighted position of lower incisors (Fig. 6.2).
- Place the lower premolars to a buccal crown torque next to zero to recreate space without changing the intercanine width (when on the occlusal picture of lower jaw, it is possible to observe the labial surface of premolars, torque correction could be achieved) (Fig. 6.3).
- Combine class III elastics to create the proper OVJ (1.2 mm) and to favor the correction of crowding also in absence of real class III relationship (Fig. 6.4).
- Create upper and lower jaw ideal shape to avoid black triangles and buccal facial corridors (Fig. 6.5).
- Plan specific attachments (see Chapter XXX) (Fig. 6.6).

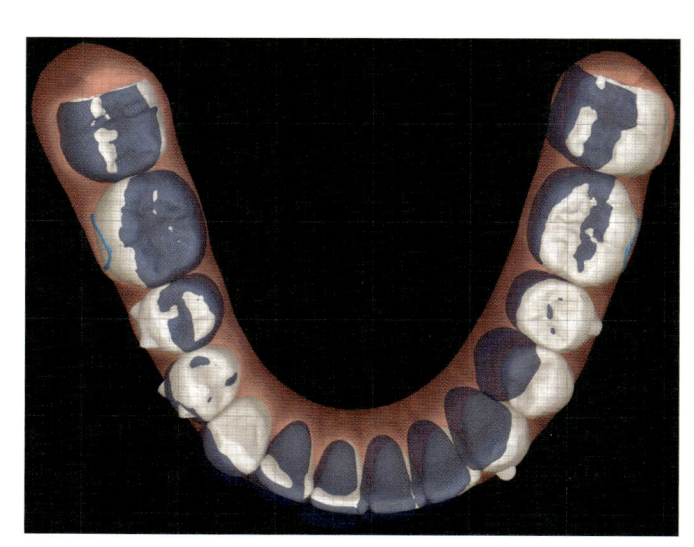

Fig. 6.2 ClinCheck tools to check incisor inclination.

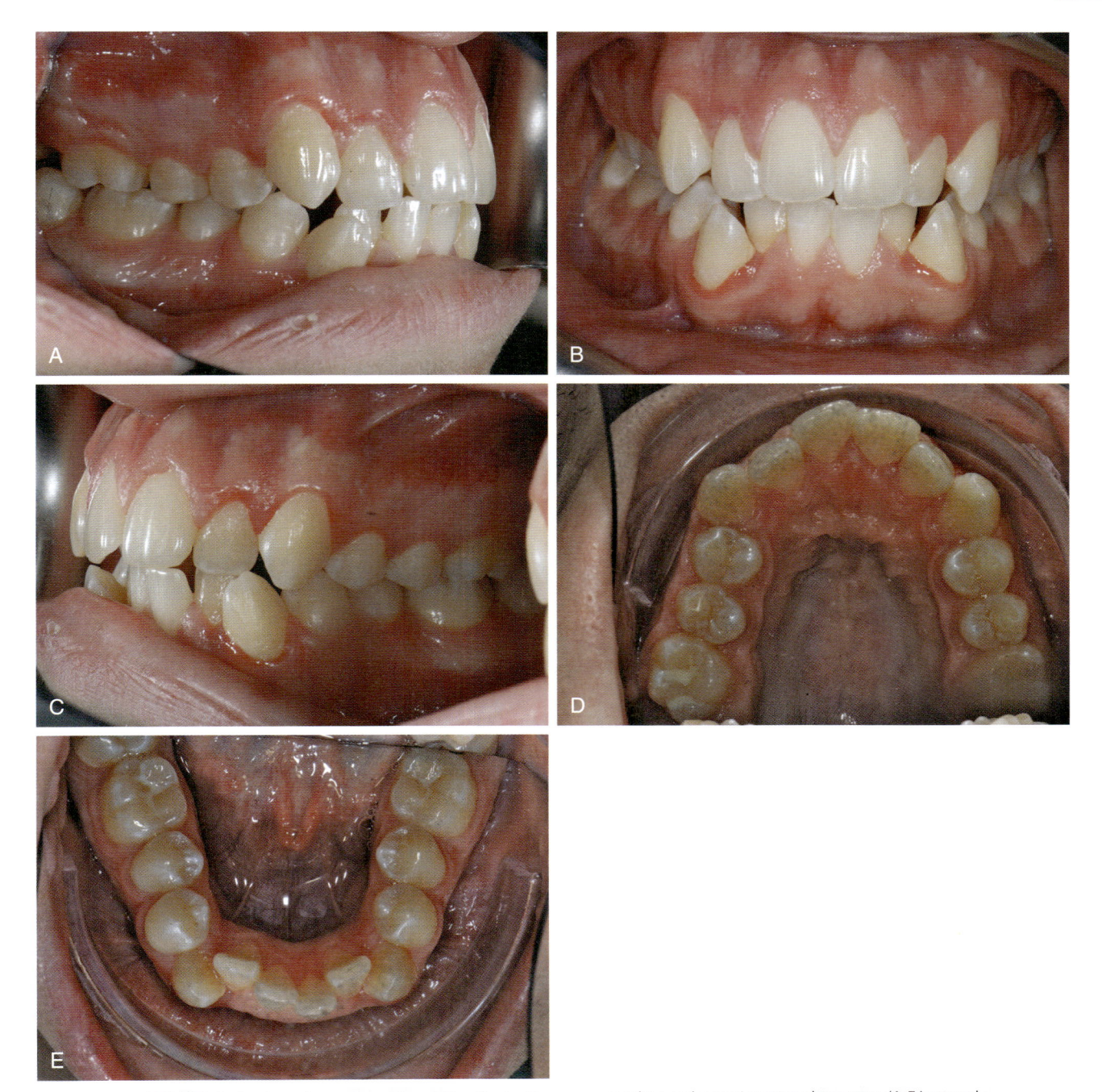

Fig. 6.3 Pretreatment records young adult patient with severe crowding and negative premolar torque. (A-E intraoral pictures)

TOOTH SIZE DISCREPANCY

The Bolton analysis is important because it allows the immediate visualization of the interarch and intraarch discrepancies. These discrepancies can affect the final overjet. Not considering the Bolton analysis in our treatment plans could lead to several unfavorable outcomes: anterior premature contacts with posterior open bite without reaching a proper class I intercuspation on both sides, excessive proclination of incisors, and uncorrected closure of upper diastemas. Therefore, the tooth size discrepancy analysis is crucial when designing orthodontic treatment. Othman and Harradine recommended a threshold of 2-mm discrepancy to be of clinical significance for restorative intervention (Figs. 6.7 and 6.8).[11-12]

Another common condition of tooth size discrepancy is represented by dental anomalies in number (bilateral or monolateral agenesis) and dental anomalies in shape (microdontia, peg-shaped lateral incisors). In the case of a monolateral agenesis in the anterior area (missing upper lateral incisor), the Bolton analysis can provide the precise dimension of the contralateral incisor helping the clinician in defining the right space that needs to be preserved for the final restoration. In case of peg-shaped contralateral incisor the Bolton analysis provides information regarding the

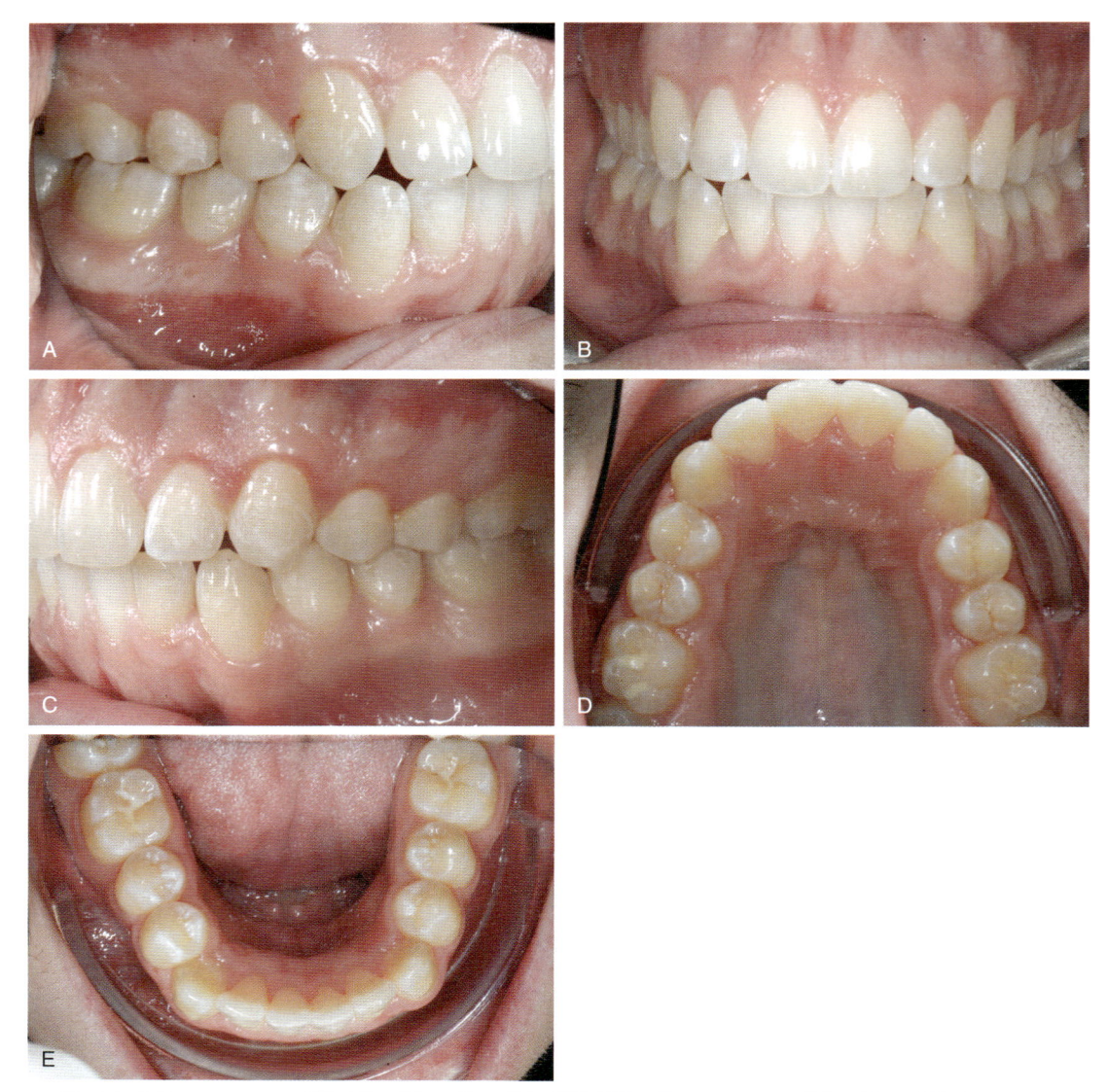

Fig. 6.4 Posttreatment records young adult patient with severe crowding and negative premolar torque treated with torque correction and interproximal reduction. (A-E intraoral pictures)

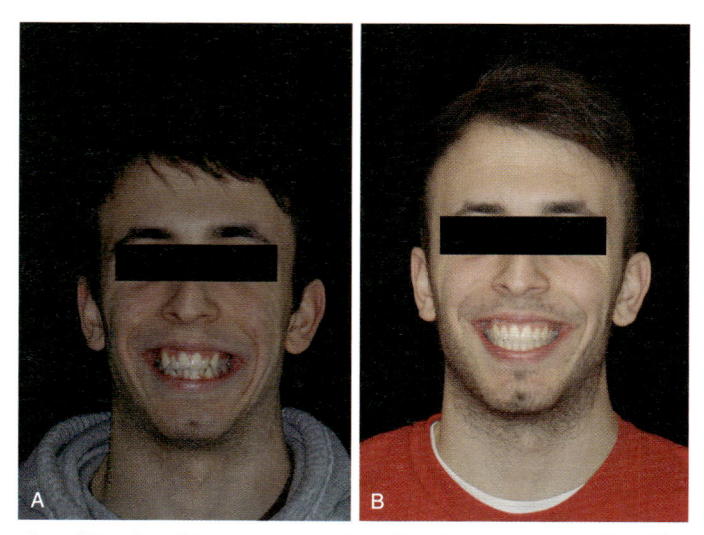

Fig. 6.5 (A) Pretreatment records young adult patient with narrow upper arch and smile black corridors. (B) Posttreatment records young adult patient with narrow upper arch and smile black corridors treated with upper expansion and lower torque correction.

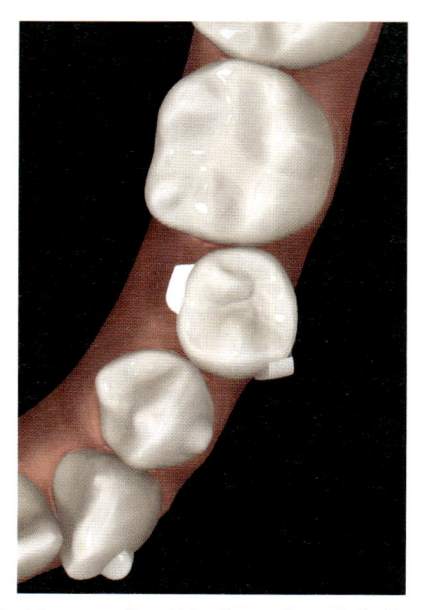

Fig. 6.6 Double conventional attachment in case of severe rotation.

6 • Class I Malocclusion   55

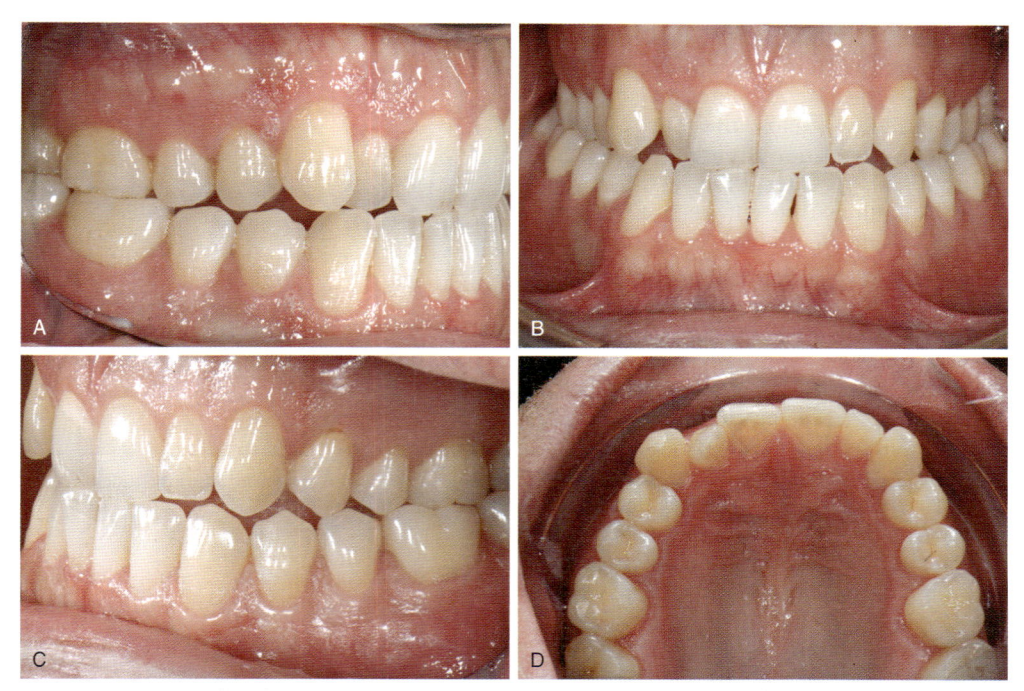

Fig. 6.7 Pretreatment records tooth size discrepancy A-D intraoral pictures.

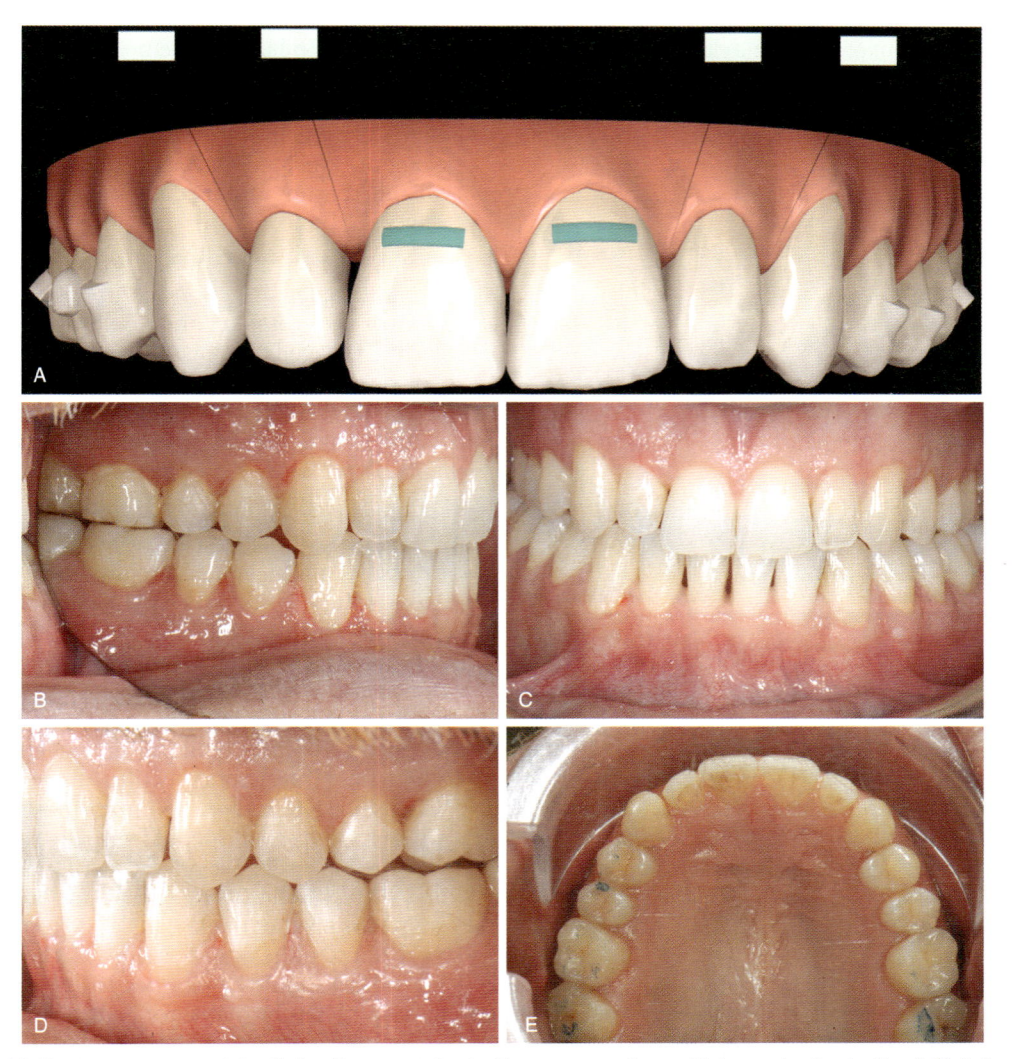

Fig. 6.8 Posttreatment records toothsize discrepancy treated by space opening and interproximal reduction A Digital project B-E intraoral pictures.

golden proportion between the anterior six teeth helping the clinician in determining the right space to be preserved for the final restorations. In the case of bilateral agenesis in which the treatment is designed to close the space of laterals with mesial movement of canines, premolars, and molars, the tooth size discrepancy values are fundamental to reduce the dimension of canines that will become laterals and to increase the dimension of premolars that will become canines.[13-15]

TRANSVERSE DISCREPANCY

One of the most duplex conditions to be treated with aligners is represented by the transverse discrepancy; the term *duplex* refers to the different complexity in the treatment of anterior crossbite and posterior crossbite, since anterior crossbite represents an elective condition to be treated with aligners while the posterior relies its possibility to be successful on the severity of posterior crossbite and on the use of supporting auxiliary devices (cross elastics) (Fig. 6.9).

The anterior crossbite (central, lateral, or canine) in bilateral or monolateral configuration is a perfect condition to be approached with Invisalign aligners since the thickness of the aligner itself avoids any need of bite turbos to create disclusion, a condition needed during traditional fixed orthodontics. For this reason, the treatment of one single element of anterior crossbite could be predictably fixed with a lite lite is the commercial name of Invisalign with reduced number of aligners. For this reason is not light but lite. Treatment if the rest of

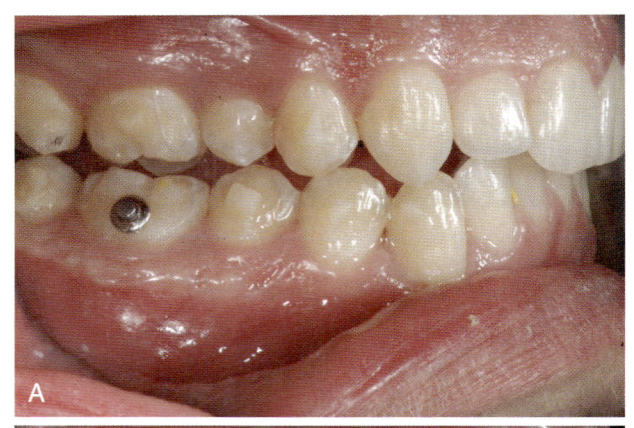

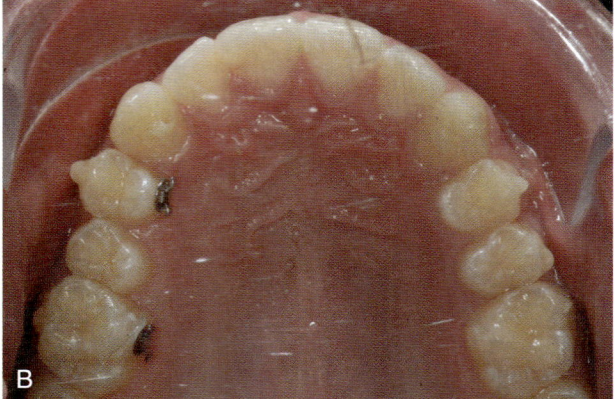

Fig. 6.9 Cross (A-B intraoral pictures) elastics to support posterior expansion.

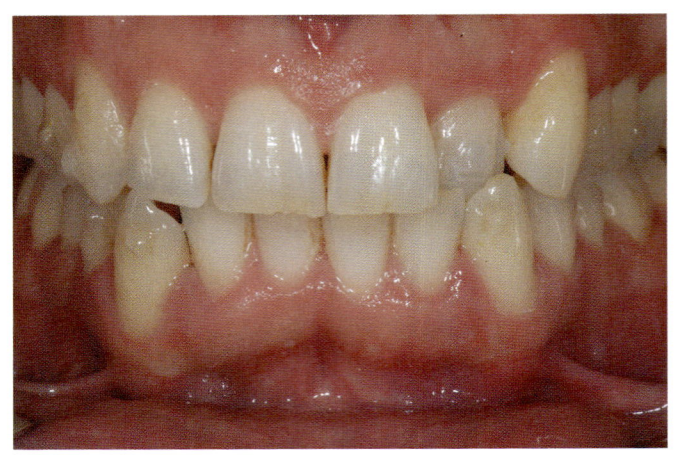

Fig. 6.10 Anterior contact during buccal movement for crossbite resolution.

malocclusion conditions permits this simplified approach. The following should be done to increase predictable results:

- During treatment the buccal movement of laterals or centrals will create an edge-to-edge contact; to overcome this traumatic contact, it may be convenient to change aligners more rapidly to reduce the time exposed to trauma (Fig. 6.10).
- Together with labial movement to fix the crossbite, some millimeters of extrusion should be planned to create normal overbite.
- Generally, in case of anterior crossbite, the apex of the element is located more buccal compared to the crown; for this reason, unparticular root movement is required (Figs. 6.11 and 6.12).

The correction of posterior crossbite represents a variable, predictable correction with aligners according to the severity of the crossbite; one single element crossbite could be easily managed only by the system, while for the correction of severe maxillary contraction with multiple elements in crossbite the use of auxiliaries is widely suggested. In particular, these indications should be followed to create a reliable correction:

- In case of single element crossbite, more crown torque should be planned instead of buccal expansion.
- In case of multielement crossbite, buttons for crisscross elastics should be planned to help the correction and support the elastic modification of the aligners by using direct bonding on the teeth and cooperation with 12 hours of elastics (6 oz, 4 mm).
- To simplify the correction, some minimal IPR in the interproximal spaces could be helpful only to remove possible initial interferences while starting the expansion.
- The use of bite ramps even in the absence of deep bite is strongly suggested. It could simplify the posterior movement creating disclusion, favoring the buccal movement and the vertical extrusion moment in combination with crisscross elastics (Figs. 6.13 and 6.14).
- According to the malocclusion, further elastics for sagittal control should be planned (class II or III) (Fig. 6.15).
- In case of severe maxillary contraction, a crown torque inclination assessment should be done to understand the amount of possible correction only with dental expansion.

6 • Class I Malocclusion 57

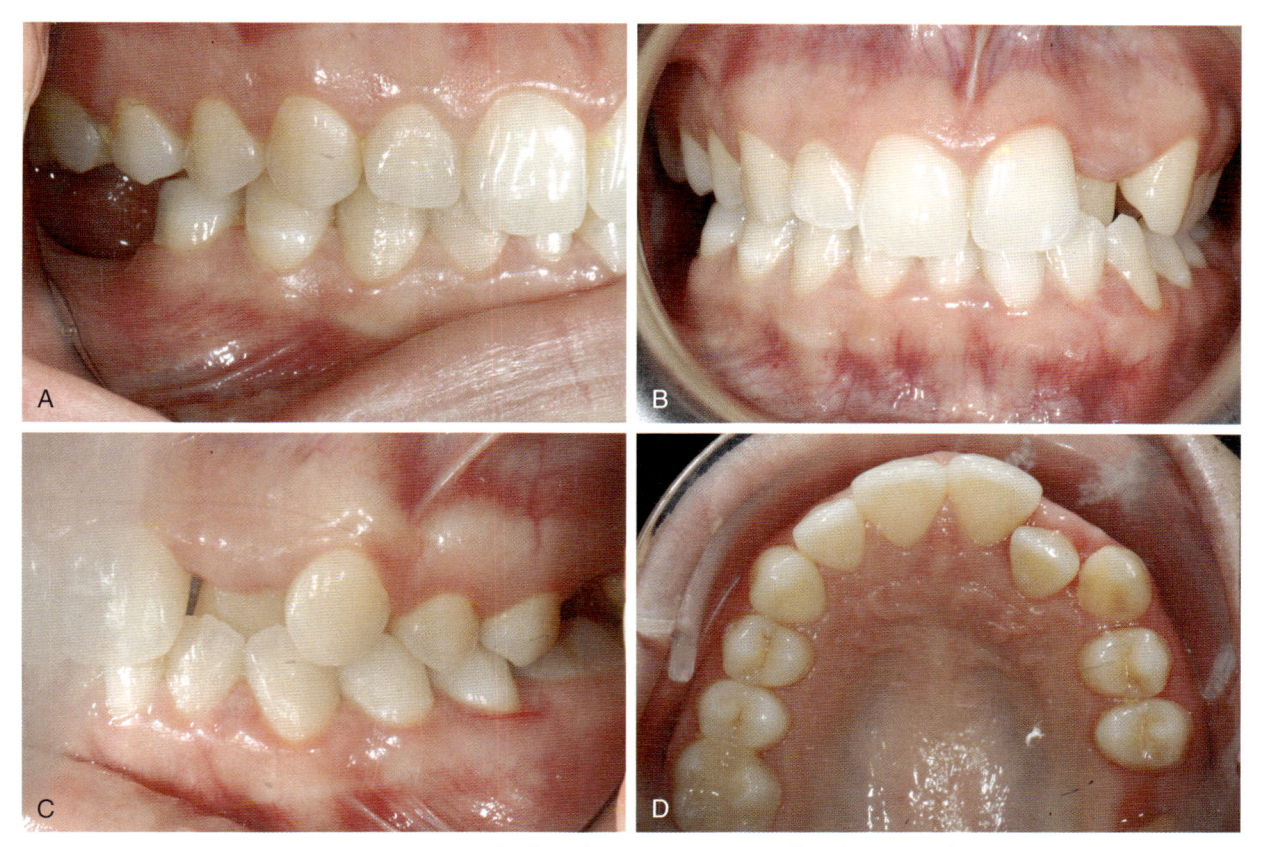

Fig. 6.11 Pretreatment records of lateral incisor in anterior crossbite. A-D intraoral pictures

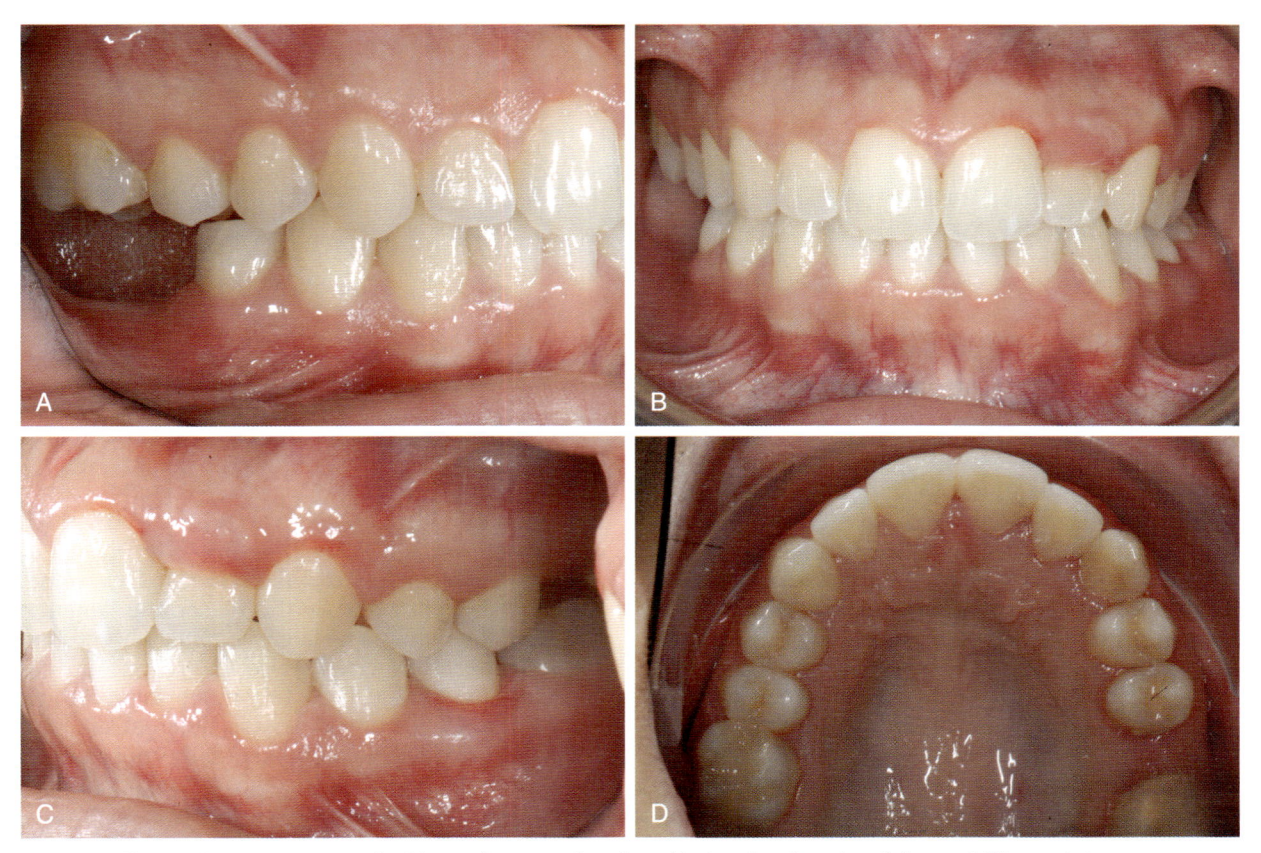

Fig. 6.12 Posttreatment records with complete correction of crossbite in reduced number of aligners. A-B intraoral pictures

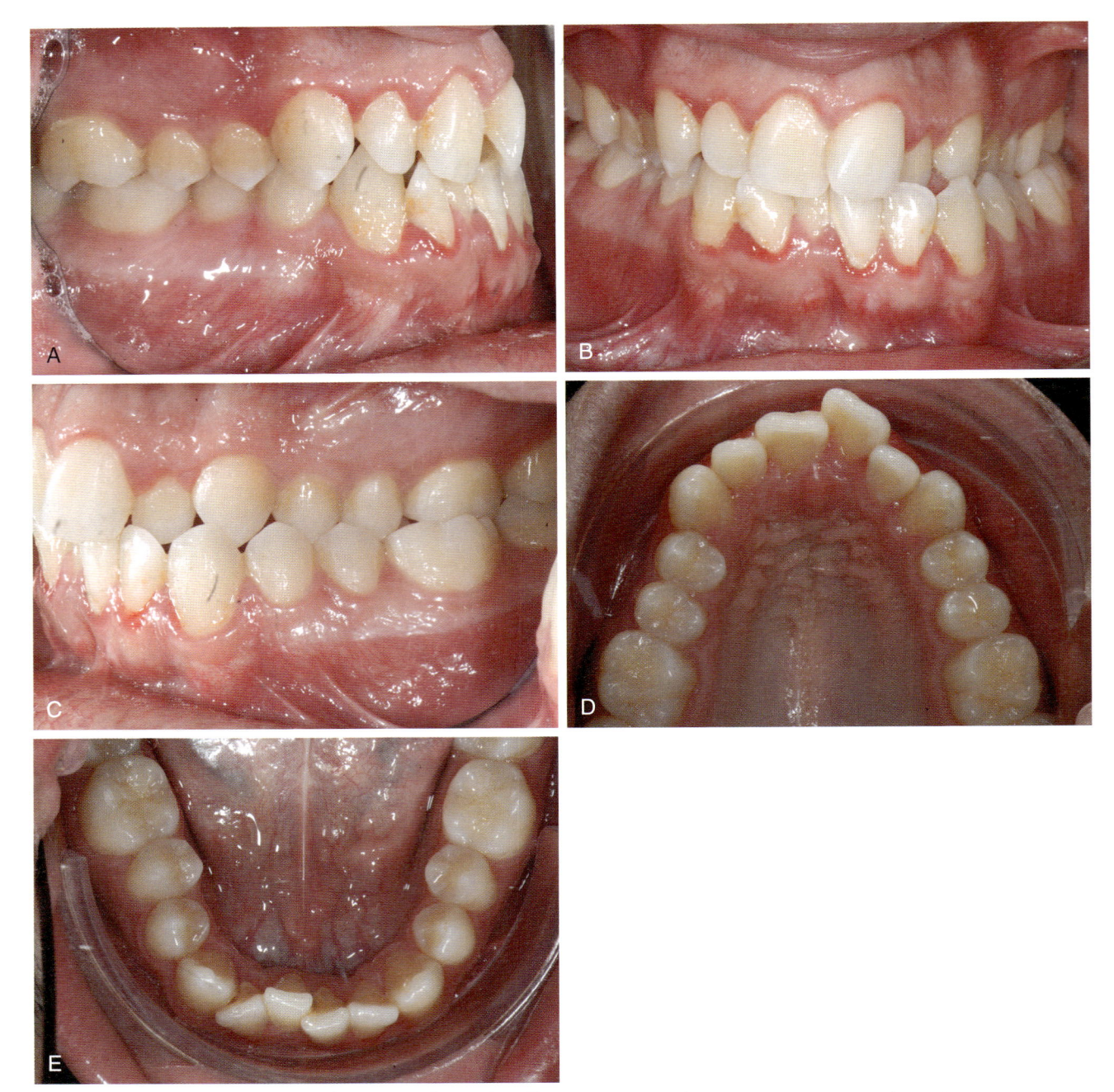

Fig. 6.13 Pretreatment records of severe posterior crossbite with maxillary contraction. A-E intraoral pictures

The predictable plan for posterior crossbite is basically focused on expansion up to 2.5/3 mm per quadrant. If the crown torque of lateral elements and the periodontal condition could allow this kind of correction, the combined use of bite ramps and crisscross elastics could predictably increase the outcome achievement.

MORPHOLOGIC DISCREPANCY

Less common conditions of class I malocclusions are represented by those situations of teeth with morphologic anomalies, such as single or multiple anterior agenesis and microdontia (conoid laterals), that affect the orthodontic treatment and ideal outcome according to the therapeutic choice.

All morphologic discrepancies are strictly connected to Bolton discrepancy, and for this reason the same approach described later should be followed to achieve proper occlusal outcome and normal overjet. Moreover, an important consideration should be done on the microesthetics and macroesthetics when teeth show a different shape.

In the case of monolateral dental morphologic anomaly (conoid or agenesis), it becomes necessary to leave the proper space to concentrate on the opposite normal shape element dimension. The Bolton button could provide information about teeth size, and on the ClinCheck it is possible

6 • Class I Malocclusion 59

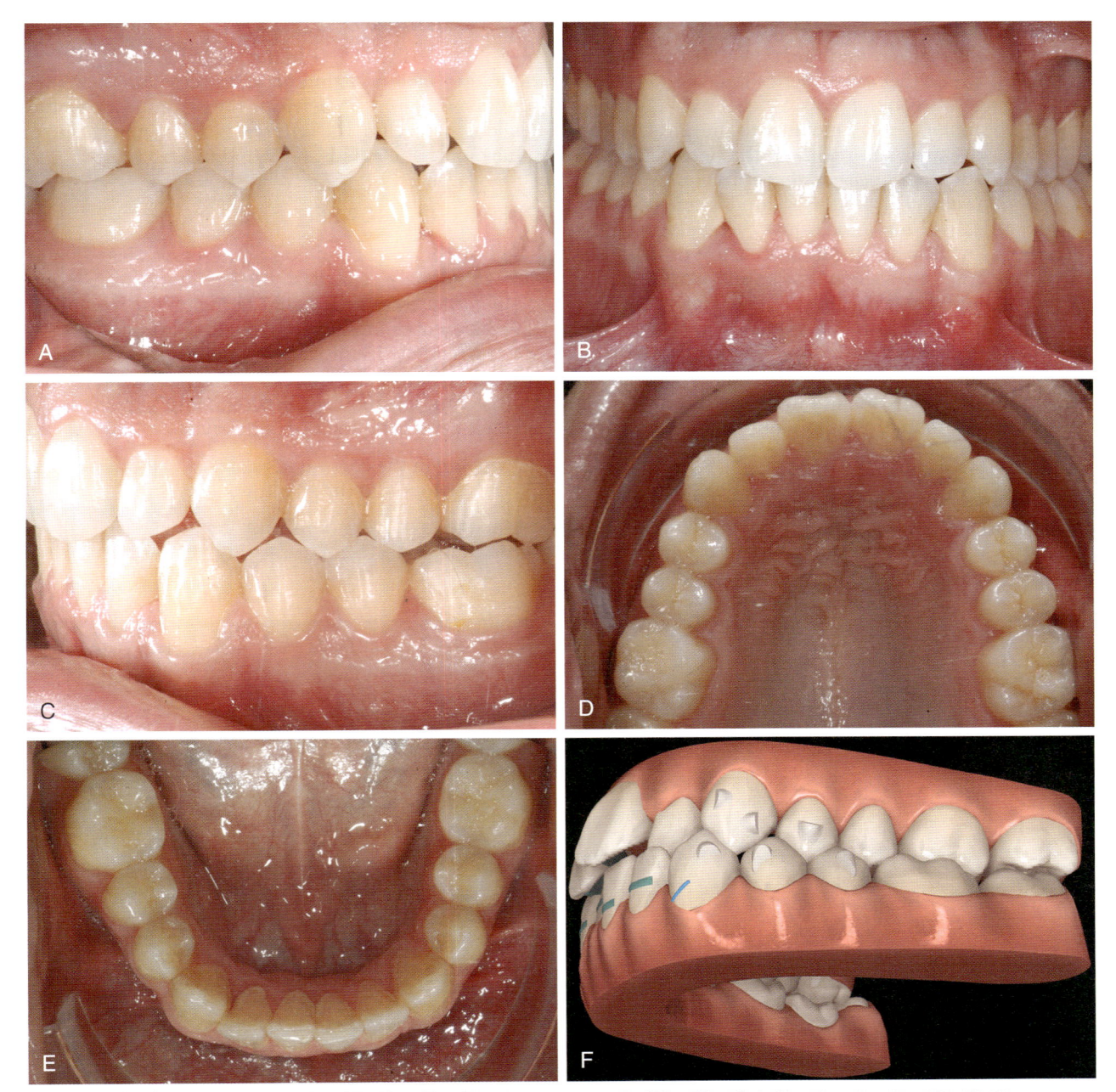

Fig. 6.14 Posttreatment records after expansion + torque correction + interproximal reduction + bite ramps. A-E intraoral pictures F Digital setup showing bite ramps for posterior disocclusion.

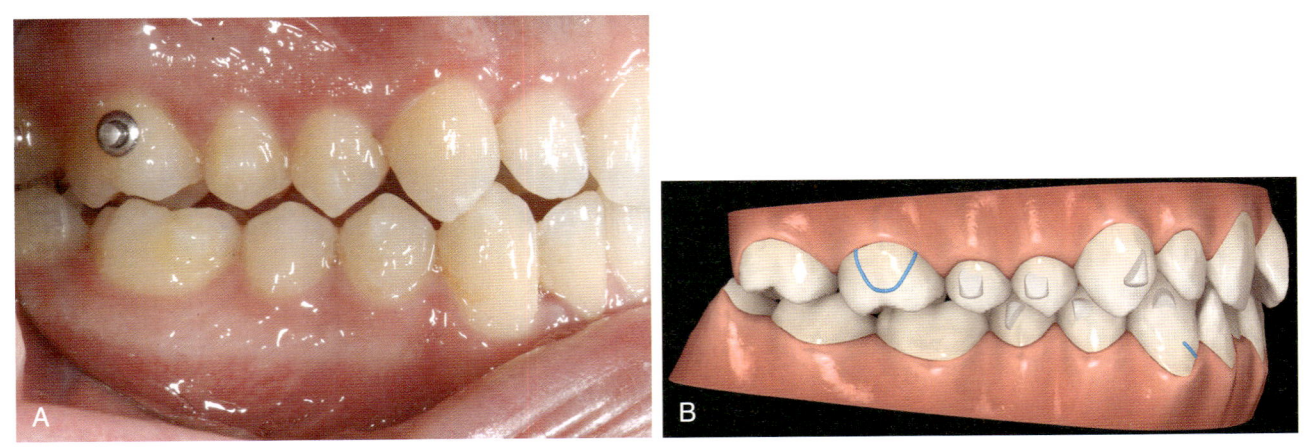

Fig. 6.15 Class III elastics. A- intraoral pictures B Digital Setup

to plan space opening mesial and distal to the conoid element to organize the final restoration (Fig. 6.16). In case of single agenesis, one further assessment should be done concerning the space between the roots. Since the final restoration will be an implant, it is fundamental to measure the space between the apexes to realize if the outcome could be achieved only with aligners or some auxiliaries will be needed. When the apical distance is around 5 mm, no other special auxiliaries will be needed, just the space opening between crowns, while when the distance is less than 5 mm, some auxiliaries (lingual sectional or power arm) could be necessary to achieve the proper space for implant insertion (Figs. 6.17 and 6.18).

In the case of agenesis of both lateral incisors, the choice of space closure with total mesial movement of posterior teeth or space opening for implant insertion has long been discussed in the literature.[12-13] Actually, in case of young patients, the ideal solution seems to be the space closure with reshaping of the canines (both additive and subtractive enamel plastic) to simulate laterals combined with reshaping of first premolars simulating canines (additive enamel plastic). The advantages of approaching with aligners are the possibility to have all the information about size of the teeth (Bolton tool), balancing IPR on canines and space opening on first premolars to create ideal anterior relationship between the six anterior teeth combined with leveling the anterior gingival margins to create a harmonic smile (Figs. 6.19 and 6.20).

PREPROSTHETIC NEED

The last common condition analyzed of class I malocclusion is strongly related to those situations in which the orthodontic treatment could be helpful in creating more favorable conditions for prosthetic solution, thus gaining space where it was missing for final restoration. Being very schematic, two conditions in adult patients with missing teeth commonly require the orthodontic support to achieve an ideal prosthetic solution, namely:

1. Tipping in the edentulous space
2. Overeruption in the edentulous space

The mesial tipping of molars, in particular the tipping of second molars because of missing first molar, represents a

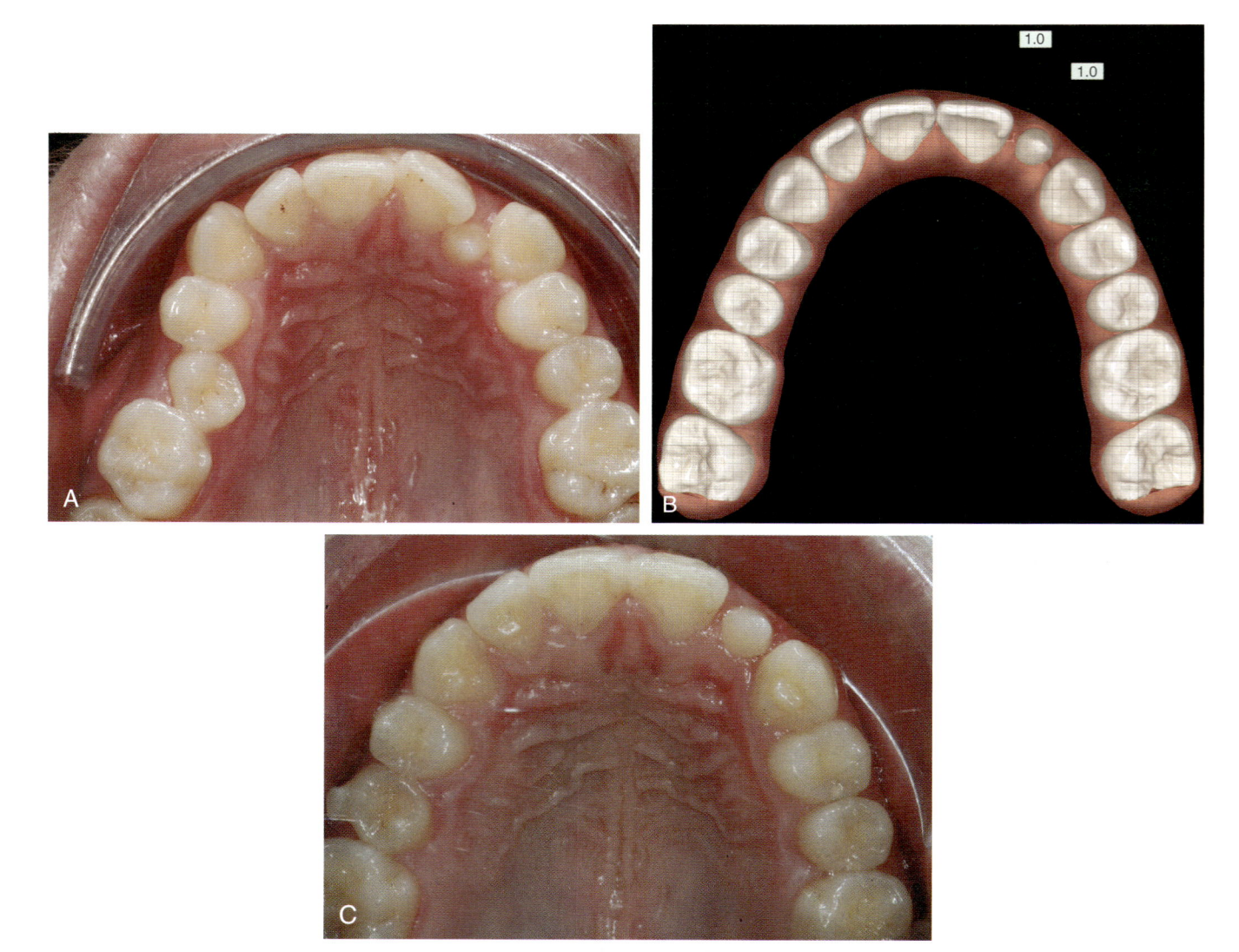

Fig. 6.16 Space opening for Peg shaped restoration. A pre-treatment B digital plan C post treatment

6 • Class I Malocclusion   61

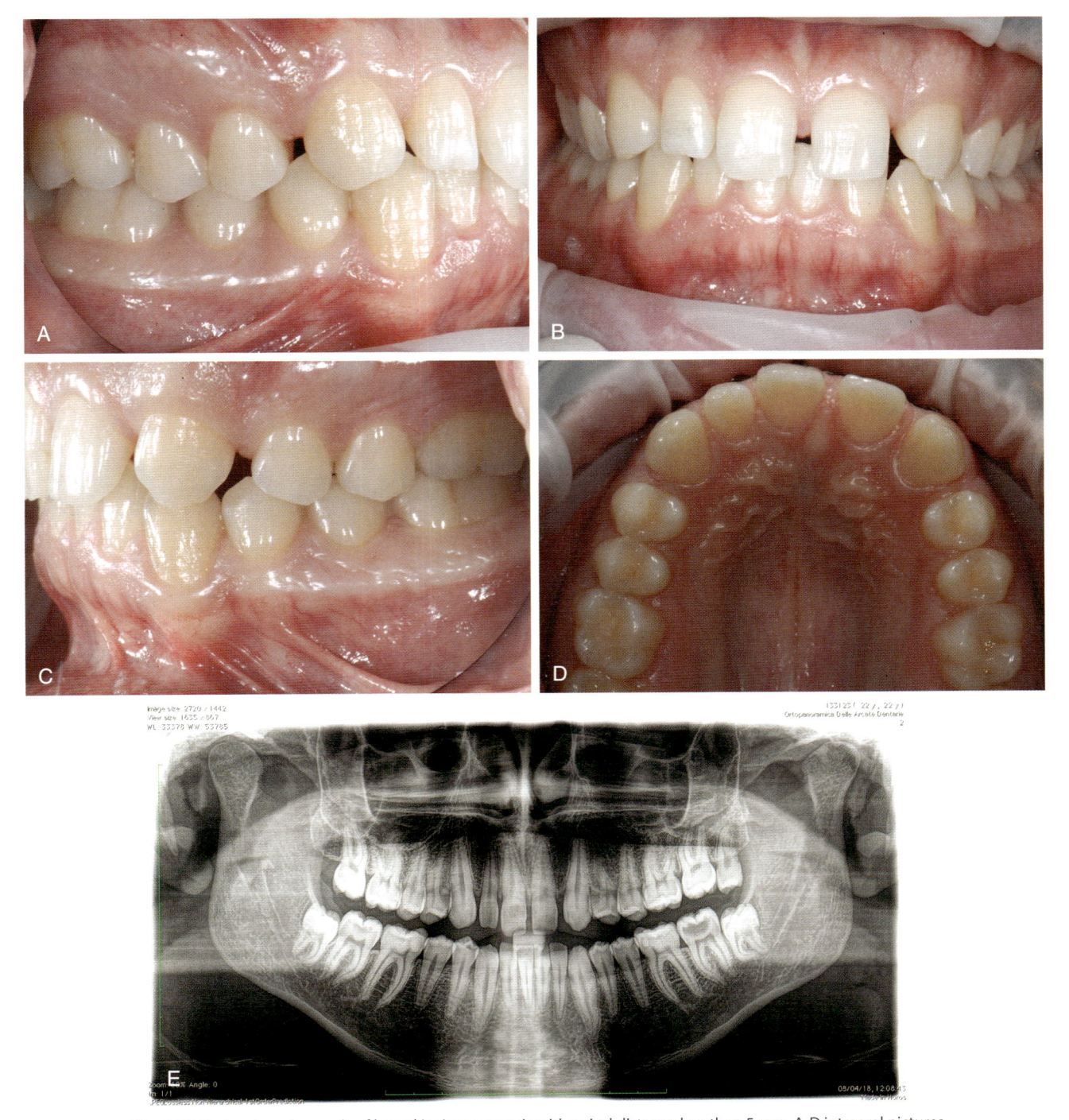

Fig. 6.17 Pretreatment records of lateral incisor agenesis with apical distance less than 5 mm. A-D intraoral pictures E panoramic x-ray

frequent condition sometimes combined with distal tipping of premolars.[16-17] Approaching this problem with the aligners is highly predictable because of the following:

- The force to upright the second molar creates a reaction force, which upright the premolars and this reciprocal force work properly together in opening the space (Fig. 6.21).
- The amount of space can be decided in advance on the software according to the dimension of the contralateral element.
- To be more efficient, it is possible to ask to avoid pontics in the edentulous area to leave the aligner to embrace more surfaces of the molar to upright delivering more homogeneous force.
- In the ClinCheck plan it is fundamental to combine distal inclination of crown with distal movement to put the center of rotation next to the apex.

For the same reason when one or more teeth are missing, the problem could happen in another dimension of the

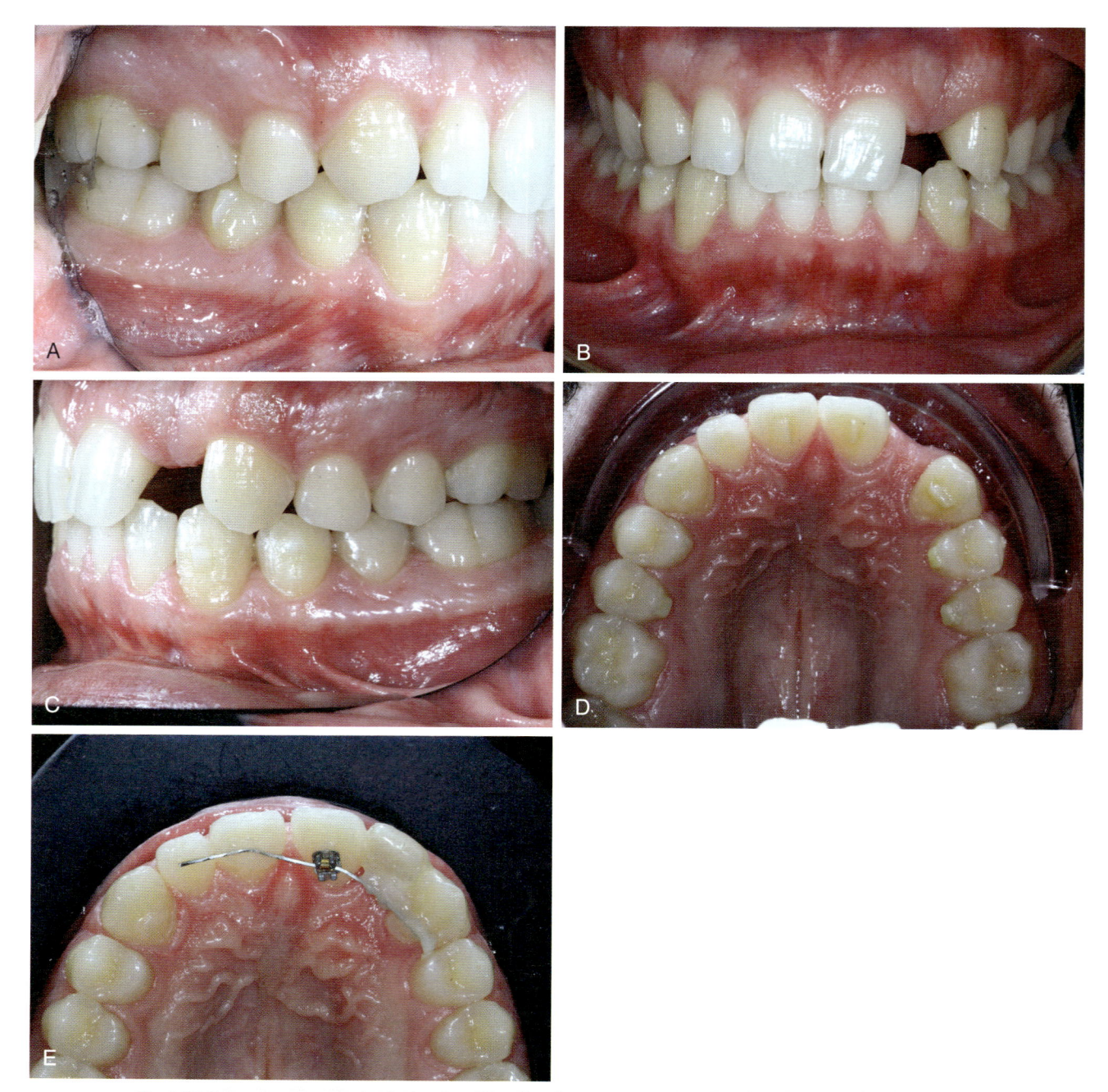

Fig. 6.18 Posttreatment records of monolateral, lateral incisor agenesis with Invisalign and fixed sectional for root control. A-E intraoral pictures

space affecting the vertical movement (overeruption) of molars.

Approaching this problem with traditional orthodontics means that an auxiliary device for skeletal anchorage in the bone will be strongly needed. The traditional biomechanics to intrude molars are highly complex for anchorage lack.[18-19] The opportunity to solve the overeruption with aligners simplifies the treatment because the vertical force of intrusion is applied to the teeth by means of labial, lingual, occlusal, and distal surface (not only on side), and it generates a reaction force that tends to extrude the adjacent tooth blocked by the occlusion and the thickness of aligners. This biomechanical system is more in balance when compared to traditional, and if no other movements in different planes are required, it can be accomplished in reduced number of aligners (Figs. 6.22 and 6.23).

6 • Class I Malocclusion   63

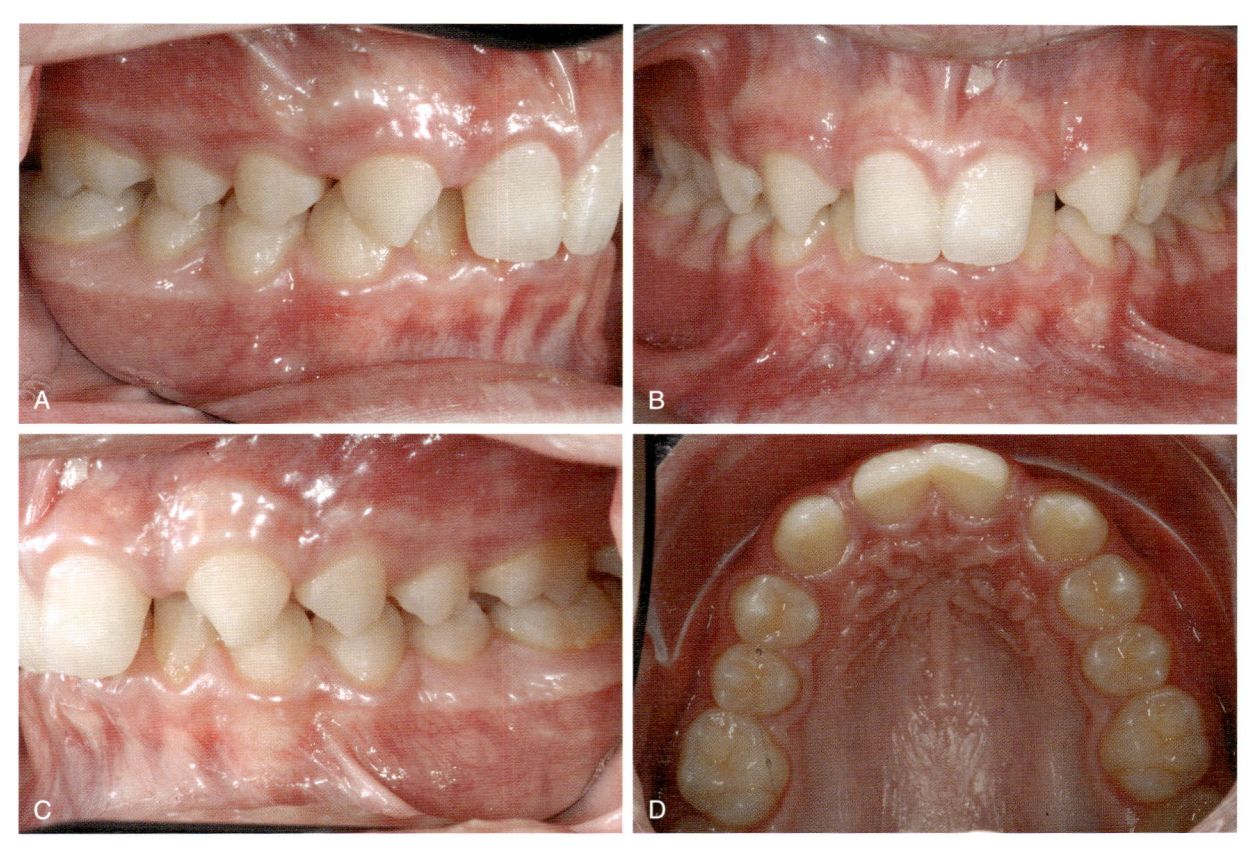

Fig. 6.19 Pretreatment records of bilateral, lateral incisors agenesis. A-D intraoral pictures

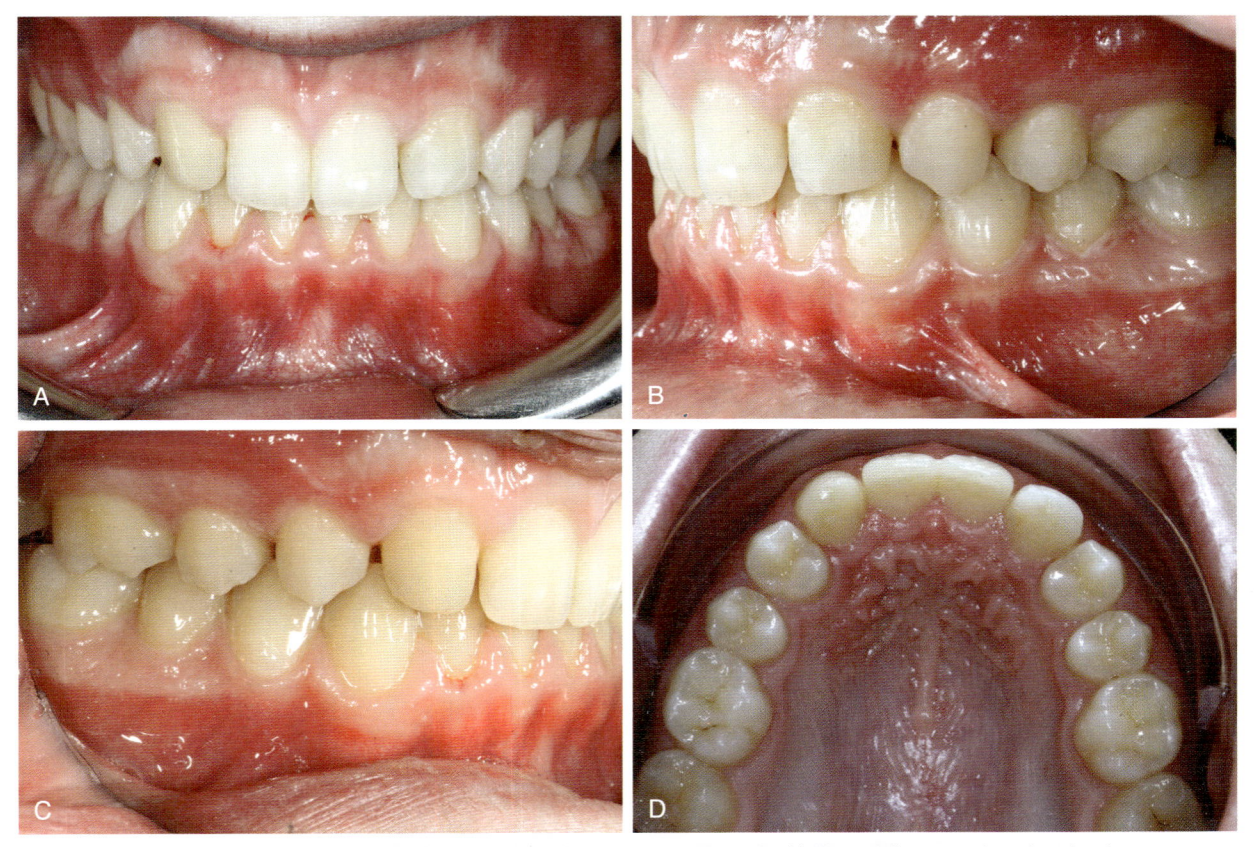

Fig. 6.20 Posttreatment records of bilateral, lateral incisors agenesis treated by space closure and teeth reshaping. A-D intraoral pictures

64 Principles and Biomechanics of Aligner Treatment

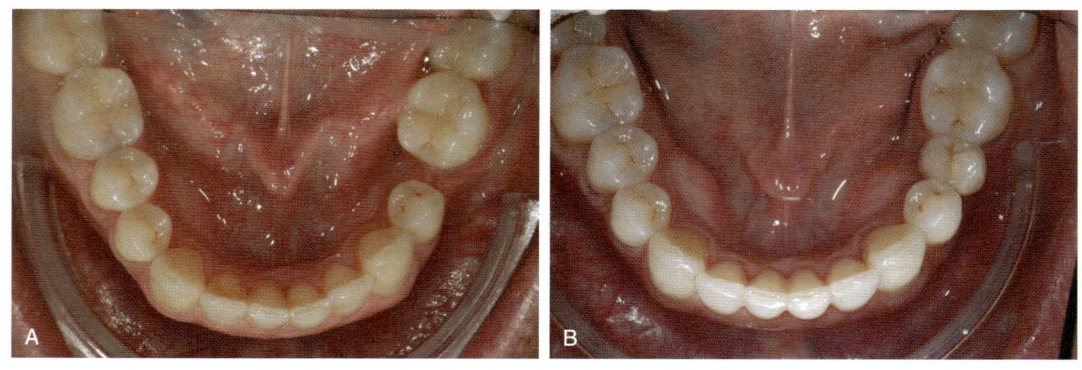

Fig. 6.21 Space opening by distal tipping of molars. A pre-treatment intraoral picture B post-treatment intraoral picture with implant inserted

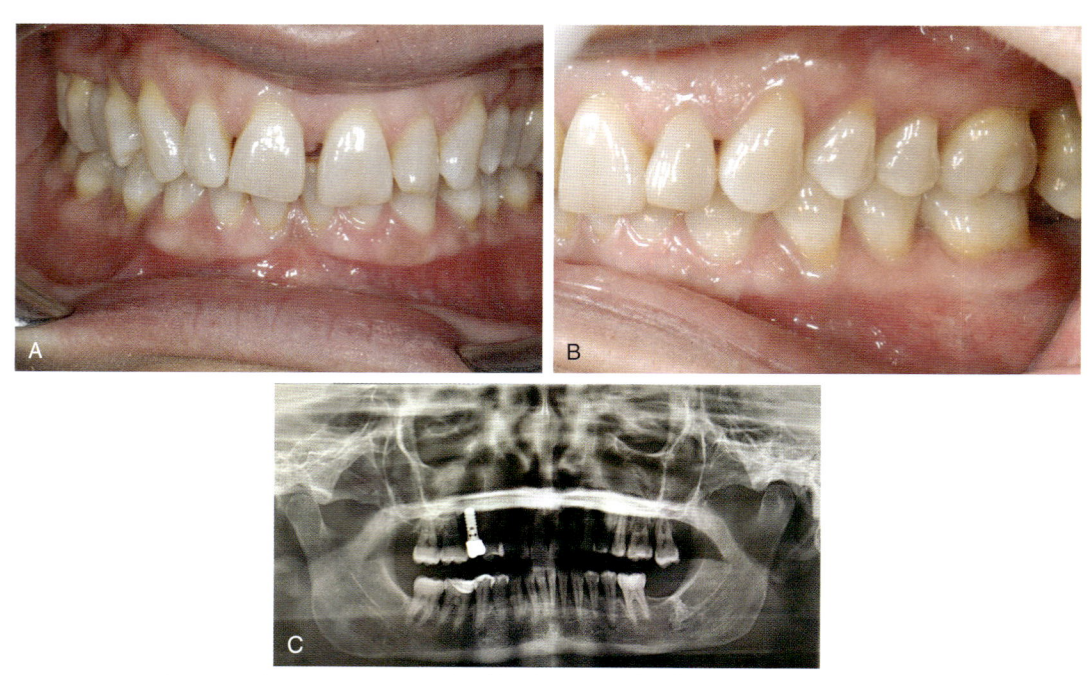

Fig. 6.22 Pretreatment records of overerupted upper second molar. A-B intraoral pictures C panoramic x-ray

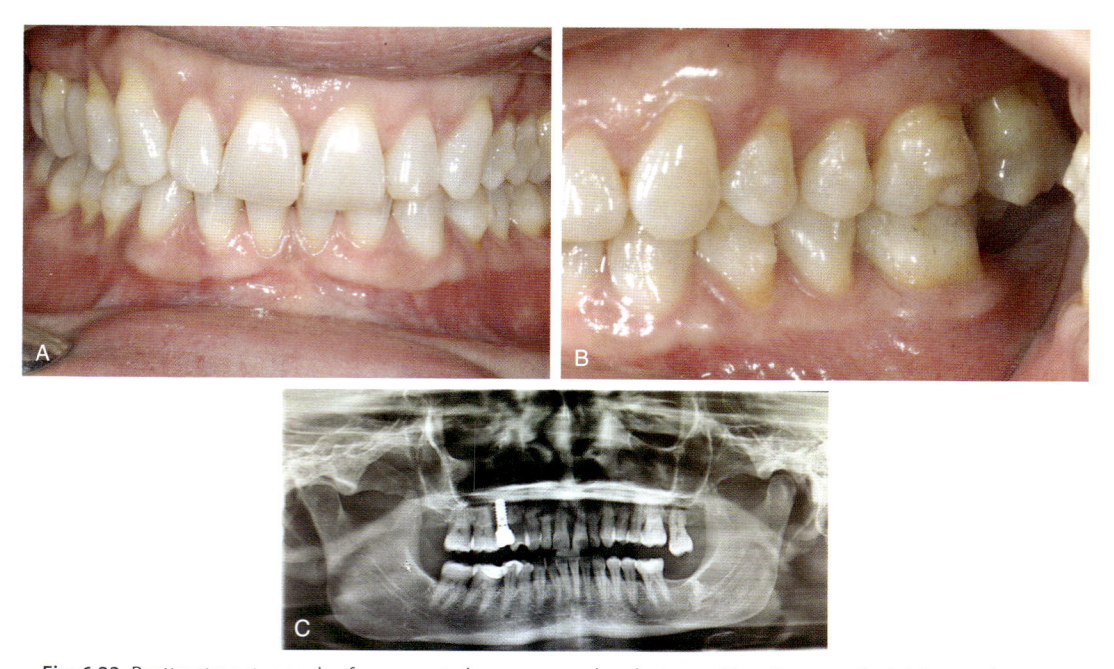

Fig. 6.23 Posttreatment records of overerupted upper second molar treated by aligners only. A-B intraoral picture C panoramic x-ray

References

1. Rossini G, Parrini S, Castroflorio T, et al. Efficacy of clear aligners in controlling orthodontic tooth movement: a systematic review. *Angle Orthod*. 2015;85(5):881-889.
2. Sachdeva R. Integrating digital and robot technologies: diagnosis, treatment planning, and therapeutics. In Graber ML, Vanarsdall RL, Vig, KWL, eds. *Orthodontics Current Principles and Techniques*. 5th ed. Elsevier; 2011.
3. Scholz RP, Sachdeva RC. Interview with an innovator: SureSmile chief clinical officer Rohit C. L. Sachdeva. *Am J Orthod Dentofacial Orthop*. 2010;138(2):231-238.
4. Simon M, Keilig L, Schwarze J, et al. Treatment outcome and efficacy of an aligner technique—regarding incisor torque, premolar derotation and molar distalization. *BMC Oral Health*. 2014;14:68.
5. Veli I, Ozturk MA, Uysal T. Curve of Spee and its relationship to vertical eruption of teeth among different malocclusion groups. *Am J Orthod Dentofacial Orthop*. 2015;147(3):305-312.
6. Tepedino M, Franchi L, Fabbro O, et al. Post-orthodontic lower incisor inclination and gingival recession—a systematic review. *Prog Orthod*. 2018;19(1):17.
7. Papadimitriou A, Mousoulea S, Gkantidis N, et al. Clinical effectiveness of Invisalign® orthodontic treatment: a systematic review. *Prog Orthod*. 2018;19(1):37.
8. Simon M, Keilig L, Schwarze J, et al. Forces and moments generated by removable thermoplastic aligners: incisor torque, premolar derotation, and molar distalization. *Am J Orthod Dentofacial Orthop*. 2014;145(6):728-736.
9. Kravitz ND, Kusnoto B, Agran B, et al. Influence of attachments and interproximal reduction on the accuracy of canine rotation with Invisalign. A prospective clinical study. *Angle Orthod*. 2008;78(4):682-687.
10. Meredith L, Farella M, Lowrey S, et al. Atomic force microscopy analysis of enamel nanotopography after interproximal reduction. *Am J Orthod Dentofacial Orthop*. 2017;151(4):750-757.
11. Othman SA, Harradine NW. Tooth-size discrepancy and Bolton's ratios: the reproducibility and speed of two methods of measurement. *J Orthod*. 2007;34(4):234-242.
12. Cançado RH, Gonçalves Júnior W, Valarelli FP, et al. Association between Bolton discrepancy and angle malocclusions. *Braz Oral Res*. 2015;29:1-6.
13. Rosa M, Zachrisson BU. Integrating space closure and esthetic dentistry in patients with missing maxillary lateral incisors. *J Clin Orthod*. 2007;41(9):563-573.
14. Rosa M, Lucchi P, Ferrari S, et al. Congenitally missing maxillary lateral incisors: long-term periodontal and functional evaluation after orthodontic space closure with first premolar intrusion and canine extrusion. *Am J Orthod Dentofacial Orthop*. 2016;149(3):339-348.
15. Jamilian A, Perillo L, Rosa M. Missing upper incisors: a retrospective study of orthodontic space closure versus implant. *Prog Orthod*. 2015;16:2.
16. Giancotti A, Farina A. Treatment of collapsed arches using the Invisalign system. *J Clin Orthod*. 2010;44(7):416-425.
17. Mampieri G, Giancotti A. Invisalign technique in the treatment of adults with pre-restorative concerns. *Prog Orthod*. 2013;14:40.
18. Arslan A, Ozdemir DN, Gursoy-Mert H, et al. Intrusion of an over-erupted mandibular molar using mini-screws and mini-implants: a case report. *Aust Dent J*. 2010;55(4):457-461.
19. Tripathi T, Kalra S, Rai P, et al. True intrusion of maxillary first molars with zygomatic and palatal miniscrew anchorage: a case report. *Aust Orthod J*. 2016;32(2):233-240.

7 Aligner Treatment in Class II Malocclusion Patients

TOMMASO CASTROFLORIO, WADDAH SABOUNI, SERENA RAVERA, and FRANCESCO GARINO

Introduction

Since the introduction of clear aligner treatment (CAT), controversy has existed over whether moderate to difficult orthodontic treatment can be routinely accomplished with aligner technique.[1] When dealing with class II malocclusions, CAT offers different possible therapeutic options:

1. Distalization
2. Molar derotation
3. Elastic jump
4. Extractions
5. Mandibular advancement
6. Orthognathic surgery

MAXILLARY MOLAR DISTALIZATION

In some nonextraction cases, maxillary molar distalization is the method of choice to gain 2 to 3 mm of space in the dental arch to obtain a class I relationship[2] in both teens and adults.

The upper molars can be distalized by means of extraoral or intraoral forces.[3] Extraoral traction with headgear has a long history of use in class II treatment since it has been designed to push distally the maxilla and the maxillary molars.[4,5] In recent years, several techniques have been developed to reduce the dependence on patient compliance, such as intraoral appliances with and without skeletal anchorage. However, even these devices can produce undesirable tipping of the maxillary molars and/or loss of anterior anchorage during distalization.[6,7] To achieve a tooth bodily movement implies that the applied force must pass through the center of resistance of the tooth or a sophisticated equivalent system of forces and moments needs to be applied to the tooth crown.[8] A recent review of the existing literature[9] assessed the efficacy of aligners in aligning and straightening the arches, with better results for mild to moderate crowding when compared to the results obtained with fixed appliances. More recently, it was stated that the overall available evidence regarding orthodontic tooth movement (OTM) control during CAT increased significantly, with three randomized controlled trials (RCTs) at grade A and an overall quality of evidence of moderate/high level, and that maxillary molar distalization of 2.5 mm and premolar extraction space closure (7 mm) are the most predictable and controlled movements with CAT.[10]

In 2014, Simon et al.[11] stated that maxillary molar distalization was the most predictable movement (88%) to perform with CAT. The authors started to focus on the key role of a correct staging of the planned movement and of the adoption of proper attachments during the whole distalization phase. Thus a highly significant element of bias in the 2012 study by Drake et al.[12] was the staging of 0.5 mm per aligner instead of the 0.25 mm recommended. In 2016, Ravera et al.[13] confirmed the results of Simon et al.[14] and demonstrated that distalization is efficiently achievable up to 2.5 mm on the first and second maxillary molars, with optimal vertical control of posterior teeth and any loss of anchorage on the anterior teeth. These results were obtained through the combination of staging, vertical rectangular attachments, and class II elastics (0.25–4.5 oz) for anchorage reinforcement.[15] The use of attachments and elastics was previously described by expert clinicians.[15] The application of composite attachments could be useful to improve the biomechanic efficiency of aligner therapy. Long vertical attachments located on the buccal aspect of the molars can create a sufficient moment to oppose the tipping movement.[16] Thus long vertical attachments can provide good tipping control while molars are moving and then can increase posterior anchorage while retracting anterior teeth.

The need for a determined attachment combination was confirmed in a 2016 RCT by Garino et al.,[17] who observed significant differences in the amount of distalization when comparing a five-attachment configuration (second and first molars, second and first premolars, and canine) with a three-attachment configuration (first molar, second and first premolars), with the first ones being most efficient. Controlling the tipping movement during molar distalization can be difficult because of the limited aligner-tooth surface in the direction of force application. The absence of long rectangular attachments on the second molar resulted in a probable loss of anchorage during the distalization of the first molar, with consequent reduced amount of distal movement of the second molar at the end of the treatment and significant tipping of the first molar. Furthermore, the absence of a proper anchorage preparation in the distal portion reduced the possibility of an adequate control of the retracting anterior teeth. As a result, the central incisors showed an uncontrolled tipping movement in the group with a three-attachment configuration.

Recently Gomez et al.[18] demonstrated that when the aligner segment was displaced distally without attachments, a clockwise moment and distal inclination were produced on the upper canine. The presence of composite attachments helped counteract this inclination, producing a countermoment that in turn favored a bodily movement. In another finite element analysis study, Comba et al.[19] demonstrated that the use of attachments on tooth surface counteracts the uncontrolled tipping during distalization through the generation of a countermoment that ends in the root uprighting. This moment is dependent from a complex force system and is generated by the active surfaces of attachments. When analyzing a couple of attachments located on the buccal surface of an upper canine, one located at the distocervical portion and the other located at the mesioincisal portion, compression areas were found on the mesial face of the cervical attachments and on the distal face of the incisal attachment. These outcomes validate Gomez findings.

The vertical pattern is an important point to consider while planning molar distalization. The distal movement measured in our study was associated with significant intrusion movements of the molars. The thickness of the aligners and the consequent occlusal force exerted on them might facilitate intrusion and explain the absence of any change of anterior vertical dimension while distalizing. Furthermore, Gomez et al.[18] reported a marked tendency of "flaring" of the buccal and palatal flanks of the aligner segment during distal displacement. This finding is interesting because it could suggest an intrusive effect on the tooth.

The aligner therapy is a customized orthodontic treatment for both the patient and the orthodontist. The presence of composite attachments for the control of the maxillary molars during the distalization process is a choice of the prescribing clinician for most of the available systems in the market.

MAXILLARY MOLAR ROTATION

Mesiopalatal rotation of the upper first molar is present in about 95% of patients with angle class II, division 1 malocclusion and in 83% of them as a whole.[15,16] Mesiopalatal rotation of upper first molars often ends up in an intraarch loss of space.[17] Frequently, this crowding occurs in the premolar and canine segments, thus potentially preventing the correct mesiodistal position of these teeth. On this basis, buccodistal rotation of maxillary molars can be considered a useful procedure to partially improve class II dental relationship. Molar rotation was indicated as one of the predictable movements controlled by aligners.[20]

THE ELASTIC EFFECT

The elastic effect can be defined as class II correction using interarch mechanics. It is simulated on virtual setups by a jumplike shift of the occlusion from class II to class I to allow easier visualization of the anticipated treatment goal. Individual tooth movements required to align teeth are set up to project the effect of this bite correction using buttons and elastics.

Elastic wear is recommended from the start of treatment, continuing until the desired anteroposterior correction has been achieved.

The effect of elastics is simulated as a one-stage anteroposterior movement at the end of treatment, which enables verification of the final arch coordination and occlusion.

Fewer aligners are required when simultaneous staging is used along with use of elastics as compared with distalization. However, a preparation phase in which all the possible interarch interferences are removed is required in the virtual setup planning to create enough room in which the class II elastics can promote their effects.

Despite the large use of class II elastics in everyday practice, little evidence is known about their effects. A recent systematic review stated that the current literature suggests using light forces (average, 2.6 oz) obtained with a 3/16-in diameter elastic and a rectangular 0.016- to 0.022-in stainless steel archwire.[21] In aligner orthodontics, the use of 1/4-in diameter 4.5 oz was recommended[13,15] on the basis of expert clinician experience. However, as shown in Chapter 5, finite element analysis has shown the need for stronger class II elastics in CAT. Because class II elastics heavily rely on patient compliance, full-time usage is recommended. It has been described as an average period of 8.5 months for the correction of the class II discrepancy with elastics only, and the correction is usually obtained with predominant dentoalveolar effects. This is the average treatment time required to correct an end-to-end class II malocclusion according to existing literature.[21]

EXTRACTIONS

Please refer to Chapter 8 for specifics on extractions.

MANDIBULAR ADVANCEMENT

Please refer to Chapter 16 for specifics on mandibular advancement.

ORTHOGNATHIC SURGERY

Orthognathic surgery consists of surgical procedures performed on the maxilla and/or the mandible to correct serious basal malocclusions and to harmonize the profile. It is beneficial in adults since the most difficult cases cannot be treated by orthopedic and orthodontic therapy alone.

Please refer to Chapter 17 for specifics on orthognathic surgery.

The Clinical Protocol

Distalization is performed to correct average to moderate class II malocclusions (<3 mm) by retracting the maxillary teeth. Distalization should be preferred in patients presenting a class II malocclusion due to maxillary protrusion or in adult patients undergoing compromise treatment.

During distalization, it is essential to use class II elastics or miniscrews to avoid loss of anchorage at the anterior teeth.[13,22,23]

Depending on the severity of the sagittal malocclusion, we can use different clinical approaches:

- For dental sagittal discrepancies where less than 3 mm of distalization are needed, we can safely perform aligner-driven sequential distalization.
- For dental discrepancies ranging between 3 and 5 mm, depending on the clinical situation, we perform sequential distalization combined, or not, with stripping, molar derotation, or an elastic effect.
- If dental discrepancy exceeds 5 mm, we opt for either extraction treatment or orthognathic surgery, once again depending on the clinical situation and the patient's decision.

Maxillary Distalization Case Reports

CASE SUMMARY 1

A 25-year-old female patient asked for an aesthetic orthodontic treatment easy to manage considering her job as a makeup artist traveling across Europe.

She presented a class II, division 1 relationship, mild crowding in the lower arch, and moderate crowding in the upper arch. The overjet was increased to 10 mm. The profile analysis revealed protruded lip position (Fig. 7.1).

Considering the aesthetics request of the patient and her refuse for surgical interventions or extractions, the treatment plan was designed to obtain a final molar and canine class I relationship through a sequential distalization of the maxillary teeth using Invisalign (Align Technology Inc., San José, CA, USA) aligners, composite attachments on all the distalizing teeth, and class II elastics[13,17,20] (Fig. 7.2).

The patient was instructed to wear the aligners and the class II elastics for at least 21 hours per day. Furthermore, she used the AcceleDent device for 20 minutes every day of the orthodontic treatment. Aligners were changed every 2 weeks until the maxillary second molars were fully distalized, then every 10 days until the first molars were in their final position, and then every 7 days until the end of treatment. The ClinCheck (Align Technology Inc., San José, CA, USA) software revealed the need for 63 aligners to obtain the prescribed results (distalization planned for

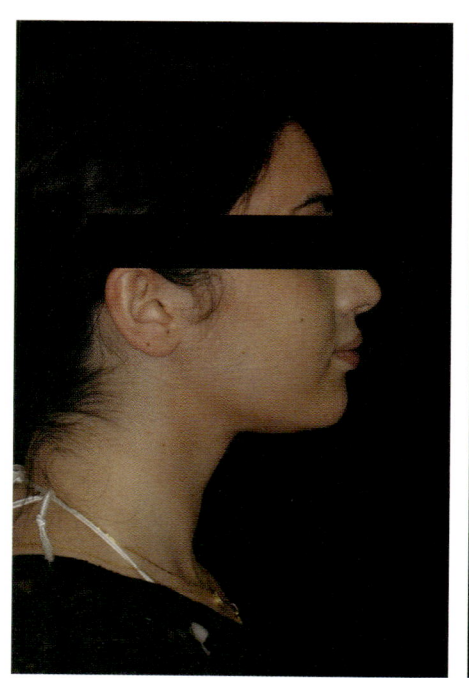

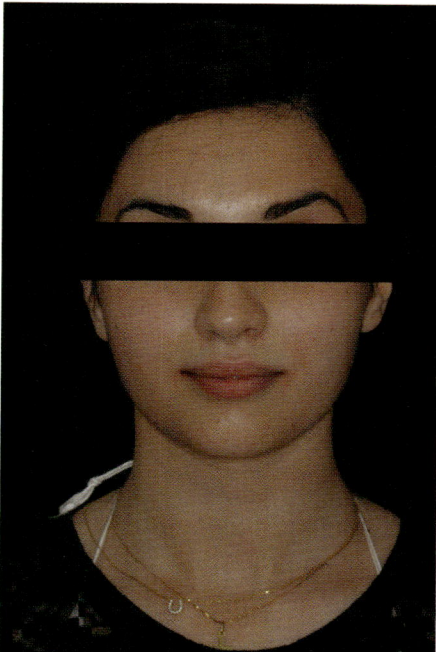

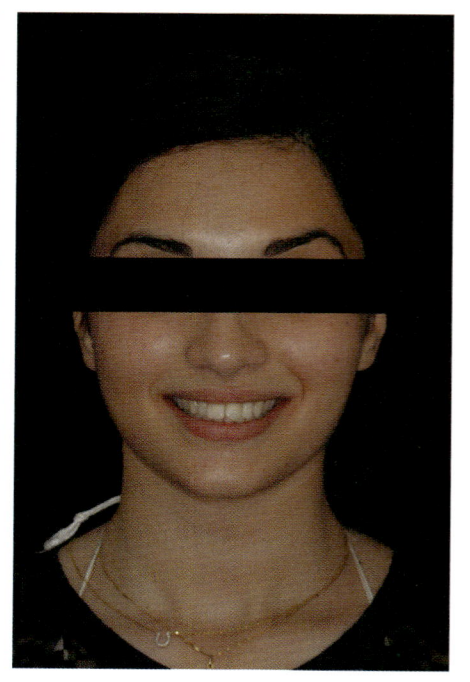

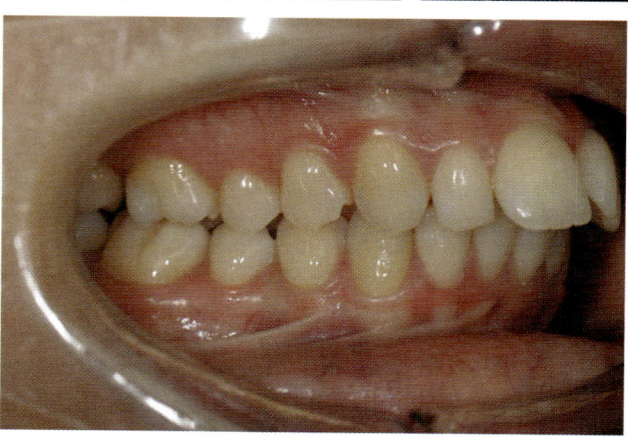

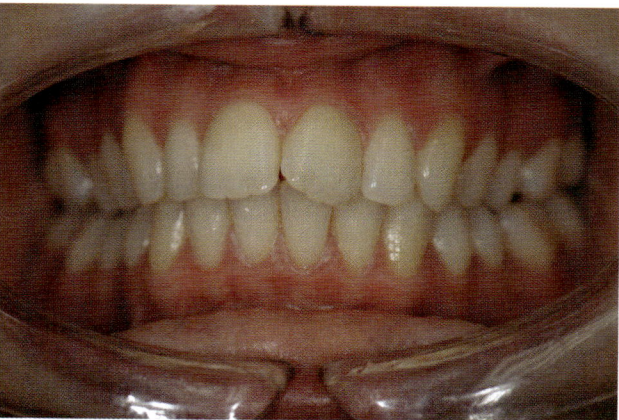

Fig. 7.1 Case 1 initial clinical and radiographic records.

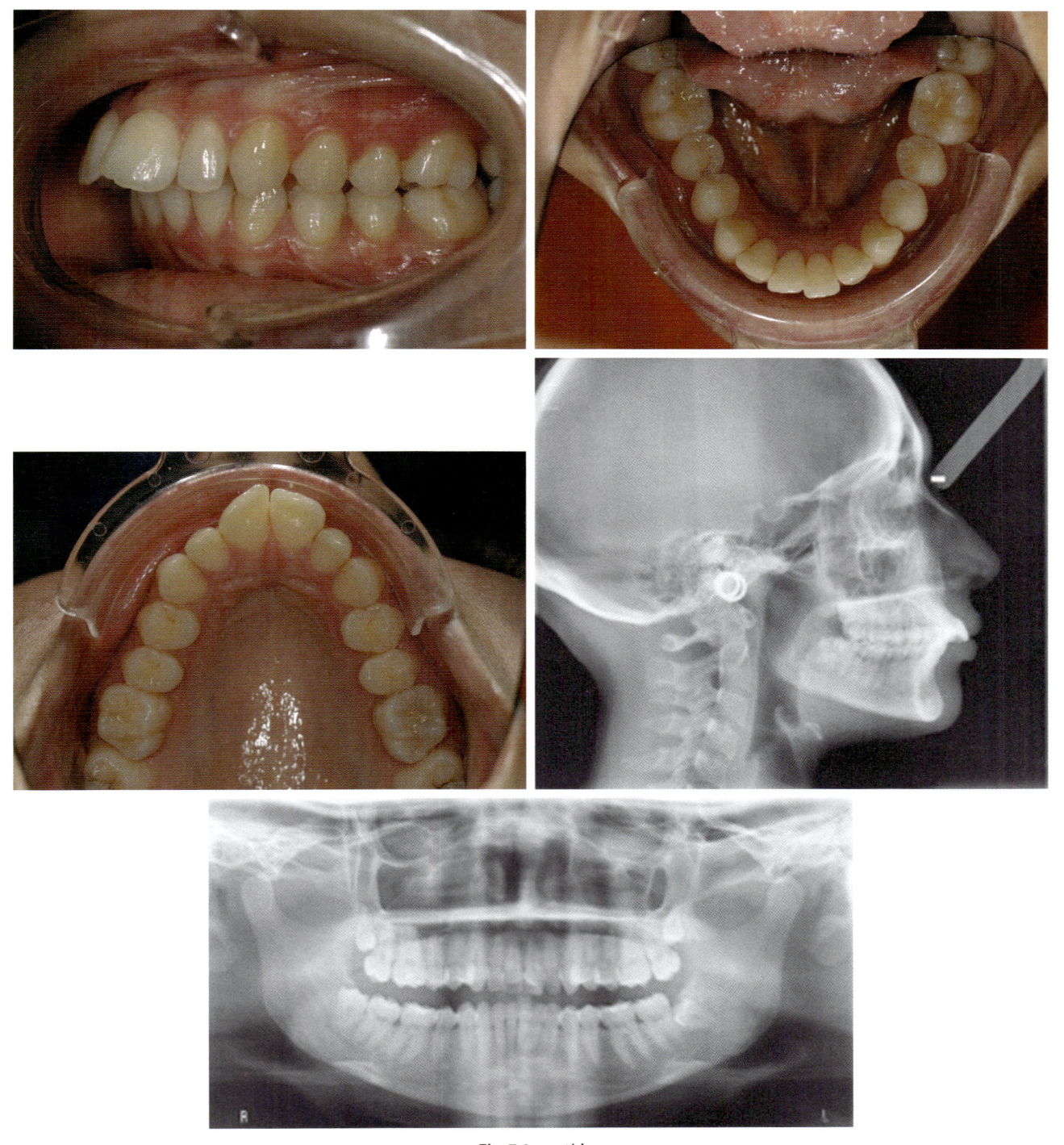

Fig. 7.1, cont'd

3 mm) with the prescribed sequence of stages, attachments, and class II elastics. Thus the estimated treatment time was approximately 30 months. The patient chose to use AcceleDent, and the case was closed in 18 months of treatment without further aligner with respect to the prescribed (Fig. 7.3).

The clinical results were excellent and revealed final molar and canine class I relationships with functional overbite and overjet. The profile of the lower third of the face was highly improved with respect to the beginning (Fig. 7.4).

The superimposition of the cephalometric tracings revealed a maxillary molar distalization of about 6 mm without significant tipping and an excellent control of the buccolingual inclination of the incisors (Fig. 7.5).

The class II elastics were responsible for a mandibular protraction of about 1.5 mm. Retention was provided by Vivera (Align Technology Inc., San José, CA, USA) retainers.

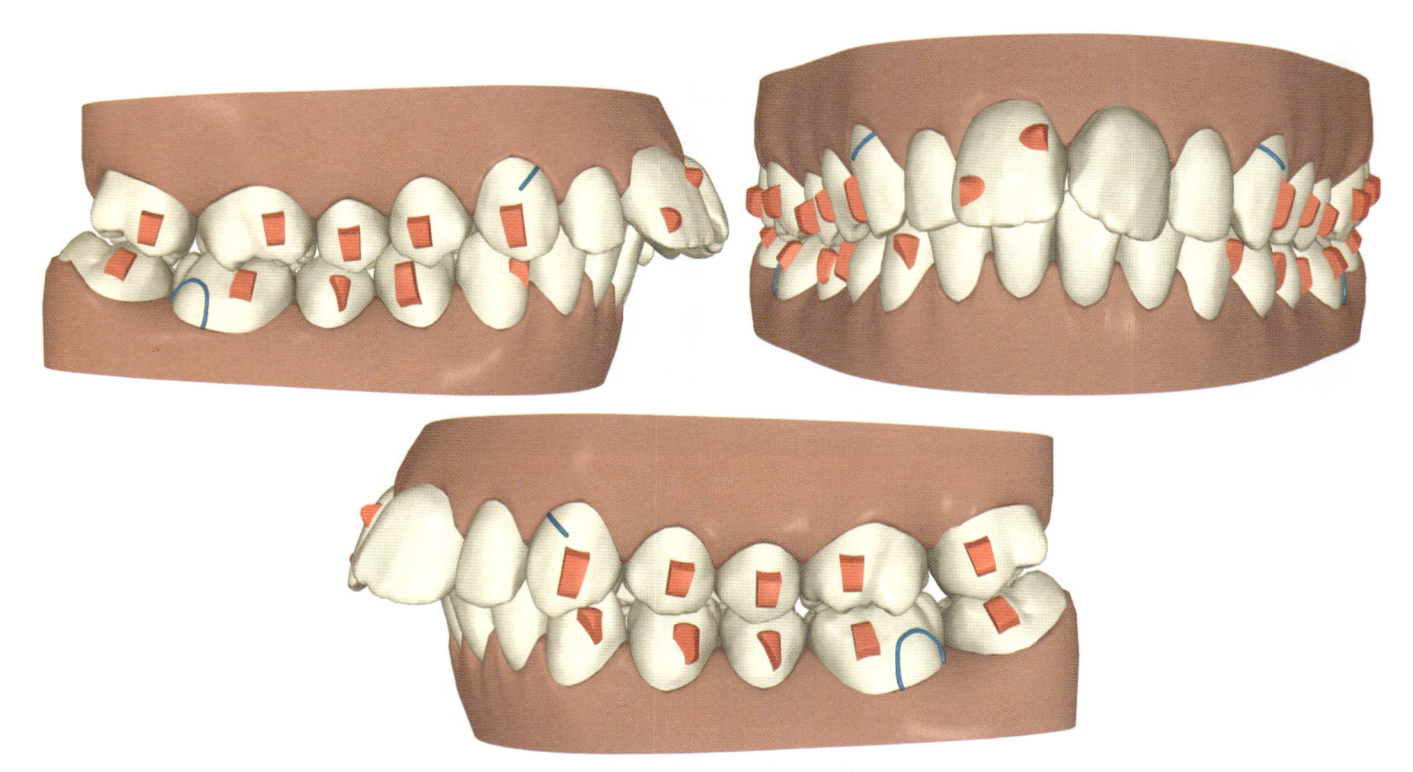

70 Principles and Biomechanics of Aligner Treatment

Fig. 7.2 Case 1 frontal and sagittal views of initial ClinCheck.

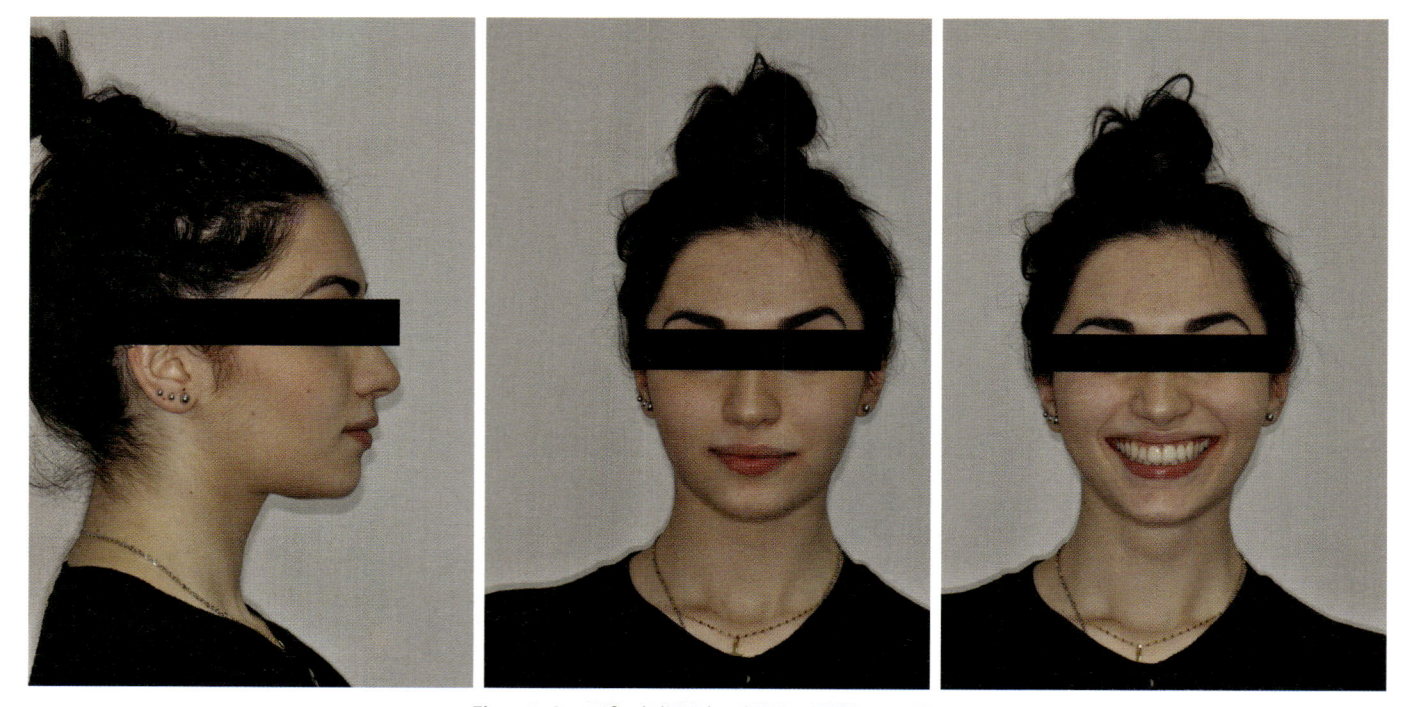

Fig. 7.3 Case 1 final clinical and radiographic records.

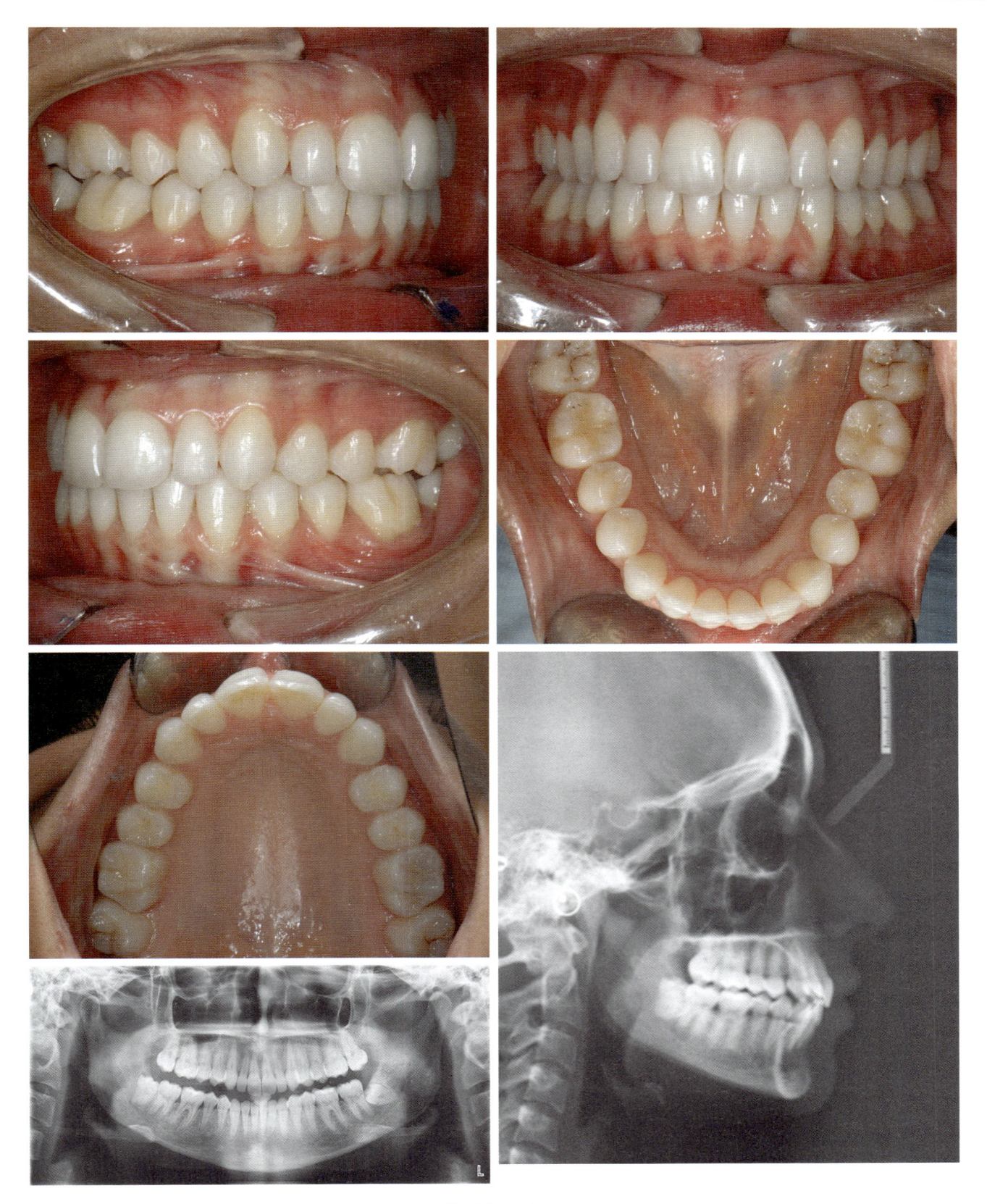

Fig. 7.3, cont'd

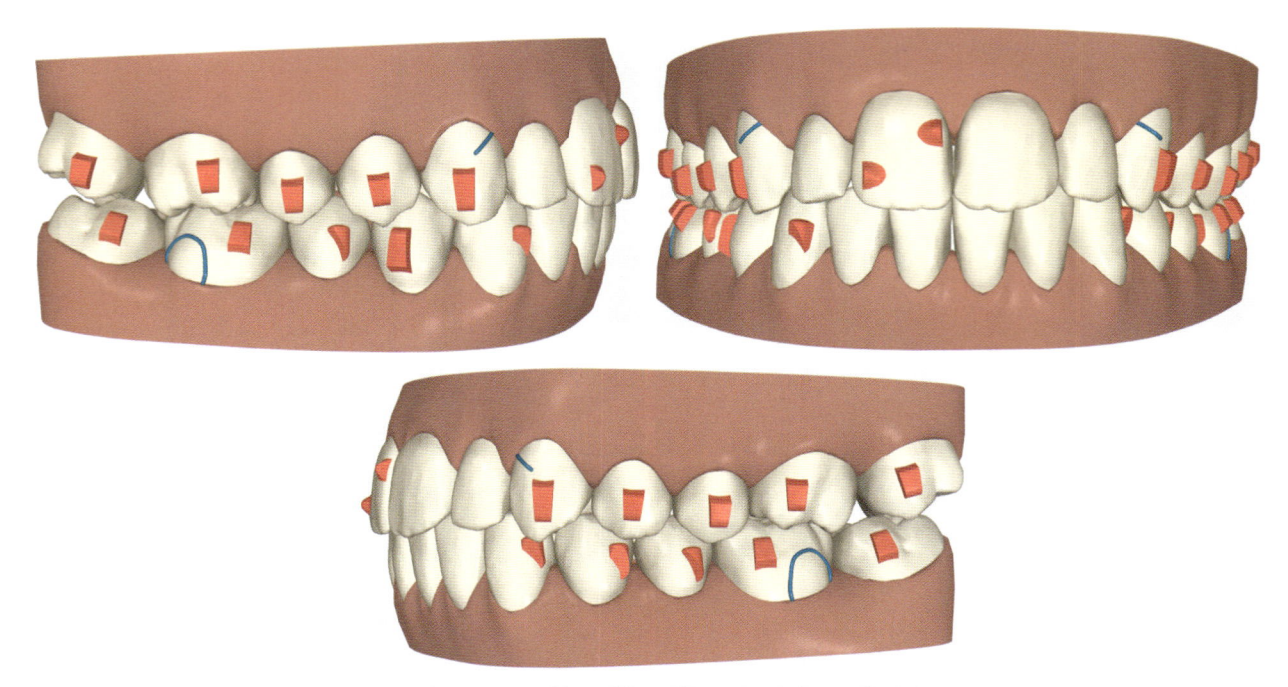

Fig. 7.4 Case 1 frontal and sagittal views of final ClinCheck.

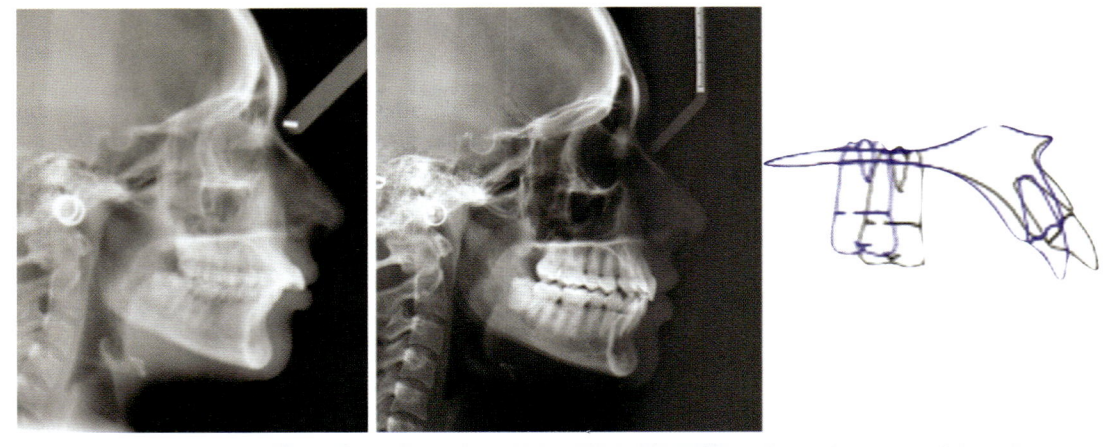

Fig. 7.5 Case 1 lateral x-ray comparison and cephalometric maxillary superimposition before and after therapy.

CASE SUMMARY 2

A 30-year-old female patient asked for an aesthetic orthodontic treatment easy to manage.

She presented a class II, division 2 relationship, moderate crowding in the upper arch, and mild crowding in the lower arch. The overjet was increased to 3 mm. The profile analysis revealed an acceptable lip position (Fig. 7.6).

Considering the aesthetics request of the patient and her refuse for orthognathic surgery, the treatment plan was designed to obtain a final molar and canine class I relationship by a sequential distalization of the maxillary teeth using Invisalign (Align Technology Inc., San José, CA, USA) aligners, composite attachments on all the distalizing teeth, and class II elastics. The average distalization movement prescribed was 2.5 mm (Fig. 7.7).

The patient was instructed to wear the aligners and the class II elastics for at least 21 hours per day. Aligners were changed every 2 weeks until the maxillary second molars were fully distalized, then every 10 days until the first molars were in their final position, and then every 7 days until the end of treatment. The ClinCheck (Align Technology Inc., San José, CA, USA) software revealed the need for 61 aligners to obtain the prescribed results with the prescribed sequence of stages, attachments, and class II elastics. The estimated treatment time was approximately 28 months.

In an intermediate phase, first outcomes of sequential distalization were clearly visible. As shown in Figs. 7.8 and 7.9, molars already distalized in a correct class I relationship were spaced apart from premolars.

The clinical results were excellent and revealed final molar and canine class I relationships with correct overbite and overjet. The profile of the lower third of the face was slightly improved with respect to the beginning, since the aesthetic analysis and cephalometric measurements showed acceptable values at the beginning of the treatment already (Figs. 7.10 and 7.11).

The superimposition of the cephalometric tracings revealed a maxillary molar distalization of about 2.5 mm without significant tipping and an excellent control of the buccolingual inclination of the incisors (Fig. 7.12).

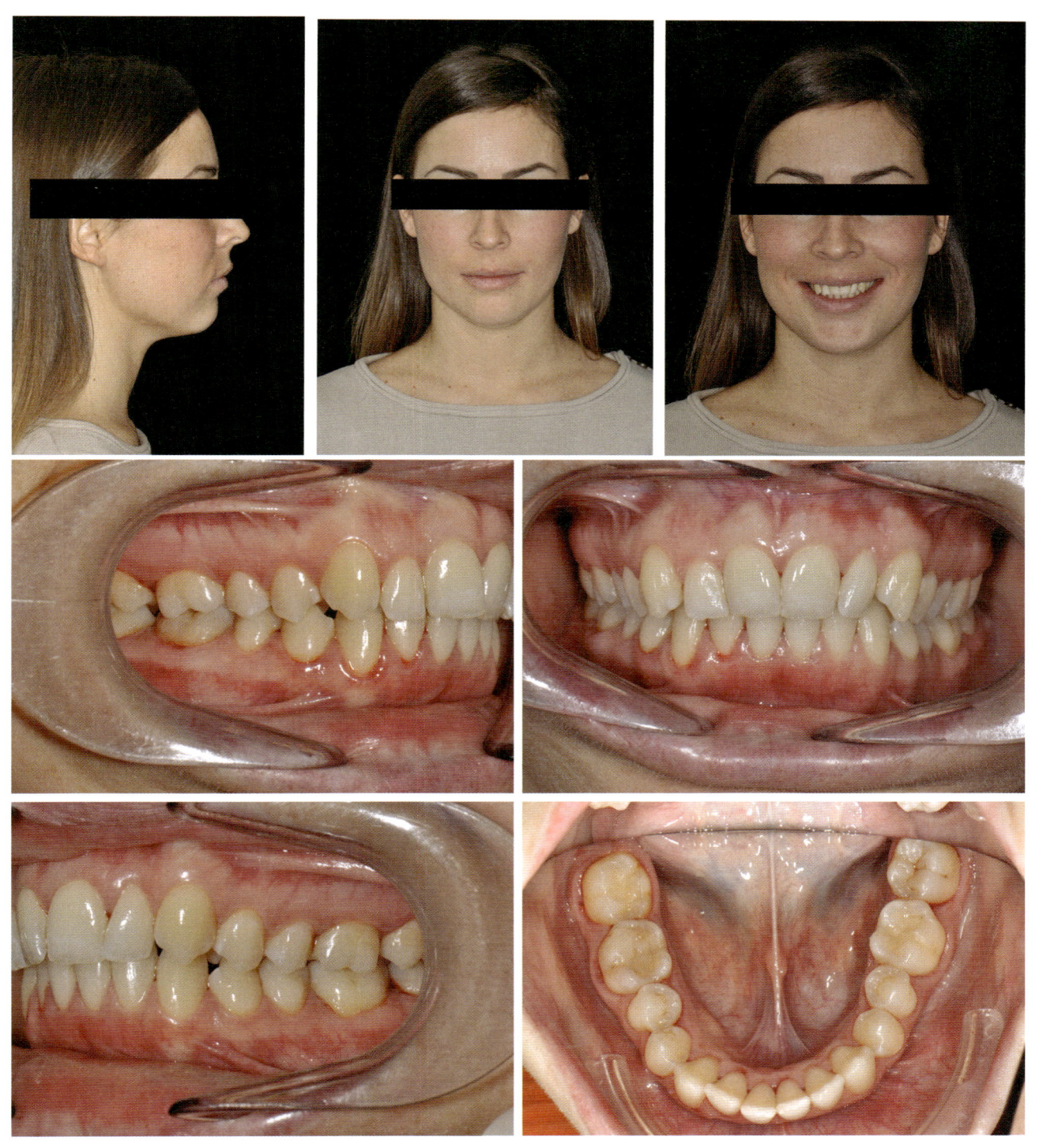

Fig. 7.6 Case 2 initial clinical and radiographic records.

Continued

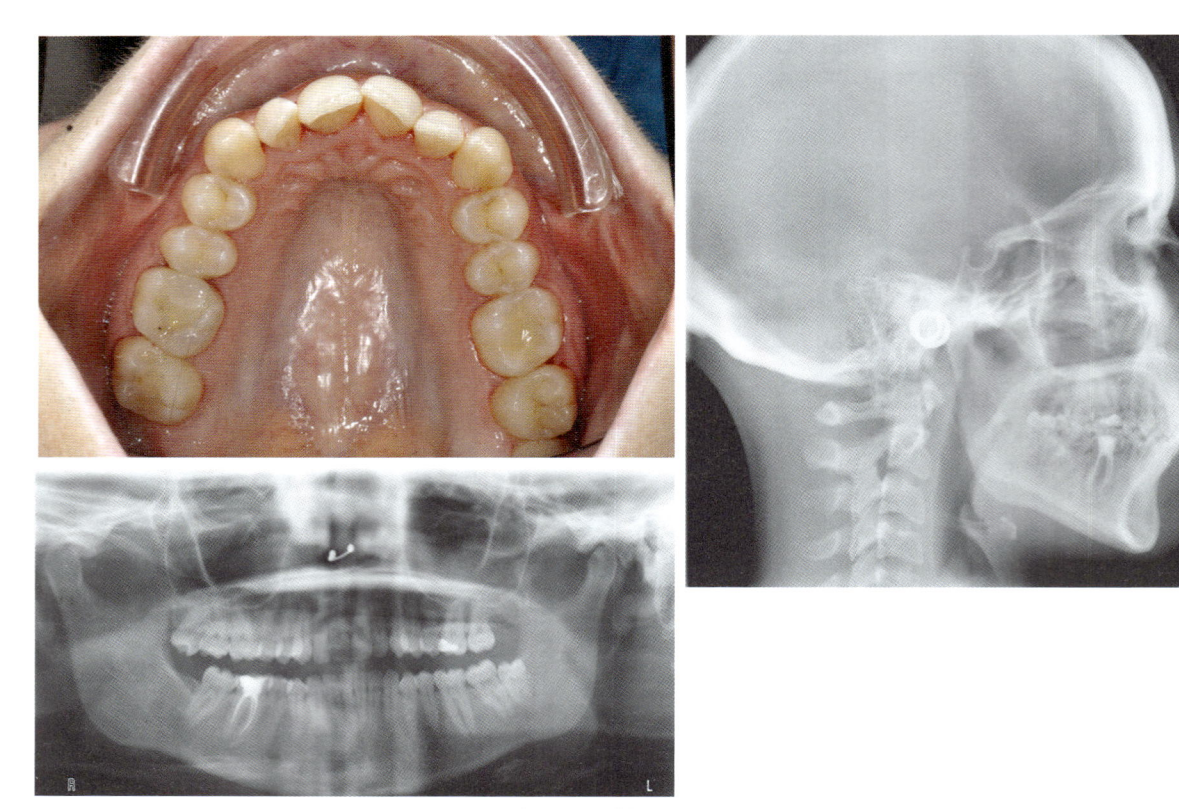

74 Principles and Biomechanics of Aligner Treatment

Fig. 7.6, cont'd

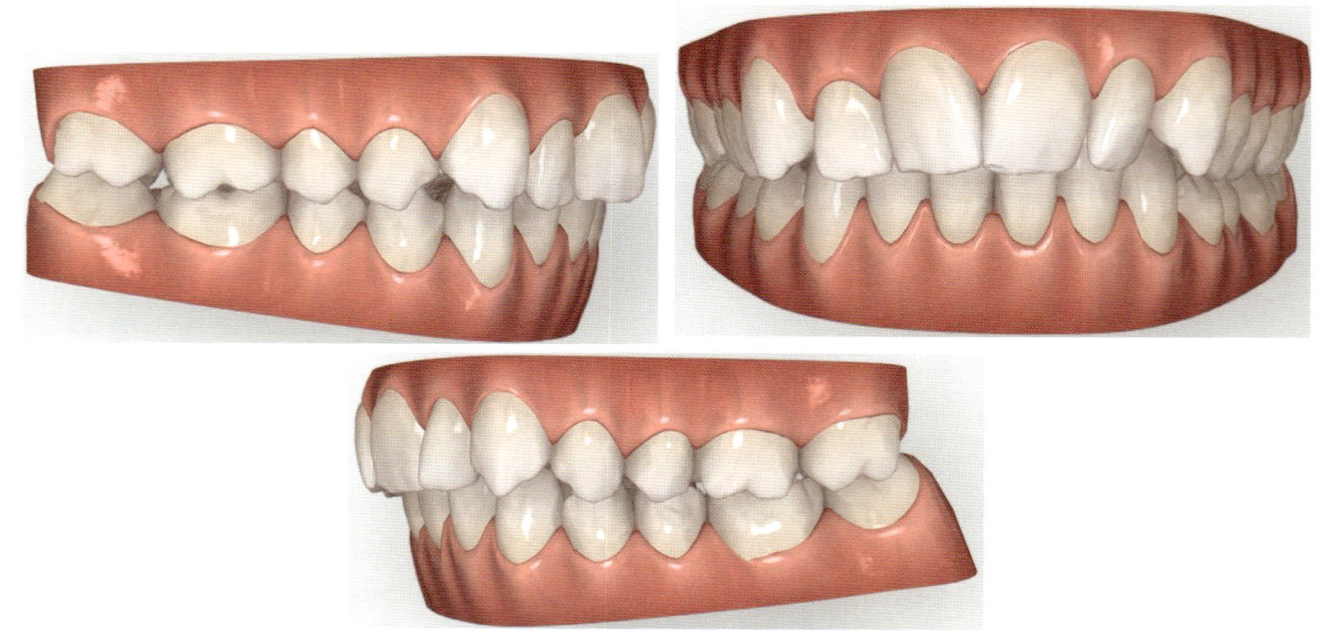

Fig. 7.7 Case 2 frontal and sagittal views of initial ClinCheck.

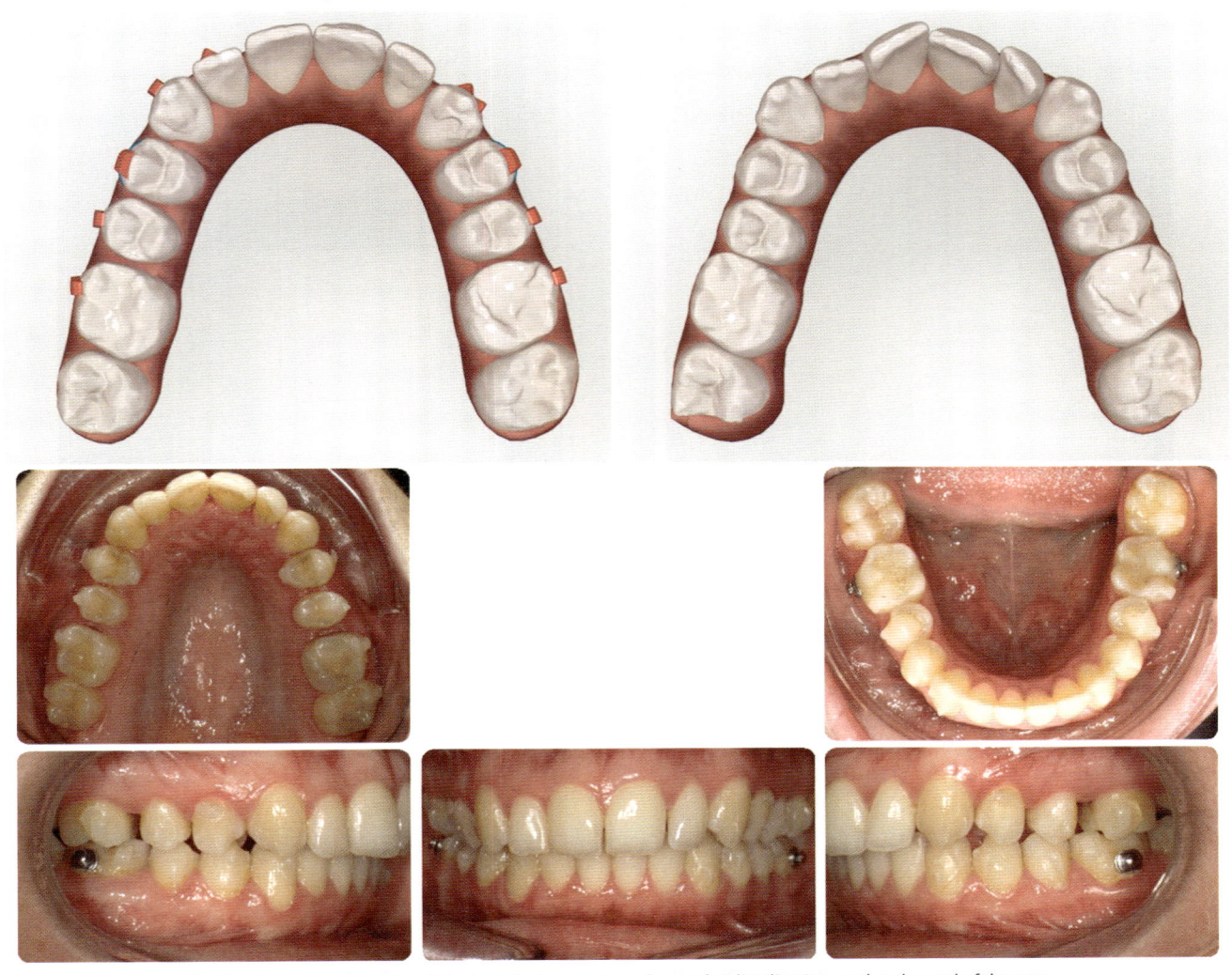

Fig. 7.8 Case 2 upper occlusal views at the beginning, after molar distalization, and at the end of therapy.

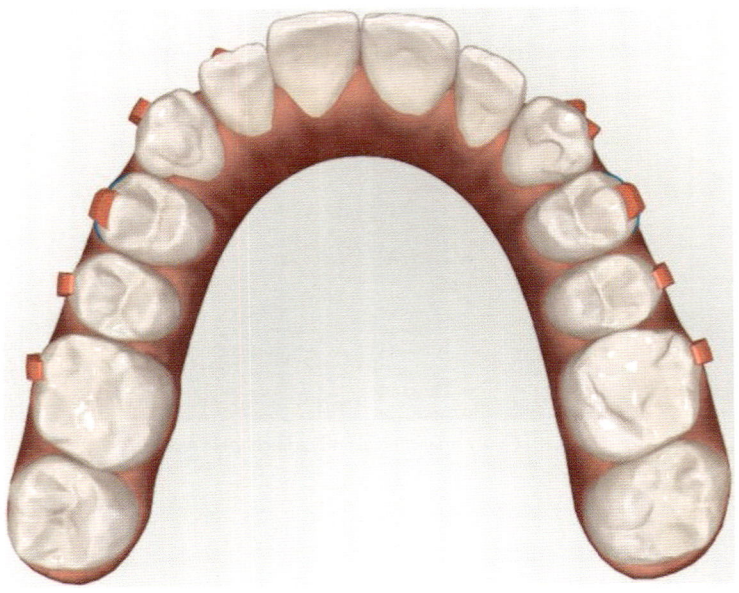

Fig. 7.9 Case 2 end of distalization; intraoral frontal, occlusal, and sagittal views.

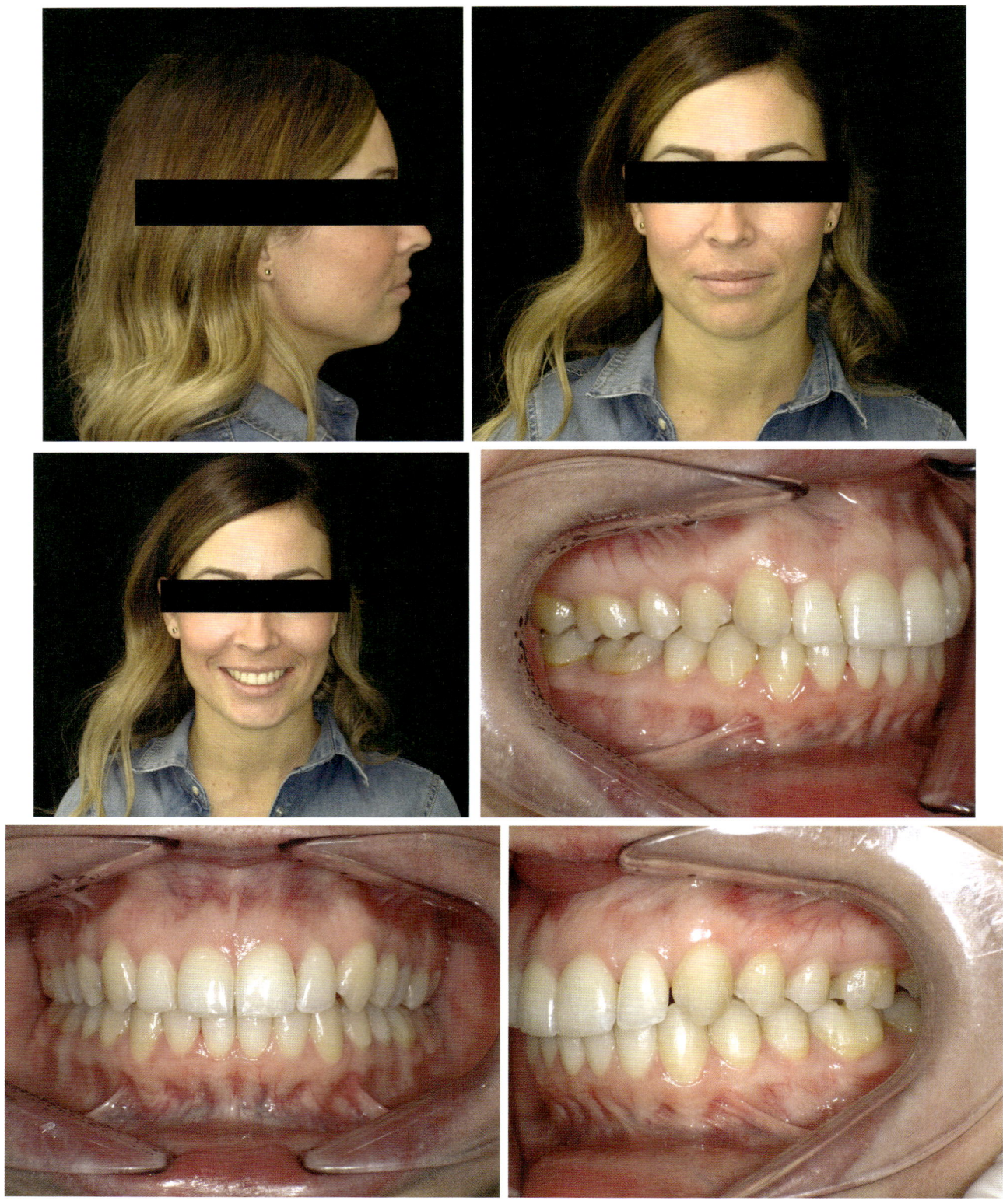

Fig. 7.10 Case 2 final clinical and radiographic records.

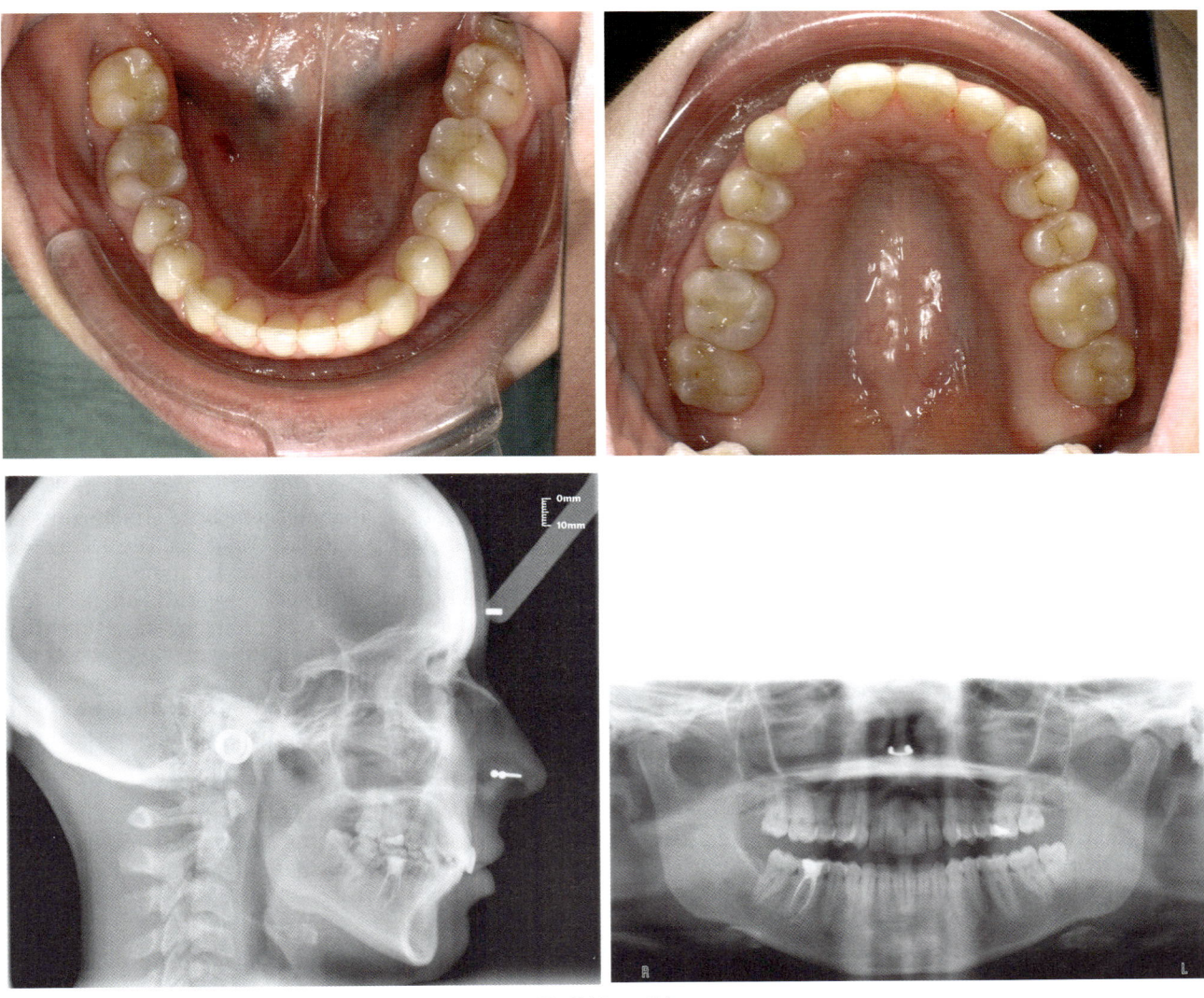

7 • Aligner Treatment in Class II Malocclusion Patients   77

Fig. 7.10, cont'd

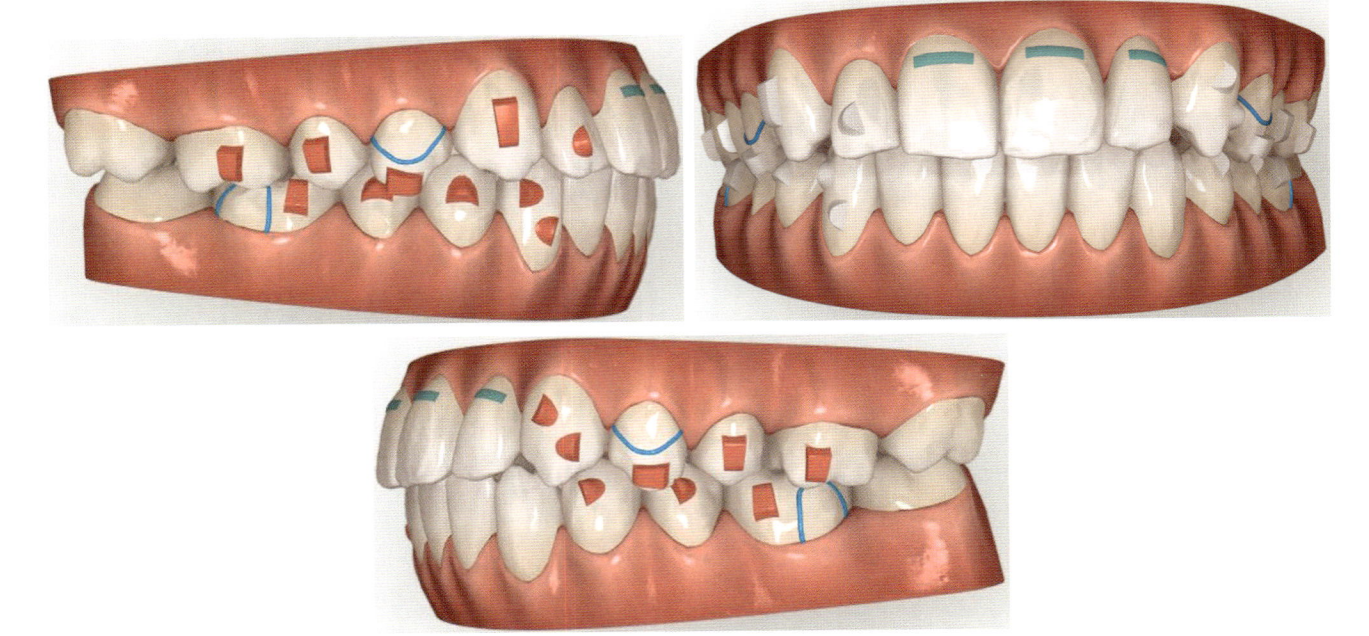

Fig. 7.11 Case 2 frontal and sagittal views of final ClinCheck.

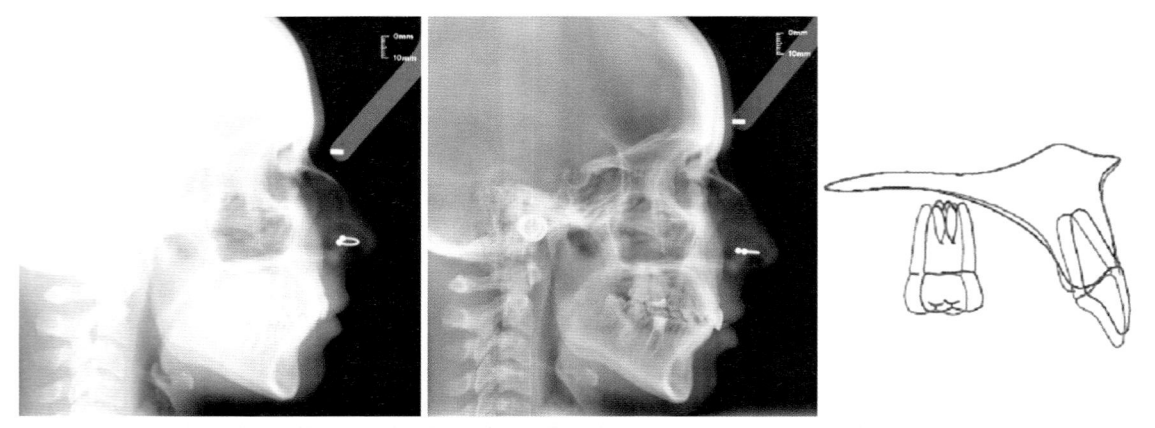

Fig. 7.12 Case 2 lateral x-ray comparison and cephalometric maxillary superimposition before and after therapy.

CASE SUMMARY 3

This 15-year-old female patient has no previous orthodontic history, a full 5-mm left- and right-side molar class II maxillary alveolar arch width deficiency, 5 mm of maxillary crowding, a 4-mm overbite, and an 8-mm overjet. Skeletally she presented a hypodivergent class II and a cervical vertebrae maturation (CVM) stage 5. Esthetically her face was harmonious in both frontal and lateral views (Fig. 7.13).

Residual growth was insufficient to consider orthopedic treatment. Consequently, taking into account the aesthetics request of the patient, the treatment plan was designed to correct the class II, achieving final molar and canine class I relationship by molar derotation, sequential distalization, and elastic jump using Invisalign (Align Technology Inc., San José, CA, USA) aligners, composite attachments on all the distalizing teeth, and class II elastics. The average distalization movement prescribed was 1.5 mm.

The patient was instructed to wear the aligners and the class II elastics for at least 21 hours per day. Aligners were changed every 2 weeks until the maxillary second molars were fully distalized, then every 10 days until the first molars were in their final position, and then every 7 days till the end of treatment. To obtain the prescribed results, 56 aligners were needed (Fig. 7.14).

The clinical results were good and showed final molar and canine class I relationships with correct overbite and overjet. The profile of the lower third of the face was improved with respect to the initial records (Fig. 7.15).

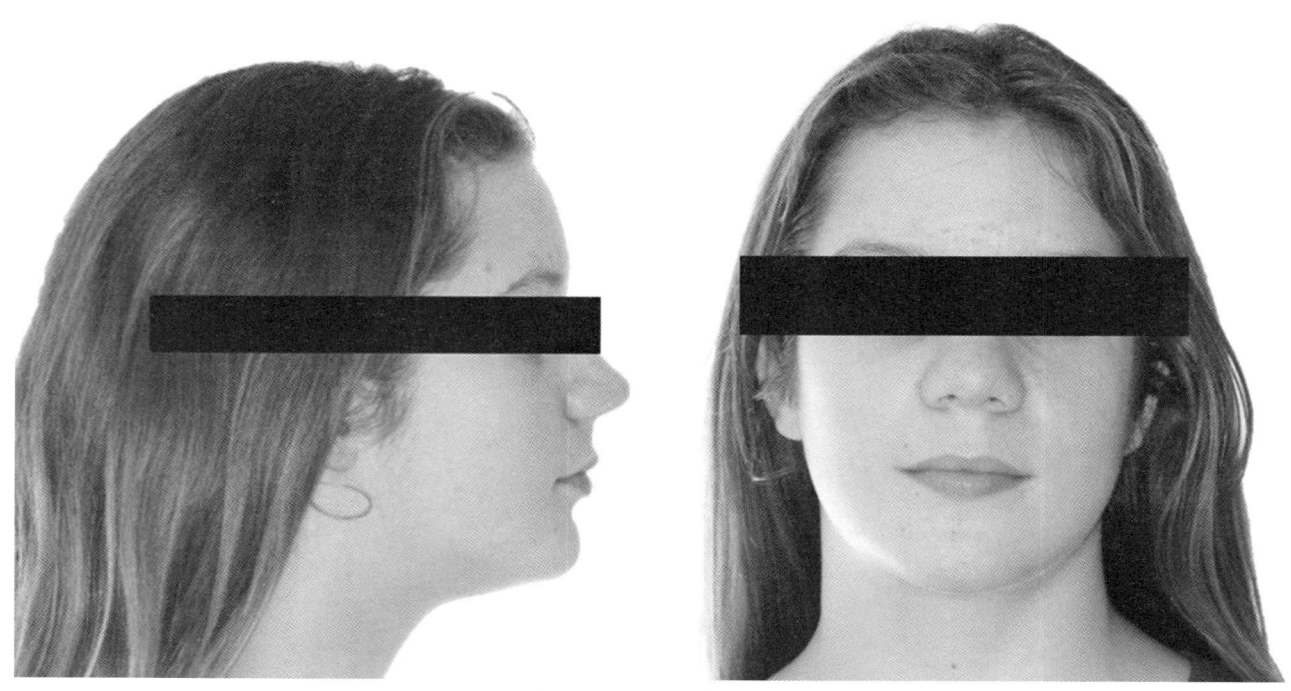

Fig. 7.13 Case 3 initial clinical and radiographic records.

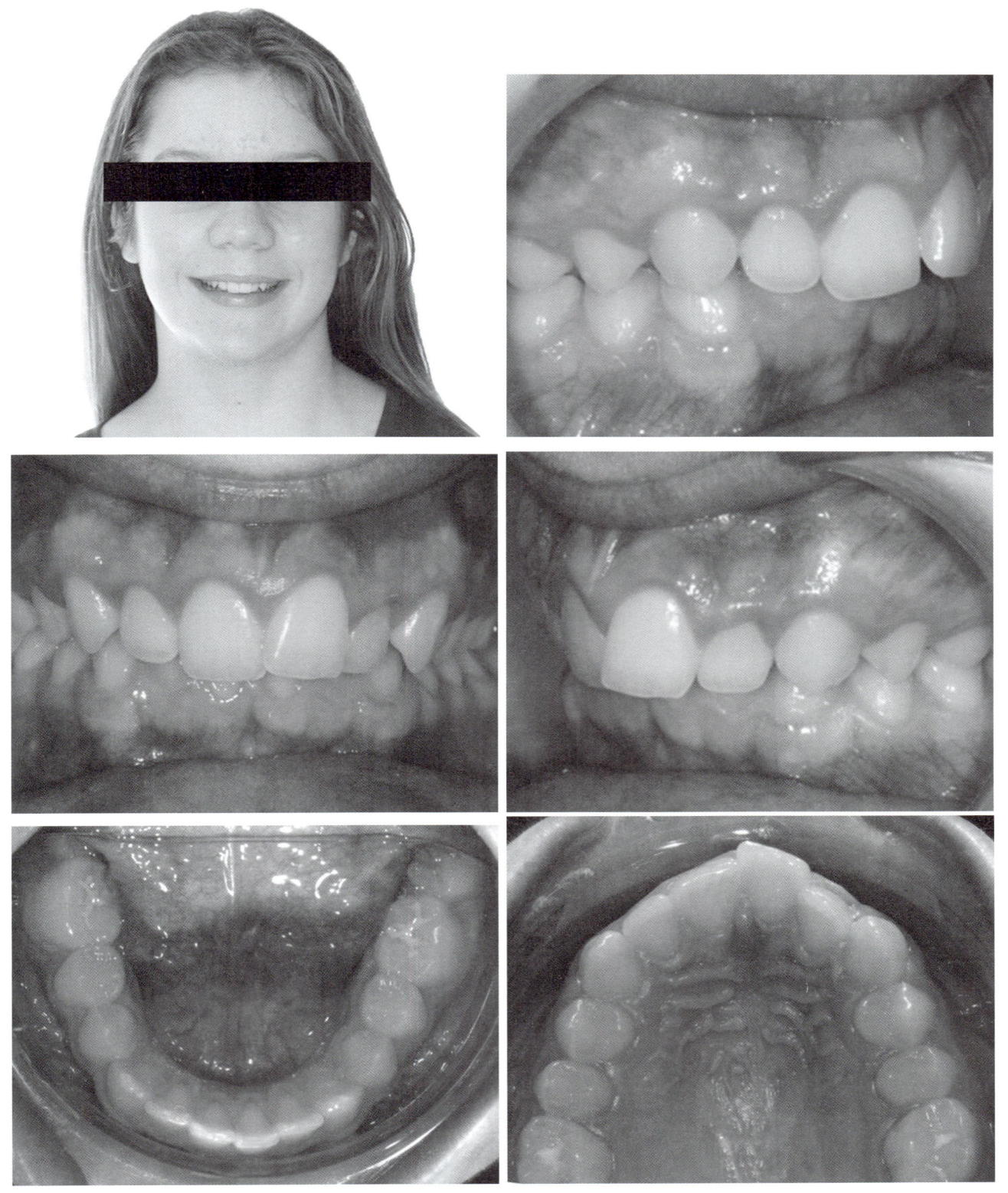

7 • Aligner Treatment in Class II Malocclusion Patients

Fig. 7.13, cont'd

Continued

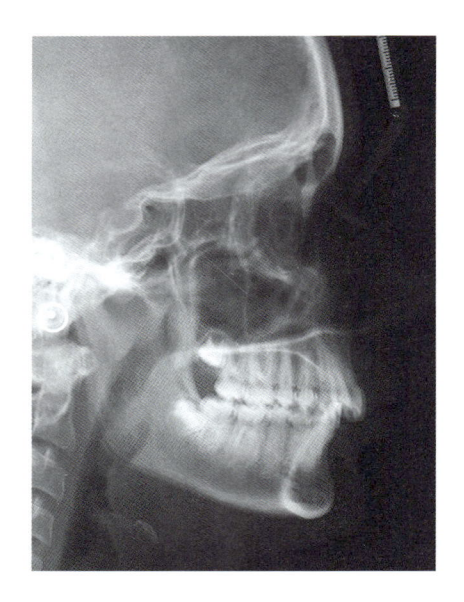

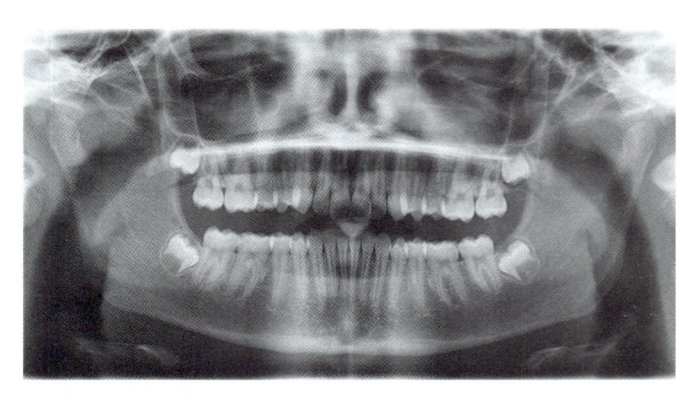

80 Principles and Biomechanics of Aligner Treatment

Fig. 7.13, cont'd

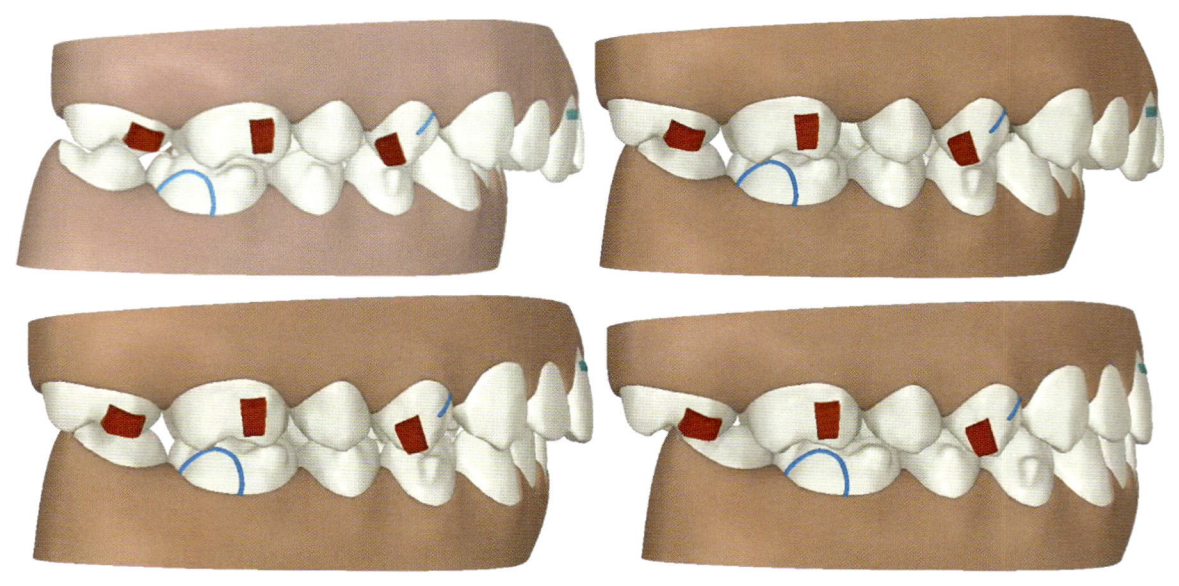

Fig. 7.14 Case 3 sagittal views of initial, intermediate, final pre- and postjump ClinCheck.

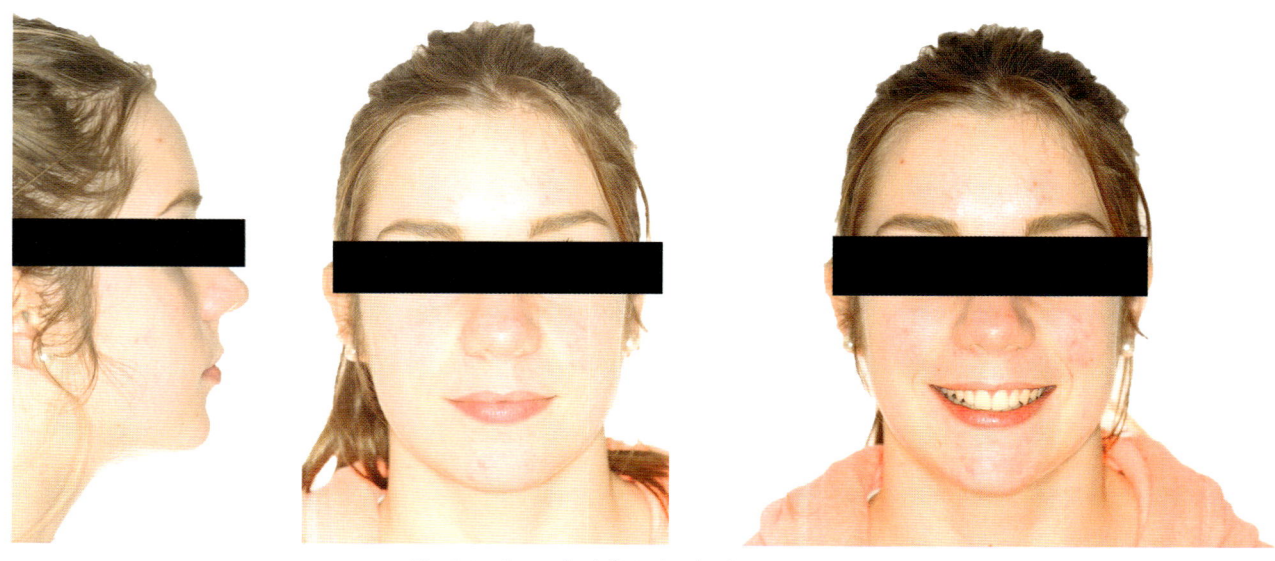

Fig. 7.15 Case 3 final clinical and radiographic records.

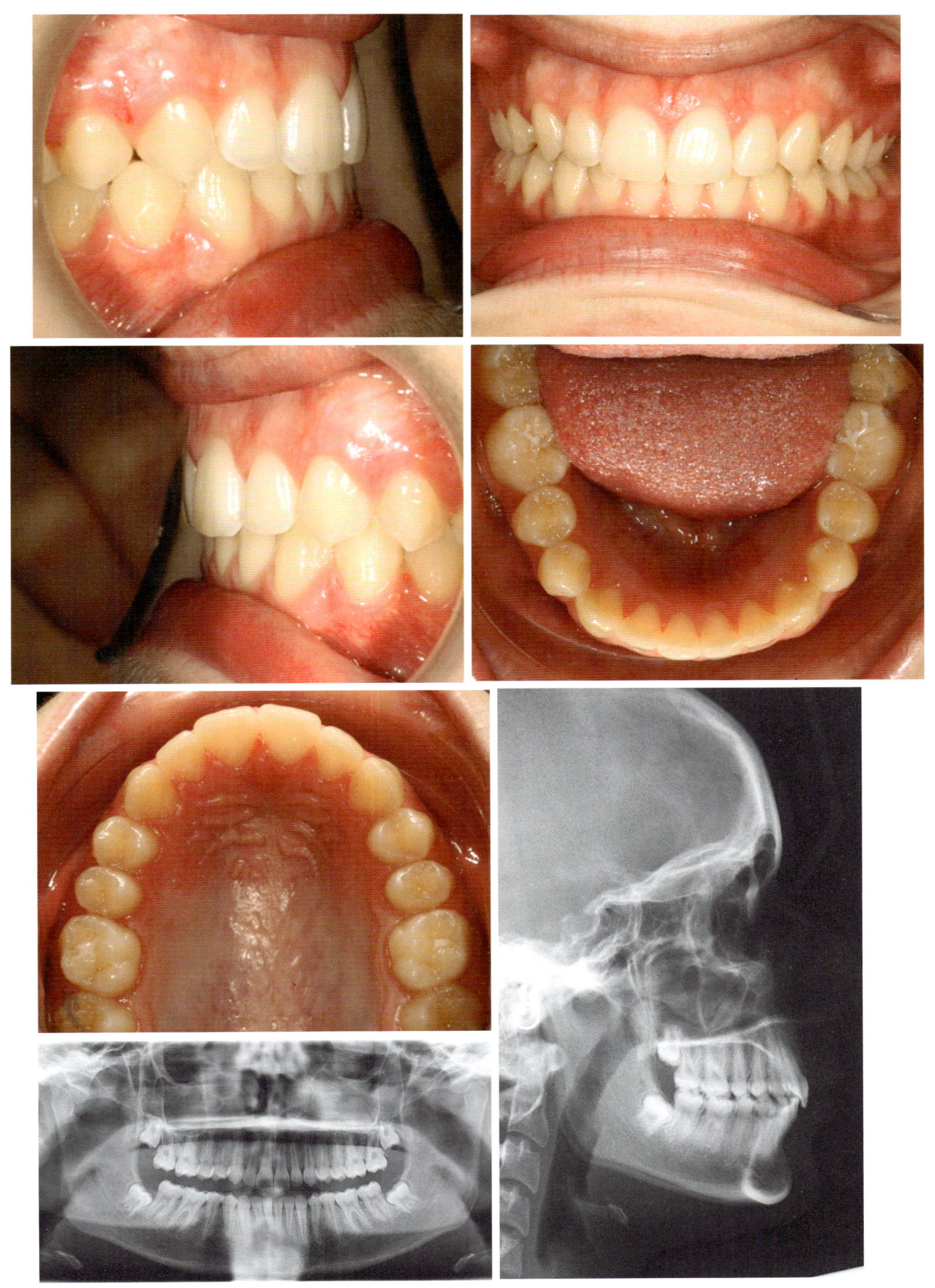

7 • Aligner Treatment in Class II Malocclusion Patients

Fig. 7.15, cont'd

References

1. Boyd RL. Esthetic orthodontic treatment using the Invisalign appliance for moderate to complex malocclusions. *J Dent Educ.* 2008;72:948-967.
2. Nanda RS, Tosun YS. *Correction of Anteroposterior Discrepancies.* Hanover Park: Quintessence Publishing Co; 2010:63-72.
3. Grec RH, Janson G, Branco NC, et al. Intraoral distalizer effects with conventional and skeletal anchorage: a meta-analysis. *Am J Orthod Dentofacial Orthop.* 2013;143:602-615.
4. Fontana M, Cozzani M, Caprioglio A. Non-compliance maxillary molar distalizing appliances: an overview of the last decade. *Prog Orthod.* 2012;13:173-184.
5. Egolf RJ, BeGole EA, Upshaw HS. Factors associated with orthodontic patient compliance with intraoral elastic and headgear wear. *Am J Orthod Dentofacial Orthop.* 1990;97:336-348.
6. Fuziy A, Rodrigues de Almeida R, Janson G, et al. Sagittal, vertical, and transverse changes consequent to maxillary molar distalization with the pendulum appliance. *Am J Orthod Dentofacial Orthop.* 2006;130:502-510.
7. Fontana M, Cozzani M, Caprioglio A. Soft tissue, skeletal and dentoalveolar changes following conventional anchorage molar distalization therapy in class II non-growing subjects: a multicentric retrospective study. *Prog Orthod.* 2012;13:30-41.
8. Kusy RP. Influence of force systems on archwire-bracket combinations. *Am J Orthod Dentofacial Orthop.* 2005;127:333-342.
9. Rossini G, Parrini S, Castroflorio T, et al. Efficacy of clear aligners in controlling orthodontic tooth movement: a systematic review. *Angle Orthod.* 2015;85:881-889.
10. Rossini G, Parrini S, Deregibus A, et al. Controlling orthodontic tooth movement with clear aligners. An updated systematic review regarding efficacy and efficiency. *J Aligner Orthod.* 2017;1:7-20.
11. Simon M, Keilig L, Schwarze J, et al. Forces and moments generated by removable thermoplastic aligners: incisor torque, premolar derotation, and molar distalization. *Am J Orthod Dentofacial Orthop.* 2014;145:728-736.
12. Drake CT, McGorray SP, Dolce C, et al. Orthodontic tooth movement with clear aligners. *ISRN Dent.* 2012;2012:657973.
13. Ravera S, Castroflorio T, Garino F, et al. Maxillary molar distalization with aligners in adult patients: a multicenter retrospective study. *Prog Orthod.* 2016;17:12.
14. Simon M, Keilig L, Schwarze J, et al. Treatment outcome and efficacy of an aligner technique—regarding incisor torque, premolar derotation and molar distalization. *BMC Oral Health.* 2014;14:68.
15. Daher S. *Dr. Sam Daher's Techniques for Class II Correction with Invisalign and Elastics.* https://s3.amazonaws.com/learn-invisalign/docs/06840000000Fp2xAAC.pdf.
16. Paquette DE. Extraction treatment with Invisalign. In Tuncay O, ed. *The Invisalign System.* New Malden: Quintessence Publishing Co; 2006:195-205.
17. Garino F, Castroflorio T, Daher S, et al. Effectiveness of composite attachments in controlling upper-molar movement with aligners. *J Clin Orthod.* 2016;50:341-347.
18. Gomez JP, Peña FM, Martínez V, et al. Initial force systems during bodily tooth movement with plastic aligners and composite attachments: a three-dimensional finite element analysis. *Angle Orthod.* 2015;85:454-460.
19. Comba B, Parrini S, Rossini G, et al. Three-dimensional finite element analysis of upper-canine distalization with clear aligners, composite attachments, and class II elastics. *J Clin Orthod.* 2017;51:24-28.
20. Solano-Mendoza B, Sonnemberg B, Solano-Reina E, et al. How effective is the Invisalign® system in expansion movement with Ex30' aligners? *Clin Oral Investig.* 2017;21:1475-1484.
21. Janson G, Sathler R, Fernandes TM, et al. Correction of class II malocclusion with class II elastics: a systematic review. *Am J Orthod Dentofacial Orthop.* 2013;143:383-392.
22. Mohamed RN, Basha S, Al-Thomali Y. Maxillary molar distalization with miniscrew-supported appliances in class II malocclusion: a systematic review. *Angle Orthod.* 2018;88:494-502.
23. Yamada K, Kuroda S, Deguchi T, et al. Distal movement of maxillary molars using miniscrew anchorage in the buccal interradicular region. *Angle Orthod.* 2009;79:78-84.

8 Aligners in Extraction Cases

KENJI OJIMA, CHISATO DAN, and RAVINDRA NANDA

Introduction

The demand for inconspicuous and natural-feeling orthodontic appliances has been rising over time. The introduction of the Invisalign system marked a significant step forward in orthodontics in that it allowed for inconspicuous orthodontic correction using appliances with a natural feel. The original Invisalign system, however, came with serious limitations: the control of root movement was not possible and it was difficult to move large teeth over significant distances.[1-10] Recent advances in the quality of materials, the use of attachments, and the introduction of a new force system have expanded the range of applications of the Invisalign system from mild crowding to more difficult extraction cases.[11-16]

As is the case with all orthodontic procedures, one of the greatest sources of dissatisfaction among adult patients with aligner therapy is the long treatment time. This report describes the treatment of a patient with severe anterior crowding who was treated with Invisalign appliances after the extraction[17-20] of her three remaining premolars. Her lower left premolar had already been removed. A photobiomodulation device was used to possibly accelerate tooth movement.

Diagnosis and Treatment Plan

When this 25-year-old female presented at our clinic, she expressed a desire to correct her maxillary anterior crowding and improve the aesthetic appearance of her smile. While the patient's facial profile was straight, both lips were slightly recessive with regard to the E-line (Fig. 8.1). An intraoral examination showed a class II molar relationship with a 2-mm overjet, a 3-mm overbite, and coincident midlines. The arch-length discrepancy was 15 mm in the maxilla and 10 mm in the mandible. Infralabioversion was noted for both upper canines and a marked buccal shift of the upper left second molar (Fig. 8.2).

Cephalometric analysis indicated a skeletal class II relationship with a steep mandibular plane angle (Fig. 8.3). The upper central incisors were slightly inclined lingually and the lower central incisors were inclined labially. The lateral gap in the mandibular head confirmed by her panoramic x-ray did not impede mandibular function. There was evidence of slight regression in the periodontal tissue around the upper canines; with no tooth mobility, the maximum pocket depth was 5 mm.

Based on these observations, the patient was diagnosed as a skeletal class II case with infralabioversion of the maxillary canines and a steep mandibular plane angle. The treatment plan called for the retraction of both upper and lower incisors: 17.8 mm of movement was required in the maxilla and 14.8 mm in the mandible. First, the two upper first premolars and lower right second premolar were extracted. Her lower left second premolar had been removed in her early teens. Therefore, to allow for mesial movement, her upper left second molar and upper right third molar were extracted, too. Because the patient expressed concern about the poor aesthetics of fixed orthodontic appliances over a potentially long period of time, the decision was made to implement the Invisalign system in conjunction with photobiomodulation (OrthoPulse) to possibly speed up treatment.[21-32]

ClinCheck software was used to analyze the location, angle, and need for the recontouring of the canine in relation to the final desired occlusion (Fig. 8.4). Adequate incisor retraction in this class II malocclusion required the 2-mm distal movement of the upper first molars and 2-mm mesial movement of the lower first molars. Even after the extractions, there was insufficient space to move the maxillary anterior teeth by premolar extraction alone. To create more space, the overexpansion of the dental arches was required. Tooth movements were simulated on the ClinCheck software (Fig. 8.5), the amount of expansion required in each arch was estimated, the positions were planned, and the shapes of the required attachments were decided.

Treatment Progress

Three third molars were removed (except the upper left third molar) before treatment. After the extraction of the upper premolars and lower left first premolar, aligner treatment was initiated. We used all the maxillary teeth from first molar to first molar as anchorage for the distalization of the second molars. In the mandible, we used all the teeth excluding the canines and second premolars as anchorage for the mesial movement of the canines. Since the root of the lower right canine was angled outward, we moved the tooth simply by tipping; the lower left canine was moved bodily along with its root. The distalization of the upper second molars was completed in 12 weeks and distal movement of the upper first molars was completed 2 weeks later. The closure of the lower extraction space continued during this period with mesial movement of the lower first molars.

After 5 months of treatment, retraction movement of the upper canines was completed, with the incisors of the midline corrected. At this point, we recalculated the retraction

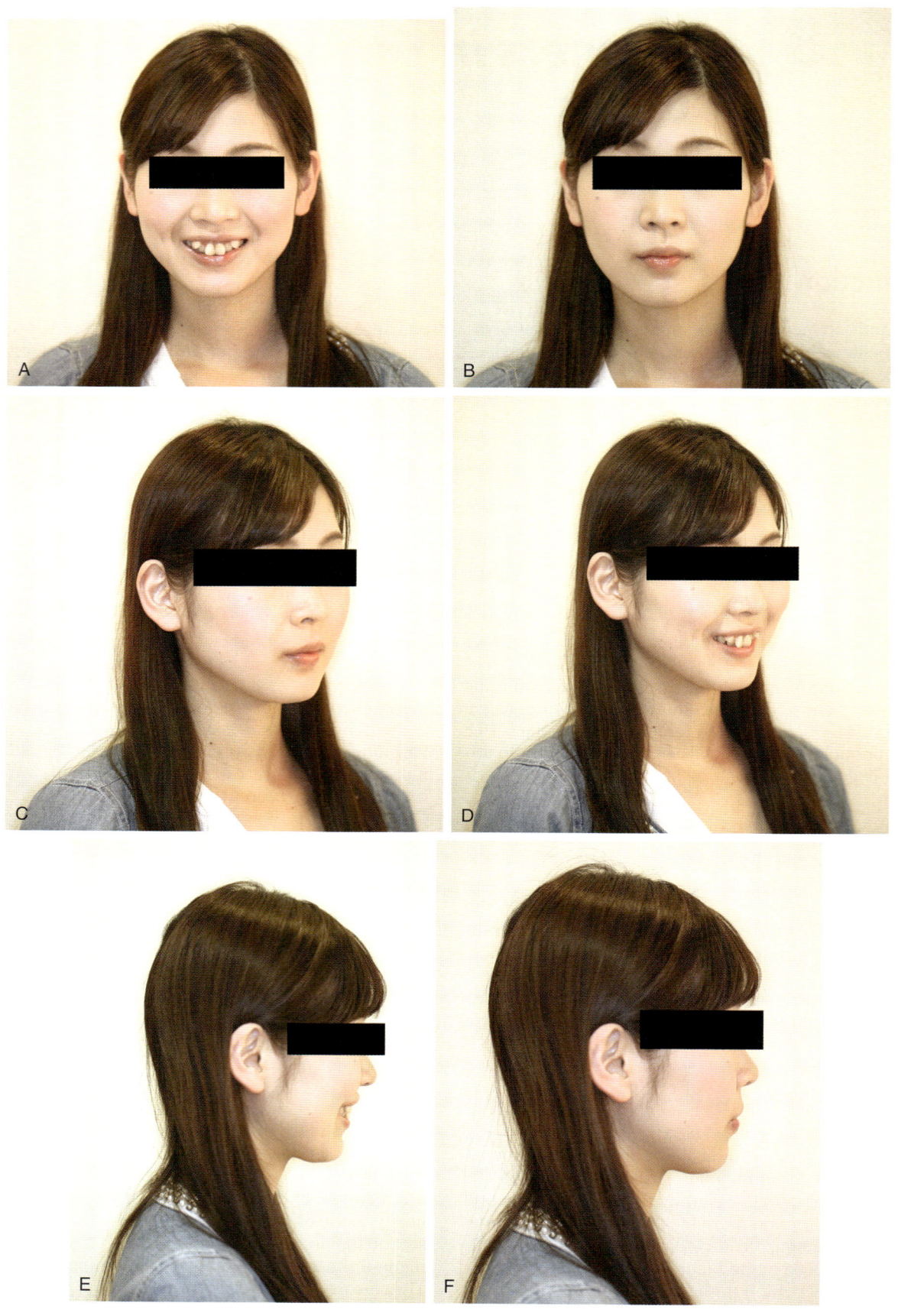

Fig. 8.1 (A) Smile appearance of the patient. (B) Frontal picture at rest. (C) Three-quarter picture at rest. (D) Three-quarter smile appearance. (E) Profile smiling. (F) Profile at rest.

8 • Aligners in Extraction Cases   85

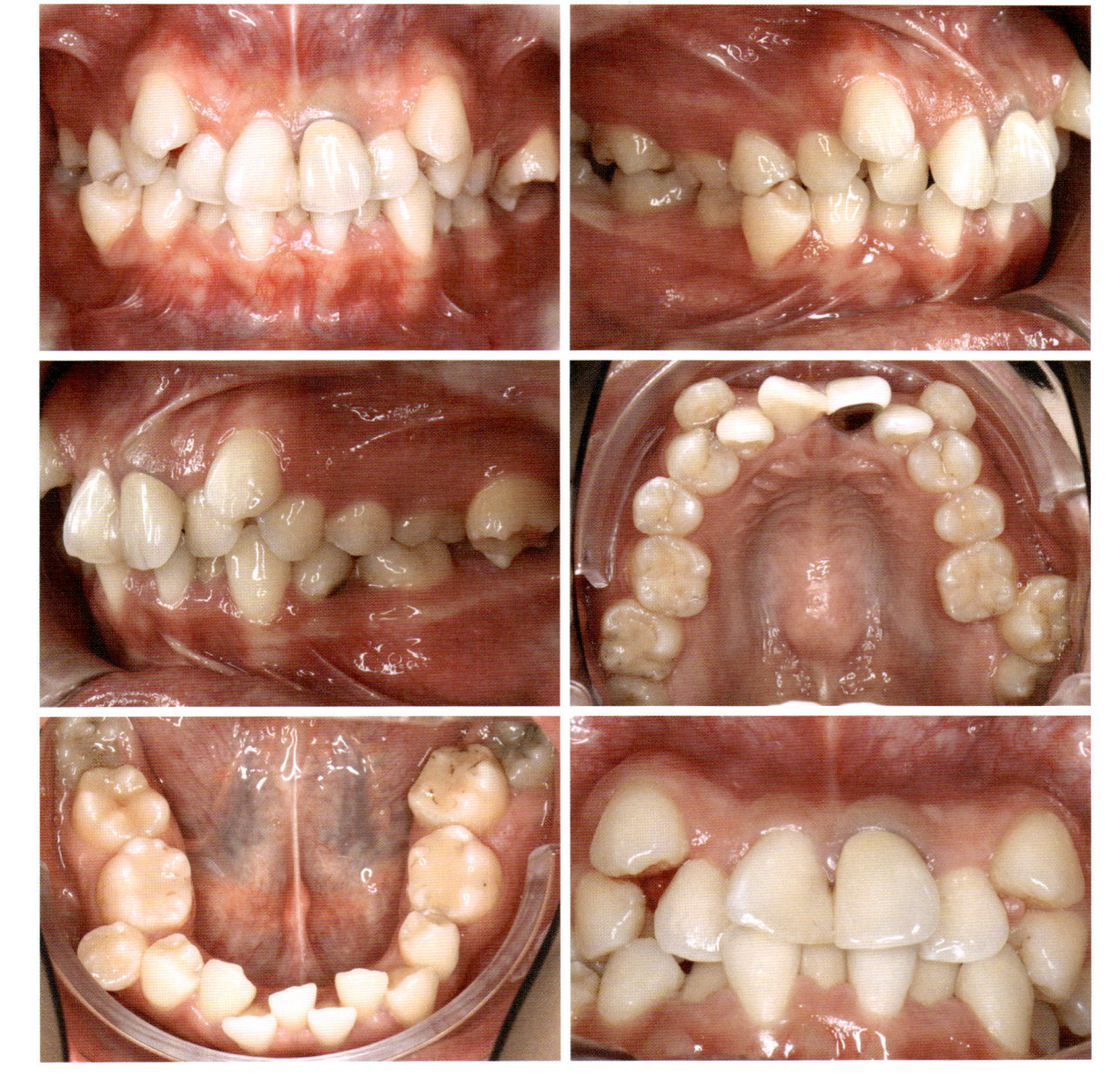

Fig. 8.2 Initial intraoral pictures.

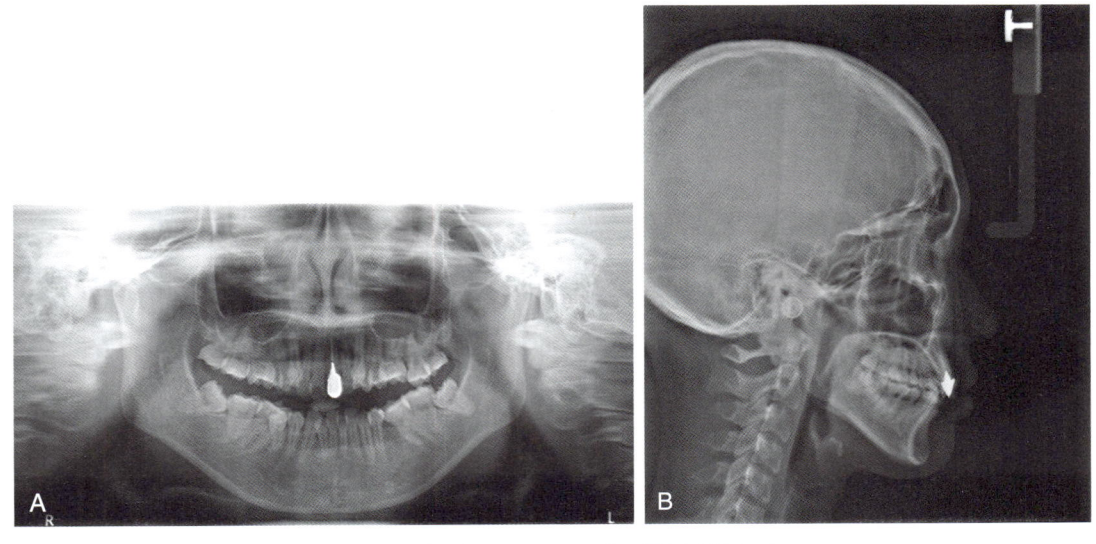

Fig. 8.3 (A) Initial orthopantomography. (B) Initial lateral x-ray.

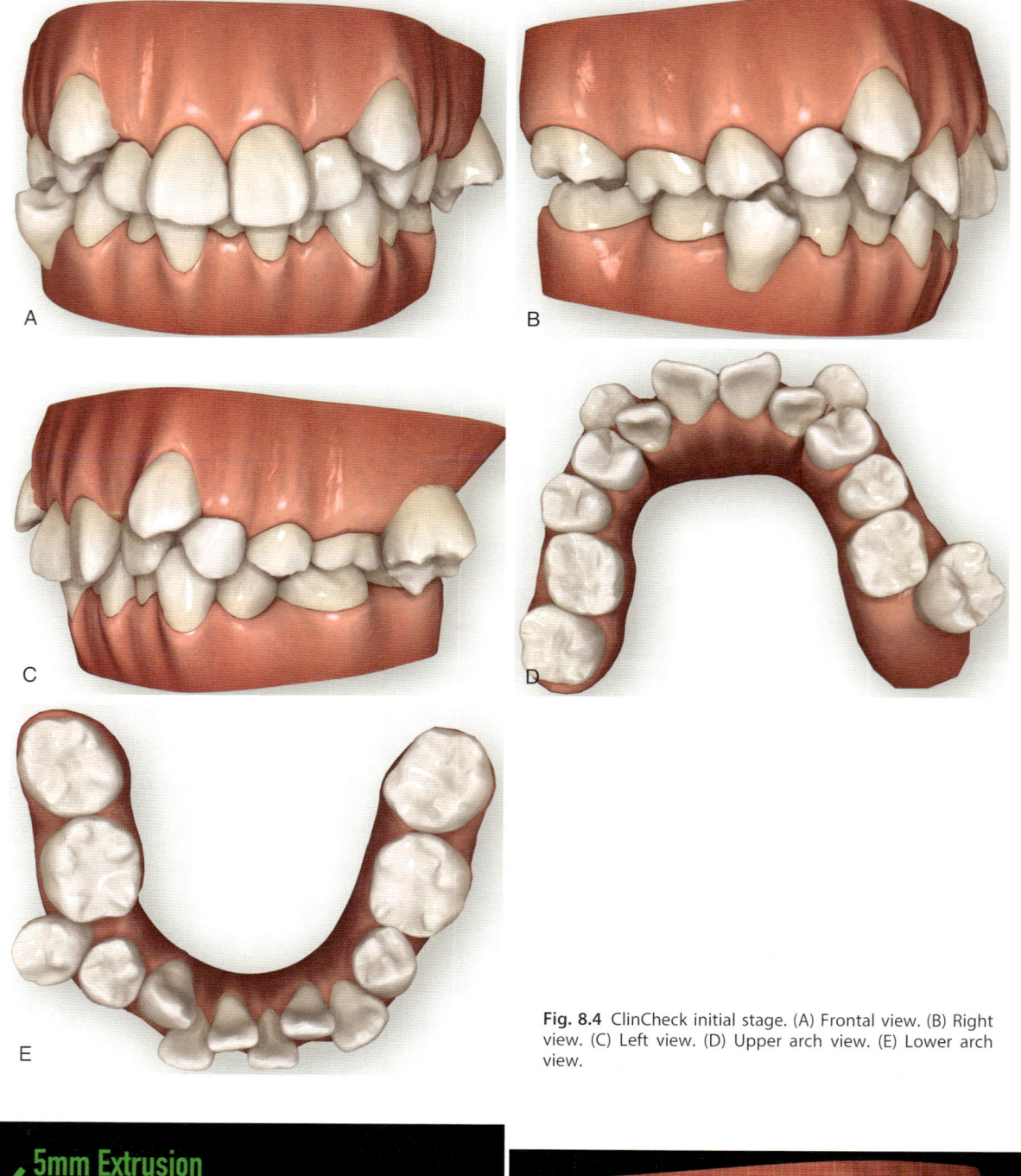

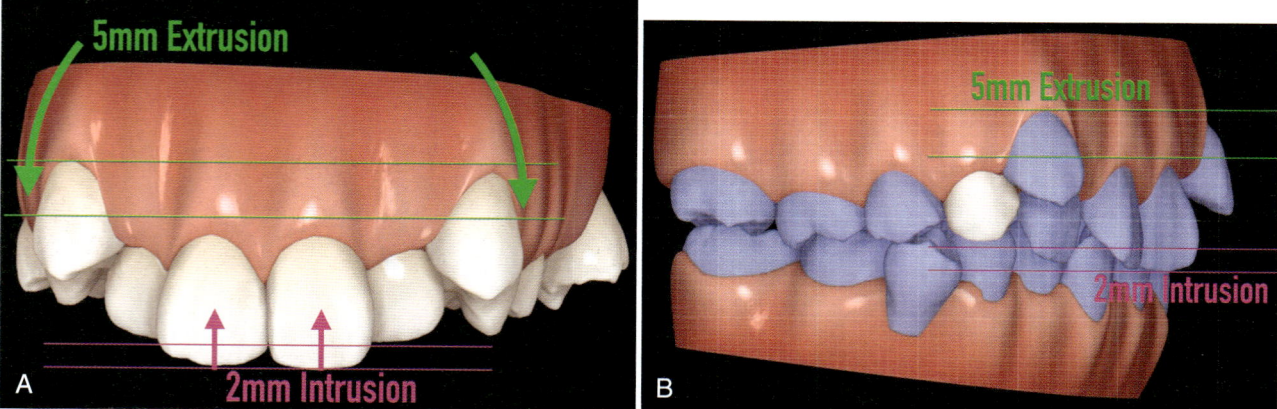

86 Principles and Biomechanics of Aligner Treatment

Fig. 8.4 ClinCheck initial stage. (A) Frontal view. (B) Right view. (C) Left view. (D) Upper arch view. (E) Lower arch view.

Fig. 8.5 Schematic representation of vertical orthodontic tooth movement design in the frontal plane (A). Amount of vertical movements for upper canines and central incisors (B).

space for the maxillary incisors by means of a panoramic x-ray. Since the mandibular extraction spaces were closed, we could use all the teeth from second premolar to second premolar, including the canines, as anchorage for the mesial movement of the lower first molars.

The aligner margins were trimmed about 3 mm to accommodate direct-bonded hooks on the upper first canines. Lingual buttons were bonded to the distobuccal edges of the lower first molars, and class II elastics (0.25 in, 6 oz) were prescribed to be worn 20 hours per day. To prevent the mesial tipping of the lower first molars, vertical rectangular attachments were added to their mesiobuccal edges (Fig. 8.6).

Improvement was seen in the anteroposterior relationship after use of the class II elastics, and a class I relationship was established in the buccal segments. The next phase involved the retraction of the upper anterior teeth. After 8 months of treatment, the first ClinCheck phase was finished (Figs. 8.7 and 8.8).

The distalization of the upper first molars was complete, with space visible at the mesial edge of the upper left first molar. The movement of the lower second premolars and canines had closed all the mandibular spaces.

The shapes and positions of the attachments were modified for the refinement phase. The crown positions were considered together with the root positions to decide the optimal conditions. After 9 months of treatment, the aligner compatibility and the crown and root positions were all consistent with the computer-simulated predictions (Figs. 8.9 and 8.10).

In the final stages of refinement, the occlusal contact of all upper and lower molars and a one-to-two-tooth occlusal relationship in the buccal segments were confirmed. Both the overbite and overjet were 1 mm.

After a total 10 months of treatment, all buttons, hooks, and attachments were removed (Fig. 8.11). The patient was instructed to wear class II elastics at night for an additional 10 months.

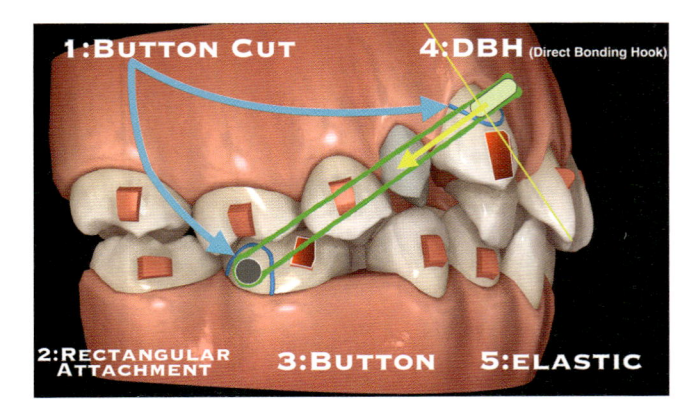

Treatment Results

The patient's chief complaint—the infralabioversion of the canines—was resolved, and the improvement in gingival esthetics yielded a pleasant smile (Figs. 8.12, 8.13, and 8.14). Due to the retraction of the maxillary incisors, the upper lip was particularly natural and relaxed, and the lips were positioned appropriately in relation to the E-line. A class I molar relationship with symmetric arches was achieved, and all spaces were closed (Fig. 8.15). The physiologically correct overbite and overjet were coincident with the dental and facial midlines.

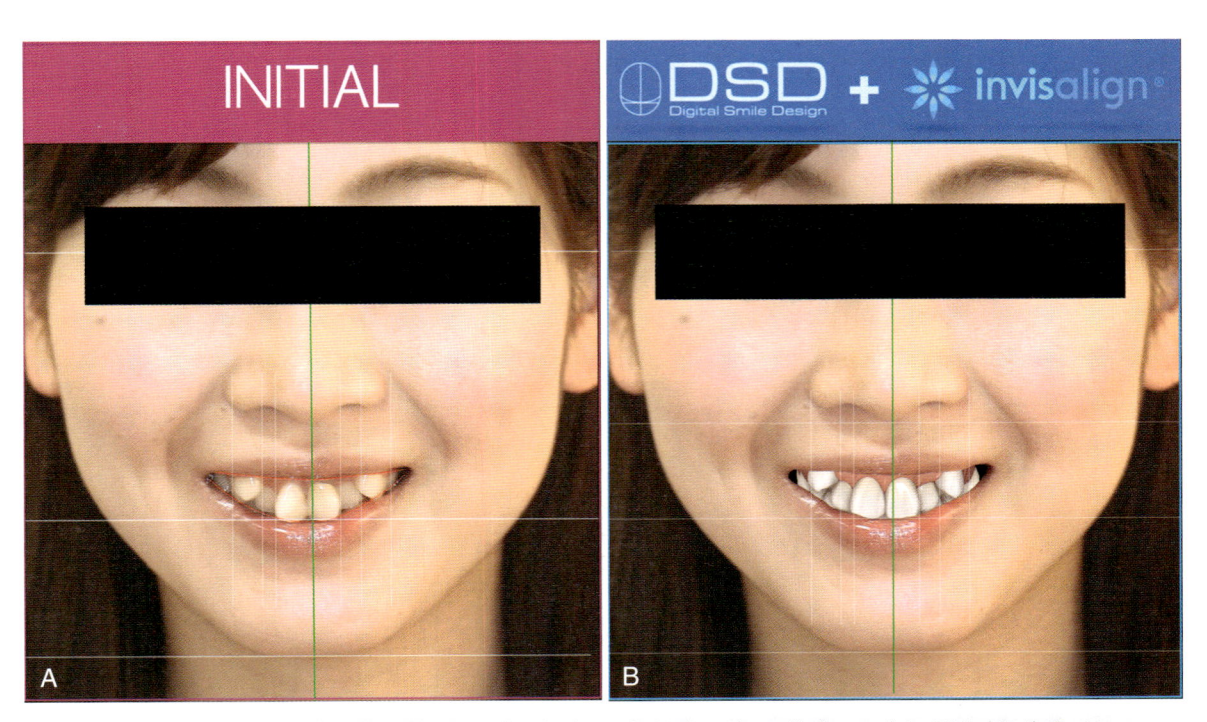

Fig. 8.6 Schematic representation of attachments and auxiliaries required in extraction cases.

Fig. 8.7 (A) Initial smile esthetic analysis. (B) ClinCheck simulation into the smile frame of the Digital Smile Design software.

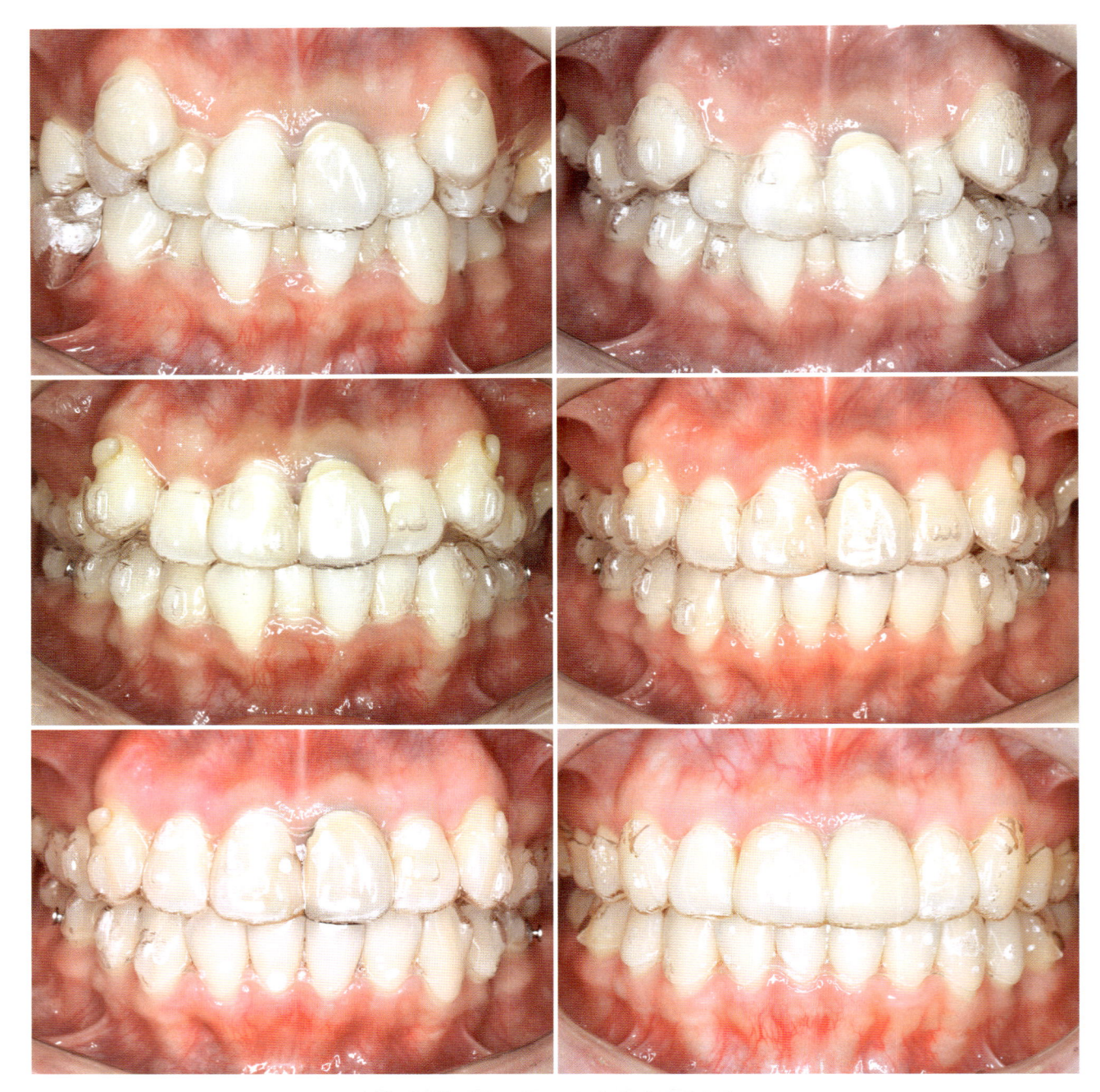

88 Principles and Biomechanics of Aligner Treatment

Fig. 8.8 Treatment progresses in the frontal view.

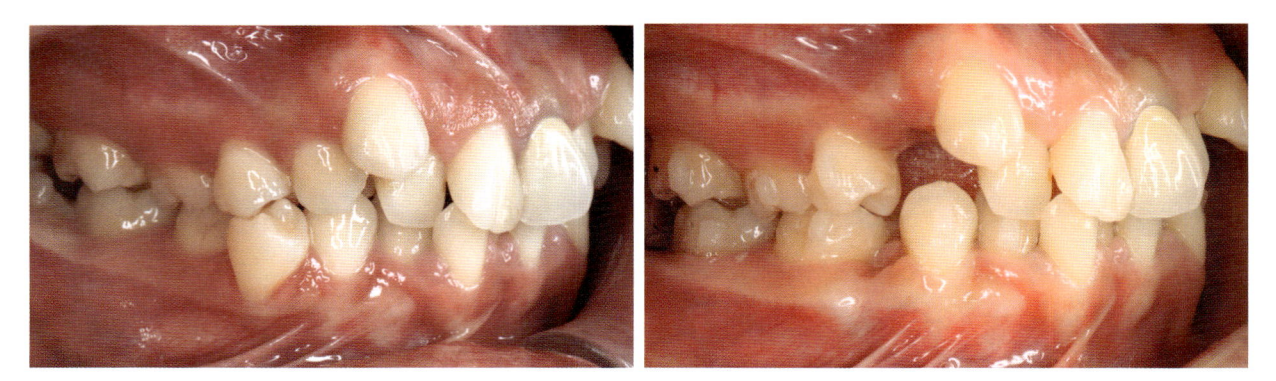

Fig. 8.9 Treatment progresses in the right view.

8 • Aligners in Extraction Cases 89

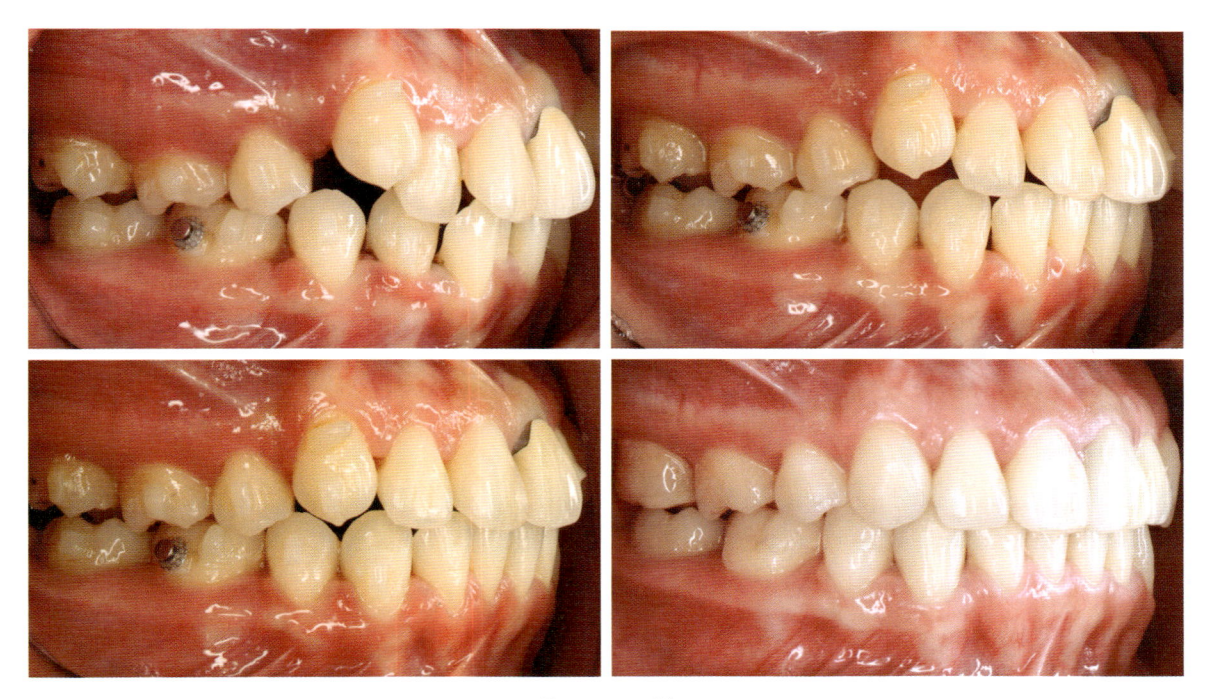

Fig. 8.9, cont'd

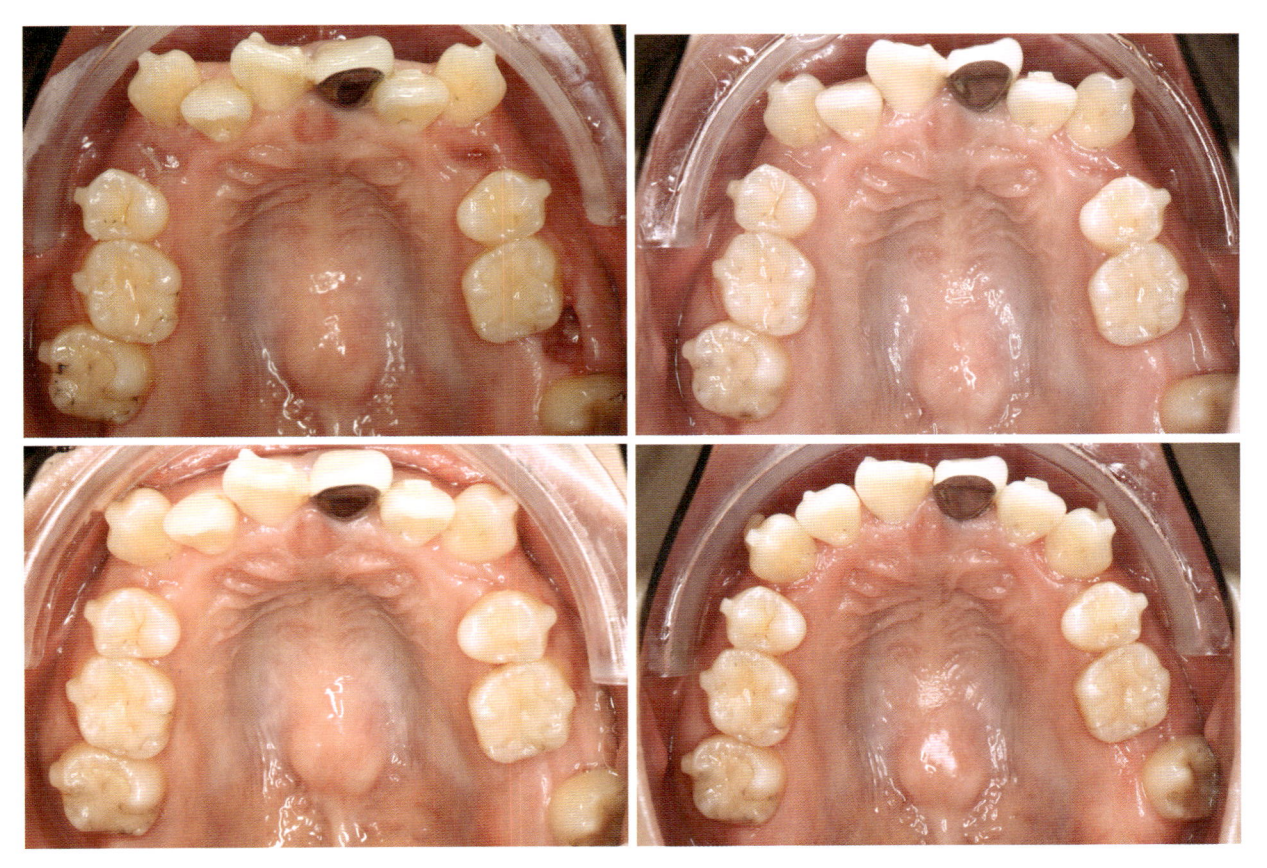

Fig. 8.10 Treatment progresses in the occlusal views.

Continued

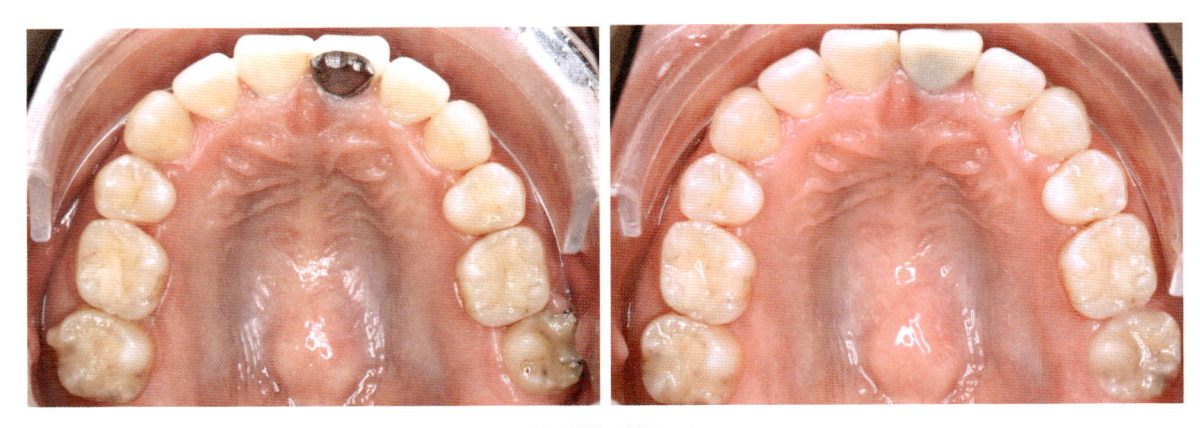

Principles and Biomechanics of Aligner Treatment

Fig. 8.10, cont'd

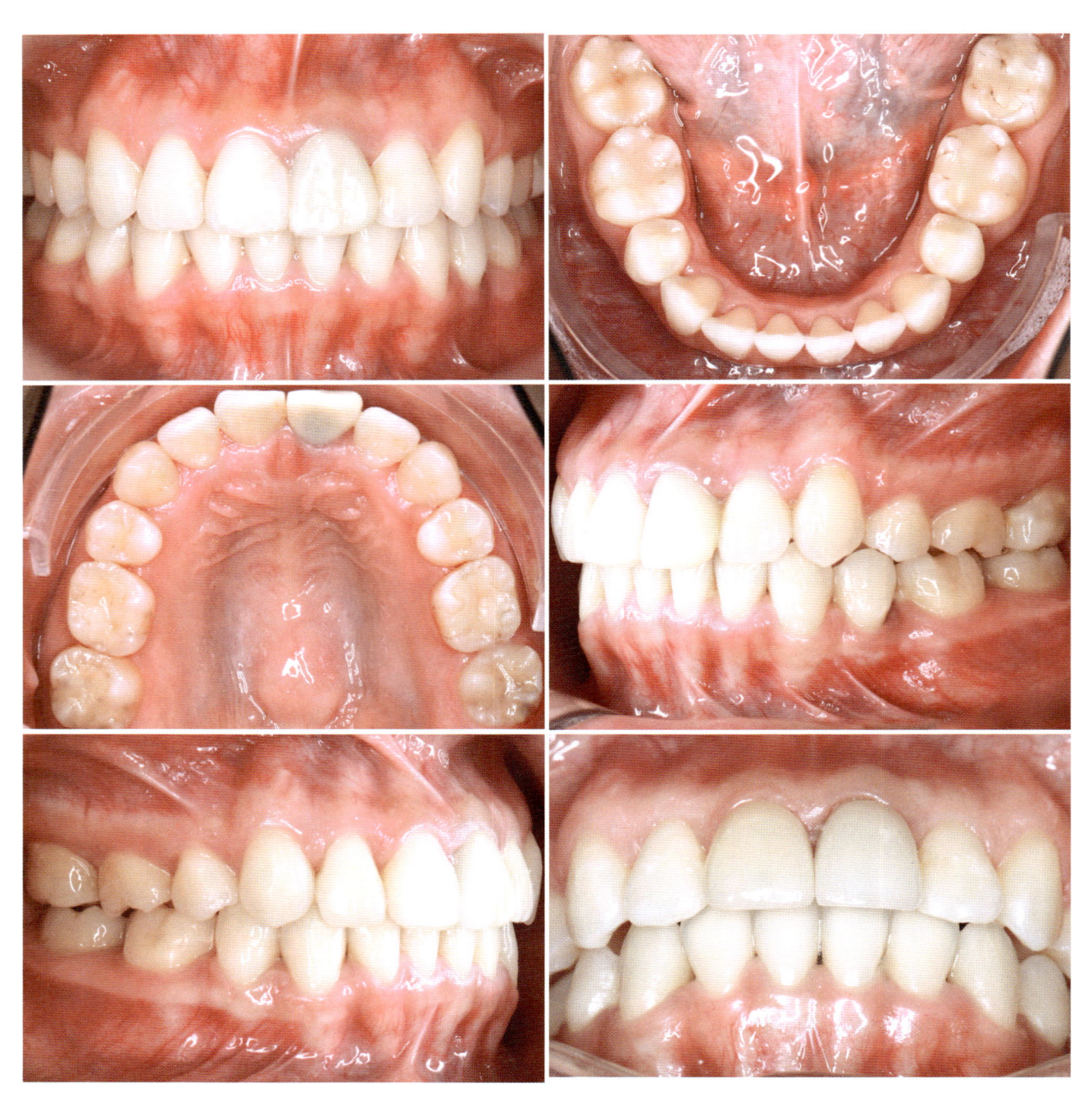

Fig. 8.11 Posttreatment pictures.

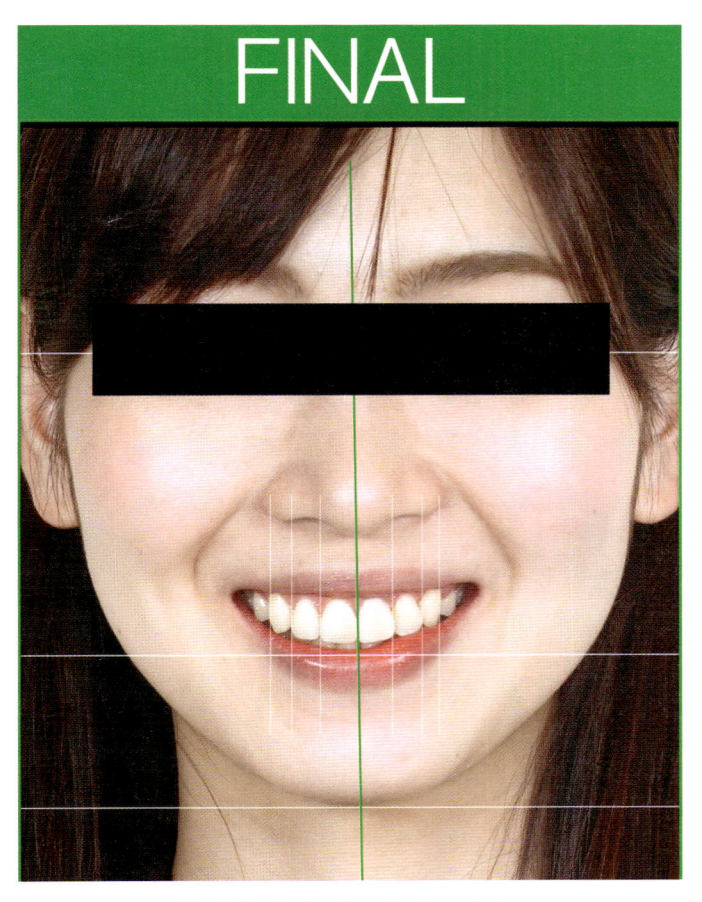

Fig. 8.12 Final smile esthetic analysis.

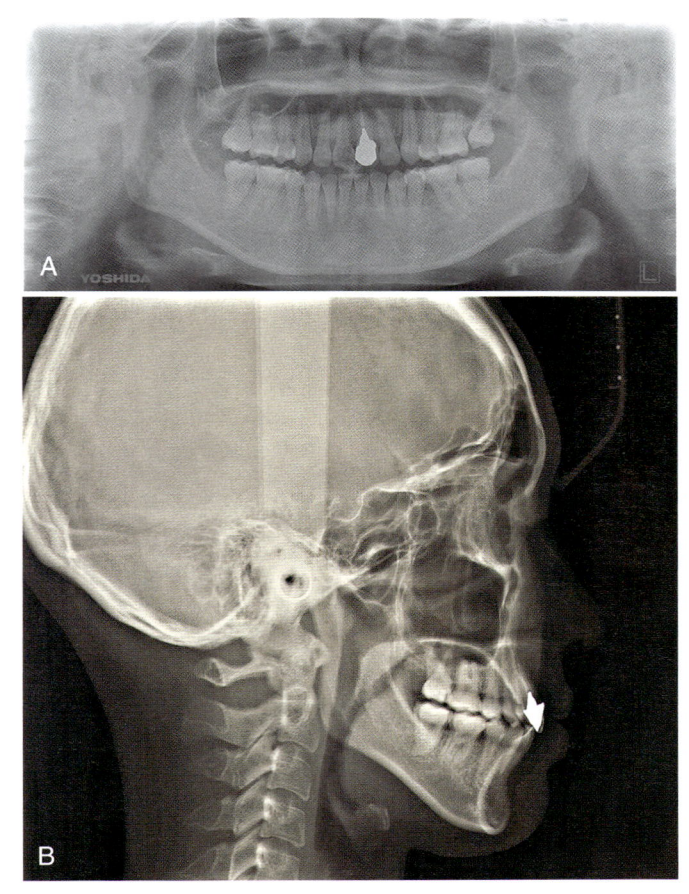

Fig. 8.13 (A) Final orthopantomography. (B) Final lateral x-ray.

The posttreatment protrusive and lateral movements of the mandible were smooth and linear. It is likely that the patient was using considerable force when biting in centric occlusion due to nervousness during the initial examination. Panoramic x-rays confirmed that there was no change in the level of the alveolar bone, which remained stable and in a healthy condition. No signs of root resorption were noted.

A cephalometric analysis indicated that the mandibular plane angle was slightly reduced. Superimpositions showed that while the upper and lower incisors were retruded, their axes were upright and closer to the norm.

Discussion

Aligners appeal to adults because of their pleasing aesthetics and their ability to produce gradual tooth movements with light forces over the course of time. The focus of previous reports has been on cases that did not require extractions or those with only partial extractions. This is perhaps due more to the difficulty of closing spaces without crown tipping than to the difficulty of moving teeth. When extraction spaces are closed with aligners, a bowing effect is often caused by the sagging of the plastic around the extraction sites. This effect can be prevented by using class II elastics to enhance intermaxillary anchorage. If an elastic is attached directly to an aligner, however, the plastic will separate from the teeth, making it more difficult to maintain control over mesial and distal tooth movements. In the case shown here, direct-bonded hooks were attached to the upper canines to allow the teeth to rotate both mesially and distally within the aligners, leaving a margin of more than 2 mm between the incisal edges and the aligners.

Rather than attach the elastics in the mandibular arch (which was serving as anchorage) directly to the aligners, they were attached to buttons on the buccal surfaces of the first molars. This kept the aligners from lifting off the teeth, while vertical rectangular attachments on the mesial edges of the molars prevented mesial angulation. This avoided the tipping of the teeth adjacent to the mandibular extraction sites.

Because the patient found the original predicted length of treatment unacceptable, OrthoPulse[33-35] was used in conjunction with the aligners to possibly accelerate treatment time. Despite the lack of published accounts of the effectiveness of this device beyond its application to fixed appliances, the patient was instructed to use it for 10 minutes every evening. We were able to shorten the interval between aligner changes to 3 days, resulting in a remarkable reduction in the treatment time to just

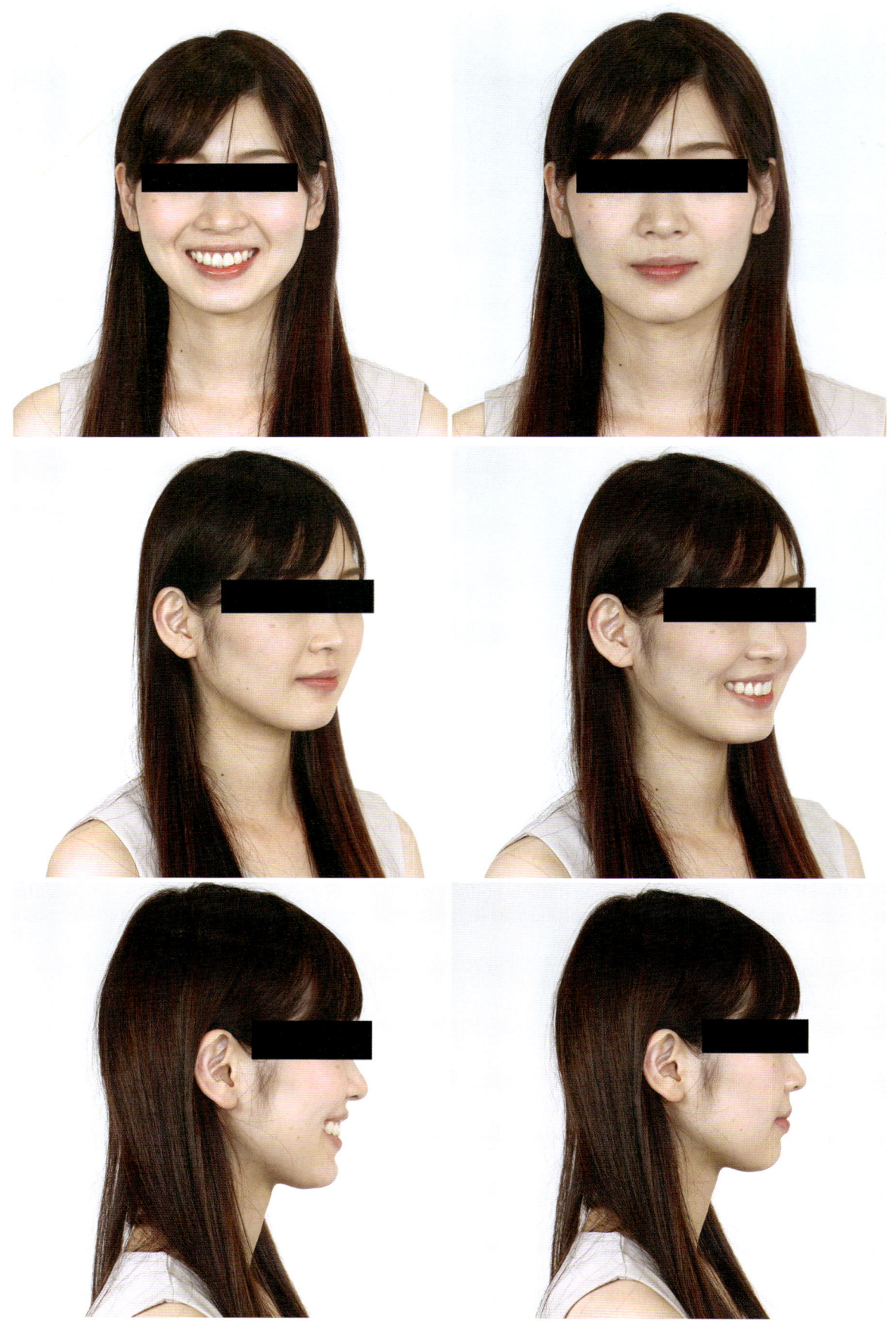

Fig. 8.14 Posttreatment extraoral pictures.

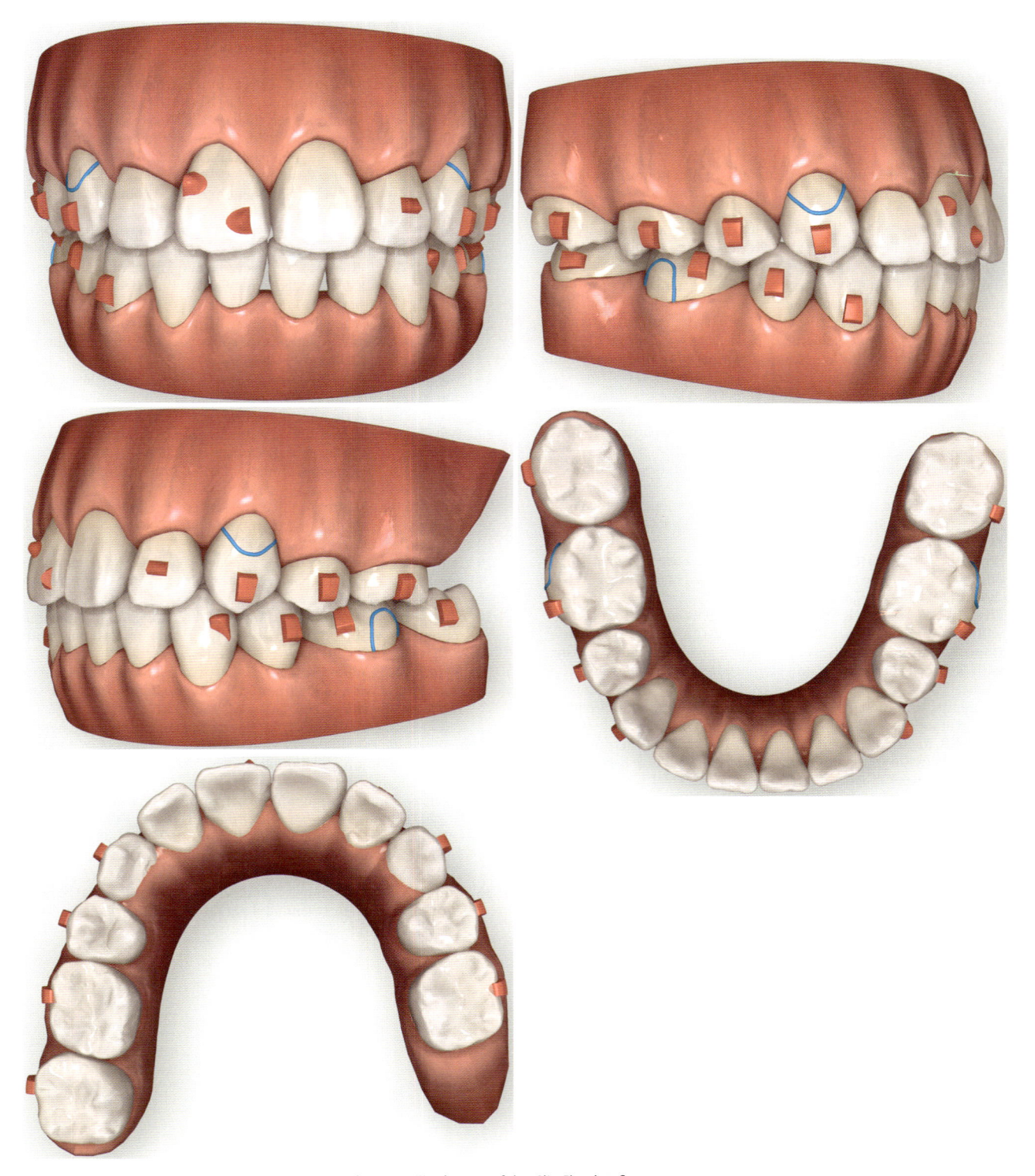

Fig. 8.15 Final stage of the ClinCheck refinement.

10 months. The patient experienced no discomfort from the OrthoPulse device or from the faster aligner changes. She finished treatment with no interferences in protrusive or lateral mandibular movements and no esthetic concerns.

Conclusion

Not only are aligners aesthetically pleasing to adult patients, but the ease with which they can be removed makes them extremely safe. In the future, aligners are likely to be used in more complex cases involving rotations, deep overbites, open bites, and unusual extractions. Further clinical investigations into the effects of accelerated tooth movement in such cases are required.

References

1. Vlaskalic V, Boyd, R. Orthodontic treatment of a mildly crowded malocclusion using the Invisalign system. *Austral Orthod J.* 2001;17:41-46.
2. Boyd RL, Miller RJ, Vlaskalic V. The Invisalign system in adult orthodontics: mild crowding and space closure cases. *J Clin Orthod.* 2000;34:203-212.
3. Giancotti A, Di Girolamo R. Treatment of severe maxillary crowding using Invisalign and fixed appliances. *J Clin Orthod.* 2009;43:583-589.
4. Schupp W, Haubrich J, Hermens E. M. glichkeiten und grenzen der schienentherapie in der kieferorthop. *die Zahnmed.* 2013:171-184.
5. Schupp W, Haubrich J, Neumann I. Treatment of anterior open bite with the Invisalign system. *J Clin Orthod.* 2010;44:501-507.
6. Guarneri MP, Oliverio T, Silvestre I, et al. Open bite treatment using clear aligners. *Angle Orthod.* 2013;83:913-919.
7. Krieger E, Seiferth J, Marinello I, et al. Invisalign treatment in the anterior region. *J Orofac Orthop.* 2012;73:365-376.
8. Giancotti A, Farina A. Treatment of collapsed arches using the Invisalign system. *J Clin Orthod.* 2010;44:416-425.
9. Sachan A, Chaturvedi TP. Orthodontic management of buccally erupted ectopic canine with two case reports. *Contemp Clin Dent.* 2012;3:123-128.
10. Boyd RL. Esthetic orthodontic treatment using the Invisalign appliance for moderate to complex malocclusions. *J Dent Educ.* 2008;72:948-967.
11. Castroflorio T, Garino F, Lazzaro A, et al. Upper-incisor root control with Invisalign appliances. *J Clin Orthod.* 2013;47:346-351.
12. Hahn W, Zapf A, Dathe H, et al. Torquing an upper central incisor with aligners: acting forces and biomechanical principles. *Eur J Orthod.* 2010;32:607-613.
13. Schupp W, Haubrich J, Neumann I. Invisalign treatment of patients with craniomandibular disorders. *Int Orthod.* 2010;8:253-267.
14. Miller KB, McGorray SP, Womack R, et al. A comparison of treatment impacts between Invisalign aligner and fixed appliance therapy during the first week of treatment. *Am J Orthod.* 2007;131:302e1-9.
15. Boyd RL. Complex orthodontic treatment using a new protocol for the Invisalign appliance. *J Clin Orthod.* 2007;41:525-547.
16. Vlaskalic V, Boyd RL. Clinical evolution of the Invisalign appliance. *J Calif Dent Assoc.* 2002;30:769-776.
17. Womack WR. Four-premolar extraction treatment with Invisalign. *J Clin Orthod.* 2006;40:493-500.
18. Ojima K, Dan C, Nishiyama R, et al. Accelerated extraction treatment with Invisalign. *J Clin Orthod.* 2014;8:487-499.
19. Bowman SJ, Celenza F, Sparaga J, et al. Creative adjuncts for clear aligners, part 3: extraction and interdisciplinary treatment. *J Clin Orthod.* 2015;49:249-262.
20. Fiorillo G, Festa F, Grassi C. Upper canine extraction in adult cases with unusual malocclusions. *J Clin Orthod.* 2012;46:102-110.
21. Domínguez A, Velásquez SA. Effect of low-level laser therapy on pain following activation of orthodontic final archwires: a randomized controlled clinical trial. *Photomed Laser Surg.* 2013;31:36-40.
22. Kau CH, Kantarci A, Shaughnessy T, et al. Photobiomodulation accelerates orthodontic alignment in the early phase of treatment. *Prog Orthod.* 2013;14:30.
23. Rojas JC, Gonzalez-Lima F. Low-level light therapy of the eye and brain. *Eye Brain.* 2011;3:49-67.
24. Eells JT, Wong-Riley MT, VerHoeve J, et al. Mitochondrial signal transduction in accelerated wound and retinal healing by near-infrared light therapy. *Mitochondrion.* 2004;4:559-567.
25. Watanabe H, Bohensky J, Freeman T, et al. Hypoxic induction of UCP3 in the growth plate: UCP3 suppresses chondrocyte autophagy. *J Cell Physiol.* 2008;216:419-425.
26. Masha RT, Houreld NN, Abrahamse H. Low-intensity laser irradiation at 660 nm stimulates transcription of genes involved in the electron transport chain. *Photomed Laser Surg.* 2013;31:47-53.
27. Wakabayashi H, Hamba M, Matsumoto K, et al. Effect of irradiation by semiconductor laser on responses evoked in trigeminal caudal neurons by tooth pulp stimulation. *Laser Surg Med.* 1993;13:605-610.
28. Kawasaki K, Shimizu N. Effects of low-energy laser irradiation on bone remodeling during experimental tooth movement in rats. *Laser Surg Med.* 2000;26:282-291.
29. Santiwong P., de la Fuente A, Skrenes D, et al. Photobiomodulation accelerates orthodontic alignment in the early phase of treatment. *Prog Orthod.* 2013;14:30.
30. Shaughnessy T, Kantarci A, Kau CH, et al. Intraoral photobiomodulation-induced orthodontic tooth alignment: a preliminary study. *BMC Oral Health.* 2016;16:3.
31. Nahas AZ, Samara SA, Rastegar-Lari TA. Decrowding of lower anterior segment with and without photobiomodulation: a single center, randomized clinical trial. *Lasers Med Sci.* 2017;32:129-135.
32. Carvalho-Lobato P, Garcia VJ, Kasem K, et al. Tooth movement in orthodontic treatment with low-level laser therapy: a systematic review of human and animal studies. *Photomed Laser Surg.* 2014;32:302-309.
33. Ojima K, Dan C, Kumagai Y, et al. Invisalign treatment accelerated by photobiomodulation. *J Clin Orthod.* 2016;50:309-317.
34. Ojima K, Dan C, Kumagai Y, et al. Upper molar distalization with Invisalign treatment accelerated by photobiomodulation. *J Clin Orthod.* 2018;52(12):675-683.
35. Ojima K, Dan C, Kumagai Y, et al. Accelerated extraction treatment with the Invisalign system and photobiomodulation. *J Clin Orthod.* 2020;54(3):151-158.

9 Open-Bite Treatment with Aligners

ALDO GIANCOTTI and GIANLUCA MAMPIERI

In recent years, aligners have shown to be an extraordinary and effective tool to correct open-bite cases. Such unexpected results make them the gold standard in the treatment of malocclusions characterized by vertical excess as in open-bite cases. Open bite is challenging to treat for its multifactorial etiology and for high incidence of relapse.

The aim of this chapter is to show strategies and protocols for the treatment of anterior open bite by clear aligners.

Diagnosis of Anterior Open Bite

Obviously, a proper diagnosis is essential in determining the appropriate corrective measures. It is possible to classify three types of open bite:

1. Dental
2. Dentoskeletal
3. Skeletal

Generally, skeletal open bite requires an orthosurgical approach. Instead, dental and dentoskeletal open-bite cases can be treated only by means of orthodontics.[1,2]

Biomechanics for Anterior Open-Bite Correction

The biomechanics for anterior open-bite correction can be achieved either by extruding the incisors or intruding the posterior teeth, or by a combination of both. For the nonsurgical treatment of adult patients, some guidelines consider extraction and retraction for dental open-bite correction.[3] A limited number of open-bite cases is suitable for such type of treatment.

Dental open-bite cases are mostly associated with the following characteristics:

- Normal craniofacial pattern
- Incisor proclination
- Undererupted anterior teeth
- Little or no gingival display on smile
- No more than 2 to 3 mm of upper incisor exposure at rest

If the anterior open bite depends only on tooth position, it is a relative open bite; the biomechanics for the correction are easy, as follows:

- Reducing incisor proclination to produce a relative extrusion
- Pure extrusion of incisors by extrusive attachments

The amount of incisal and gingival display needs to be assessed clinically prior to deciding if pure extrusion is desired from a smile esthetics point of view.

When dentoskeletal factors are important in determining the cause of open bite, it is often caused by posterior dentoalveolar excess as well as by both downward and backward mandibular rotation.[4-10] These types of open bite with a skeletal component caused by heredity and/or supererupted posterior teeth require complex orthodontic treatments with active molar intrusion or even major orthognathic surgery.[3,11]

In case of a dentoskeletal open bite, specific procedures have been designed to intrude posterior teeth or, at least, prevent molar eruption or extrusion in the attempt to reduce or control anterior facial height, especially during the growing age (high-pull headgear, lower transpalatal arch with resin button, and posterior bite blocks). The introduction of temporary anchorage devices (TADs) has allowed an active intrusion of posterior teeth also in adult patients with a consequent mandibular counterclockwise rotation and improvement of anterior open bite.

Extraction of posterior teeth is another strategic approach to correct anterior open bite. Indeed, when indicated, molar extraction for caries or periodontal reasons could be highly effective in reducing facial height. Forward movement of the terminal molars allows the mandible to hinge upward and forward. It has been postulated that 1 mm of intrusive vertical movement of the molars results in approximately 2 to 3 mm of bite closure by mandibular counterclockwise rotation.[12]

In the treatment of a dentoskeletal open-bite case, one shall observe some biomechanical principles. Any procedure meant to increase facial height by means of extrusion of posterior teeth must be avoided. Leveling the arches is usually not to be considered appropriate, and the maintenance or creation of a curve of Spee would be desirable. Furthermore, banding of second molars should be avoided to prevent any extrusion movement when molars are engaged on the arch wire.[13]

The abovementioned scenario can be easily avoided by using aligners, which allow for nonextrusion and represent a great advantage during open-bite treatment. This is why a number of researchers consider aligners as the gold standard.[14]

Aligner Protocols for Open-Bite Treatment

CLINCHECK SOFTWARE DESIGN

The clear aligner treatment of open-bite cases depends on the type of malocclusion requiring correction, and specific biomechanics have to be requested by checking the appropriate boxes on the prescription form of the ClinCheck software program to generate a predictable ClinCheck plan.

Dental open bite, also known as relative open bite, clinically features excessive incisor proclination; it can be treated only by reducing incisor proclination, producing a relative extrusion of anterior teeth. For these movements, attachments are not strictly required.

The first step consists of recovering the needed space in both arches. Space can be gained by arch expansion and/or interproximal reduction (IPR). The decision depends on the shape of the arches, tooth dimension, periodontal structure, and condition. Aligners can easily modify the shape of the arch, and it is later possible to retract the incisors obtaining enough relative extrusion in mild open bite to solve the issue.

ATTACHMENTS IN OPEN-BITE CORRECTION

In case of more severe dental open bites, anterior teeth extrusion can be strategic. Undoubtedly, extrusion is the most difficult movement to reproduce with aligners. In such conditions, attachments play an important role to determine tooth extrusion. Attachments and anchorage optimized anterior extrusive attachments are automatically placed on the incisors by the software when pure extrusion of 0.5 mm or more is detected (Figs. 9.1 and 9.2). Conventional extrusion attachments have a rectangular shape with beveled edge toward the gingiva to allow for optimal pressure from the aligner and then achieve proper extrusion (Fig. 9.3). These attachments could be positioned also on the palatal surface if aesthetic reasons are a priority (Fig. 9.4). Our experience suggests that the use of rectangular-shaped attachments with beveled edge toward the gingiva with the largest possible dimensions in relation to the incisor and most incisal possible allowed for an optimal control of relative and absolute incisor extrusion.

Anchorage attachments can have different shapes and dimensions, according to the type and/or number of teeth involved.

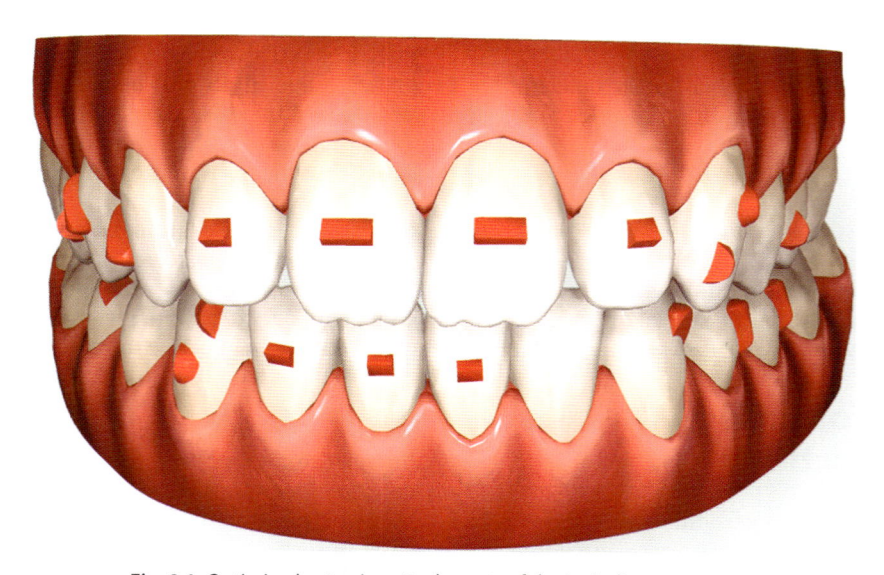

Fig. 9.1 Optimized extrusive attachments of the Invisalign system.

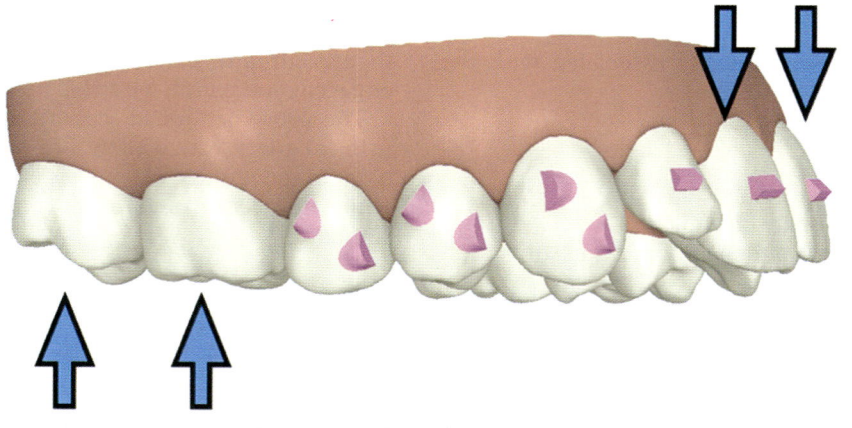

Fig. 9.2 The anterior extrusive forces and reciprocal posterior intrusive forces work in synergy to correct the anterior open bite.

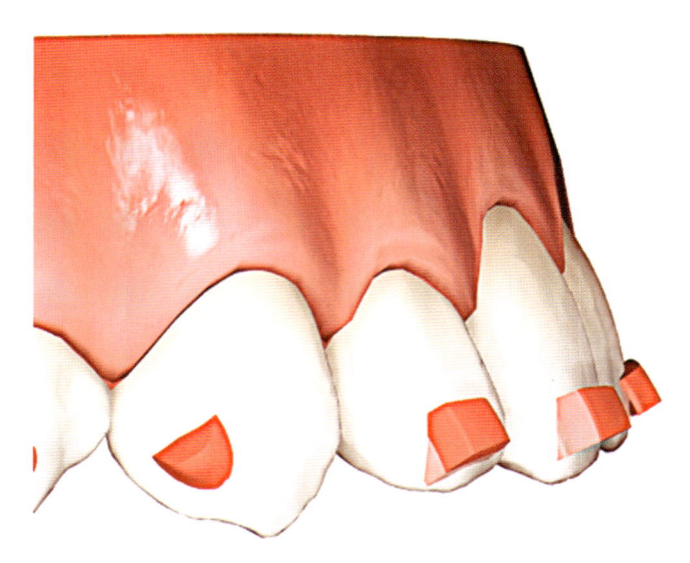

Fig. 9.3 Rectangular shape attachments with beveled edge toward gingiva.

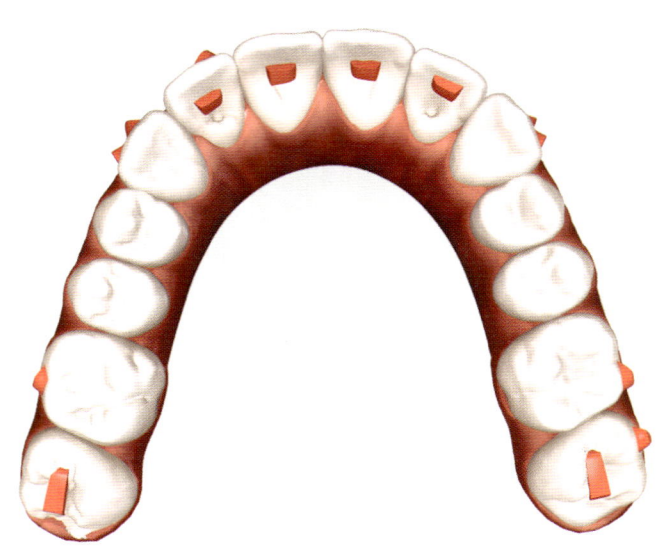

Fig. 9.4 Palatal attachments and occlusal attachments on upper molars.

The dentoskeletal open-bite treatment complies to a more complex protocol to correct the malocclusion. Indeed, in this type of open bite, the skeletal structure shows a dentoalveolar posterior vertical excess, which is responsible for an increased lower facial height.

For this reason, anterior tooth extrusion alone is not enough for correction, and one shall reduce the posterior vertical excess by dental intrusion.

Posterior dental intrusion results in a mandibular counterclockwise rotation mainly responsible for the open bite's correction, which can be verified by final cephalometric values. The anterior extrusive forces and reciprocal posterior intrusive forces work in synergy to close the anterior open bite (see Fig. 9.2).

The amount of posterior intrusion may range from less than 0.5 mm to a maximum of 1.0 mm. Beyond the range of predictability for aligner movements, it may be necessary to use TADs.

Molar intrusion can be planned with aligners, and therefore we define it as selective intrusion. The first and second molars in the upper arch and first molars and bicuspids in the lower arch are involved in the plan. The protocol related to attachment placement for anchorage usually envisages rectangular attachments on the molars and optimized ones on bicuspids. As for intrusion teeth, the official Invisalign protocol does not include the use of attachments. Some experienced clinicians prefer to add occlusal rectangular attachments to increase intrusive components and thus increase effectiveness (see Fig. 9.4).

In more severe open-bite malocclusions, some clinicians prefer to stage posterior intrusion sequentially for a more predictable clinical outcome: first the maxillary second molars, then the first molars, and then the second premolars.[15]

An important aspect to make predictable planning with aligners is to design an overcorrection. In the ClinCheck we have to see the final virtual occlusion with heavy anterior occlusal contacts and at least 2 mm of positive overbite.

Our point of view concerning dental intrusion is that the most important effect of aligners in reducing posterior vertical excess is the bite-block effect, which is caused by two layers of aligner material between posterior teeth.[14] It allows to effectively intrude posterior teeth, hence enabling subsequent autorotation of the mandible and reducing anterior facial height.

The bite-block effect cannot be quantitatively priorly planned or displayed in the virtual digital setup by ClinCheck, but we can routinely observe it clinically, especially in patients with a normal or larger mandible.

In final, to guarantee the maintenance of the result over time, it is essential to use Vivera, the clear retainer produced by Align, because the posterior occlusal coverage will prevent the reeruption of posterior teeth.

Case Report 1

CASE SUMMARY

A 29-year-old female patient presented a severe crowding, an unpleasant smile, as well as speech issues. Clinical extraoral examination showed a convex skeletal soft tissue profile due to a retrognathic mandible and incompetent lips at rest with mentalis and lip strain when the lips were pursed together. Intraoral examination evidenced class II canine and class I molar relationship on both sides, an anterior open bite, an excessive incisor proclination, and crowding on both arches (Fig. 9.5; Table 9.1).

Cephalometric analysis showed increased mandibular plane angle and increased lower anterior facial height (see Table 9.6 later). Posterior maxillary dentoalveolar heights were defined as excessive (Fig. 9.6).

Fig. 9.5 Case Study 1: Initial clinical records.

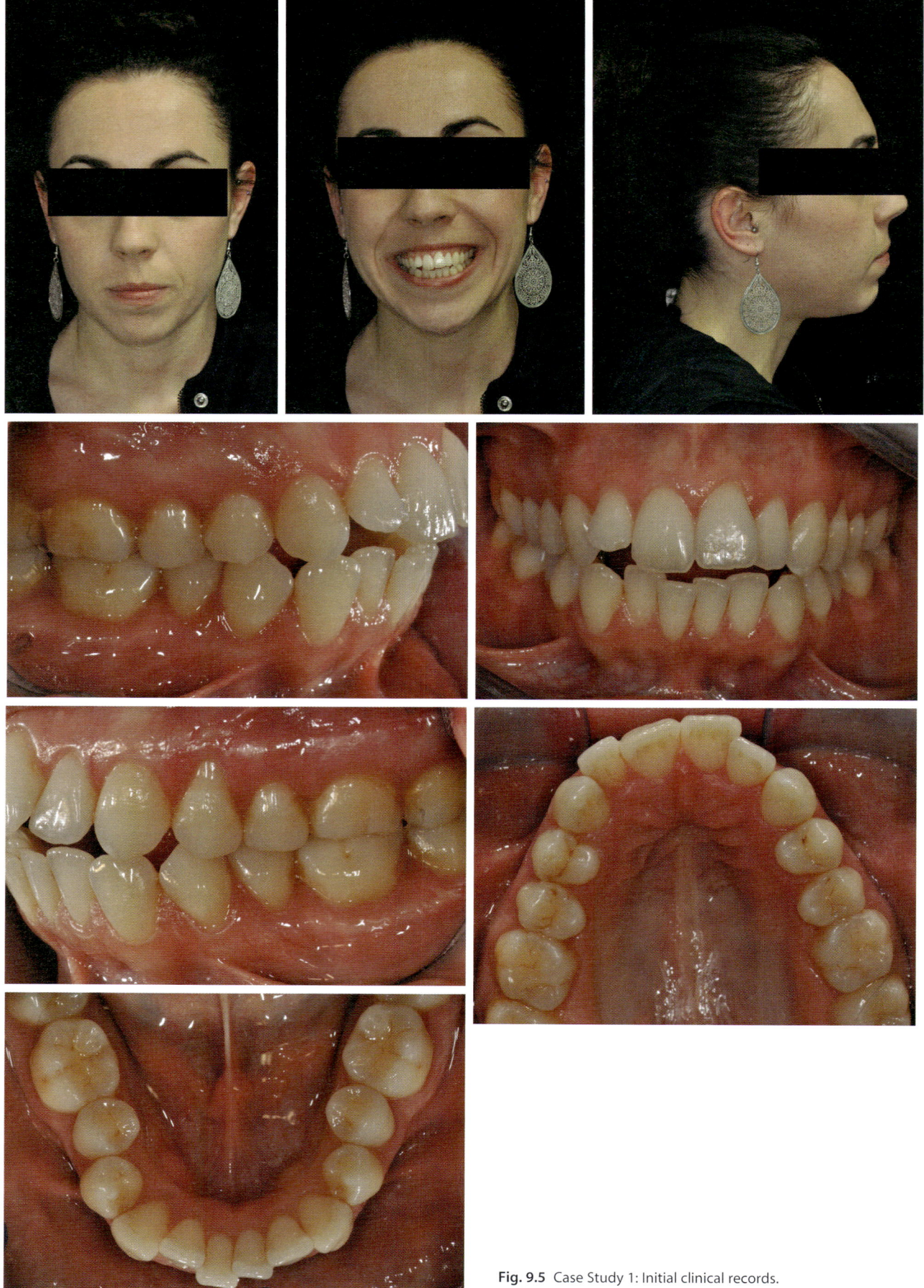

PROBLEM LIST

Table 9.1 Case Study 1: Problem List

Dimension	Skeletal	Dental	Soft Tissue
Anteroposterior	- Convex skeletal profile due to retrognathic mandible - Skeletal class II	- Class II canine relationship - Excessive incisor proclination	- Retrusive lower lip and chin
Vertical	- Increased lower anterior facial height - Increased mandibular plane angle - Increased maxillary posterior dentoalveolar heights	- Overbite: -3 mm - Narrow upper arch	- Mentalis muscle strain at rest - Incompetent lips
Transverse		- Narrow upper and lower arch	

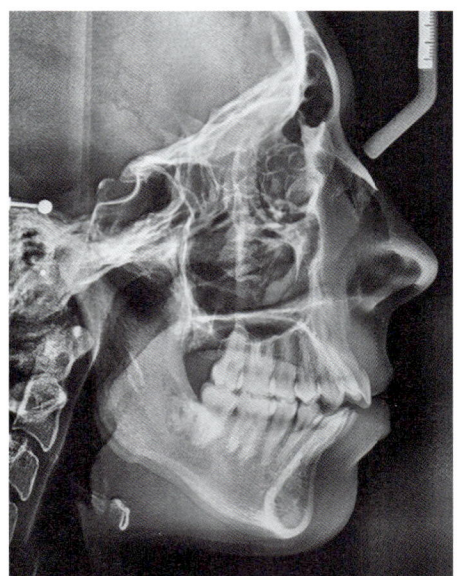

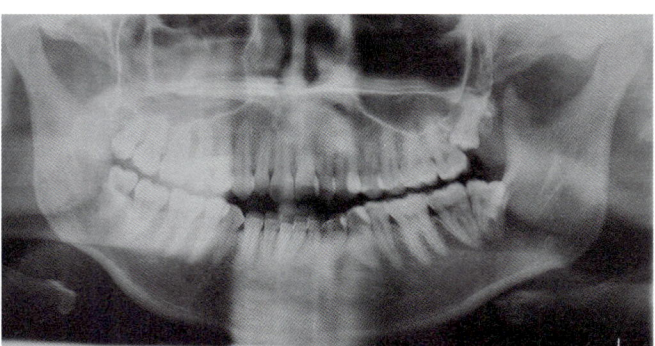

Fig. 9.6 Case Study 1: Pretreatment x-ray records.

TREATMENT OBJECTIVES

The main treatment objectives were to close the anterior open bite, obtain class I canine relationships, correct the excessive incisor proclination, and improve smile arc (Table 9.2).

TREATMENT PLAN

The treatment of dentoskeletal open bite requires closure of anterior open bite through a combination of retraction and extrusion of the upper incisors and by intrusion of posterior maxillary dentition to enable subsequent autorotation of the mandible with an improvement of vertical and sagittal relationship.

Additional treatment goals included leveling and aligning, optimizing the posterior occlusion, aiming at class I canine relationships, as well as ideal overbite and overjet to improve the facial profile and obtain natural lip competence without mentalis strain.

TREATMENT ALTERNATIVES

The treatment alternatives consisted of the following:

1. Orthosurgical treatment, including a LeFort I osteotomy with posterior maxillary impaction
2. Conventional treatment with intrusion of the posterior maxillary dentition by using TADs for skeletal anchorage
3. Extraction treatment to reduce the vertical dimension while easing reduction of the anterior protrusion and mandibular crowding

TREATMENT SEQUENCE

Correction was achieved by means of the expansion of the upper arch by 4 mm that allowed tooth alignment and the correction of upper incisor proclination. In the lower arch, molar and premolar torque was corrected. The optimized attachments on cuspids and first bicuspids in the upper arch were programmed to perform the anchorage unit necessary

Table 9.2 Case Study 1: Treatment Objectives

Dimension	Skeletal	Dental	Soft Tissue
Anteroposterior	■ Reduce skeletal convexity with autorotation of the mandible	■ Improve class II canine relationship by autorotation of the mandible	■ Improve soft tissue profile
Vertical	■ Reduce lower facial height and mandibular plane angle by intruding the maxillary and mandibular posterior teeth and autorotating the mandible	■ Improve anterior overbite and smile arc by intruding upper posterior teeth and maintaining the vertical position of the anterior teeth.	■ Reduce interlabial gap ■ Improve the profile by intruding maxillary dentoalveolar sites. ■ Achieve lip closure without activation of mentalis muscles
Transverse		■ Expand upper and lower arch	

to achieve the required reduction of incisor proclination gaining enough space by means of IPR and arch expansion. Intrusion of posterior teeth determined by aligners would have favored a counterclockwise rotation of the mandible, thus promoting the anterior open-bite correction (Fig. 9.7). Open-bite correction occurred by means of a first phase of 25 aligners and a finishing stage including 12 aligners. In addition, the expansion, together with the correction of the tipping of cuspids and bicuspids, allowed for coordination of both arches and a slight mesial mandibular repositioning with an optimization of the occlusal relationships and correction of class II canine malocclusion.

TREATMENT RESULTS

After 12 months of therapy, treatment objectives set in the pretreatment plan were achieved. The anterior open bite had been completely closed, a proper overbite and overjet had been corrected, and class I canine relationship had been established (Fig. 9.8).

The extraoral records show an evident improvement in the patient's smile. The pre- and posttreatment cephalometric showed 2 mm of intrusion of the upper molars determined by aligners. Such dental movement resulted in a mandibular counterclockwise rotation mainly responsible for the closure of the anterior open bite and the reduction of vertical skeletal values in the final cephalometric assessment. Caused by two layers of aligner material between the posterior teeth, molar intrusion is identified by clinicians as the bite-block effect and enables not only the correction of anterior open bite by means of the mandible's counterclockwise rotation, but also an improvement of the class II relationship, thanks to mandibular repositioning (Fig. 9.9; Table 9.3).

Follow-up after 24 months showed the great stability of the results ensured by means of Vivera retainers. The use of aligners for retention provides a long-term posterior intrusive

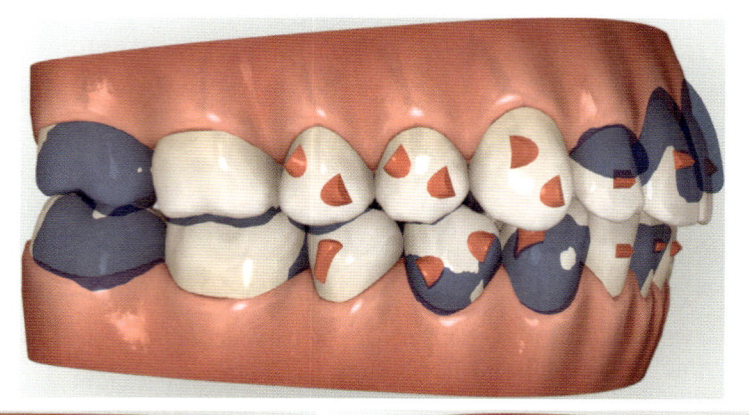

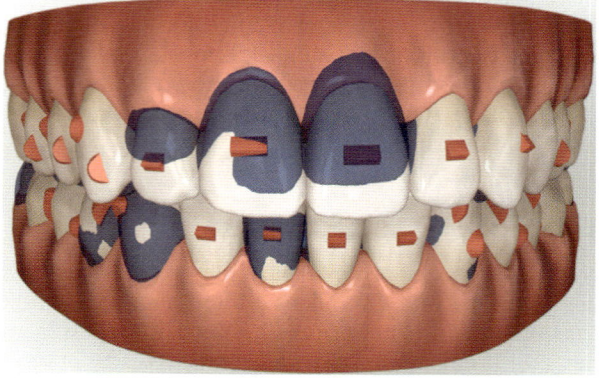

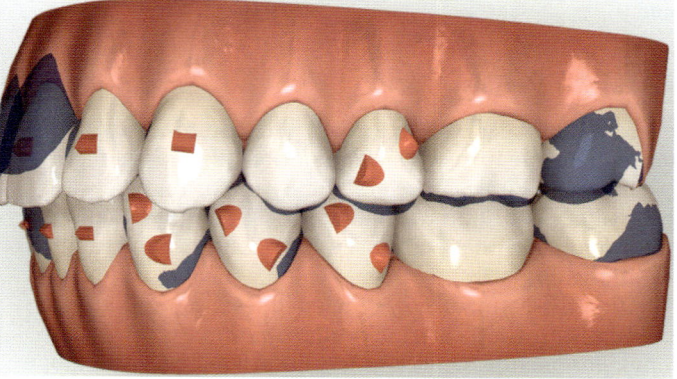

Fig. 9.7 Case Study 1: Pre- and post-ClinCheck superimposition.

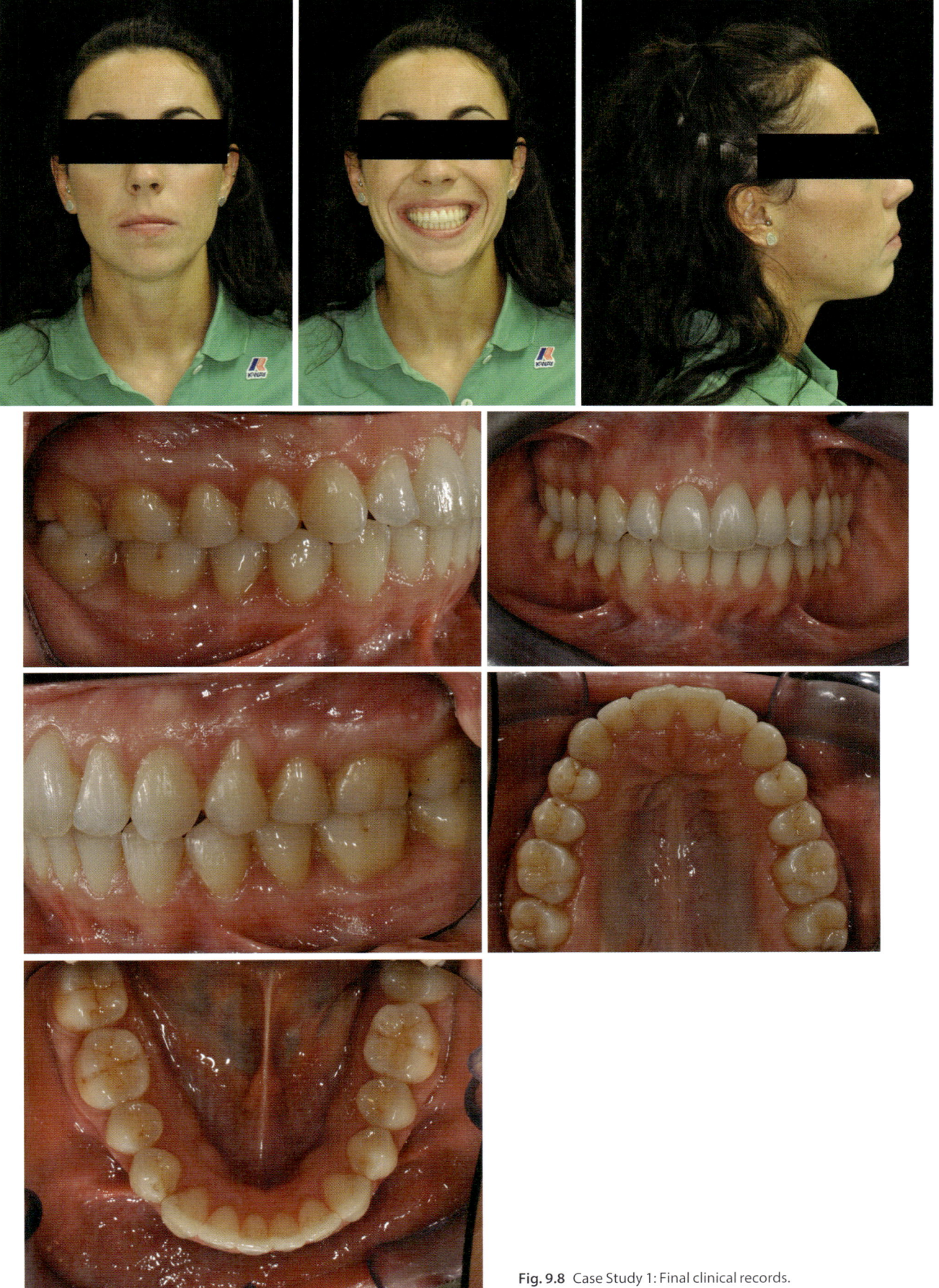

9 • Open-Bite Treatment with Aligners   101

Fig. 9.8 Case Study 1: Final clinical records.

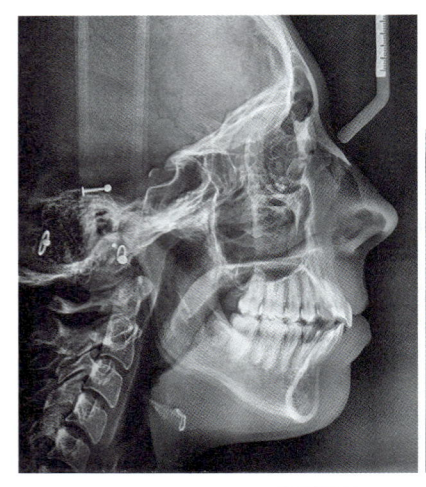

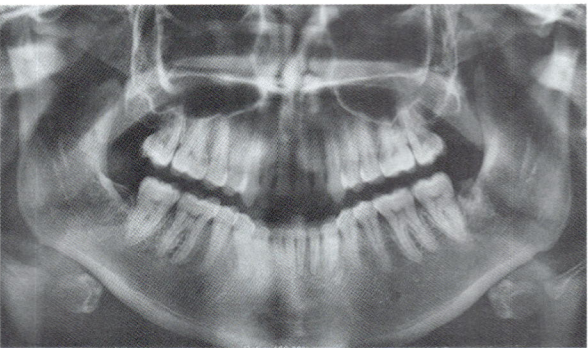

Fig. 9.9 Case Study 1: Posttreatment x-ray records.

Table 9.3 Case Study 1: Summary of Cephalometric Changes

Cephalometric Morphologic Assessment	Mean SD	Pretreatment	Posttreatment
SAGITTAL SKELETAL RELATIONS			
Maxillary position S-N-A	82° ± 3.5	72°	74°
Mandibular position S-N-B	80° ± 3.5	66°	69°
Sagittal jaw relation A-N-B	2° ± 2.5	6°	5°
VERTICAL SKELETAL RELATIONS			
Maxillary Inclination S-N/ANS-PNS	8° ± 3.0	14°	14°
Mandibular inclination S-N/GO-GN	33° ± 2.5	46°	42°
Vertical jaw relation ANS-PNS/GO-GN	25° ± 6.0	30°	29°
DENTOBASAL RELATIONS			
Maxillary incisor inclination 1/ANS-PNS	110° ± 6.0°	119°	106°
Mandibular incisor inclination 1/Gog-Me	90° ± 5.0°	97°	96°
Mandibular incisor compensation 1/A-PG (MM)	2 ± 2.0	4	4
DENTAL RELATIONS			
Overjet (MM)	3.5 ± 2.5	4	2
Overbite (MM)	2 ± 2.5	-3	2
Interincisal angle 1/1	132° ± 6.0	97°	120°

force similar to that of posterior bite blocks, which is recommended for vertical control after anterior open-bite treatment.[1]

Case Report 2

CASE SUMMARY

A 21-year-old female presented with a mild skeletal class II, division 1 malocclusion, moderate lower and mild upper crowding, moderate anterior open bite, a severely hyperdivergent skeletal pattern, and an unbalanced transverse relationship. Clinical examination indicated excessive lower facial height with a gummy smile and a typical long-face appearance (Fig. 9.10; Table 9.4). The patient had a 3-mm anterior open bite, with posterior occlusion only on the second molars. Radiographic examination confirmed the vertical excess in the lower face (Fig. 9.11). Two treatment options were presented: surgical correction or aligner therapy with TADs.

9 • Open-Bite Treatment with Aligners 103

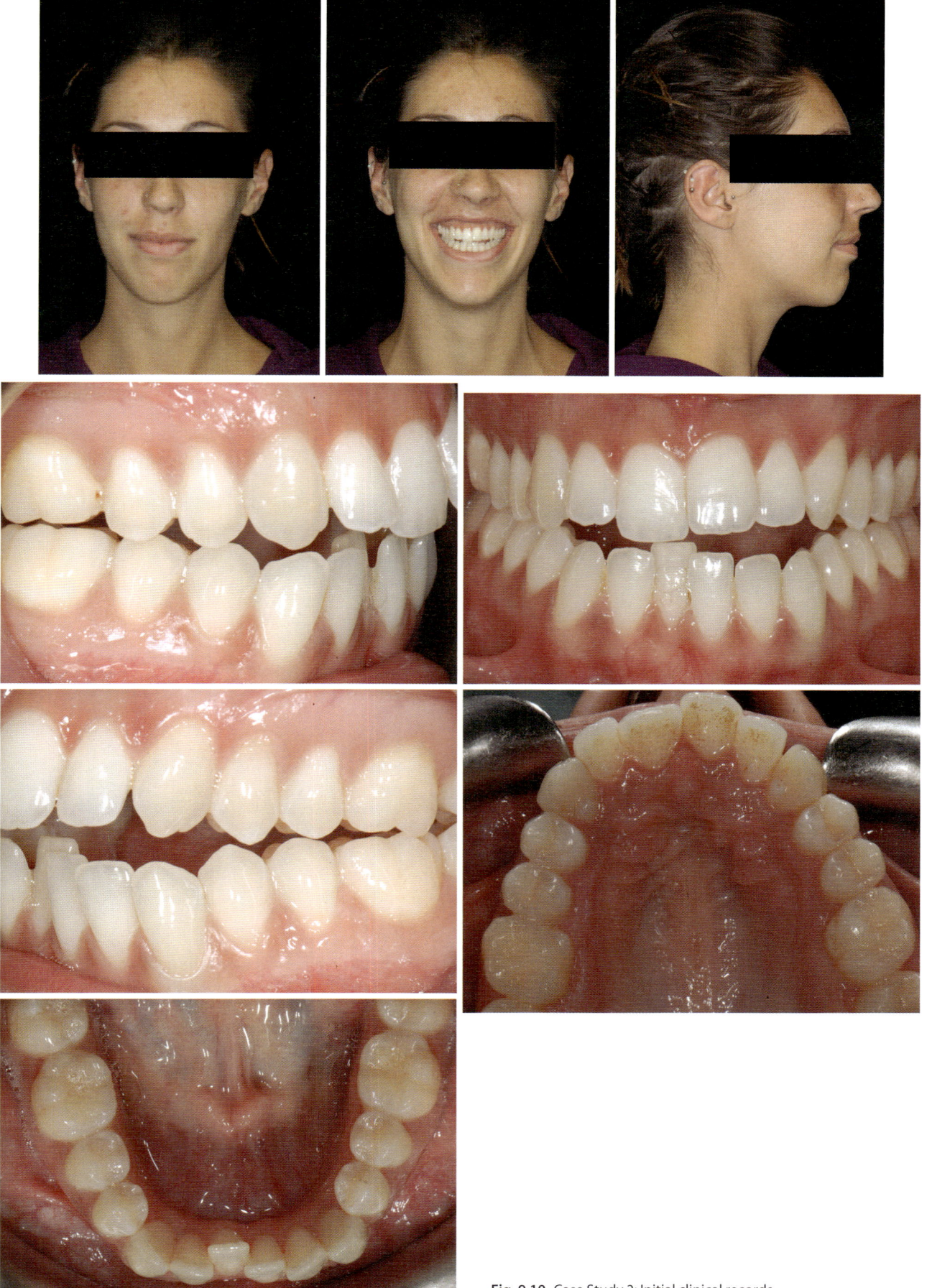

Fig. 9.10 Case Study 2: Initial clinical records.

PROBLEM LIST

Table 9.4 Case Study 2: Problem List

Dimension	Skeletal	Dental	Soft Tissue
Anteroposterior	• Skeletal class II, division 1 malocclusion	• Occlusal contacts only on the second molars • Excessive incisors proclination	• Retrusive lower lip and chin
Vertical	• Increased lower anterior facial height • Excessive maxillary posterior growth • Severe hyperdivergent pattern	• Moderate anterior open bite (-3mm)	• Long face type • Gummy smile • Mentalis muscle strain at rest
Transverse	• Transversal skeletal deficiency	• Moderate lower and mild upper crowding • Unbalanced occlusion relationships	

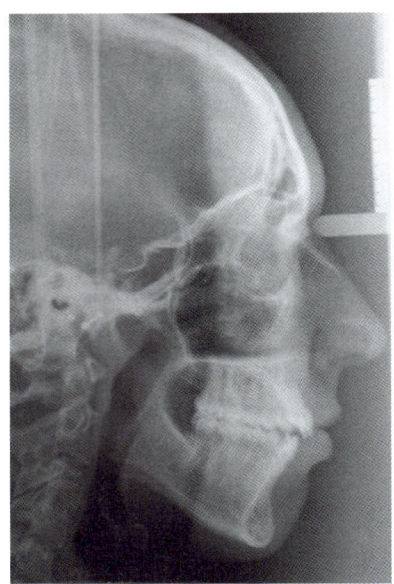

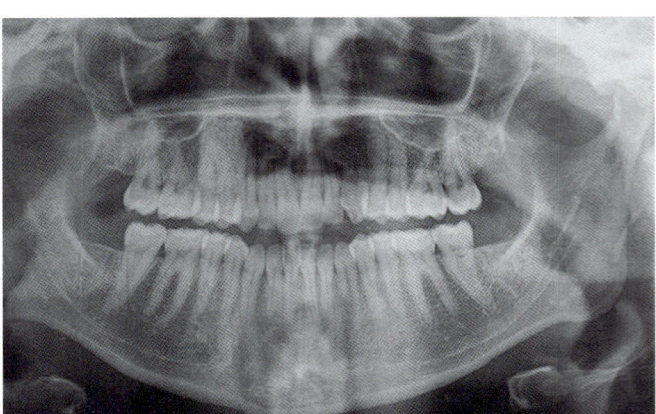

Fig. 9.11 Case Study 2: Pretreatment x-ray records.

TREATMENT OBJECTIVES

The treatment aim was to close anterior open bite, correct excessive vertical facial height, obtain balanced occlusal contacts with a class I molar relationship, and improve patient's smile (Table 9.5).

TREATMENT PLAN

The skeletal class II and the anterior open bite required correction by counterclockwise rotation of the mandible allowed by maxillary molar intrusion, without moving the vertical position of anterior teeth. Such upward and forward rotation would reduce facial height and improve vertical and sagittal relationships with proper dental torque and inclination.

The treatment also included the achievement of class I molar relationships, dental alignment and leveling, optimization of posterior transversal occlusion, as well as reaching ideal overbite and overjet to improve the facial profile and smile arc. The pre- and postvirtual plan is shown in Fig. 9.12.

TREATMENT ALTERNATIVES

The treatment alternatives consisted of the following:

1. Invisalign therapy with intrusion of the posterior maxillary and mandibular dentition by using TADs as skeletal anchorage
2. Orthosurgical treatment including a LeFort I osteotomy with posterior maxillary impaction

9 • Open-Bite Treatment with Aligners

Table 9.5 Case Study 2: Treatment Objectives

Dimension	Skeletal	Dental	Soft Tissue
Anteroposterior	Improve class II by counterclockwise mandibular rotation induced by molar intrusion	Improve class II molar relationship and incisor inclination by counterclockwise mandibular rotation induced by molar intrusion	Improve soft tissue profile
Vertical	Reduce lower facial height, maxillary downward clockwise rotation, and hyperdivergent pattern by intruding upper posterior teeth and consequent autorotation of the mandible	Improve anterior overbite and smile arc by intruding upper posterior teeth and maintaining the vertical position of the anterior teeth	Improve the profile by intruding maxillary dentoalveolar sites
Transverse	Expand maxillary arch dentally	Improve balanced occlusion relationships by mandible autorotation	
		Reduce upper and lower crowding by contact points stripping	

TREATMENT SEQUENCE

The patient chose the second option. Posterior maxillary dentoalveolar intrusion for vertical correction was achieved by miniscrew mechanics. Buccal 3 mm × 8 mm Spider Pin miniscrews were placed mesially to each maxillary first molar. An auxiliary 0.018 in × 0.022 in stainless steel sectional wire was placed on each side of the working cast coated at the ends with composite resin for easier placement in the mouth. A surgical hook was crimped at each first molar and 150-g nickel titanium coil springs were tied from these to the TADs. To avoid the development of undesirable molar labial torque due to the force application on the buccal side only, the plan included use of upper and lower aligners to control it. The digital treatment plan was designed for alignment, IPR, and, if needed, tooth retrusion. Instead, posterior intrusion and anterior extrusion, or other vertical movements as in Case 1, were carefully avoided because the difference between TAD and aligner mechanics could lead to imperfect aligner fit and inadequate torque control (Fig. 9.13). The aligner treatment consisted of 13 upper and lower aligners, plus 10 upper and lower refinement aligners. Customized, precise cuts of the aligners were designed on the ClinCheck to accommodate the auxiliary wires, usually affecting two or three teeth on each side.

TREATMENT RESULTS

Adequate intrusion and consequent closing of open bite were achieved in 6 months with dental alignment and leveling (Fig. 9.14).

Goals set in the pretreatment plan were totally reached after 15 months of therapy (Fig. 9.15; Table 9.6). The anterior open bite had been completely corrected, resulting in a proper overbite and overjet. A class I molar relationship had been established.

Patient's smile positively changed by improving vertical lower facial height and gummy smile. The values in the final cephalometric assessment show a 3-mm intrusion of the upper molars and reduction of the vertical skeletal determined by aligners (Fig. 9.16; see Table 9.6).

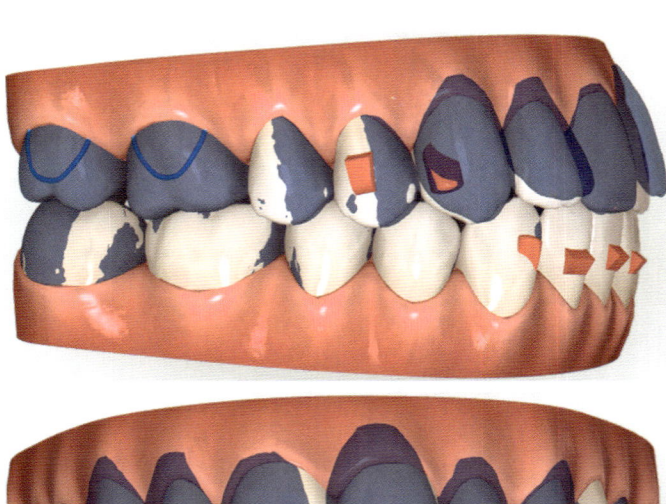

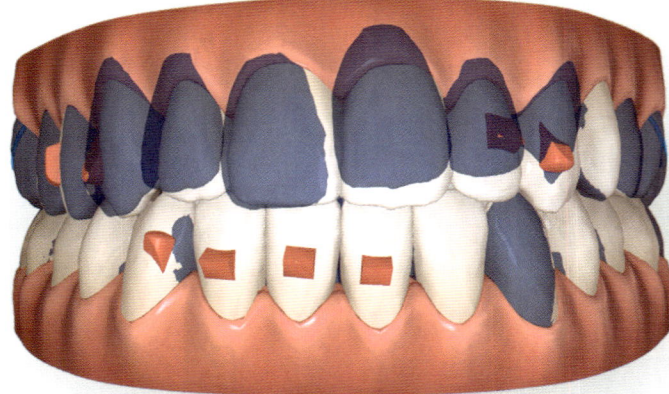

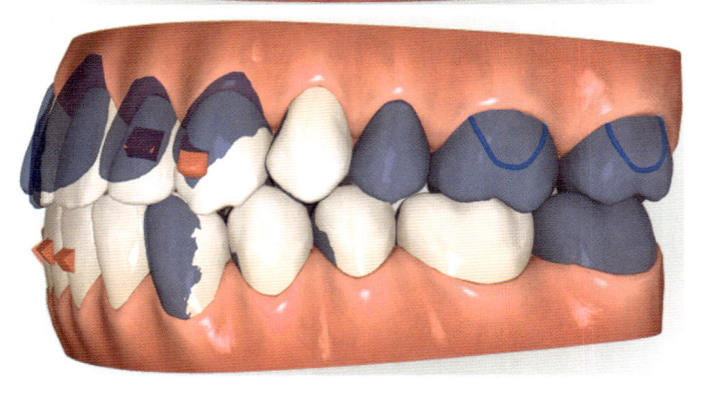

Fig. 9.12 Case Study 2: Pre- and post-ClinCheck superimposition.

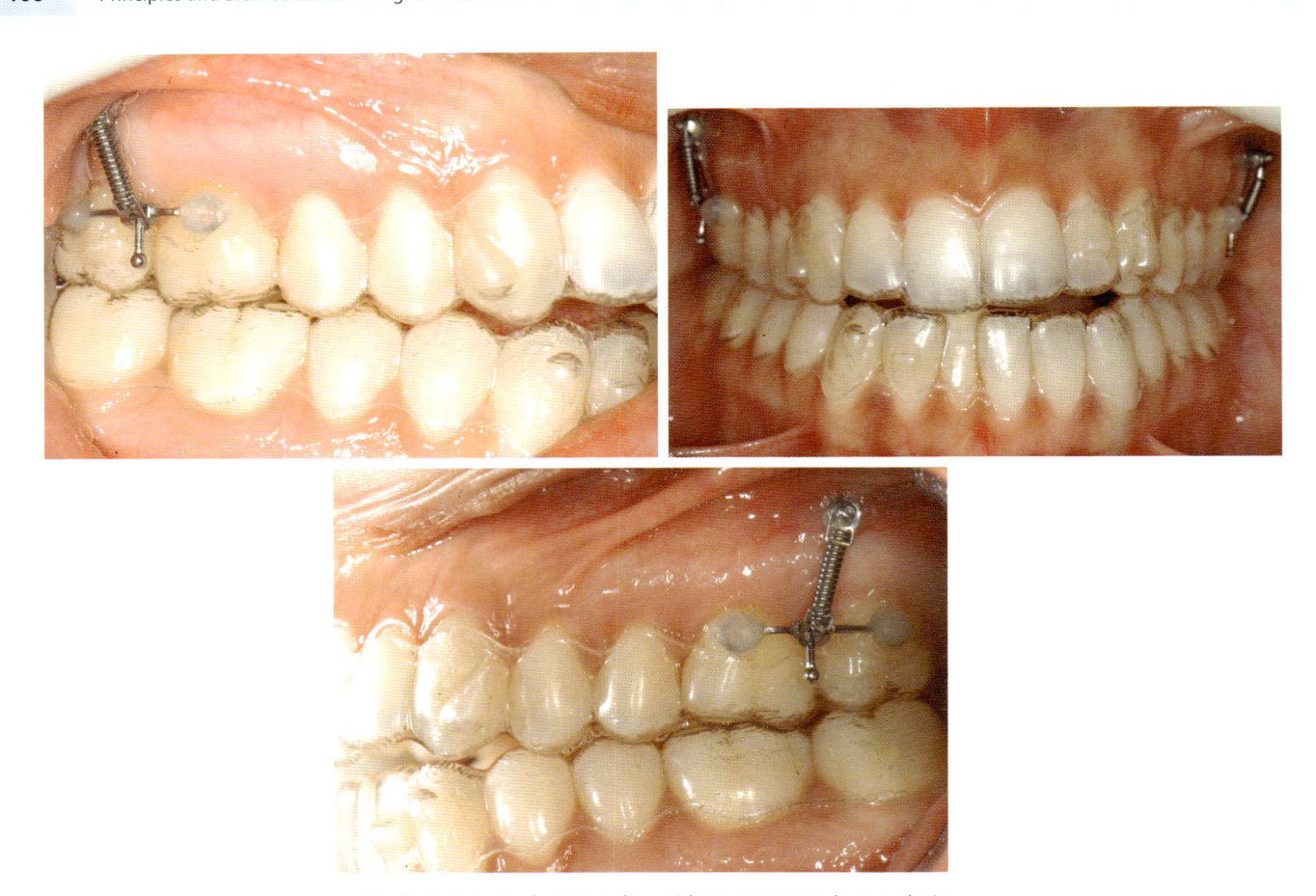

106 Principles and Biomechanics of Aligner Treatment

Fig. 9.13 Case Study 2: Invisalign with temporary anchorage devices for posterior intrusion.

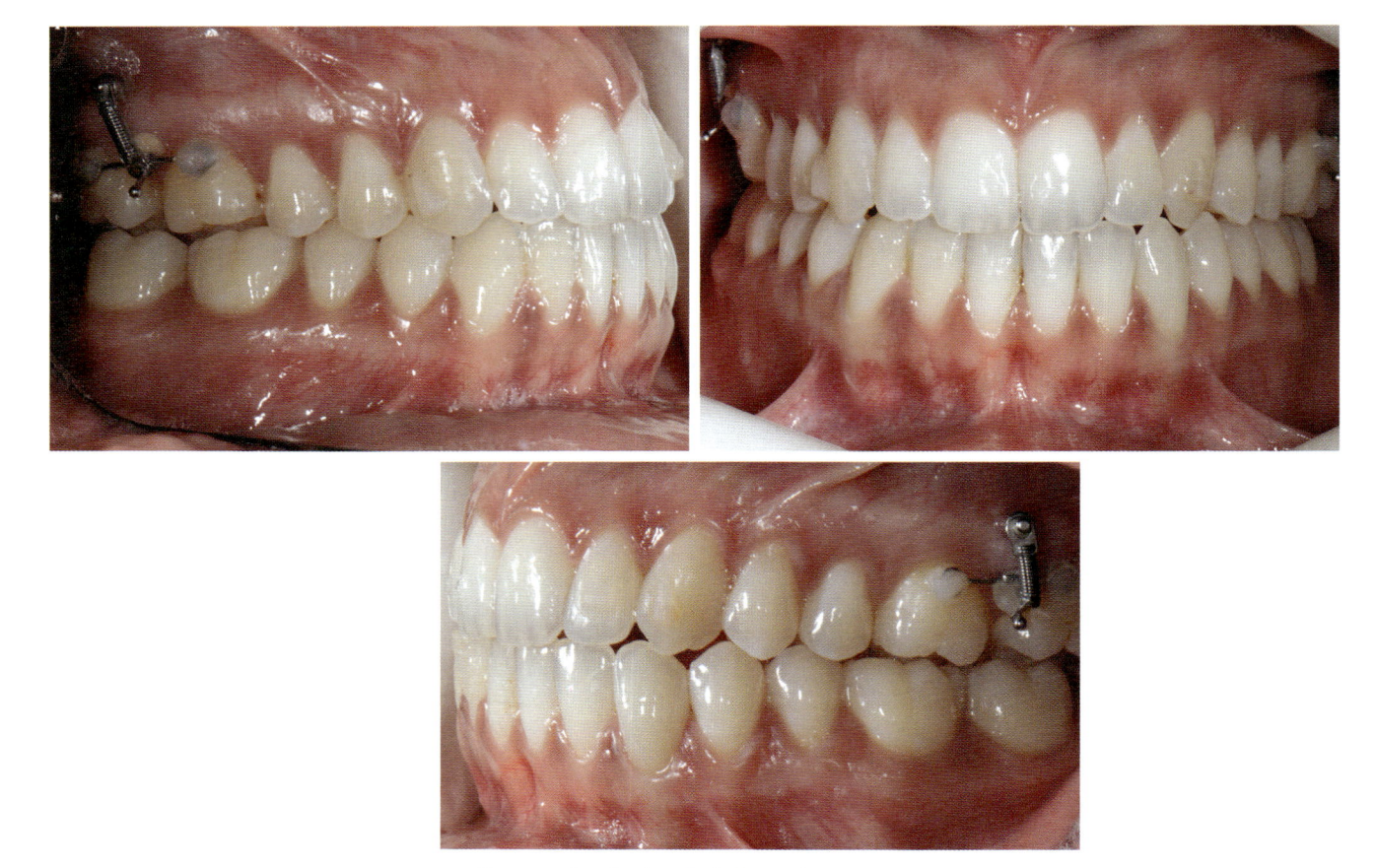

Fig. 9.14 Case Study 2: End of posterior intrusion.

9 • Open-Bite Treatment with Aligners   107

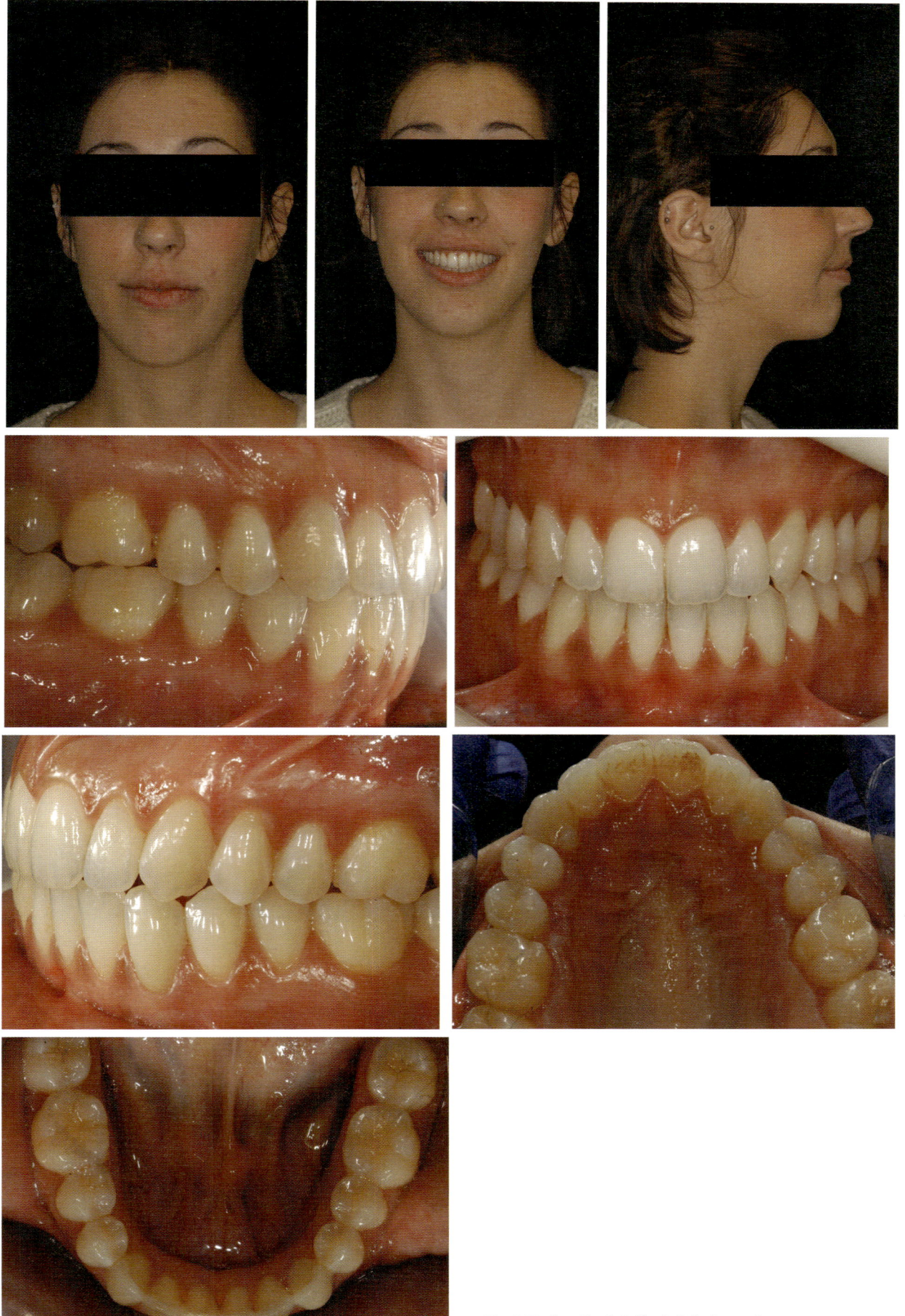

Fig. 9.15 Case Study 2: Final clinical records.

Table 9.6 Case Study 2: Summary of Cephalometric Changes

Cephalometric Morphologic Assessment	Mean SD	Pretreatment	Posttreatment
SAGITTAL SKELETAL RELATIONS			
Maxillary position S-N-A	82° ± 3.5	72°	72°
Mandibular position S-N-PG	80° ± 3.5	70°	70,5°
Sagittal jaw relation A-N-PG	2° ± 2.5	2°	1,5°
VERTICAL SKELETAL RELATIONS			
Maxillary inclination S-N/ANS-PNS	8° ± 3.0	9°	9°
Mandibular inclination S-N/GO-GN	33° ± 2.5	41°	38°
Vertical jaw relation ANS-PNS/GO-GN	25° ± 6.0	30°	29°
DENTOBASAL RELATIONS			
Maxillary incisor inclination 1/ANS-PNS	110° ± 6.0	109°	102°
Mandibular incisor inclination 1/GO-GN	94 ± 7.0	97°	96°
Mandibular incisor compensation 1/A-PG (MM)	2 ± 2.0	4	4
DENTAL RELATIONS			
Overjet (MM)	3.5 ± 2.5	5	2
Overbite (MM)	2 ± 2.5	-2	1
Interincisal angle 1/1	132° ± 6.0	125°	132°

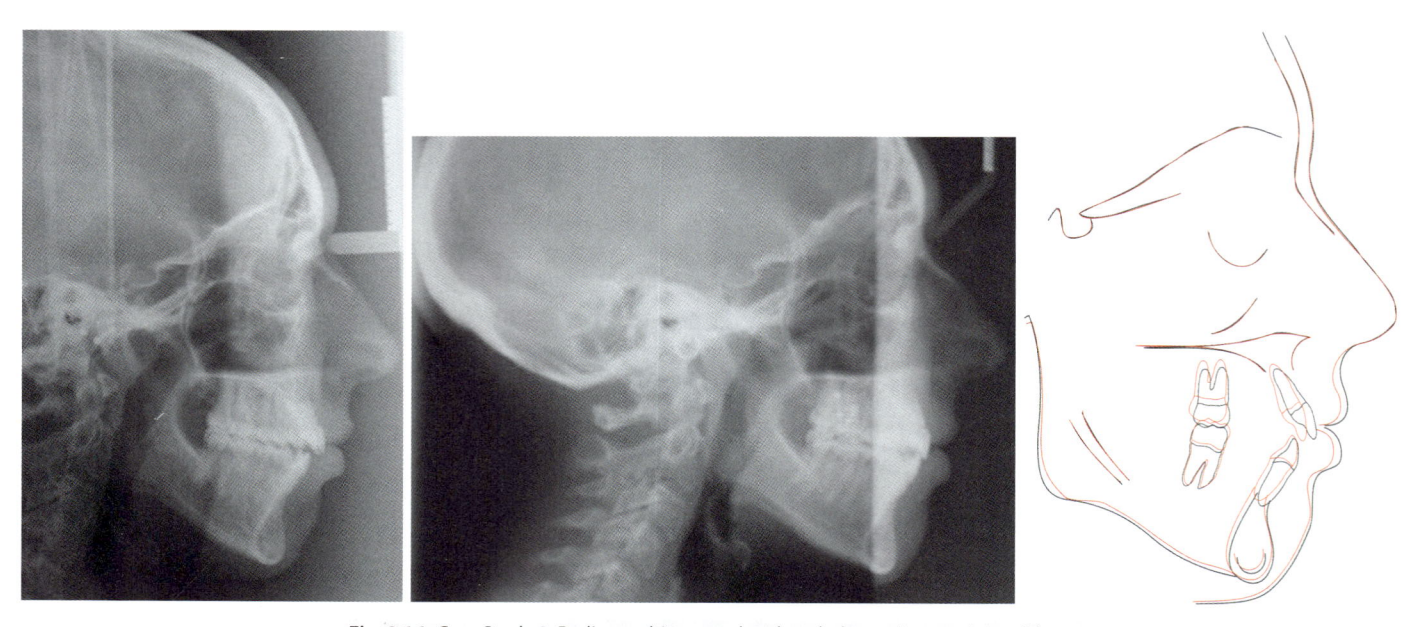

Fig. 9.16 Case Study 2: Radiographic control and cephalometric superimposition.

References

1. Ngan P. Fields HW. Open bite: a review of etiology and management. *Pediatr Dent.* 1997;19:91-98.
2. Subtelny HD, Sakuda M. Open bite: diagnosis and treatment. *Am J Orthod.* 1964;50(5):337-358.
3. Cangialosi TJ. Skeletal morphologic features of anterior open bite. *Am J Orthod.* 1984;85:28-36.
4. Lopez-Gavito G, Wallen TR, Little RM, et al. Anterior open-bite malocclusion: a longitudinal 10-year post-retention evaluation of orthodontically treated patients. *Am J Orthod.* 1985;87:175-186.
5. Nanda SK. Patterns of vertical growth in the face. *Am J Orthod Dentofacial Orthop.* 1988;93:103-116.
6. Cozza P, Mucedero M, Baccetti T, et al. Early orthodontic treatment of skeletal open bite malocclusion: a systematic review. *Angle Orthod.* 2005;75(5):707-713.
7. Betzenberger D, Ruf S, Pancherz H. The compensatory mechanism in high angle malocclusions: a comparison of subjects in the mixed and permanent dentition. *Angle Ortho.* 1999;69:27-32.
8. Sarver DM, Weissman SM. Nonsurgical treatment of open bite in nongrowing patients. *Am J Orthod Dentofacial Orthop.* 1995;108:651-659.
9. Kuhn R. Control of anterior vertical dimension and proper selection of extraoral anchorage. *Angle Orthod.* 1968;38:340-349.
10. Pearson LE. Treatment of vertical backward rotating type growth pattern patients in todays' environment. Meeting of Southern Assoc of Orthodontists, Birmingham, AL, October 20-23, 1996 (confirmed by personal communication).
11. Nahoum HI. Vertical proportions: a guide for prognosis and treatment in anterior open bite. *Am J Orthod.* 1977;72:128-146.
12. Neilsen IL. Vertical malocclusions: etiology, development, diagnosis and some aspects of treatment. *Angle Orthod.* 1991;61:247-260.
13. Haralabakis NB, Yiagtzis SC, Toutounzakis NM. Cephalometric characteristics of open bite in adults: a three-dimensional cephalometric evaluation. *Int J Adult Orthod Orthognath Surg.* 1994;9:223-231.
14. Giancotti A, Garino F, Mampieri G. Use of clear aligners in open bite cases: an unexpected treatment option. *J Orthod.* 2017;20:1-12.
15. Kay S. *Clear Aligner Technique.* Batavia, IL: Quintessence Publishing; 2018.

10 Deep Bite

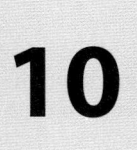

LUIS HUANCA, SIMONE PARRINI, FRANCESCO GARINO, and TOMMASO CASTROFLORIO

Introduction

Deep bite is defined as an increase of the overbite, and it is measured as vertical overlap of the incisors perpendicular to the occlusal plane.[1,2] It can be divided into dentoalveolar origin (overeruption of frontal teeth) and skeletal origin (decreased lower face height, low mandibular plane angle).[3] Deep bite prevalence varies from 8% to 51% depending on the threshold values applied, ethnic group, and gender.[4–6]

A correlation between deep bite and sagittal molar malocclusion was described. In particular, class II molar malocclusion is significantly associated with increased overbite compared with class I malocclusion.

Regarding treatment strategies in deep bite patients, there is not a complete consensus in the existing literature. A 2017 review published by Millet et al.[7] assessed that it is not possible to provide any evidence-based guidance to recommend or discourage any type of orthodontic treatment to correct class II, division 2 malocclusion in children.

As assessed by Nanda,[1] it is possible to adopt three different therapeutic strategies: extrusion of posterior teeth, intrusion of upper and/or lower incisors, and flaring of anterior teeth (also known as relative intrusion). All these effects can be obtained together depending on the clinical case.

By using clear aligners instead of fixed appliance, the orthodontist can start correcting the overbite on both arches from the beginning rather than wait a few months to bond the lower arch after the upper teeth have been flared/intruded to open the bite. The alternative would be to bond bite ramps since the beginning, but these may prove uncomfortable for patients and require adjustments and extra cleanup at some point in the future.

Leveling of the Curve of Spee

A deep curve of Spee is often associated with severe anterior deep bite. By extruding posterior teeth, mainly premolars, and intruding anterior teeth, it is possible to flatten the arches and achieve an ideal overbite.[1]

It is difficult to define the net contribution of molar and premolar extrusion versus canine and incisor intrusion to the overall curve of Spee flattening, as they act as a reciprocal source of anchorage. Whenever attempting to extrude the premolars, canines and incisors will serve as an anchorage unit, and they will pay the price of a most welcome intrusion side effect. On the contrary, every time clinicians would love to achieve intrusion of the anterior teeth, the premolars represent the primary source of anchorage, and they may extrude a beneficial side effect of anterior intrusion. Even if, by using clear aligners and an attentive planification of tooth movements, clinicians may be persuaded that they can achieve specific tooth movements (i.e., intrusion of the anteriors only/extrusion of the posteriors only), they should be aware that Newton's third law of physics (action and reaction) plays an important role in distinguishing the real world from the virtual on-screen world of setup, where the laws of physics are often violated.

It is a common belief that deep bite correction and curve of Spee flattening is easier to achieve in growing patients, as extrusion of molars and premolars can be supported by vertical growth while grow is still happening.[8]

On the contrary, curve of Spee correction in adults may be much harder, as the orthodontist cannot hope in any influence or help from the vertical skeletal dimension. Furthermore, curve of Spee tends to deepen with aging,[9] with supererupted lower incisors and canines that may also show lingual inclination (upper incisors can also show lingual inclination as a consequence). This becomes clinically evident in a two-step mandibular occlusal plane with a net step between the first premolars and canines. Excessive wearing of the incisal edges may also be evident in such circumstances. While planning deep bite correction in an adult, the orthodontist should also plan any eventual restorative treatment that is needed to reestablish the proper crown anatomy.

Align Technology has created a proprietary protocol for deep bite correction called Invisalign G5. This protocol involves incisor and canine intrusion through a combination of intrusion forces exerted by the aligners on the occlusal edge of the teeth and a pressure area on the lingual surface (Figs. 10.1 and 10.2). This combination of force systems exerts a final intrusive force that is supposed to be parallel to the tooth long axis. To achieve the desired intrusion on the anterior teeth, an adequate anchorage should be provided in the premolar and molar area. G5 retention attachments have been specifically designed for premolars, and they may serve as pure anchorage attachments or as active extrusion attachments in case of extrusion of the premolars. Both movement of anterior intrusion and posterior extrusion are automatically activated if the threshold of movement is more than 0.5 mm. Molar anchorage should be provided with conventional attachments (rectangular and horizontal) to counteract the occlusal movement of the aligner determined by the anterior intrusion design.

Clinicians working with other clear aligner systems than Invisalign, or those who feel the need for alternative approaches even when using Invisalign aligners, may create a similar protocol using standard attachments and a personalized staging of intrusion.

Gingival beveled attachments may be used as an alternative to G5 retention attachments on premolars to achieve retention and extrusion. When planning extrusion, it is

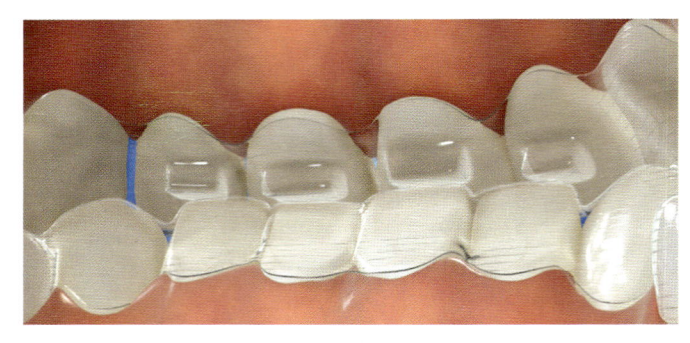

Fig. 10.1 Schematic representation of the optimized bite ramps designed by Align Technology (San José, CA, USA) and embedded into aligners. They change shape and positioning along the treatment to provide optimal support to lower incisors at every stage of treatment.

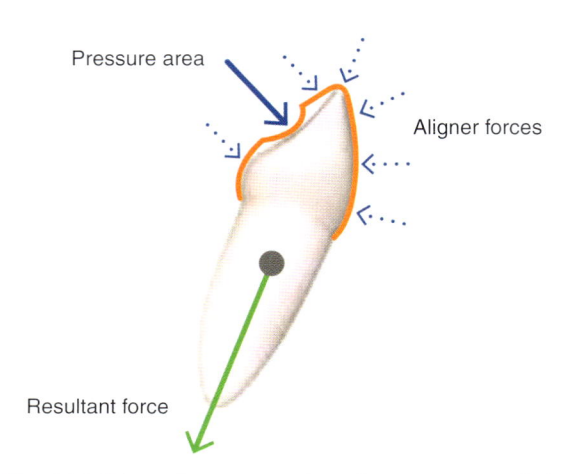

Fig. 10.2 Schematic representation of pressure areas designed by Align Technology (San José, CA, USA) and incorporated into the aligner to redirect the intrusive force along the long axis of the incisor.

useful to ask for a slower extrusion rate (e.g., 0.15 mm per stage instead of the classic 0.20 mm) to avoid lack of tracking within the aligner by respecting the physiologic tolerance of the periodontal ligament.

Some clinicians recommend a superiorly convex (reverse) curve of Spee as final objective of the alternative. While this is not the real clinical goal, the assumption behind this prescription is that the elasticity and resilience of the plastic material will very unlikely allow a full expression of the prescribed movement. By the way the lack of expression of certain movements can be compensated by this requested hypercorrection, that is the aligner equivalent of the reverse curve NiTi wires.[10] The clinician who has the feeling that the hypercorrection is really happening may always stop the use of the aligners to avoid unwanted side effects.

Curve of Spee correction should always begin with lower incisor proclination to obtain a relative intrusion and start to recover the space required during the real intrusion movement. Since the expression of the lingual root torque information on lower incisors has not yet been investigated, it can be useful to prescribe extra lingual root torque. Again, it is important to remember that interproximal spacing may help the intrusion movements.

A paper by Liu and Hu[11] explained how force changes as a consequence of different intrusion strategies for deep bite correction with clear aligners. With the same activation (0.2 mm of intrusion) and rectangular attachments placed on the premolars and first molars, the canines experienced the largest intrusive force when intruded alone. When applying contemporary intrusion of canines and incisors, the canines received a larger intrusive force than incisors. The incisors received similar forces of intrusion if intruded alone or together with canines. First premolars experienced the largest extrusive forces when all anterior teeth were intruded. Extrusion forces were exerted also on canines and lateral incisors when differential staging for intrusion of canines and incisors was used. It is not surprising that the intrusive force exerted by clear aligners is higher when less elements are involved, and it is partially lost when multiple elements are intruded at the same time. The incisors show an overall scarce tendency to feel intrusion forces. This may lead to the clinical suggestion of a staggered approach, alternating canine and incisor intrusion to exert higher and more specific forces on canines and incisors.

Therefore, a clinical suggestion in prescribing anterior intrusion with any clear aligner system could consider the following:

1. Intrusion from canine to canine at a rate of 0.15 mm per stage (first create an extra space of 0.5 mm to hold until the movement has been completed)
2. Horizontal rectangular beveled gingival attachments on lower bicuspids; those attachments should be 4 mm wide, 1.5 mm high, 1.25 mm thick at the gingival margin, and tapered to 0.25 mm thickness at the occlusal margin
3. Horizontal rectangular beveled occlusal attachments on lower canines; those attachments should be 4 mm wide, 1.5 mm high, 1.25 mm thick at the occlusal margin, and tapered to 0.25 mm at the gingival margin
4. Horizontal rectangular attachments on molars to increase anchorage
5. Alternate intrusion of canines and incisors
6. Place the attachments occlusally avoiding any interarch interferences

Leveling the Upper Incisors

Clinical observation of patient face and smile and gingival display guide the clinician in the choice of how to correct an excessive overbite.[12] In fact, in many clinical cases, a pure lower posterior extrusion/curve of Spee flattening may not be the best option, but the mechanics in the lower arch should be accompanied by vertical movements on the upper anteriors. During treatment planning with aligner orthodontics, it is possible to prescribe a selective upper or lower incisor intrusion.

It is not surprising that when trying to correct an excessive overbite, the upper smile arch needs special care, as Dr. David Sarver taught to the whole profession. The intrusion of the upper incisors should be limited to preserve convexity of the smile and enough crown exposure to preserve a youthful smile while aging.

Upper incisors and canines may be intruded by relative intrusion (i.e., by providing vestibular crown torque, some intrusion happens as a geometric consequence of this movement). To allow a full expression of this movement, it is strongly suggested to prescribe an extra lingual root torque. Power Ridge (Align Technology, San Josè, CA, USA) at the gingival third of the crown may also help in achieving labial crown torque. Simon et al.[13] demonstrated that even a buccal attachment on upper incisors could provide lingual root torque control.

Upper relative intrusion and incisor crown vestibularization is often needed in those adults who have a very deep curve of Spee, where the correction starts with labial movement of the lower incisors. Enough clearance (anterior overjet with no contacts) should be provided to avoid posterior disclusion due to hard collisions among upper and lower incisors due to occlusal interferences.

Once achievement of the correct amount of relative intrusion occurs, pure intrusion can be applied. With Align Technology G5 protocol, when the intrusion request overpasses the 0.5-mm threshold, a lingual pressure area will be added to enhance the parallelism of the final vector of intrusive force to the long axis of the tooth.

Bite ramps may be added on the lingual part of the teeth to help during deep bite correction (see Fig. 10.1). They are optimized—in other words, they can change shape and position during the different stages of treatment to keep contact with the lower incisors as a consequence of upper incisor buccal crown torque (they get longer while the upper incisor crowns get flared). When bite ramps are present, no palatal pressure areas can be added at the same time on the same tooth as the two features need some space on the lingual surfaces of incisors and/or canines. There are some claims of a possible intrusive effect of bite ramps on upper incisors because of the imposed precontact. While this claim may answer a logical thought, it is important to remember that we pass most of the time in a discluded position of the jaw respecting our vertical freeway space. As a consequence, patients bite over the bite ramps for a few seconds per day only when swallowing, thus the real effect of bite ramps as booster of upper intrusion is questionable. The way bite ramps keep the jaws constantly discluded is the same principle of many functional appliances, whose main objective is to enhance lower posterior extrusion by providing an anterior precontact. In this sense, bite ramps, supported by class II elastics, may favor lower posterior teeth extrusion, especially in growing patients. It is important to notice that, with aligners, elastics are recommended to boost posterior extrusion, as the clear aligner is otherwise creating a self-limiting barrier that can limit posterior extrusion. On the contrary with functional appliances, where the molars and premolars are left free to erupt, the posterior vertical correction happens naturally.

Reviewing the existing literature about deep bite correction with aligners, Khosravi et al.[14] showed that in their sample of 40 deep bite patients treated with Invisalign aligners, the cephalometric analyses performed to determine the mechanism by which the Invisalign appliance corrects deep bites suggest that proclination of mandibular incisors, along with intrusion of maxillary incisors and extrusion of mandibular molars, is the primary source of deep bite correction with the Invisalign appliance.

Case Report 1

The patient presented at the age of 16 with a severe overbite, a deep curve of Spee associated with lower crowding, and important lingualization of the lower right canine (Figs. 10.3 and 10.4). His chief complaint was to avoid the

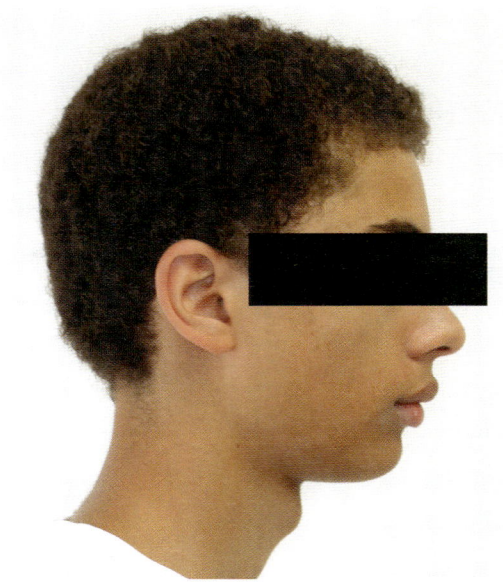

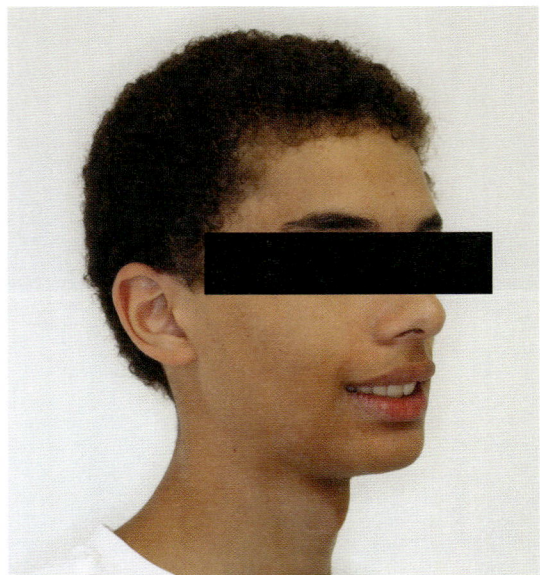

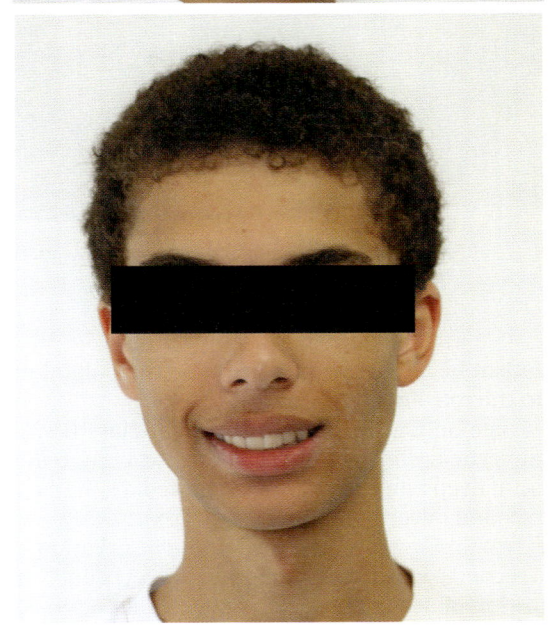

Fig. 10.3 Initial extraoral photos.

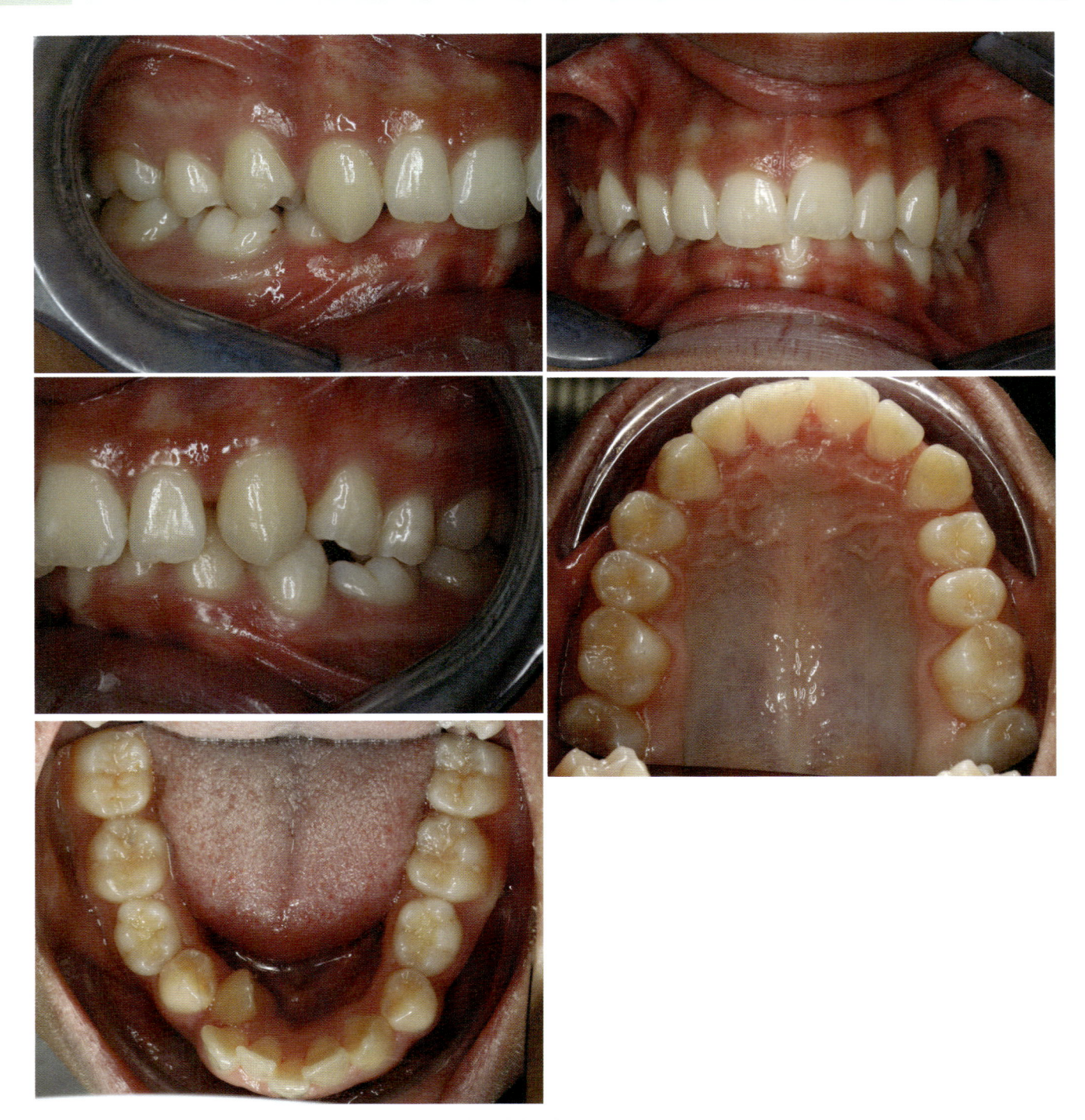

Fig. 10.4 Initial intraoral photos.

traumatism he felt every time he bit on the palatal mucosa close to the retroincisal papilla.

As visible on tracings, he had a slight class II while the skeletal vertical dimension was not as severely reduced as the dental deep bite could have suggested. He had agenesis of the second lower premolars (Fig. 10.5).

The treatment plan included the preservation of the lower second deciduous molars and eventual implant-substitution of second premolars later in life.

The treatment lasted 24 months with four sets of corrections of decreasing length. The length of the treatment was due to the severe curve of Spee that needed a big effort to be flattened. Aligner change was planned every 7 days from the beginning. The curve of Spee flattening was obtained first with proclination of the lower incisor and relative intrusion, then space was created mesial and distal to lower incisors and canines, and maintained while performing intrusion with staggered alternate movements (frog protocol) (Fig. 10.6). Anchorage attachments (rectangular horizontal) were used on the premolars but also on the canines, as at moments they served as anchorage unit for incisor intrusion (Fig. 10.7).

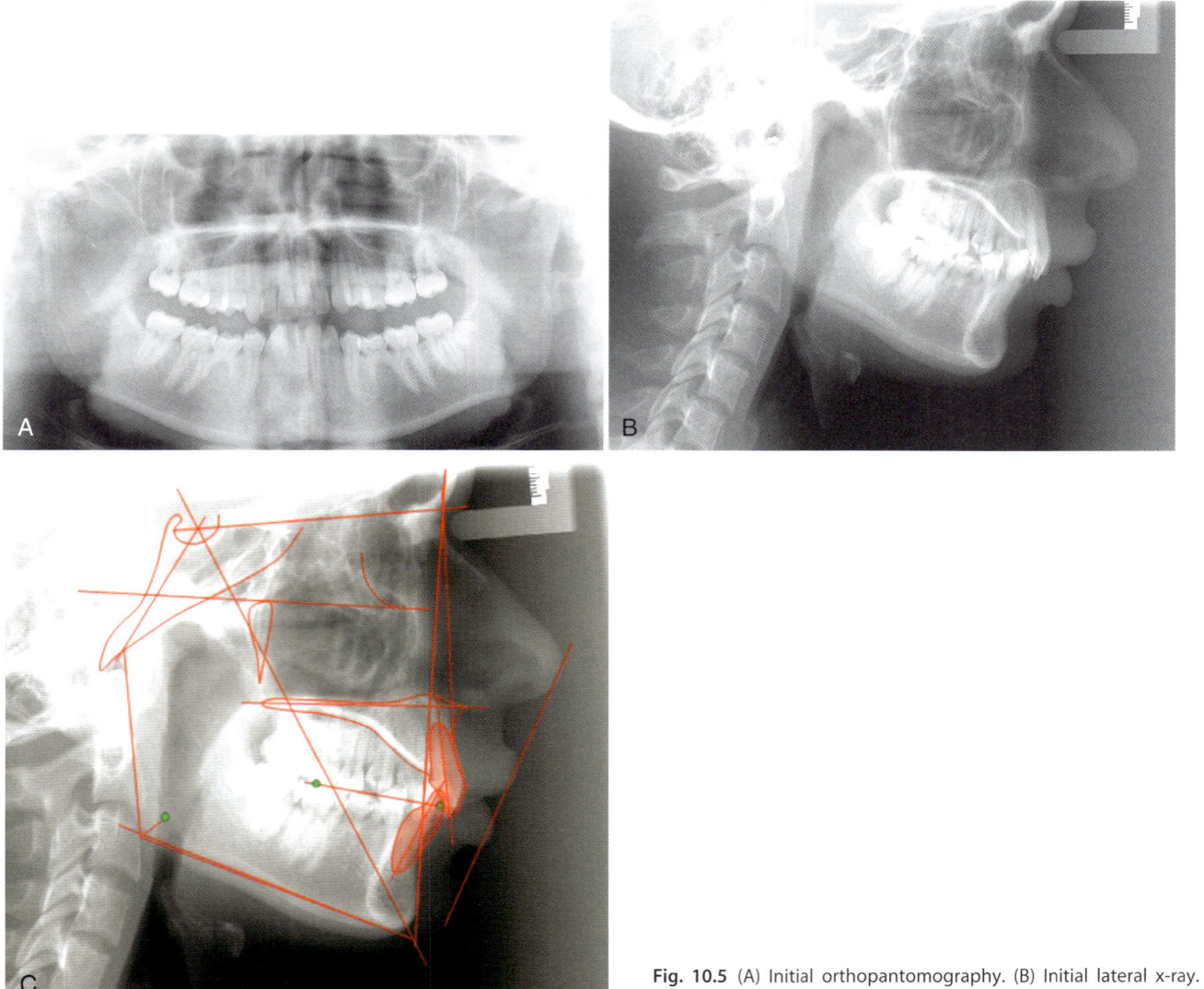

10 • Deep Bite   113

Fig. 10.5 (A) Initial orthopantomography. (B) Initial lateral x-ray. (C) Initial tracing.

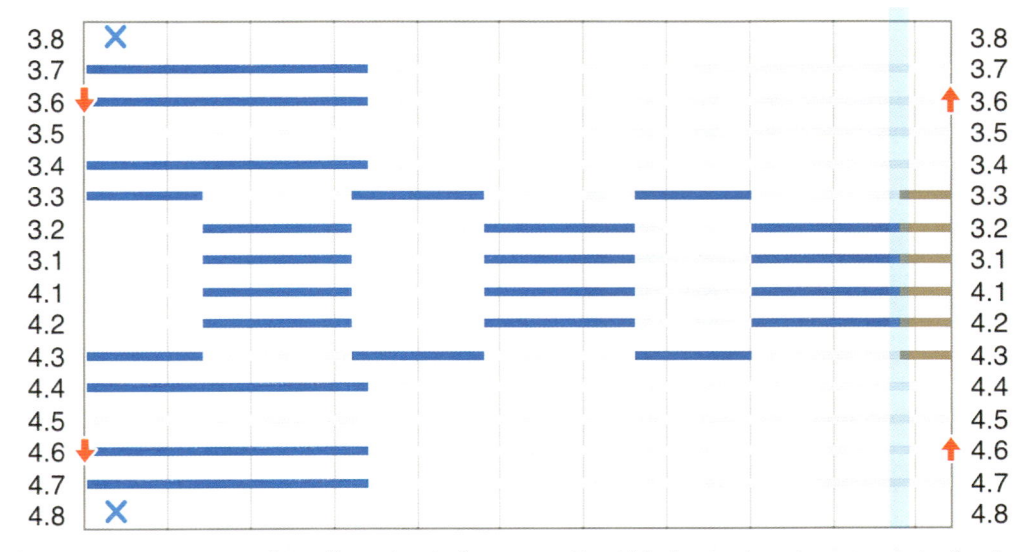

Fig. 10.6 Treatment stages scheme illustrating the frog protocol in which alternate intrusion movements of canines and incisors are planned. On the Y axis teeth are displayed, while on the X axis treatment stages are displayed: every stage corresponds to five aligners. The *blue lines* indicate active movements, *brown lines* indicate overcorrection stages. *Red arrows down* indicate when attachments should be placed, while *red arrows* up indicate when attachments should be removed.

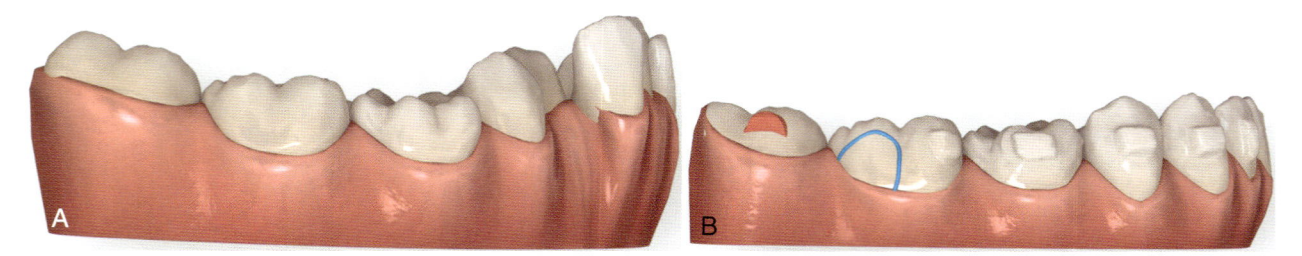

Fig. 10.7 (A) Initial curve of Spee. (B) Final curve of Spee.

The deep bite was fully corrected on the lower arch (Figs. 10.8, 10.9, and 10.10), as superimpositions on the Sella-Nasion plane (Fig. 10.11) show an unaltered vertical position of the upper incisors. An important intrusion of the lower incisors is associated with a slight advancement of the B point of the mandible probably due to the use of class II elastics.

Due to the presence of the lower deciduous molars, the patient ended into a canine class I and molar head-to-head relationship. The lower right deciduous molar responded perfectly to the therapy, while the left one was quite unresponsive to vertical movement, and a slight underbite was left at this level. The patient's chief complaint of retroincisal traumatism was fully achieved.

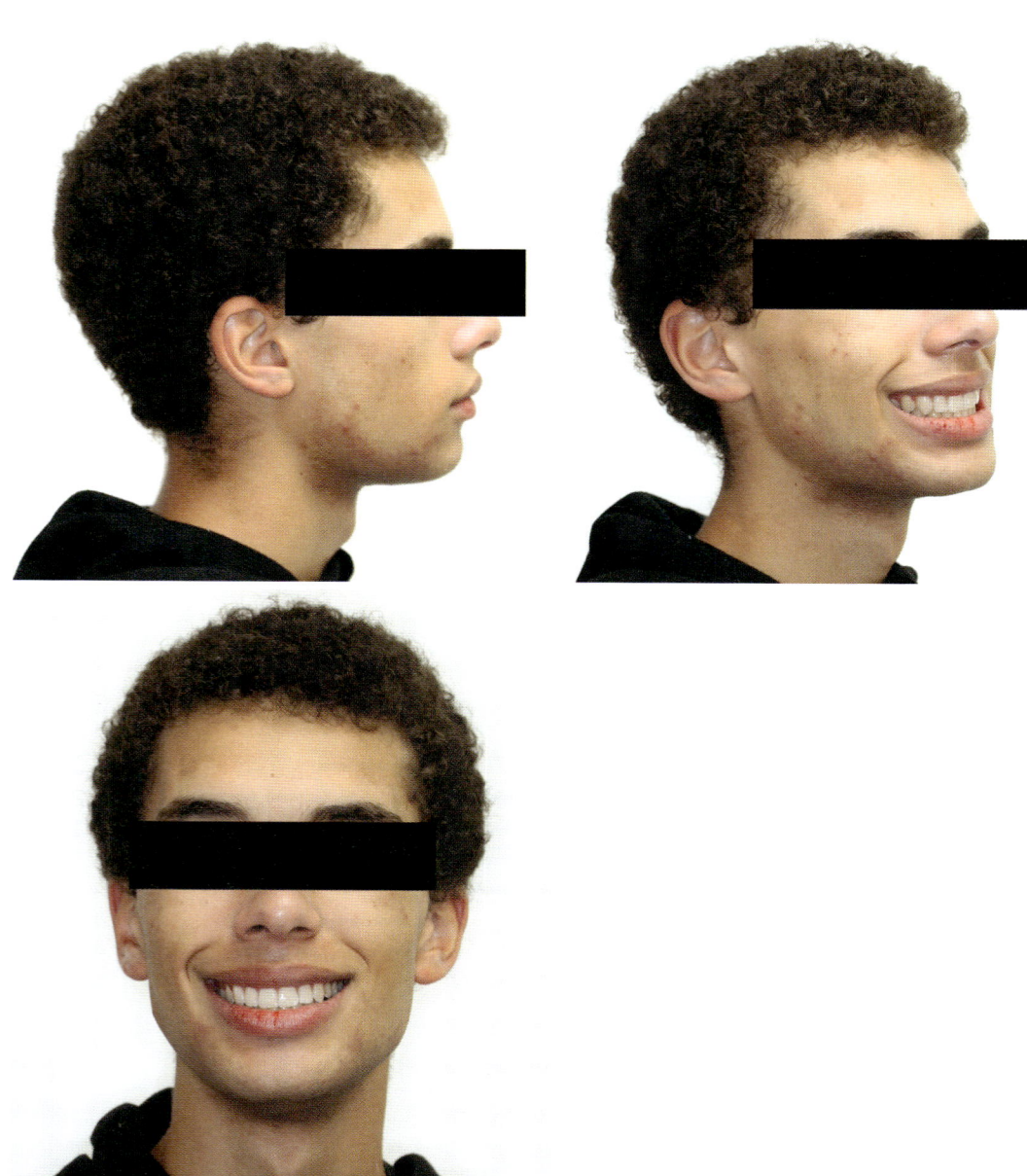

Fig. 10.8 Final extraoral photos.

Fig. 10.9 Final intraoral photos.

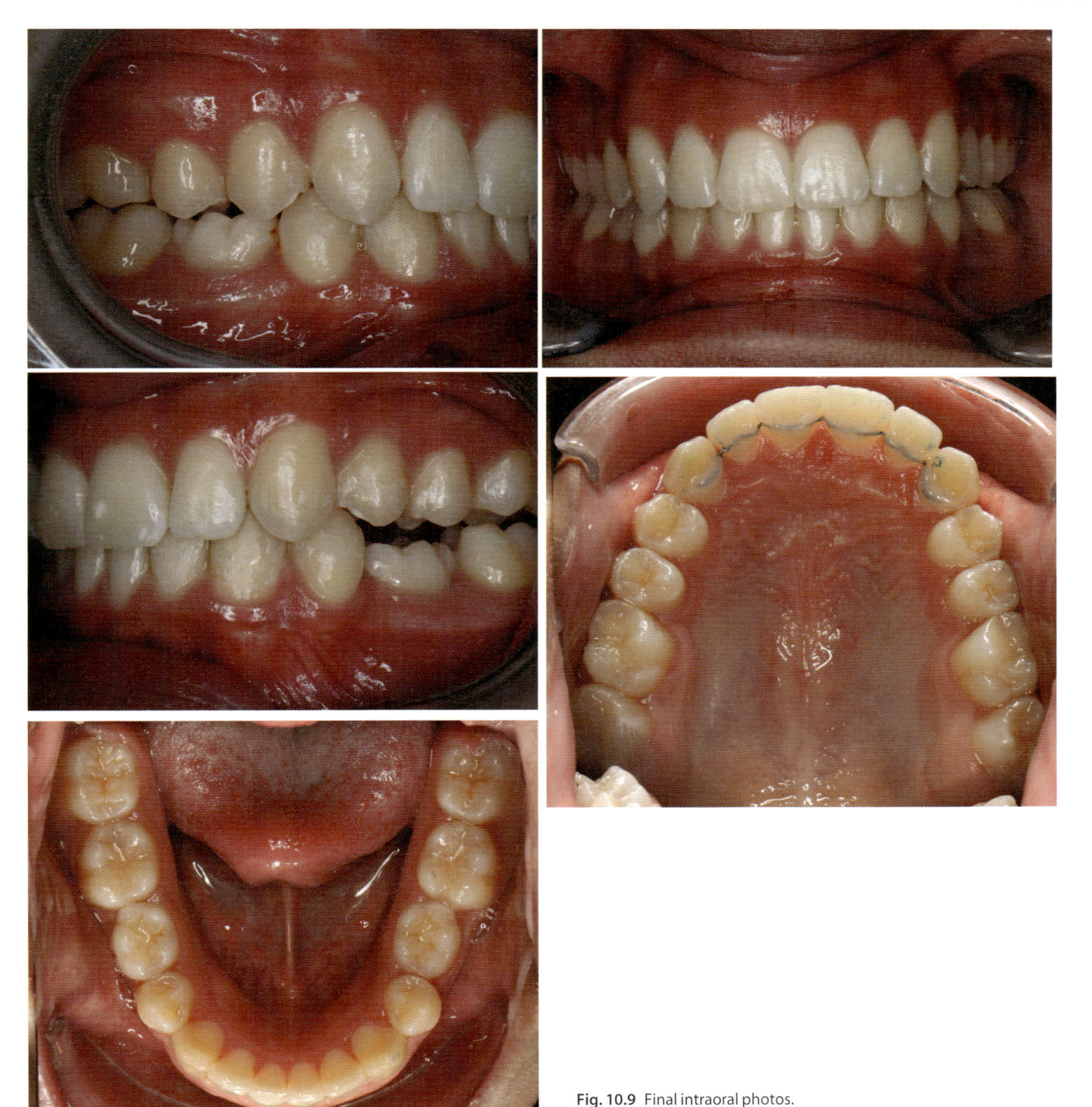

Case Report 2

An 18-year-old male patient presented with molar class II malocclusion, skeletal class II, low mandibular plane angle, deep bite with an increased curve of Spee, and crowding in the incisor area (Figs. 10.12 and 10.13). Patient's main concern was the deep overbite and crowding in the upper incisors area.

The treatment plan was designed to obtain bodily distal movements of upper molars, premolars, and canines to achieve a dental molar and canine class I.

A 50% sequential distalization protocol was applied together with the use of class II elastics (0.19 in, 4.5 oz) during the distalization process (see Chapter 7).

Attachments were placed on all distalizing teeth to control bodily distal movements (Figs. 10.14 and 10.15).

The deep bite was corrected mainly through intrusion of the lower anterior teeth, using the G5 protocol, and the presence of bite ramps on the upper incisors.

The amount of lower intrusion in the incisor area was 3.1 mm, and to reinforce the posterior anchorage, attachments were placed on bicuspids.

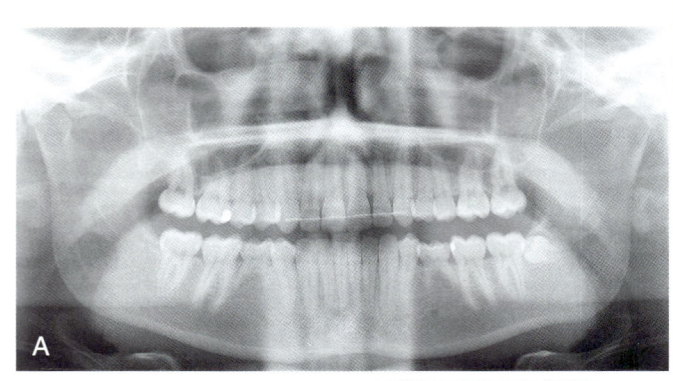

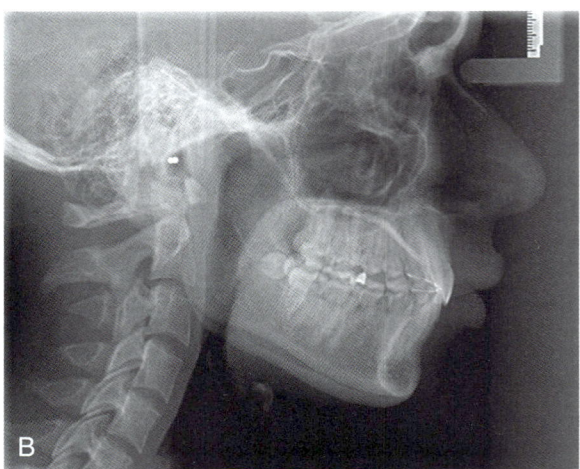

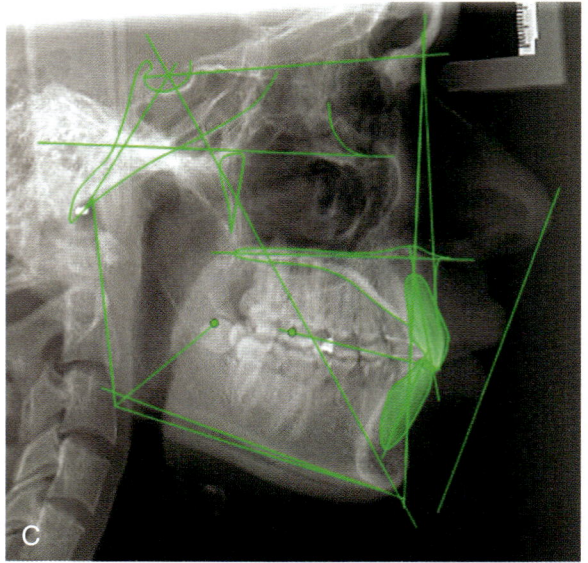

Fig. 10.10 (A) Final orthopantomography. (B) Final lateral x-ray. (C) Final tracing.

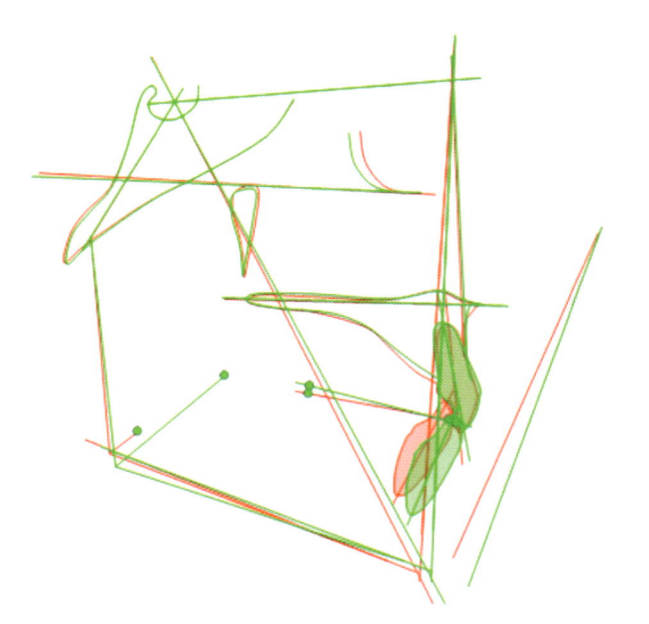

Fig. 10.11 Tracing superimposition.

A set of 45 Invisalign aligners was produced to perform the distalization movements on the upper arch and to correct the lower curve of Spee. Aligner change was planned every 2 weeks at the beginning of treatment, every 10 days after 3 months of treatment, then every 7 days after 8 months of treatment. During the distalization phase, the patient was instructed to wear class II elastics (0.25 in, 4.5 oz) bilaterally to reinforce anterior anchorage while distalizing premolars. To anchor class II elastics, hooks were planned on upper canines while buccal tubes were bonded on the lower first molars.

An additional set of 15 upper and lower aligners was requested to finalize the treatment obtaining good final intercuspation in the molar and bicuspid areas and a final overjet of 2 mm.

The treatment was concluded with bilateral class I molar and canine relationship, excellent upper and lower alignment, and good leveling of the curve of Spee (Figs. 10.16, 10.17, and 10.18).

The total treatment duration was 24 months.

10 • Deep Bite 117

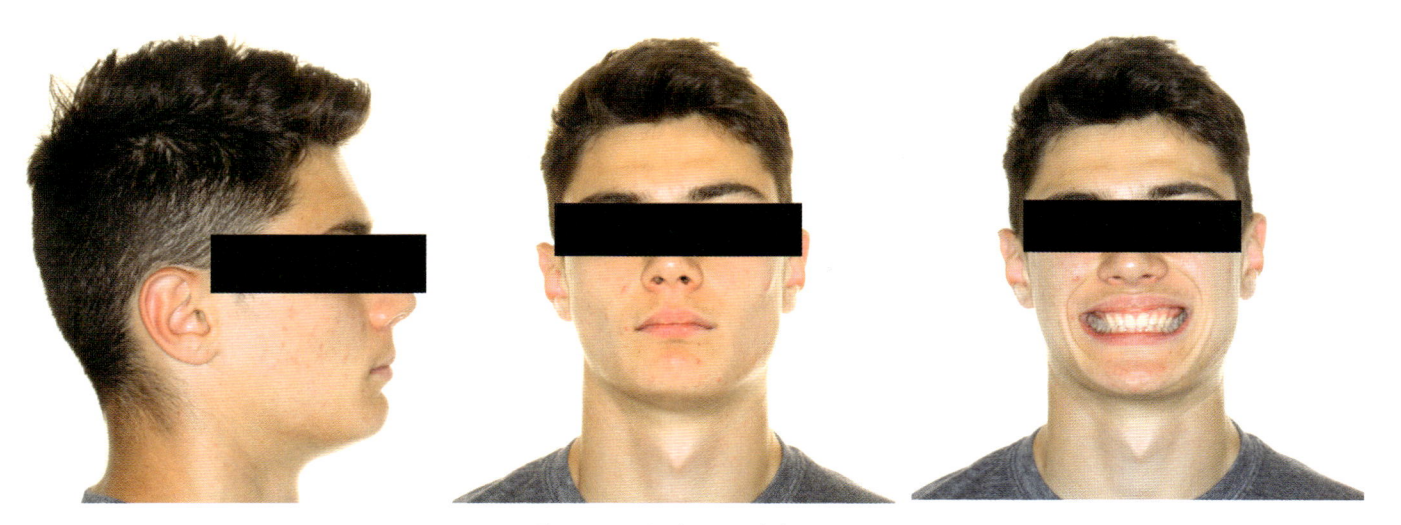

Fig. 10.12 Initial extraoral photos.

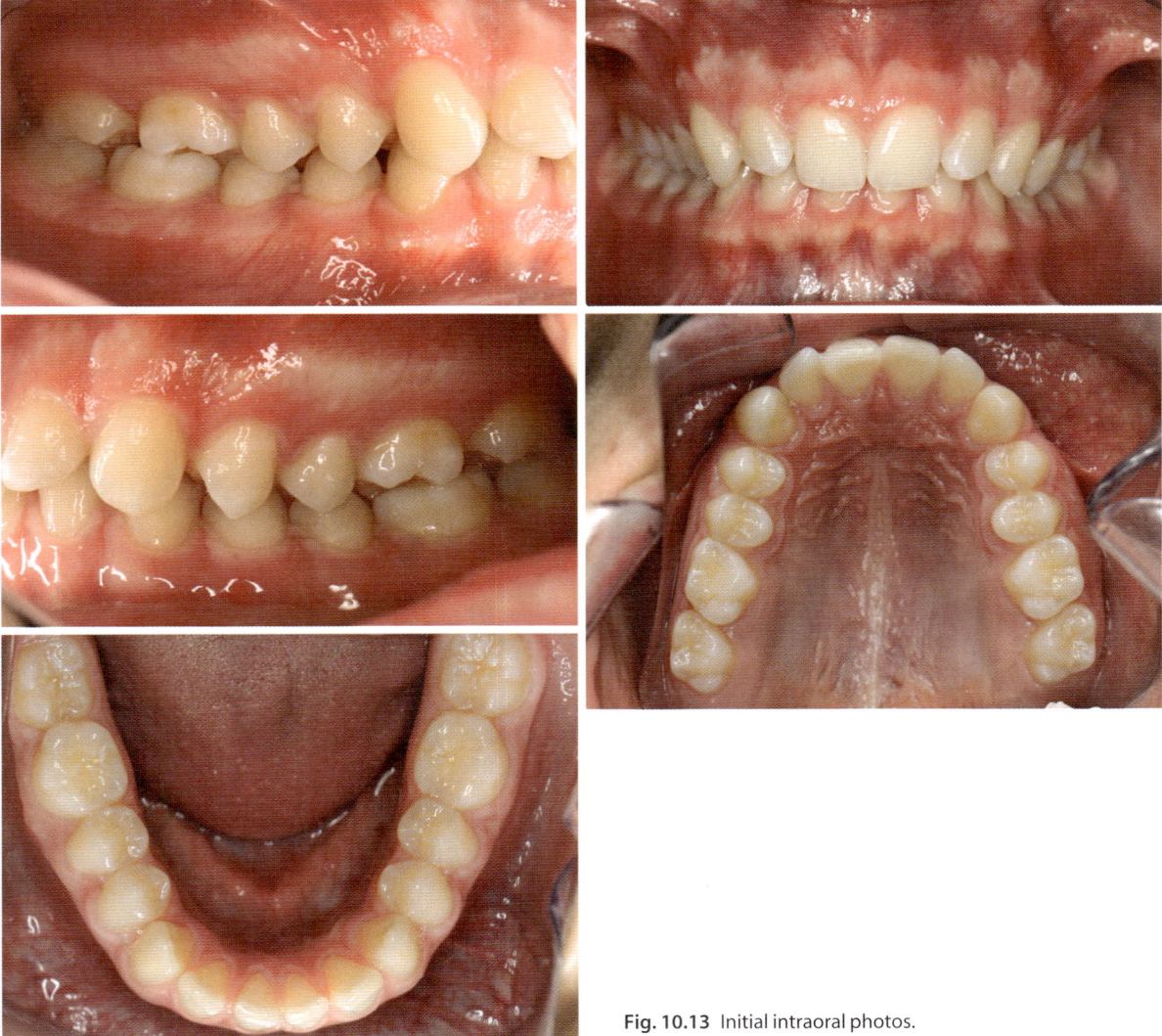

Fig. 10.13 Initial intraoral photos.

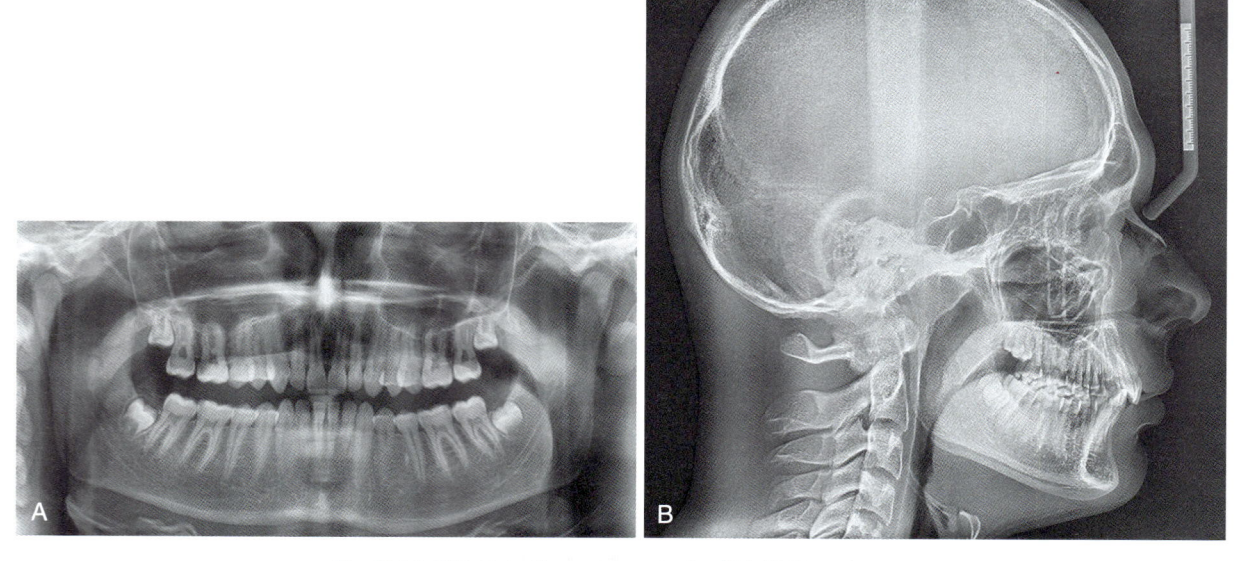

118　Principles and Biomechanics of Aligner Treatment

Fig. 10.14 (A) Initial orthopantomography. (B) Initial lateral x-ray.

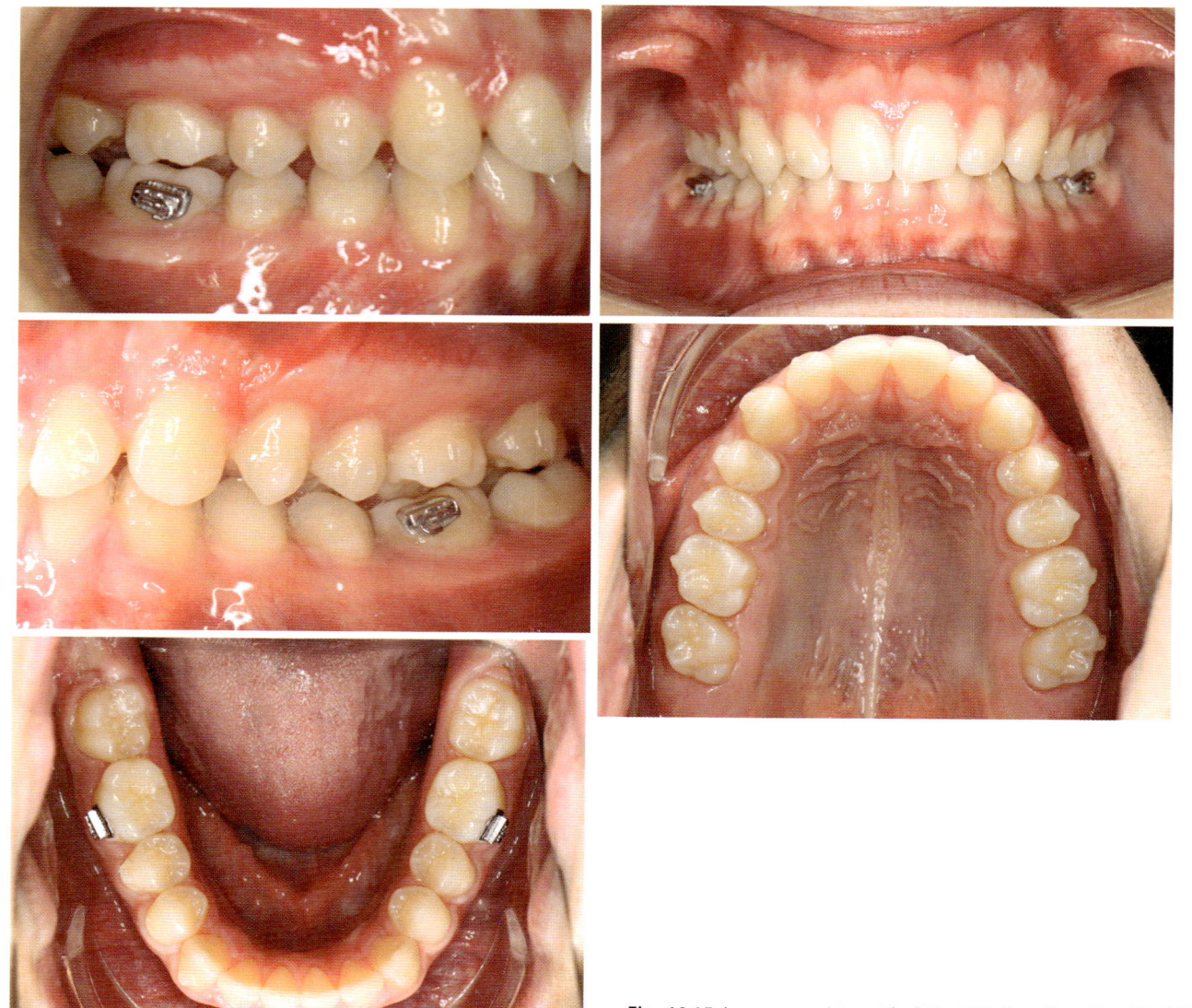

Fig. 10.15 In progress intraoral photos. Molar tubes were used on lower first molars for class II elastic anchorage.

10 • Deep Bite

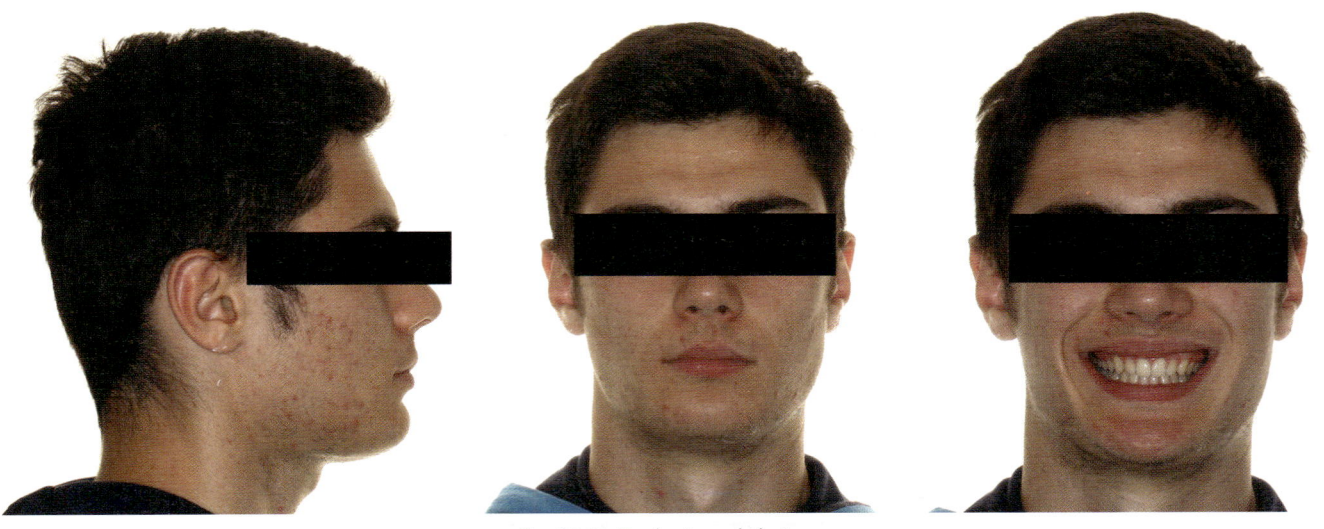

Fig. 10.16 Final extraoral photos.

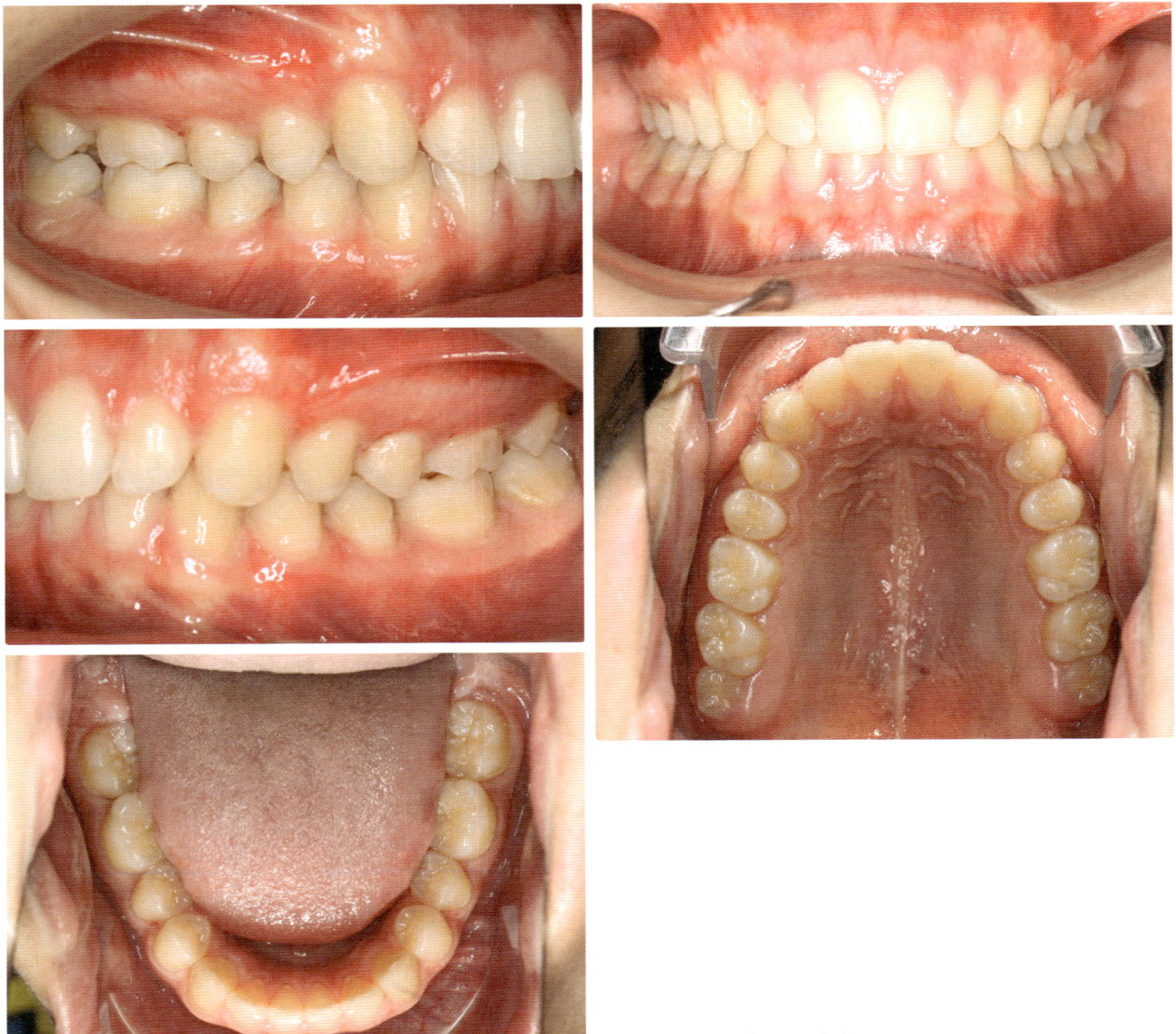

Fig. 10.17 Final intraoral photos.

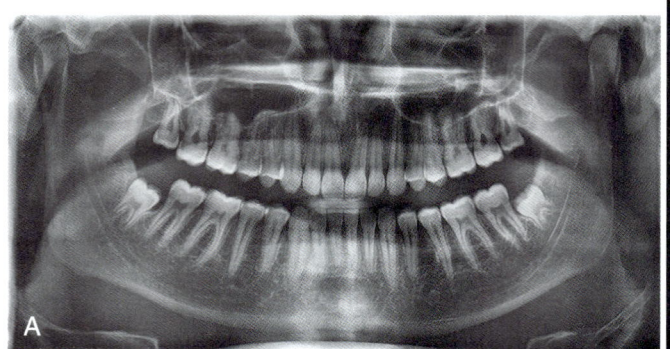

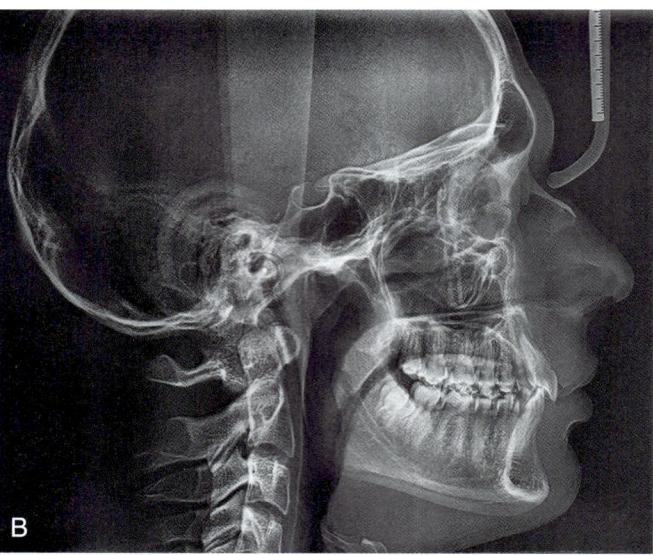

Fig. 10.18 (A) Final orthopantomography. (B) Final lateral x-ray.

References

1. Nanda R. *Biomechanics and Esthetic Strategies in Clinical Orthodontics.* Saunders; 2005.
2. Danz J, Greuter C, Sifakakis I, et al. Stability and relapse after orthodontic treatment of deep bite cases—a long-term follow-up study. *Eur J Orthod.* 2012;36:522-530.
3. Nielsen IL. Vertical malocclusions: etiology, development, diagnosis and some aspects of treatment. *Angle Orthod.* 1991;61(4):247-260.
4. Lux C, Dücker B, Pritsch M, et al. Occlusal status and prevalence of occlusal malocclusion traits among 9-year-old schoolchildren. *Eur J Orthod.* 2009;31:294-299.
5. Proffit Jr W, Fields H, Sarver D. *Contemporary Orthodontics.* 6th ed. Elsevier; 2018.
6. Tausche E, Luck O, Harzer W. Prevalence of malocclusions in the early mixed dentition and orthodontic treatment need. *Eur J Orthod.* 2004;26(3):237-244.
7. Millett DT, Cunningham SJ, O'Brien KD, et al. Orthodontic treatment for deep bite and retroclined upper front teeth in children. *Cochrane Database Syst Rev.* 2018;(2):CD005972.
8. Hans M, Enlow D. *Essential of Facial Growth.* Needham Press; 1996.
9. Marshall SD, Caspersen M, Hardinger RR, et al. Development of the curve of Spee. *Am J Orthod Dentofac Orthop.* 2008;134(3):344-352.
10. Clifford PM, Orr JF, Burden DJ. The effects of increasing the reverse curve of Spee in a lower archwire examined using a dynamic photo-elastic gelatine model. *Eur J Orthod.* 1999;21(3):213-222.
11. Liu Y, Hu W. Force changes associated with different intrusion strategies for deep-bite correction by clear aligners. *Angle Orthod.* 2018;88(6):771-778.
12. Sarver DM. The importance of incisor positioning in the esthetic smile: the smile arc. *Am J Orthod Dentofac Orthop.* 2001;120(2):98-111.
13. Simon M, Keilig L, Schwarze J, et al. Treatment outcome and efficacy of an aligner technique—regarding incisor torque, premolar derotation and molar distalization. *BMC Oral Health.* 2014;14:68.
14. Khosravi R, Cohanim B, Hujoel P, et al. Management of overbite with the Invisalign appliance. *Am J Orthod Dentofac Orthop.* 2017;151(4):691-699,e2.

11 Interceptive Orthodontics with Aligners

TOMMASO CASTROFLORIO, SERENA RAVERA, and FRANCESCO GARINO

Introduction

Early orthodontic treatment is still a debated argument. According to the existing literature, the usefulness of interceptive orthodontics is controversial even if many sagittal, vertical, and transversal malocclusions are clearly visible and diagnosed in the early mixed dentition.[1]

Some authors recommend interceptive treatment because many malocclusions tend to worsen with age.[2] Some other studies have underlined that orthodontic treatment during the pubertal phase may positively influence malocclusion improvements, contributing to the stability of final results.[3]

However, a recent review stated that removable functional appliances can produce short-term good dentoalveolar effects rather than skeletal improvements.[4] Furthermore, a recent update of a Cochrane review claimed that on the basis of low to moderate quality evidence, providing early orthodontic treatment for children with prominent upper front teeth is more effective for reducing the incidence of incisal trauma than providing one course of orthodontic treatment in adolescence. There appear to be no other advantages of providing early treatment when compared to late treatment.[5]

The reduction of upper incisor proclination should not be underestimated because the smile appearance is important among overall esthetics for adolescents as well as for children younger than 10 years of age. Correcting smile alterations, even in young children, may be fundamental in preventing bullying or teasing from others and in improving the quality of social interactions, preserving healthy psychologic development.[6]

Interceptive orthodontics could be also recommended when detecting bad oral habits as atypical swallowing and mouth breathing have been found to be strictly related to malocclusion worsening.[7] Moreover, early orthodontic treatment mainly consisting in maxillary expansion and mandibular advancement has been indicated to treat pediatric sleep apnea patients.[8]

The controversial results deriving from the existing literature in terms of effectiveness of interceptive orthodontics are mainly related to the lack of specific indicators of the right biologic timing of intervention. Although no skeletal maturity indicator may be considered to have a full diagnostic reliability in the identification of the maxillary growth peak and of the pubertal growth spurt or mandibular growth peak, treatment timing according to available indicators (mainly hand and wrist maturation [HWM] and cervical vertebral maturation [CVM] methods) has yielded more favorable outcomes. The use of the HWM or CVM methods (or others) may still be recommended for treatment planning, even though large individual responsiveness and dentoalveolar compensations have been reported, even in pubertal patients.[9]

In this chapter, we focus on clear aligner interceptive orthodontics of class II retrognathic patients and of patients with maxillary constrictions, highlighting the recommendations for case selection and treatment planning, showing some case reports.

Maxillary Expansion

Transverse maxillary constriction and maxillary crowding in children are problems commonly encountered and treated by orthodontists.[10-12] Interceptive orthodontics with maxillary expansion (ME) is one of the treatment options recommended for children with transverse deficiencies with the intent to increase the transverse widths of the maxilla. This approach is particularly important in children with posterior crossbite because it has been shown to determine abnormal chewing patterns and the development of skeletal asymmetries.[13,14]

Expansion is especially desirable for young class II division I patients who have constricted maxillae because the transverse deficiency does not self-correct between the deciduous, mixed, and permanent dentitions.[15] Increasing maxillary arch width could improve class II with retrognathic mandible, inducing a spontaneous forward repositioning of the mandible, even if there is still a lack of general consensus on this issue.[16,17] Maxillary arches are also expanded routinely to solve anterior crowding and improve the smile esthetics of kids.[6,18-20] Crowding of the permanent incisors, with associated rotations and/or anterior crossbite, is commonly observed during eruption of the permanent lateral incisors. The rationale of interceptive treatment in the early mixed dentition is to generate adequate space for the spontaneous alignment of the permanent upper lateral incisors prior to complete eruption. When crowding is limited to a few millimeters, normal growth could provide adequate space, but when the palate is narrow and the crowding exceeds this amount, maxillary expansion could represent an effective procedure.[21] As stated by Rosa et al.,[21] when planning interceptive rapid maxillary expansion (RME) in absence of posterior crossbite, the clinician should consider that first permanent molars are often tilted buccally, and a further buccal movement will produce periodontal problems and posterior occlusal interferences related to the deepening of the Wilson curve. Furthermore, the amount of anterior expansion could not be enough to solve the anterior crowding. Ideally the expansion should be limited to the anterior region of the arch, while permanent molars should move in a palatal direction.

Considering these aspects, maxillary expansion by anchorage on deciduous teeth has been proposed. The benefit of anchoring the expander on second deciduous molars and deciduous canines was the gain of 5 to 6 mm in upper arch perimeter. The gained space is sufficient to solve anterior crowding without tilting buccally permanent molars. However, those teeth spontaneously follow the buccal movement of deciduous molars for about 60% of their movement.

When thinking about differences between several activation protocols for maxillary expansion, a recent systematic review[22] helps us to understand some outcomes comparing slow maxillary expansion (SME) and RME; there is moderate evidence showing that maxillary transverse diameters increase significantly within both groups in the short-term,[23] but SME protocol is more predictive of bodily upper molar movement, while the RME protocol produces more tipping movement in the molar region.[24]

RME uses heavier interrupted forces to maximize orthopedic effects, and slow palatal expansion uses lighter continuous forces to move teeth at rates purported to be more physiologic.[11] Aligners use intermittent light forces to move teeth, and intermittent forces are able to produce orthodontic tooth movement with less cell damage in the periodontium.[25] Since it has been stated that light, continuous forces seem to be perceived as intermittent forces by the periodontium due to its viscoelastic nature,[26] the expansion produced by aligners could be described as SME.

A clear aligner maxillary expansion protocol has been recently proposed (Invisalign First, Align Technology, Inc., San José, CA, USA). Aligners could overcome some of the limitations presented by palatal expander particularly in non-crossbite cases. With these appliances, it is possible to control the movement of all the teeth in the maxillary arch, aiming to produce an initial alignment and leveling while expanding the arch. Aligners can be really helpful in controlling maxillary first molars not only on the frontal plane but on the horizontal and sagittal planes, too, avoiding all the issues mentioned earlier in relation to potential periodontal problems. Furthermore, aligners can control the expansion limited to the anterior region of the arch to generate adequate space for the spontaneous alignment of the permanent upper lateral incisors prior to complete eruption.

Because of the short clinical crowns of deciduous teeth, specific attachment shapes were designed to increase aligner retention and control the tipping movement to obtain torque compensation and avoid a deepening of the curve of Wilson (Fig. 11.1).

Regarding staging, two options are available at the moment: (1) Permanent molars (if required by the treatment plan) will be moved buccally, using the rest of the arch as anchorage, and only once they have reached their final position will the deciduous molars and canines be moved buccally using permanent molars and incisors as anchorage units. (2) Permanent molars and deciduous teeth are moved buccally in a simultaneous manner (Fig. 11.2). Because of the geometry of the aligners, their distal portions are not stiff enough to support a predictable buccal movement of so many teeth at the same time, making this staging not the first-line treatment option.

Timing is another important factor to be considered. The best timing to expand maxillary arch is during the early mixed dentition, before upper permanent lateral incisor eruption and after the permanent molars are fully erupted and in occlusion. This timing is favorable as the midpalatal suture is more immature.[27] In young children, up to age 8 or 9 years, little force is needed. Up to that age, a transpalatal

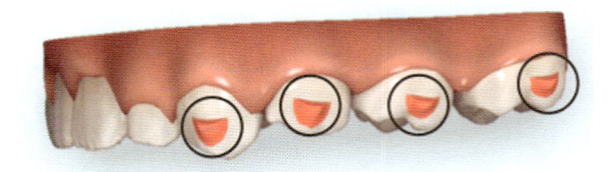

Fig. 11.1 Invisalign First optimized attachments for maxillary expansion.

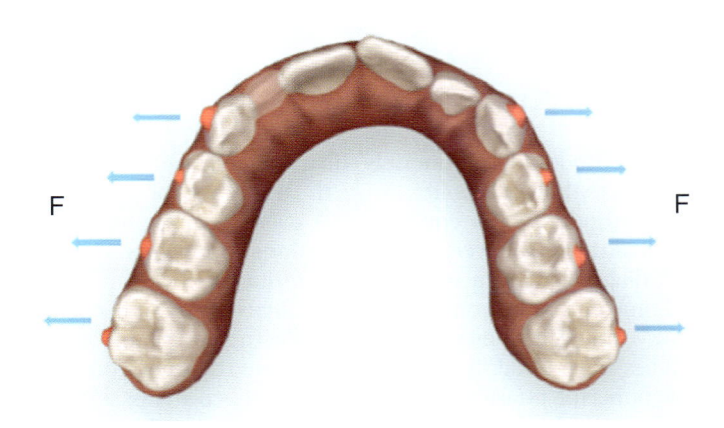

Fig. 11.2 Invisalign First maxillary expansion protocol staging.

lingual arch releasing light continuous forces for dental expansion also will open the midpalatal suture.[28] Therefore, it can be assumed that intermittent forces released by aligners can be sufficient in children up to 8 or 9 years of age to act on the transversal dimension of the maxilla.

A recent clinical trial conducted at the University of Torino (Torino, Italy) in which clear aligners and RPE effects in patients with maxillary constriction were measured on digital models, suggests that:

- A significant increase in palatal volume, so as in the other parameters, has been proved for both treatments.
- The RPE slightly outperform clear aligners considering all the parameters tested.
- The compliance and the clinical condition could affect the potential results achievable by the clear aligners.

The Clear Aligners demonstrated a reasonable ability to achieve palatal expansion. Since the materials have improved over the last years, so as the academic efforts to better understand the potential of CAT, substantial advances can be expected in the near future.[58]

Expansion Case Reports

For the following case reports, three-dimensional (3D) evaluation of upper arch and palate morphology was performed according to a previous study by Bizzarro et al.[29] The upper arches were scanned using a 3D scanner (iTero Element). The 3D data were imported to a reverse modeling software package called Geomagic Studio (3D Systems, Inc).[30] Intermolar, intersecond deciduous molar, and intercanine transverse widths at the cusps and gingival levels were measured (Fig. 11.3), as well as anterior and posterior palatal depths at the cusp level, palatal surface area (Fig. 11.4), and volume (Fig. 11.5).

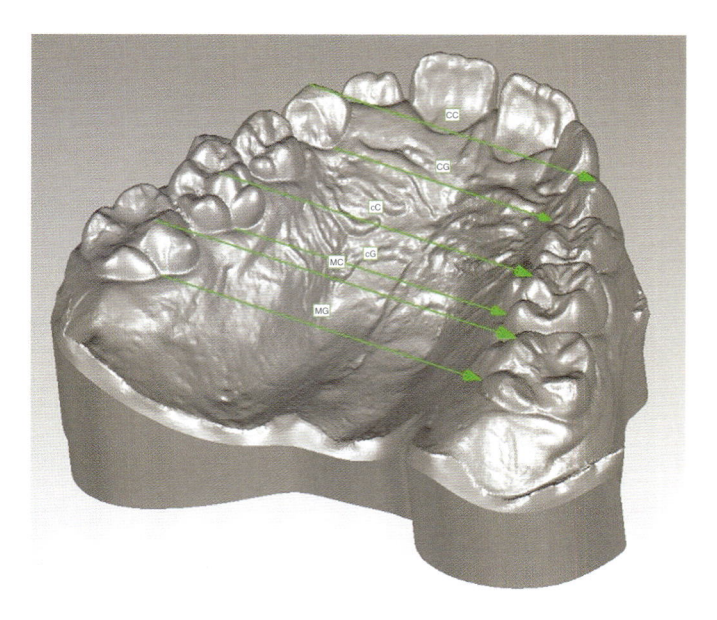

Fig. 11.3 CG intercanine widths assessed at gingival level, CC intercanine widths assessed at cusp level, cG inter-E widths assessed at gingival level, cC inter-E widths assessed at cusp level, MG intermolar widths assessed at gingival level, MC intermolar widths assessed at cusp level.

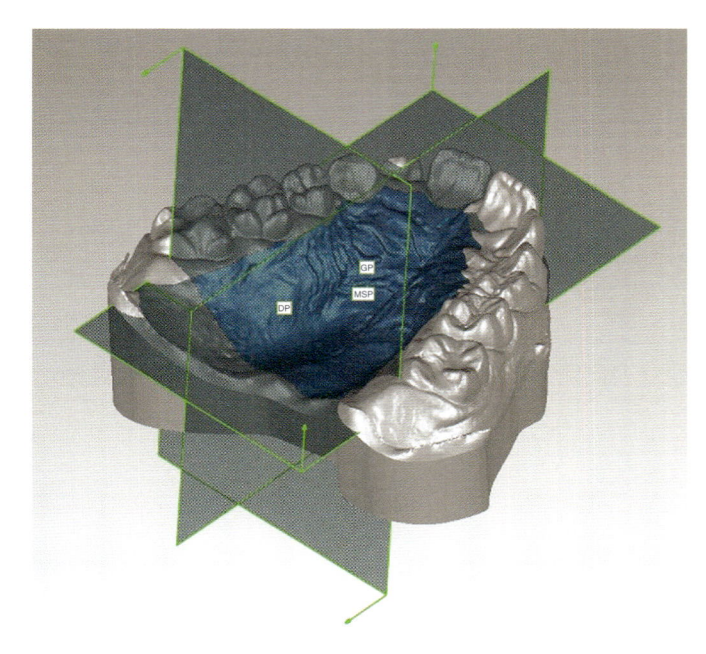

Fig. 11.4 The anterior and posterior depth of the palatal vault is defined as the vertical distance from the contact line between the cusp of the right and left canine and mesiopalatal cusp tips of the right and left first molars to the palatal vault, respectively. The palatal volume was defined by the median sagittal, distal, and gingival planes as boundaries of the palate. The distal plane *(DP)* passed through two points at the distal of the first upper permanent molars. The gingival plane *(GP)* was created by intersecting the distal and median sagittal planes *(MSP)* through the center of incisive papilla, which is considered a stable point structure.[31] All planes were perpendicular to each other.

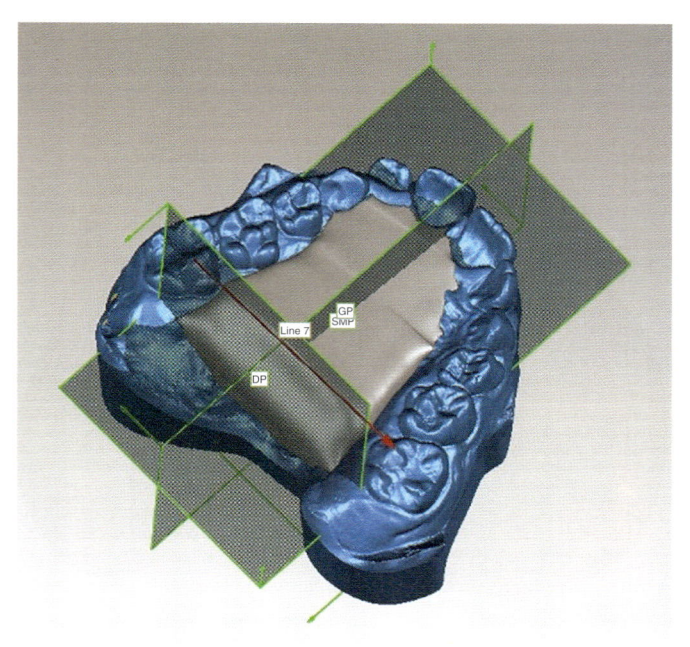

Fig. 11.5 The palatal surface area was defined by the median sagittal *(MSP)*, distal *(DP)*, and gingival *(GP)* planes as boundaries of the palate. The distal plane *(DP)* passed through two points at the distal of the first upper permanent molars.

CASE STUDY 1

Consider an 8-year-old boy with upper central incisor protrusion, mild upper anterior crowding, and palatal tipping of deciduous teeth. Invisalign First was adopted, and sequential expansion of molars first and then deciduous teeth was planned within the ClinCheck, along with alignment of central and lateral incisors. The patient was instructed to change the aligners every week, and control examinations were planned every 6 weeks. Pre- and postexpansion scan screenshots are shown in Fig. 11.6. The expansion phase lasted 8 months. The palatal volume increased from 3843.54 mm³ to 5330.89 mm³ due not only to the vestibular dental tipping but also increased interarch widths measured at both gingival and a cuspal levels. Quantitative evaluations of intraarch widths, palatal areas, and volumes for this case are summarized in Table 11.1 as Case 1 reports.

CASE STUDY 2

Consider a 9-year-old girl with upper anterior crowding and deep bite. Invisalign First was adopted, and sequential expansion of molars first and then deciduous teeth was planned within the ClinCheck, along with the alignment of central and lateral incisors. The patient was instructed to change the aligners every week and control examinations were planned every 2 months. Pre- and postexpansion scan screenshots are shown in Fig. 11.7. The expansion phase lasted 6 months. The palatal volume increased from 4342.64 mm³ to 6948.68 mm³ due not only to the vestibular dental tipping but also increased interarch widths measured at both a gingival and a cuspal level. Quantitative evaluations of intraarch widths, palatal areas, and volumes for this case are summarized in Table 11.1 as Case 2 reports.

Class II Malocclusion

Class II malocclusion is the most frequent skeletal sagittal disharmonies in the white population.[32] Diagnosis using

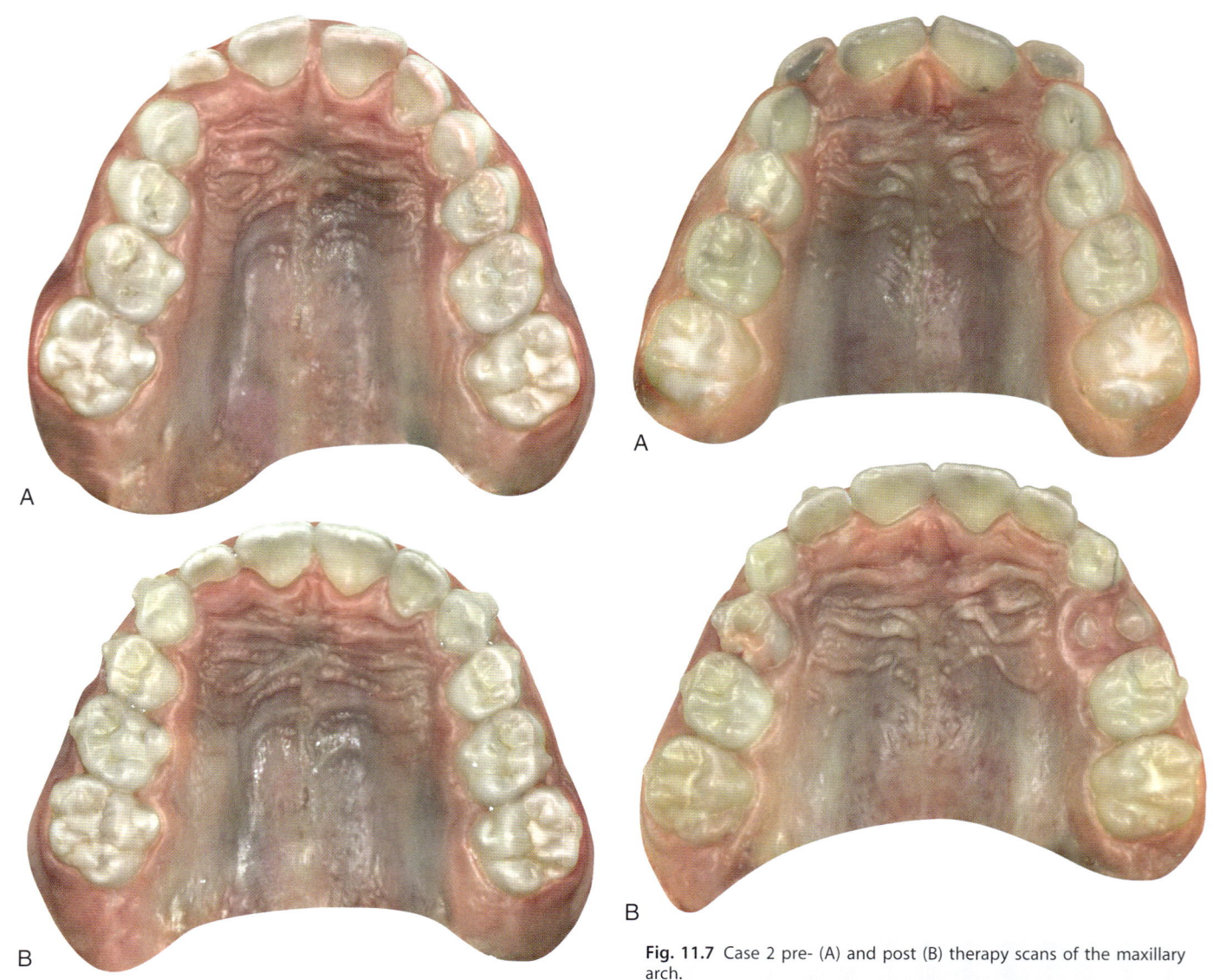

124 Principles and Biomechanics of Aligner Treatment

Fig. 11.6 Case 1 pre- (A) and post (B) therapy scans of the maxillary arch.

Fig. 11.7 Case 2 pre- (A) and post (B) therapy scans of the maxillary arch.

Table 11.1 Pre- and post-treatment volumetric and linear measurements obtained in the reported cases.

	A mm²	V mm³	CG mm	CC mm	cG mm	cC mm	MG mm	MC mm
Case 1 pre	1105.91	3843.54	22.6	29.1	28.2	32.2	32.6	36.8
Case 1 post	1316.57	5330.89	27.6	36.7	33.4	39.7	36	42.1
Case 2 pre	1111.67	4342.64	24.4	32.1	29.8	34.5	35.1	39.7
Case 2 post	1478.69	6948.68	26.3	37.5	32.9	39.5	35.4	42.1

A, Palatal surface area; *CC*, intercanine widths assessed at cusp level; *cC*, inter-E widths assessed at cusp level; *CG*, intercanine widths assessed at gingival level; *cG*, inter-E widths assessed at gingival level; *MC*, intermolar widths assessed at cusp level; *MG*, intermolar widths assessed at gingival level; *V*, palatal volume.

cephalometric tracings may highlight different dental or skeletal components of class II malocclusion: upper incisor proclination, lower incisor retroclination, mandibular retrognathia, ipomandibulia, maxillary protrusion, ipermaxillia, or different combinations of these components.

Mandible retrusion has been found to be the main factor in most basal class II malocclusions.[33,34] One orthopedic approach developed to treat mandibular skeletal retrusion in growing patients is the forward repositioning of the mandible,[35,36] even if a general consensus about the efficacy and efficiency of this approach is still missing[36,37] (probably for inconsistent evidence of homogeneous interventions,[37,38] wide variations in individual responsiveness,[39] and different timings in orthodontic intervention[9]), and undergoing mandibular advancement in specific growth phases has been reported to have a key role in successful treatment outcomes.

Several studies have shown that the optimal biologic timing for the achievement of skeletal effects is the circumpubertal growth period,[40-43] when the greater mandibular growth response occurs, so that treatment can start in the early mixed dentition.[41] The pubertal peak can be identified by several growth indicators, including skeletal maturation (cervical vertebrae maturation method, hand-wrist radiographs), dental maturation, and chronologic age,[42,44,45] and more recently the reliability of gingival crevicular fluid (GCF) biomarkers specific for growth spurt characterization has been under investigation.[46,47]

A morphologic predictive factor in successful mandible repositioning with functional appliances is the pretreatment mandibular angle (Co-Go-Me angle <125.5 degrees). As shown by Franchi and Baccetti[39] as well as previous animal and human studies,[43] a small mandibular angle is correlated with an enhanced responsiveness to mandibular forward positioning, and vice versa.

The usual main limitation for removable functional appliances is patient noncompliance, rated by O'Brien as 18% in children, raising to 30% in adolescence.[48] Noncompliance can depend on bulky and invasive devices, difficulties in speech, impact on social life, esthetics, and public perception, not precise and predicted orthodontic tooth movements. To overcome these limitations, aligner therapy may be considered a good, reliable, and comfortable alternative. The use of the compliance indicators embedded in the aligner represents a good attempt to monitor patient compliance.[49] More recently artificial intelligence has been introduced in the orthodontic field to remote monitor patient compliance (Dental Monitoring, Paris, France).

Functional treatment of growing class II patients during their pubertal growth spurt can bring about significant skeletal and dentoalveolar modifications. According to Cozza et al.,[37] the twin block is the most efficient removable functional appliance because it can stimulate 0.23 mm/month of mandibular growth (for a total of 3.4 mm in 13 months), followed by the Bionator (0.17 mm/month, total 2.8 mm in 12 months), and then the Frankel II (0.09 mm/month, total 2.8 mm in 18 months). The mechanism behind the Clark twin block is based on the presence of an inclined plane, which pushes the mandible forward, liberates the arches, and redirects the occlusal forces to drive the mandibular advancement and arrest maxillary growth.[50]

Two companies (Align Technology Inc, San José, CA, USA and Leone SPA Company, Sesto Fiorentino, Firenze, Italy) have developed a new feature within aligner appliances,[51] combining the twin block and the aligner advantages to stimulate growth of the mandible while aligning and leveling in growing patients.

The Leone company appliance called Runner (Fig. 11.8) consists of a series of clear aligners with incorporated occlusal blocks for mandibular advancement, joining the

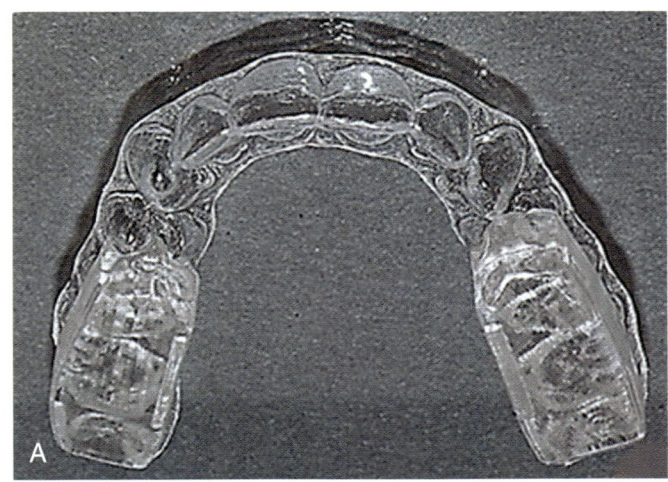

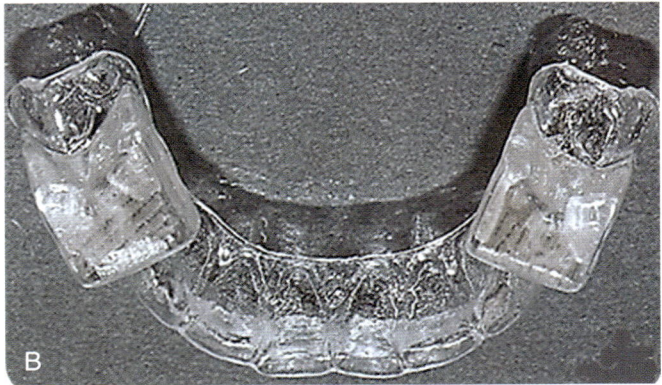

Fig. 11.8 Runner appliance. Upper arch aligner (A) and lower arch aligner (B). (From Arreghini A, et al. Class II treatment with the Runner in adolescent patients: combining twin block efficiency with aligner aesthetics. *J World Fed Orthod*. 2014;3[2]:71–79.)

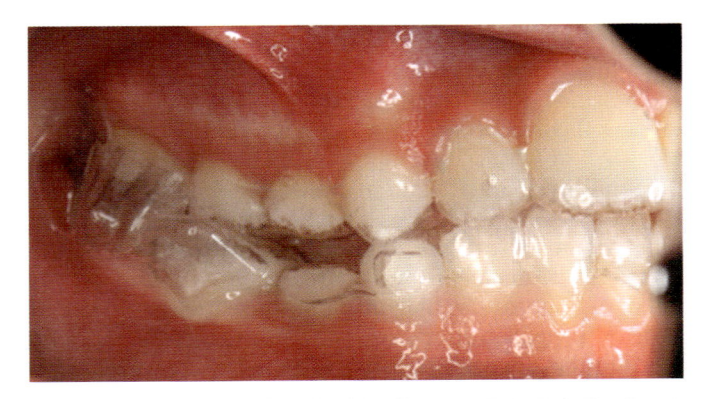

Fig. 11.9 Intraoral Invisalign First with mandibular advancement feature.

efficiency of the twin block with the esthetics and low bulk of clear aligners.[52]

The Align Technology company appliance is the Invisalign aligner incorporating lateral wings (Figs. 11.9 and 11.10) engaging the mandible in a forward position.

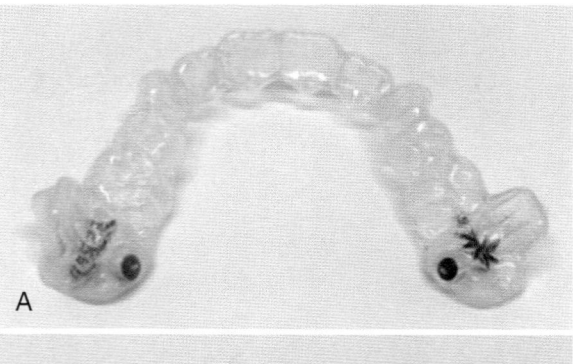

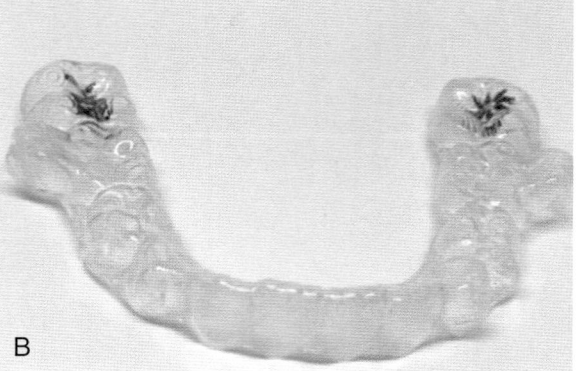

Fig. 11.10 Invisalign First with mandibular advancement feature. Upper arch aligner (A) and lower arch aligner (B)

The mandibular advancement system is divided into three clinical phases:

- *Pre–mandibular advancement phase:* the occlusal locks, which prevent expression of mandibular growth, are removed (correction of overbite, maxillary molar rotations, and overjet)
- *Mandibular advancement phase:* 2-mm advancement every eight aligners is performed
- *Transition phase (or stabilization phase):* maintains the class II correction

Mandibular advancement can be reached only if other eventual occlusal features have been modified (i.e., maxillary molar derotation, dentoalveolar expansion of the upper arch, deep bite and consequent leveling of the curve of Spee, and retroclination of the incisors), so that a prior preparation phase is required before starting mandibular advancement. While the Runner appliance, the twin block, and other functional appliances are built with a single jump repositioning the mandible, the Invisalign appliance is designed to obtain progressive advancement of the mandible with steps of 2 mm every eight aligners. The progressive advancement of the mandible has been demonstrated to be more effective in producing skeletal outcomes both in animal[53,54] and human studies.[55]

At the end of treatment, mandibular advancement is maintained by arch coordination and anterior interference removal.

In class II treatments, assessment of skeletal age and auxologic potential and predicting the direction of mandibular growth constitute strategic factors determining treatment efficacy.

Concerning the importance of right timing to choose the beginning of the interceptive class II correction phase, recent perspective-controlled studies by the University of Turin (Italy) aim to compare dental and skeletal effects of 12 months of therapy with the mandibular advancement feature by Invisalign, when performed on growing patients both at CVM2 and CVM3. When used in the pre-pubertal stage of growth, Invisalign® aligners, with Mandibular Advancement feature, have mainly dentoalveolar effects in the short-term period. When used in the pubertal growth phase, the short-term effects of Mandibular Advancement feature are dento-skeletal, with an annual rate of change comparable to what has been previously described for the Twin Block appliance.[59]

According to the existent literature, early treatment of class II division I malocclusion should be provided only to reduce the risk of incisal trauma.[56] Additionally, dental injuries have been reported to have a negative impact on the emotional and social domains of the oral health–related quality of life. Since this impact is considerable especially for children having active lifestyles, parents will consider that early orthodontic treatment is worth the financial costs and burden of care.[57]

Furthermore, there are young patients for whom the malocclusion is esthetically distressing, and they are bullied for this reason. The use of aligners provided for functional and orthopedic adjuncts can have a positive impact on the self-esteem of those patients even during the orthodontic treatment, providing excellent orthodontic care for such children.

Mandibular Advancement Case Reports

CASE STUDY 3

Consider a 9-year-old girl, in mixed dentition, with molar class II relationship, deep bite, proclined upper incisors, and retruded mandible. Cephalometric analysis shows a moderate skeletal class II malocclusion, with an ANB angle value of 5 degrees, and Wits value of 7 mm (Fig. 11.11–11.13). According to Baccetti et al.,[42] the patient was in a pubertal growth spurt, which is why the treatment plan was designed to focus on mandibular advancement. An Invisalign Teen treatment with the mandibular advancement feature was performed (Fig. 11.14).

The appliance was prescribed to determine an advancement of the mandible together with deep bite correction. The ClinCheck plan forecasted 2 mm of advancement every eight stages, and aligners were changed every week. After 6 months of treatment, a bilateral class I molar relationship was achieved (Figs. 11.15–11.16 and 11.17), and dentoskeletal improvements were achieved.

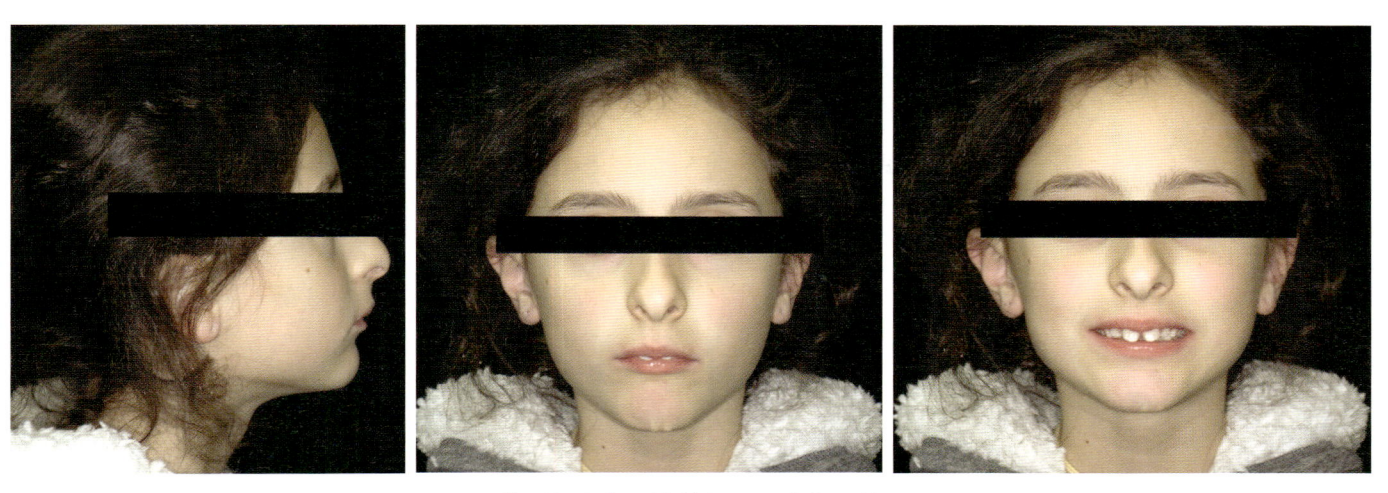

11 • Interceptive Orthodontics with Aligners 127

Fig. 11.11 Case 3 Initial extraoral pictures.

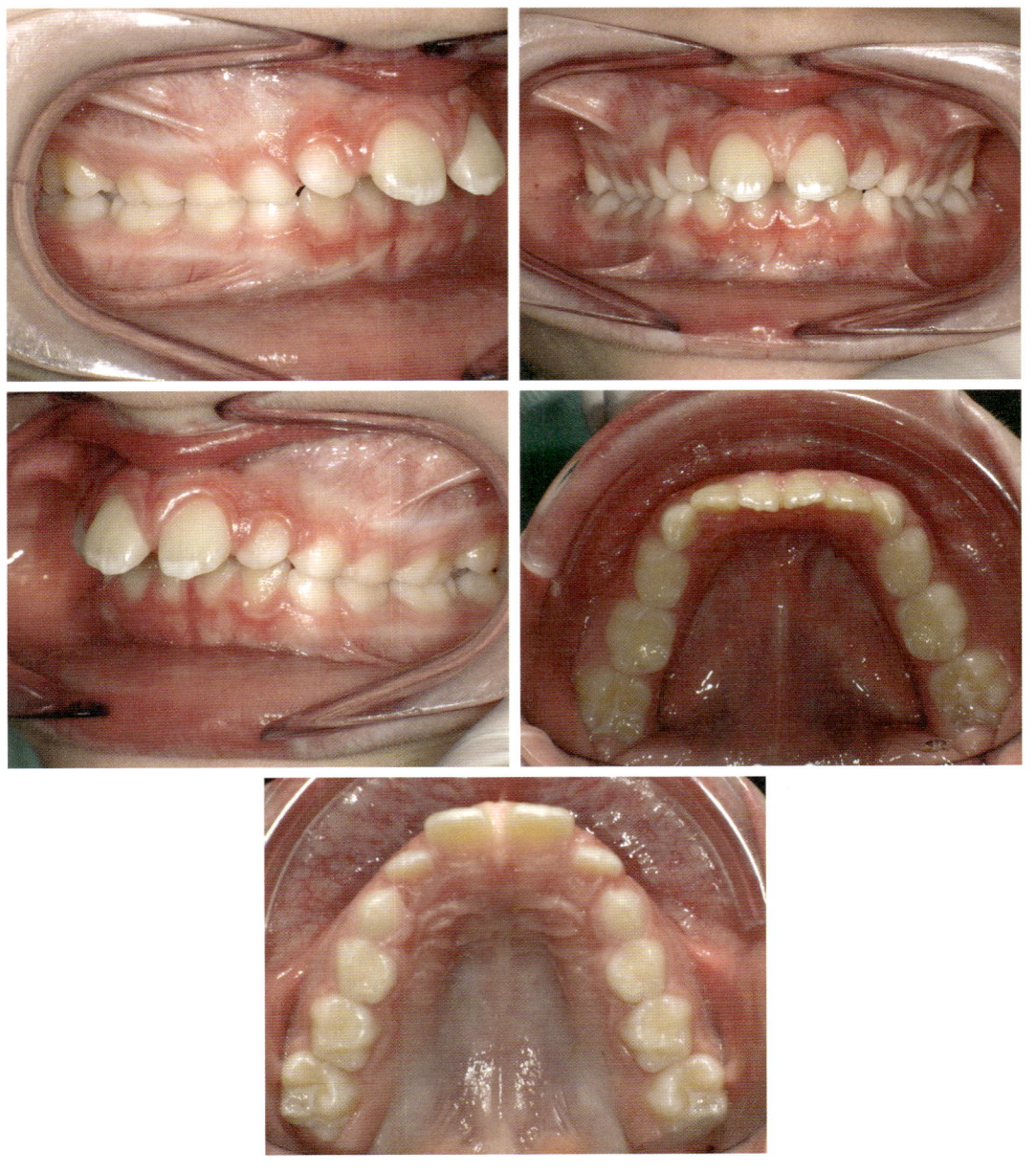

Fig. 11.12 Case 3 initial intraoral pictures.

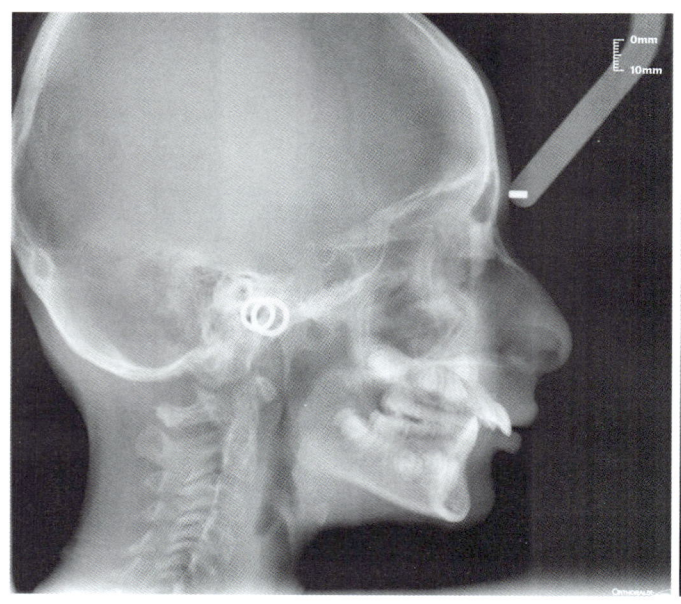

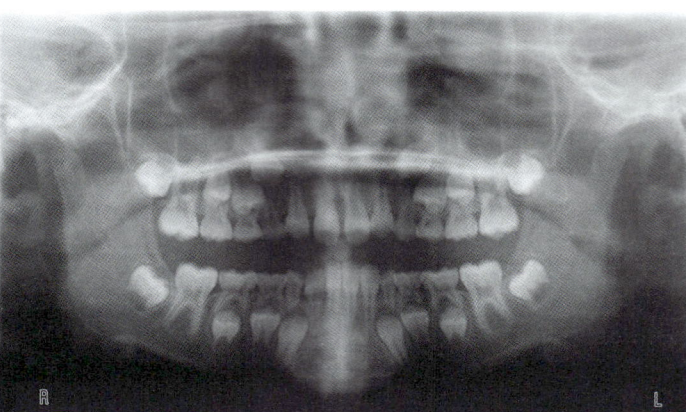

128 Principles and Biomechanics of Aligner Treatment

Fig. 11.13 Case 3 initial radiographic records.

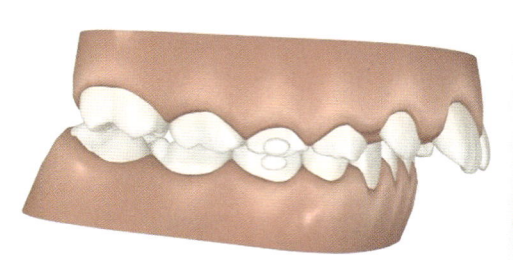

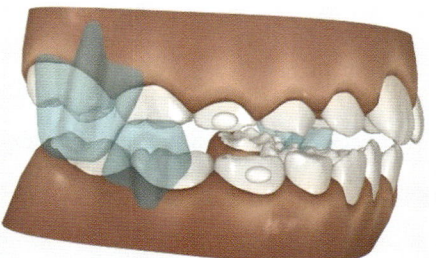

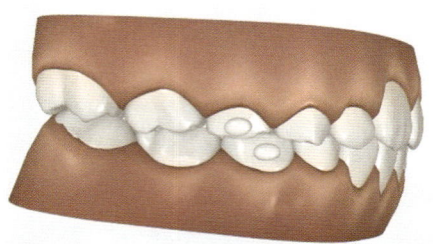

Fig. 11.14 Case 3 sagittal view of ClinCheck.

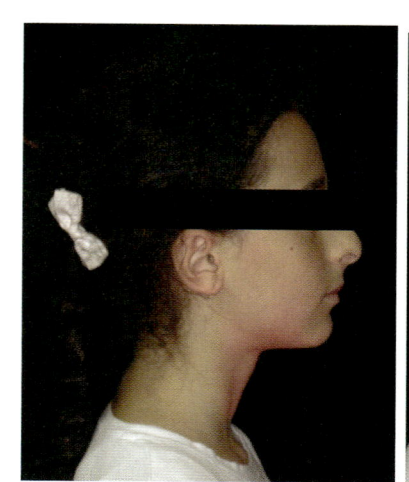

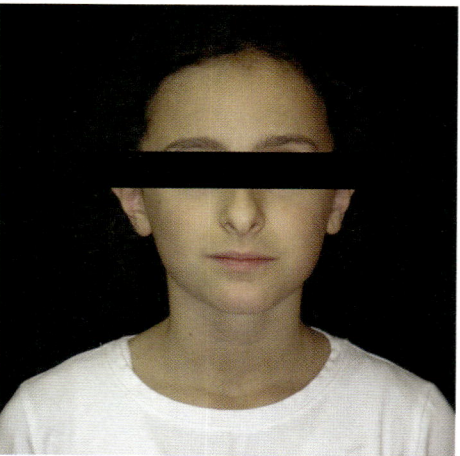

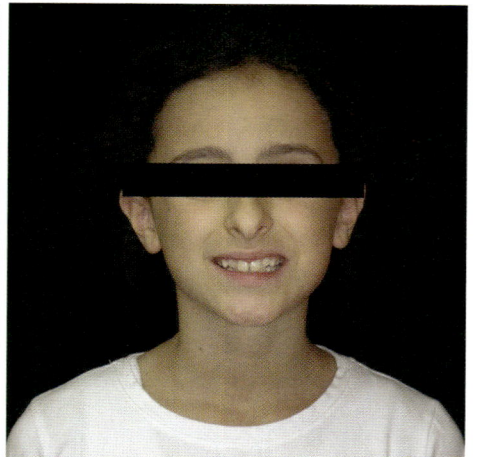

Fig. 11.15 Case 3 final clinical records.

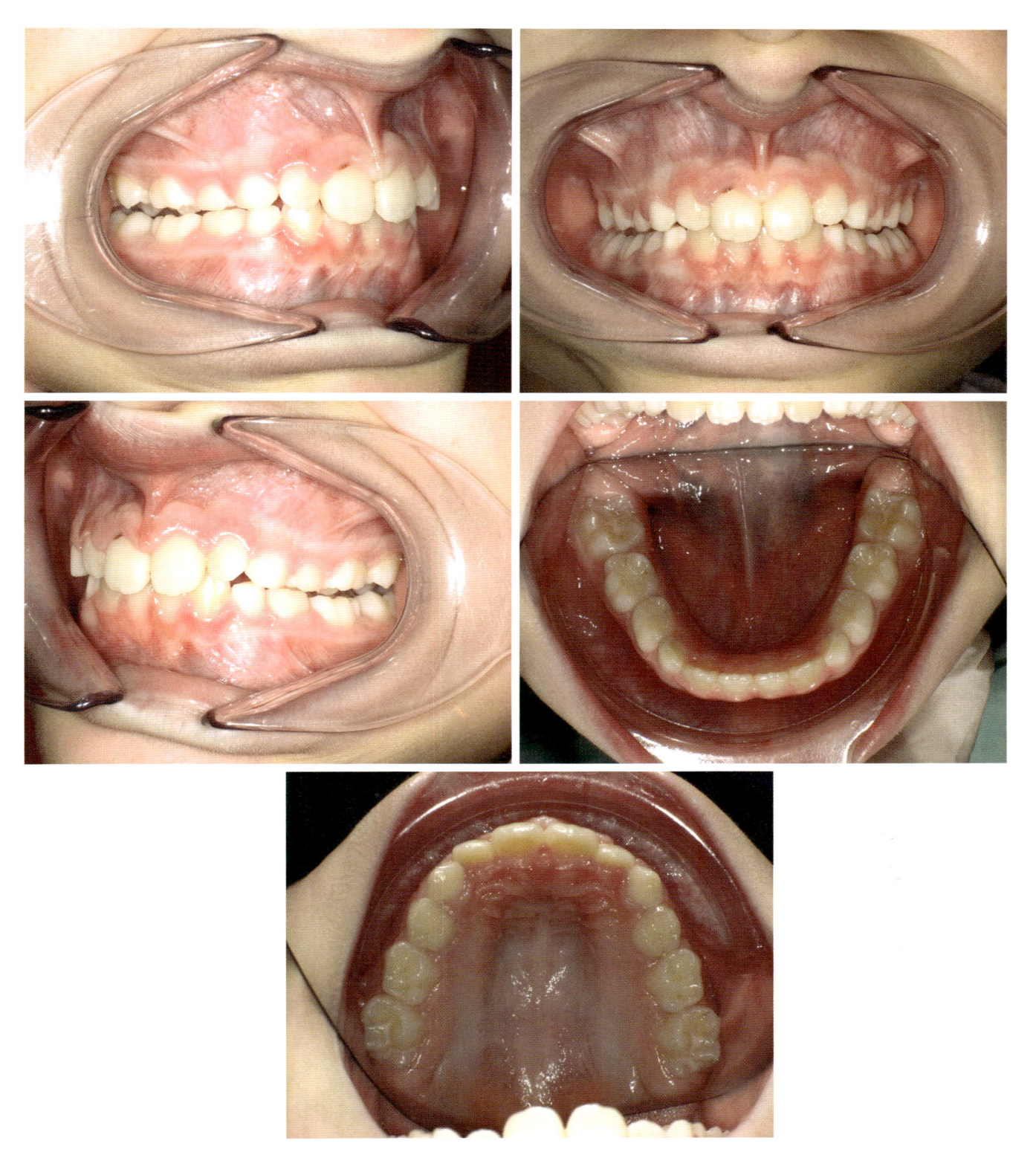

Fig. 11.16

CASE STUDY 4

Consider a 10-year-old girl in mixed dentition with psychological issues, reporting bullying episodes due to the protrusion of upper incisors and the retrusion of the mandible. The clinical examination showed a molar class II relationship, severe deep bite, skeletal class II with ANB angle of 6 degrees, and Wits value of 5 mm (Fig. 11.18–11.20).

Analyzing the cervical vertebrae maturation on the lateral x-ray, the patient resulted in a CVM3 phase, according to Baccetti et al,[42] and is therefore in a phase of accelerated condylar growth. Since the girl was psychologically stressed because of her bad-looking teeth, an additional stress due to a bulky appliance would not have been the best choice. Thus Invisalign Teen with the mandibular advancement feature was adopted (Fig. 11.21).

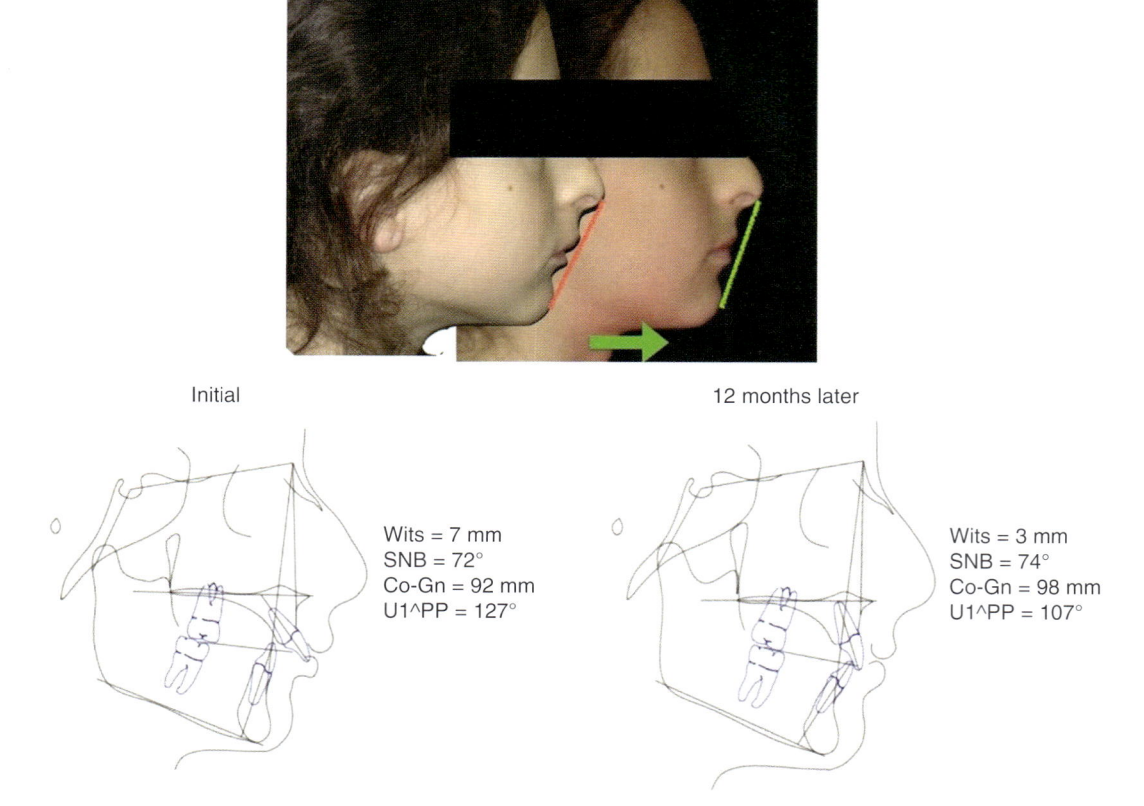

130 Principles and Biomechanics of Aligner Treatment

Initial — 12 months later

Wits = 7 mm
SNB = 72°
Co-Gn = 92 mm
U1^PP = 127°

Wits = 3 mm
SNB = 74°
Co-Gn = 98 mm
U1^PP = 107°

Fig. 11.17 Case 3 changes of mandibular profile and cephalometric values before and after therapy.

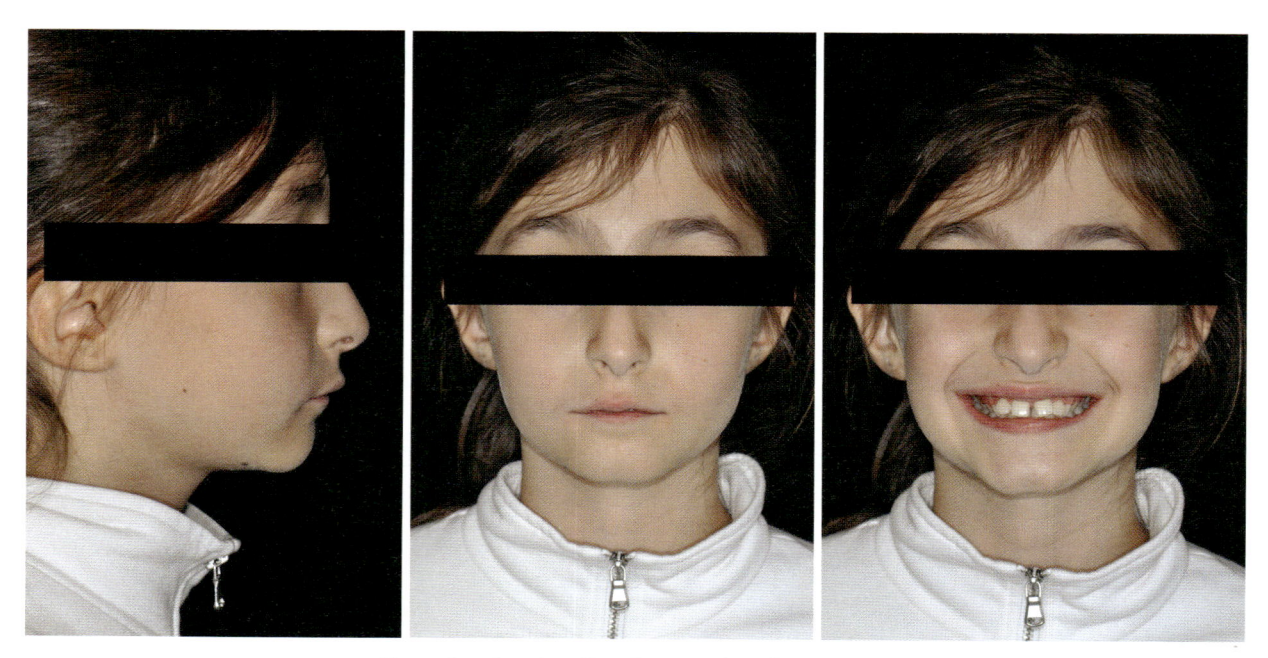

Fig. 11.18 Case 4 initial clinical and radiographic records.

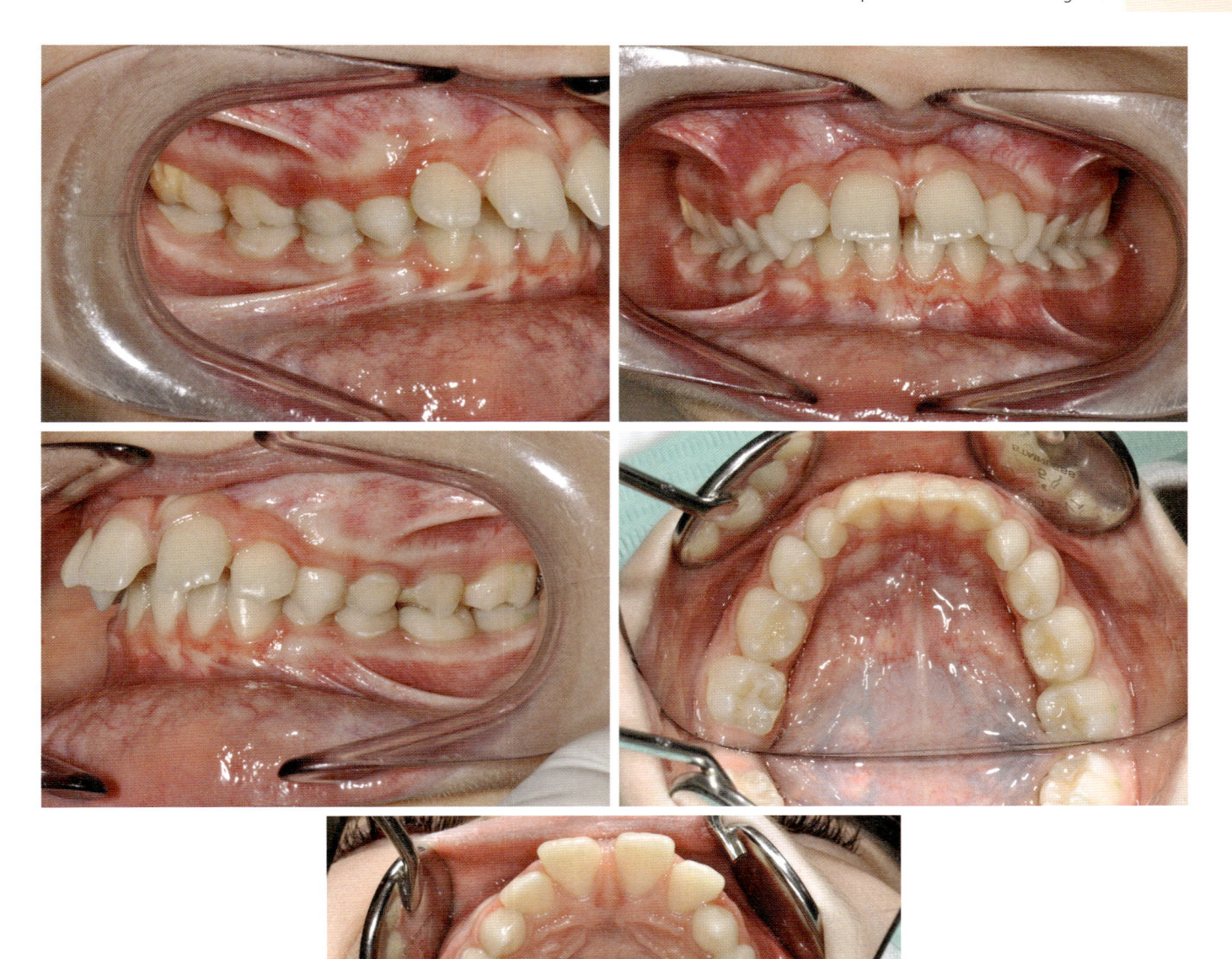

11 • Interceptive Orthodontics with Aligners   131

Fig. 11.19

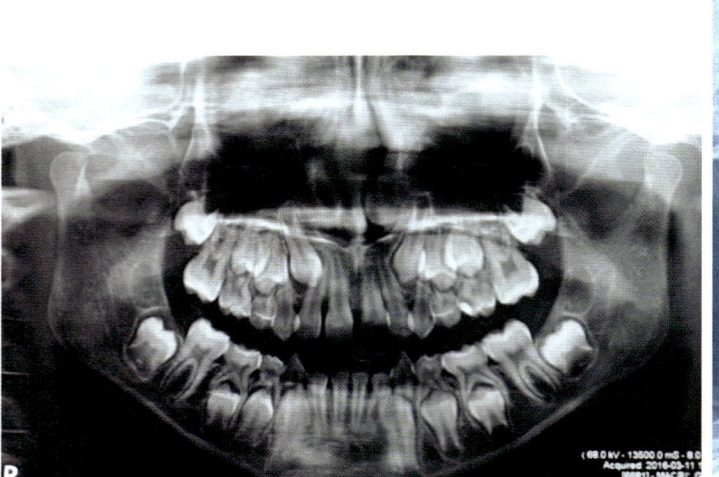

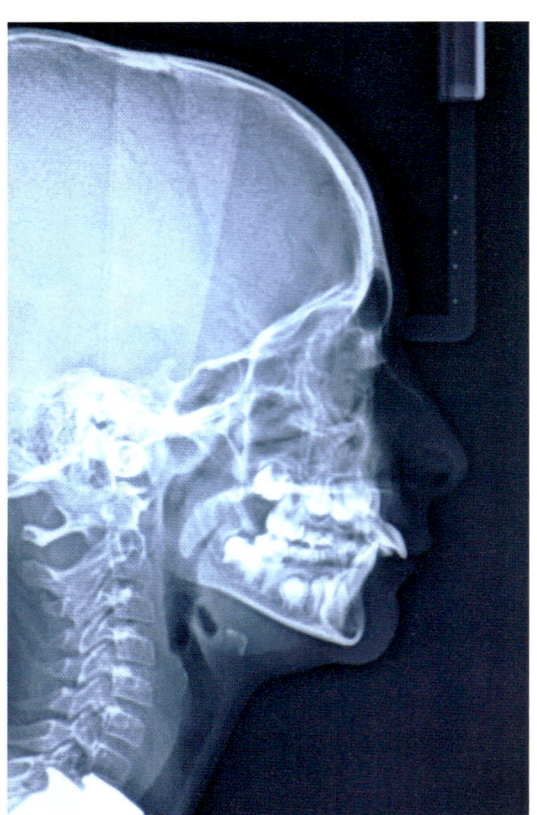

Fig. 11.20

In 6 months of treatment, an important correction of the molar relationship and of the proclination of upper incisors was obtained. During the mandibular advancement phase treatment, improvement of the facial profile was the most important motivational factor acting on the patient's and the parents' compliance (Figs. 11.22–23 and 11.24).

Conclusions

The timing of orthodontic treatment has long been debated. Among the proposed benefits of early intervention are the potential for improved response to growth modification. Transversal alterations are frequently seen in general dental practices. Aligners can control the expansion limited to the

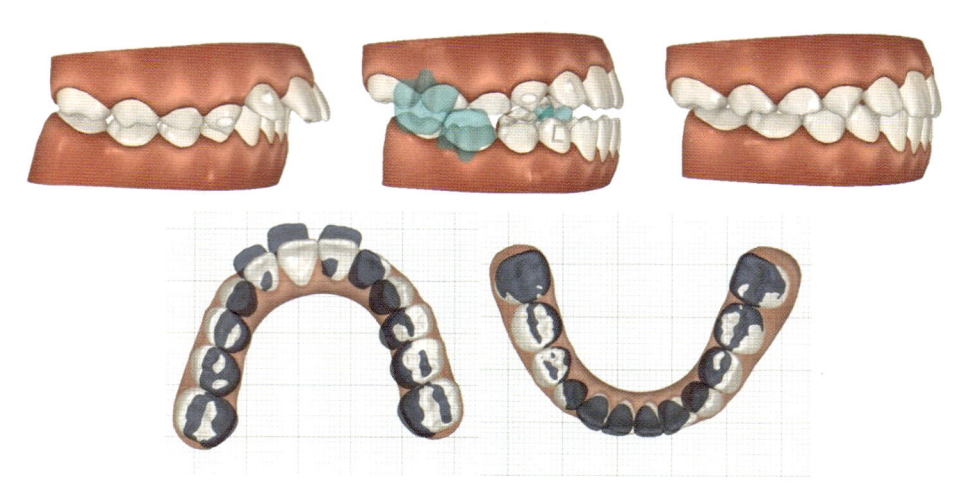

Fig. 11.21 Case 4 sagittal view of ClinCheck and superimposition of initial ClinCheck with final ClinCheck (occlusal view).

11 • Interceptive Orthodontics with Aligners   133

anterior region of the arch to generate adequate space for the spontaneous alignment of the permanent upper lateral incisors prior to complete eruption, helping the future arch development. Researchers in the fields are recommended to define possibilities and limitations of the approach.

Routine early treatment for class II division I malocclusion with retrognathic mandible should not be provided according to the existing quality of evidence. However, there are patients for whom the malocclusion is so esthetically distressing and/or who are bullied significantly because of it that treatment is certainly indicated. In those cases, the use of a discrete and noninvasive appliance like an aligner with mandibular forward repositioning wings or planes could represent an excellent possibility. Another group of patients for whom the early treatment could be indicated is represented by children with active sports schedules and lifestyles, putting them at risk of incisal trauma because of their large overjet.

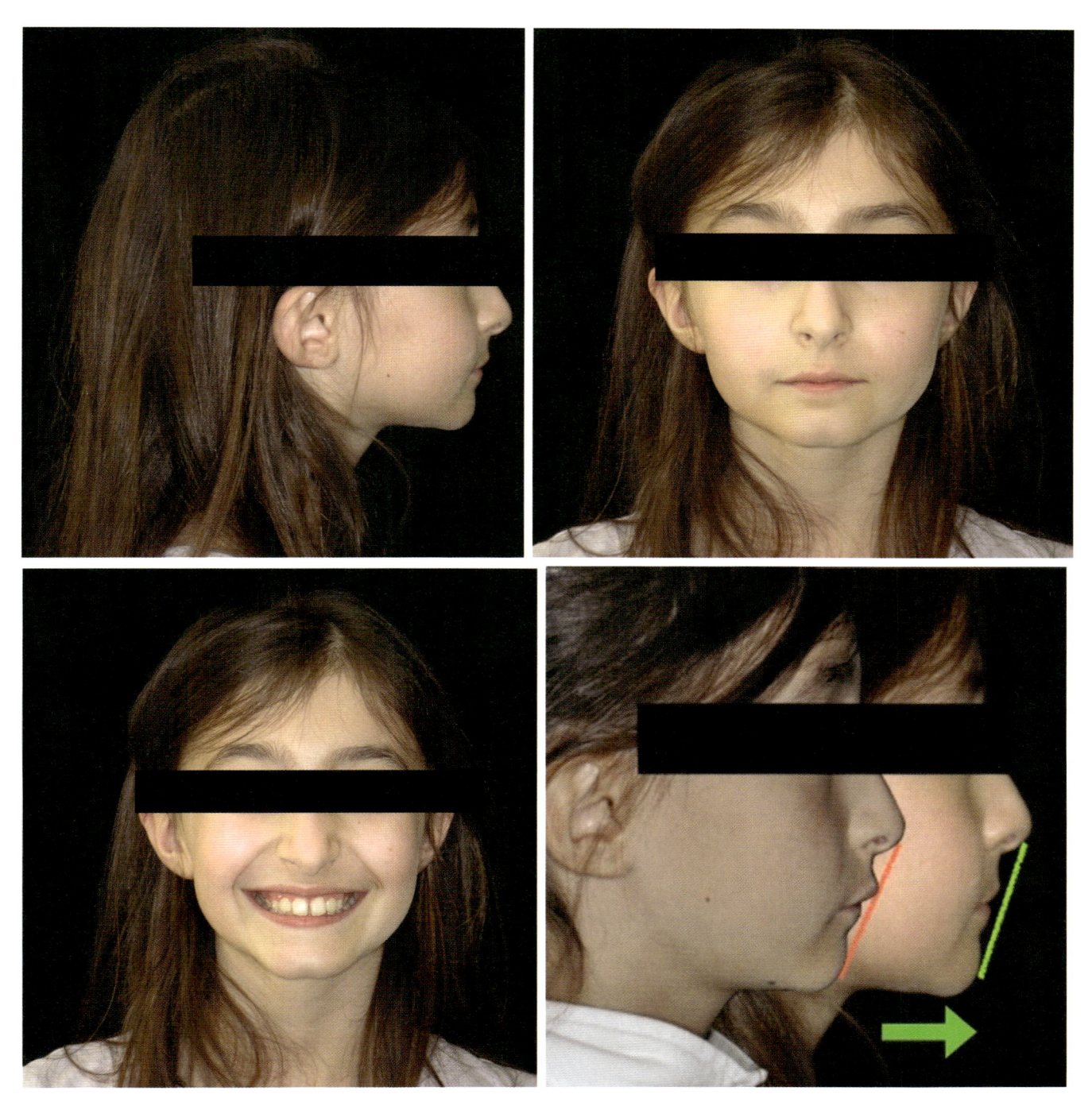

Fig. 11.22 Case 4 final clinical records and changes of mandibular profile.

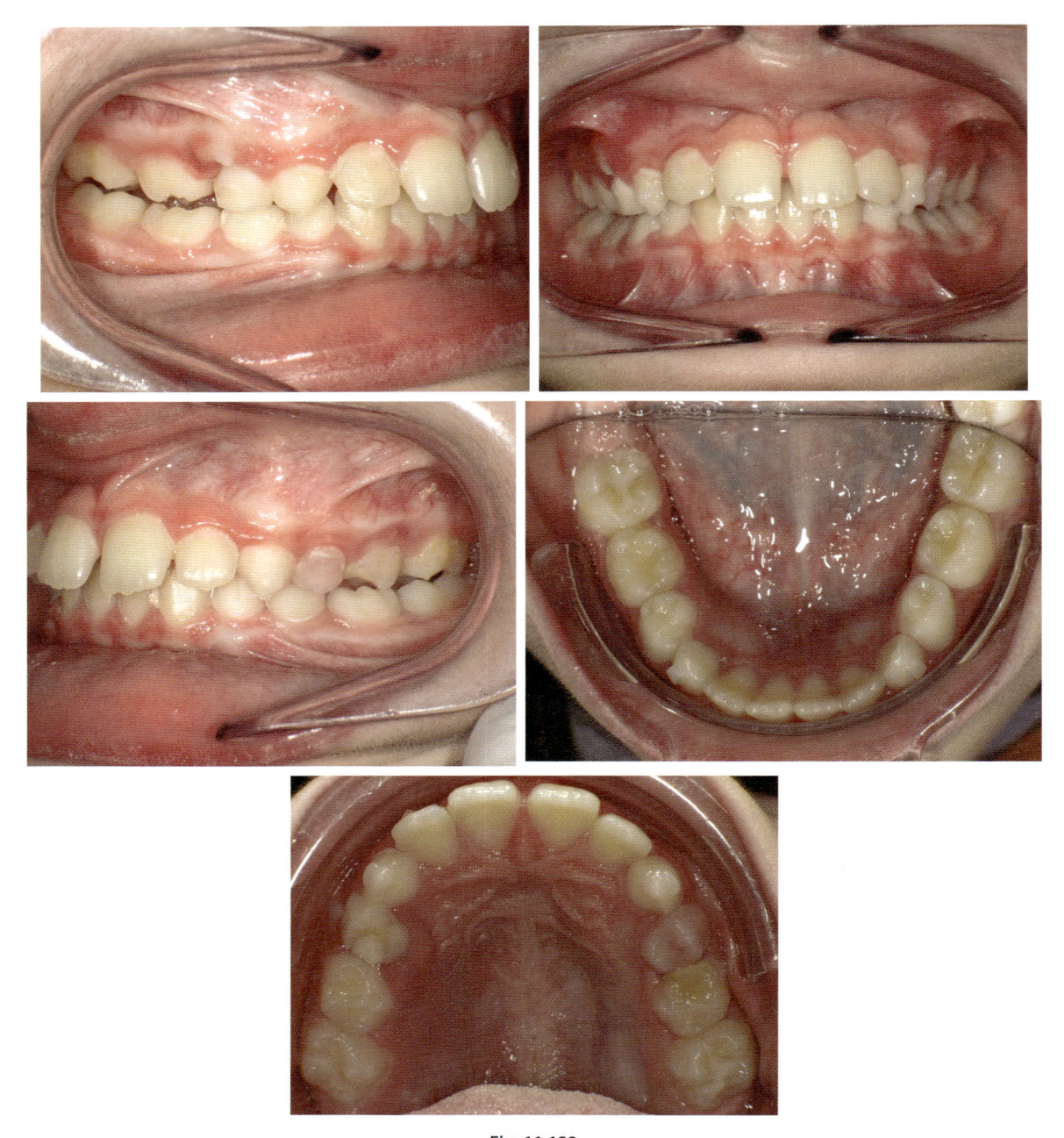

134 Principles and Biomechanics of Aligner Treatment

Fig. 11.123

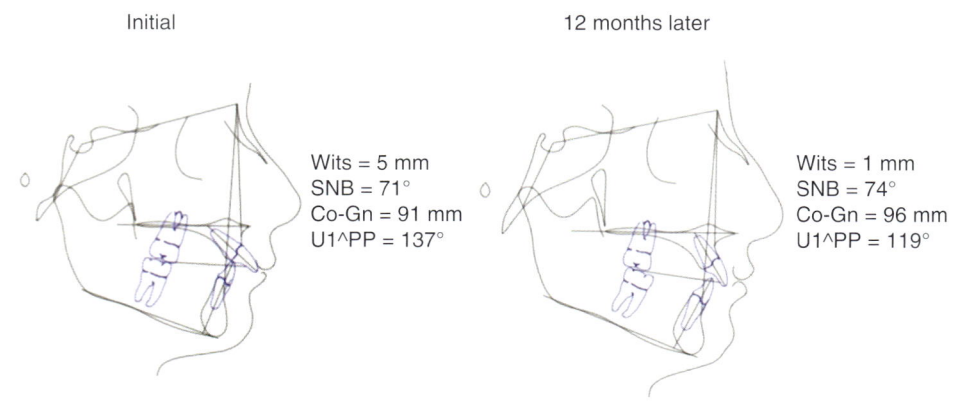

Initial

Wits = 5 mm
SNB = 71°
Co-Gn = 91 mm
U1^PP = 137°

12 months later

Wits = 1 mm
SNB = 74°
Co-Gn = 96 mm
U1^PP = 119°

Fig. 11.24 Case 4 cephalometric values before and after therapy.

References

1. Keski-Nisula KLR, Lusa V, Keski-Nisula L, et al. Occurrence of malocclusion and need of orthodontic treatment in early mixed dentition. *Am J Orthod Dentofacial Orthop.* 2003;124(6):631-638.
2. Tausche E, Luck O, Harzer W. Prevalence of malocclusions in the early mixed dentition and orthodontic treatment need. *Eur J Orthod.* 2004;26:237-244.
3. Pavlow SS, McGorray SP, Taylor MG, et al. Effect of early treatment on stability of occlusion in patients with class II malocclusion. *Am J Orthod Dentofacial Orthop.* 2008;133(2):235-244.
4. Koretsi V, Zymperdikas VF, Papageorgiou SN, et al. Treatment effects of removable functional appliances in patients with class II malocclusion: a systematic review and meta-analysis. *Eur J Orthod.* 2015;37(4):418-434.
5. Thiruvenkatachari B, Harrison J, Worthington H, et al. Early orthodontic treatment for class II malocclusion reduces the chance of incisal trauma: results of a Cochrane systematic review. *Am J Orthod Dentofacial Orthop.* 2015;148(1):47-59.
6. Rossini G, Parrini S, Castroflorio T, et al. Children's perceptions of smile esthetics and their influence on social judgment. *Angle Orthod.* 2016;86(6):1050-1055.
7. Grippaudo C, Paolantonio EG, Antonini G, et al. Association between oral habits, mouth breathing and malocclusion. *Acta Otorhinolaryngol Ital.* 2016;36(5):386-394.
8. Huang YS, Guilleminault C. Pediatric obstructive sleep apnea: where do we stand? *Adv Otorhinolaryngol.* 2017;80:136-144.
9. Perinetti G, Primožič J, Franchi L, et al. Treatment effects of removable functional appliances in pre-pubertal and pubertal class II patients: a systematic review and meta-analysis of controlled studies. *PLoS One.* 2015;10(10):e0141198.
10. Salzmann JA. An assessment of the occlusion of the teeth of children 6–11 years, United States: National Center for Health Statistics Vital and Health Statistics, Series 11, no. 130, DHEW Publication no. (HRA) 74–1612, Health Resources Administration, Department of Health Education and Welfare. Washington, DC, 1974, US Government Printing Office. *Am J Orthod Dentofacial Orthop.* 1974;66(4):462-463.
11. Corbridge JK, Campbell PM, Taylor R, et al. Transverse dentoalveolar changes after slow maxillary expansion. *Am J Orthod Dentofacial Orthop.* 2011;140(3):317-325.
12. Ciuffolo F, Manzoli L, D'Attilio M, et al. Prevalence and distribution by gender of occlusal characteristics in a sample of Italian secondary school students: a cross-sectional study. *Eur J Orthod.* 2005;27(6):601-606.
13. Pirttiniemi P, Kantomaa T, Lahtela P. Relationship between craniofacial and condyle path asymmetry in unilateral cross-bite patients. *Eur J Orthod.* 1990;12(4):408-413.
14. Piancino MG, Talpone F, Dalmasso P, et al. Reverse-sequencing chewing patterns before and after treatment of children with a unilateral posterior crossbite. *Eur J Orthod.* 2006;28(5):480-484.
15. Bishara SE, Bayati P, Jakobsen JR. Longitudinal comparisons of dental arch changes in normal and untreated class II, division 1 subjects and their clinical implications. *Am J Orthod Dentofacial Orthop.* 1996;110(5):483-489.
16. Feres MFN, Raza S, Alhadlaq A, et al. Rapid maxillary expansion effects in class II malocclusion: a systematic review. *Angle Orthod.* 2015;85(6):1070-1079.
17. Lione R, Brunelli V, Franchi L, et al. Mandibular response after rapid maxillary expansion in class II growing patients: a pilot randomized controlled trial. *Prog Orthod.* 2017;18(1):36.
18. Haas AJ. Palatal expansion: just the beginning of dentofacial orthopedics. *Am J Orthod.* 1970;57(3):219-255.
19. Martin AJ, Buschang PH, Boley JC, et al. The impact of buccal corridors on smile attractiveness. *Eur J Orthod.* 2007;29(5):530-537.
20. Maulik C, Nanda R. Dynamic smile analysis in young adults. *Am J Orthod Dentofacial Orthop.* 2007;132(3):307-315.
21. Rosa M, Lucchi P, Manti G, et al. Rapid palatal expansion in the absence of posterior cross-bite to intercept maxillary incisor crowding in the mixed dentition: a CBCT evaluation of spontaneous changes of untouched permanent molars. *Eur J Paediatr Dent.* 2016;17(4):286-294.
22. Algharbi M, Bazargani F, Dimberg L. Do different maxillary expansion appliances influence the outcomes of the treatment? *Eur J Orthod.* 2017;40(1):97-106.
23. Martina R, Farella CM, Leone P, et al. Transverse changes determined by rapid and slow maxillary expansion–a low-dose CT-based randomized controlled trial. *Orthod Craniofac Res.* 2012;15(3):159-168.
24. Brunetto M, Andriani JDA, Ribeiro GL, et al. Three-dimensional assessment of buccal alveolar bone after rapid and slow maxillary expansion: a clinical trial study. *Am J Orthod Dentofacial Orthop.* 2013;143(5):633-644.
25. Nakao K, Goto T, Gunjigake KK, et al. Intermittent force induces high RANKL expression in human periodontal ligament cells. *J Dent Res.* 2007;86(7):623-628.
26. Cattaneo PM, Dalstra M, Melsen B. Strains in periodontal ligament and alveolar bone associated with orthodontic tooth movement analyzed by finite element. *Orthodo Craniofac Res.* 2009;12(2):120-128.
27. Melsen B. Palatal growth studied on human autopsy material: a histologic microradiographic study. *Am J Orthod.* 1975;68(1):42-54.
28. De Clerck HJ, Proffit WR. Growth modification of the face: a current perspective with emphasis on class III treatment. *Am J Orthod Dentofacial Orthop.* 2015;148(1):37-46.
29. Bizzarro M, Generali C, Maietta S, et al. Association between 3D palatal morphology and upper arch dimensions in buccally displaced maxillary canines early in mixed dentition. *Eur J Orthod.* 2018;40(6):592-596.
30. Martorelli M, Maietta S, Gloria A, et al. Design and analysis of 3D customized models of a human mandible. *Procedia CIRP.* 2016;49:199-202.
31. Shah M, Verma AK, Chaturvedi S. A comparative study to evaluate the vertical position of maxillary central incisor and canine in relation to incisive papilla line. *J Forensic Dent Sci.* 2014;6(2):92-96.
32. Alhammadi MS, Halboub E, Fayed MS, et al. Global distribution of malocclusion traits: a systematic review. *Dental Press J Orthod.* 2018;23(6):40.e1-40.e10.
33. Li P, Feng J, Shen G, et al. Severe class II division 1 malocclusion in an adolescent patient, treated with a novel sagittal-guidance twin-block appliance. *Am J Orthod Dentofacial Orthop.* 2016;150(1):153-166.
34. McNamara Jr JA. Components of class II malocclusion in children 8–10 years of age. *Angle Orthod.* 1981;51(3):177-202.
35. Marsico E, Gatto E, Burrascano M, et al. Effectiveness of orthodontic treatment with functional appliances on mandibular growth in the short term. *Am J Orthod Dentofacial Orthop.* 2011;139(1):24-36.
36. Chen JY, Will LA, Niederman R. Analysis of efficacy of functional appliances on mandibular growth. *Am J Orthod Dentofacial Orthop.* 2002;122(5):470-476.
37. Cozza P, Baccetti T, Franchi L, et al. Mandibular changes produced by functional appliances in class II malocclusion: a systematic review. *Am J Orthod Dentofacial Orthop.* 2006;129(5):599.e1-12; discussion e1-6.
38. Antonarakis GS, Kiliaridis S. Short-term anteroposterior treatment effects of functional appliances and extraoral traction on class II malocclusion: a meta-analysis. *Angle Orthod.* 2007;77(5):907-914.
39. Franchi L, Baccetti T. Prediction of individual mandibular changes induced by functional jaw orthopedics followed by fixed appliances in class II patients. *Angle Orthod.* 2006;76(6):950-954.
40. Perinetti G, Contardo L, Primozic J. Diagnostic accuracy of the cervical vertebral maturation method. *Eur J Orthod.* 2018;40(4):453-454.
41. McNamara JA, Brudon WL, Kokich VG. *Orthodontics and Dentofacial Orthopedics.* Needham Press; 2001.
42. Baccetti T, Franchi L, McNamara Jr JA. The cervical vertebral maturation (CVM) method for the assessment of optimal treatment timing in dentofacial orthopedics. *Semin Orthod.* 2005;11(3):119-129.
43. Petrovic A, Stutzmann J, Lavergne J. Mechanism of craniofacial growth and modus operandi of functional appliances: a cell-level and cybernetic approach to orthodontic decision making. Craniofacial growth theory and orthodontic treatment. *Monograph.* 1990;23:13-74.
44. Beit P, Peltomäki T, Schätzle M, et al. Evaluating the agreement of skeletal age assessment based on hand-wrist and cervical vertebrae radiography. *Am J Orthod Dentofacial Orthop.* 2013;144(6):838-847.
45. Franchi L, Baccetti T, McNamara Jr JA. Mandibular growth as related to cervical vertebral maturation and body height. *Am J Orthod Dentofacial Orthop.* 2000;118(3):335-340.
46. Perinetti G, Baccetti T, Contardo L, et al. Gingival crevicular fluid alkaline phosphatase activity as a non-invasive biomarker of skeletal maturation. *Orthod Craniofac Res.* 2011;14(1):44-50.

47. de Aguiar MC, Perinetti G, Capelli Jr J. The gingival crevicular fluid as a source of biomarkers to enhance efficiency of orthodontic and functional treatment of growing patients. *Biomed Res Int.* 2017;2017:3257235.
48. O'Brien K, Wright J, Conboy F, et al. Early treatment for class II division 1 malocclusion with the twin-block appliance: a multi-center, randomized, controlled trial. *Am J Orthod Dentofacial Orthop.* 2009;135(5):573-579.
49. Tuncay OC, Bowman SJ, Nicozisis JL, et al. Effectiveness of a compliance indicator for clear aligners. *J Clin Orthod.* 2009;43(4):263-268.
50. Clark WJ. The twin block technique. A functional orthopedic appliance system. *Am J Orthod Dentofacial Orthop.* 1988;93(1):1-18.
51. Rossini G, Parrini S, Castroflorio T, et al. Efficacy of clear aligners in controlling orthodontic tooth movement: a systematic review. *Angle Orthod.* 2014;85(5):881-889.
52. Arreghini A, Carletti I, Ceccarelli MC, et al. Class II treatment with the Runner in adolescent patients: combining twin block efficiency with aligner aesthetics. *J World Fed Orthod.* 2014;3(2):e71-e79.
53. Wang S, Ye L, Li M, et al. Effects of growth hormone and functional appliance on mandibular growth in an adolescent rat model. *Angle Orthod.* 2018;88(5):624-631.
54. Kim JY, Jue S-S, Bang H-J, et al. Histological alterations from condyle repositioning with functional appliances in rats. *J Clin Pediatr Dent.* 2018;42(5):391-397.
55. Aras I, Pasaoglu A, Olmez S, et al. Comparison of stepwise vs single-step advancement with the functional mandibular advancer in class II division 1 treatment. *Angle Orthod.* 2017;87(1):82-87.
56. Batista KB, Thiruvenkatachari B, Harrison JE, et al. Orthodontic treatment for prominent upper front teeth (class II malocclusion) in children and adolescents. *Cochrane Database Syst Rev.* 2018;3(3):CD003452.
57. Brierley CA, DiBiase A, Sandler PJ. Early class II treatment. *Aust Dent J.* 2017;62:4-10.
58. Bruni A. (2021). Clear aligner treatment for transverse maxillary deficiency: in vitro study and randomized controlled trial. Doctoral Dissertation, University of Torino, Torino, Italy.
59. Ravera S, Castroflorio T, Galati F, Cugliari G, Garino F, Deregibus A, Quinzi V. Short term dentoskeletal effects of mandibular advancement clear aligners in Class II growing patients. A retrospective controlled study according to STROBE Guidelines. *Eur J Paediatr Dent.* 2021 Jun; 22(2):119-124.

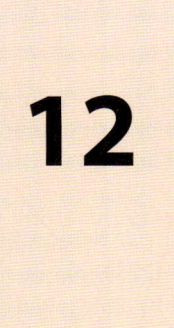

12 The Hybrid Approach in Class II Malocclusions Treatment

FRANCESCO GARINO, TOMMASO CASTROFLORIO, and SIMONE PARRINI

Introduction

Several protocols have been proposed for treatment of class II malocclusions. In nonextraction protocols, maxillary molar distalization can be used to correct molar relationships in patients with maxillary dentoalveolar protrusion and minor skeletal discrepancies.[1]

The upper molars can be distalized by means of extraoral or intraoral forces.[2] In recent years, several techniques have been developed to reduce the dependence on patient compliance, such as intraoral appliances with and without skeletal anchorage. However, even these devices can produce undesirable tipping of the maxillary molars and/or loss of anterior anchorage during distalization.[3]

In the last decades, increasing numbers of adult patients have sought orthodontic treatment and expressed a desire for esthetic and comfortable alternatives to conventional fixed appliances. Clear aligner therapy (CAT) was introduced to answer this request.

In a review by Rossini et al. it has been stated that maxillary molar distalization up to 2.5 mm is one of the most predictable movements with CAT.[4,5] This high predictability was obtained through combination of staging, the use of proper attachment configuration,[5] and full-day class II elastics (0.25 in, 4.5 oz) (see Chapters about Class II treatment and see Chapters 5 and 7). These results confirm what every orthodontist knows: Treatment success requires technical knowledge from the orthodontist as well as the cooperation of the patient.[6] Class II treatments with CAT require mean treatment times of 18 to 20 months during which class II elastics need to be used all day from treatment beginning until class I canine relationship has been established.[3,7] Corrective devices should be comfortable, provide rapid and effective treatment, and favor patient compliance with orthodontic treatment. Clear aligners are comfortable and aesthetically acceptable as already discussed in the previous chapters,[8,9] and require strong patient compliance since they are removable. The existing literature showed that the mean duration of objectively measured wear was considerably lower than stipulated wear time among all removable appliances. Furthermore, compliance was found to be better in the early stages of treatment.[10]

Starting from these premises, the possible combined use of aligners and other orthodontic devices aimed to optimize patient adherence to therapy reducing the time required to wear class II elastics has been proposed. This kind of combined approach has been named hybridization of aligner therapy. Among others, temporary anchorage devices (bone-borne hybrid approach [see Chapter about miniscrews]) and tooth-borne distalization devices are the most popular hybridization approaches in CAT.

The application of forces in such distalizing appliances could be from buccal region, palatal region, or both, and they could be based on sliding mechanics or be friction free (e.g., in the Pendulum appliance).

Tooth-Borne Hybrid Approach With Distalizing Device

Various types of molar distalization appliances are available and presented in the orthodontic literature, such as the Pendulum device, the Distal Jet, and the Carriere Motion 3D Appliance (CMA) (Henry Schein Orthodontics, Carlsbad, CA, USA).

These appliances are considered easy to install and can promote distal movement of the maxillary molars without the effect of maxillary orthopedic restriction.[11] However, most of these intraoral devices show undesirable reciprocal anchorage loss in the premolars and incisors during distal molar movement.[12] Furthermore, molar tipping is frequently observed in most of the cases.

The Distal Jet appliance is composed of two bilateral tubes connected to a Nance appliance. A bayonet wire is inserted into the lingual sheath of the first molar bands. On the tube there is a stainless steel coil spring and a clamp. The clamp can slide toward the molar and be tightened to compress the coil. The force exerted by the spring begins at 150 g and decreases as space is opened.[13]

The Pendulum appliance was introduced by Hilgers in 1992[14] and is still one of the most used distalizing devices.[14] It is a fixed appliance composed of a plastic pad–contacted palatal rugae. The distalizing force is produced by beta-titanium springs that extend from the palatal acrylic and fit into lingual sheaths on the molar tube, which gives greater control of these teeth.[15]

Both the Distal Jet and Pendulum appliances produce an increase in vertical dimension due to a backward rotation of the mandible.[16-18] These vertical changes comprise a slight opening of the mandibular plane angle (about 1 degree) and an increase in lower anterior facial height (2.2–2.8 mm).[19] Ghosh and Nanda reported that the increase in lower anterior facial height was significantly greater in patients with higher pretreatment mandibular plane angles.[20] The increased lower facial height and mandibular plane angle could have resulted from driving the molars back into the "wedge." These results suggest that the Pendulum may be contraindicated in patients with excessive lower facial height and/or minimal overbite.[18] Similar results were reported for the Distal Jet appliance.[16]

The maxillary molar distalization obtained with those appliances is characterized by a great amount of molar distal tipping (in average >10 degrees).[12]

Whereas the Distal Jet produces a labial tipping of the upper incisors as a result of the uncontrolled counterforce acting on the premaxillae, the Pendulum appliance showed a more controlled inclination of the upper incisors with a mild crown buccal tipping.

CMA consists of two rigid bars bonded bilaterally to the maxillary canines and first molars. The canine pad with a built-in mesial hook used for placement of intermaxillary elastics is bonded to the anterior third of the clinical crown. Posteriorly, the molded pad with a ball-and-socket joint is bonded to the first molar at the center of its clinical crown to facilitate molar derotation and distalization.[21-23]

The activation of the appliance is obtained by the use of two types of elastics: the first one being 0.25 in, 6 oz; the second one 0.19 in, 8 oz, to be used from the second month of treatment until the molar and canine class I relationships are established. Elastics should be worn 22 hours per day, changing elastics three times per day.[24]

The principle of this appliance is similar to a cantilever-based fixed appliance previously shown by Nanda.[25] The author described that system as an effective way to correct molar class II in nongrowing patients. An active cantilever with information of molar tipback was applied at the upper arch, while in the lower arch the author used a multi-bracket fixed appliance and class II elastics. The undesired effects of class II elastics were controlled by the fixed appliance in lower arch and by the activation of the cantilever in upper arch.

Previous retrospective clinical studies demonstrated the possibility of obtaining a maxillary molar distalization between 1.6 and 5.1 mm[24] with the mean amount of molar tipping not exceeding 3.7 degrees when CMA was used in combination with fixed appliances as anchorage units on the lower arch.[24] Furthermore the treatment time had a mean duration of about 4 to 5 months.[24]

There is a lack of high-quality evidence supporting or contrasting the use of CMA. In another retrospective study in which CMA effects were compared to other class II correction methods, CMA showed the same results obtained with class II elastics in terms of molar distalization but in less time.[26]

One clinically and statistically relevant effect of treatment with CMA occurred in lower anterior facial height that was associated with a significant increase in the mandibular plane angle.[27]

Proclination of the lower incisors resulting from the class II elastics mechanics was observed and resulted in a significant amount (4.2 degrees).[24]

All the tooth-borne appliances mentioned earlier produce some side effects that need to be controlled during the hybrid aligner treatment. Excessive upper and lower incisor proclination could be difficult to control with aligners. According to Rossini et al., buccolingual tipping and torque control of upper incisors have a mean accuracy of about 50% of the planned movement.[4] The proclination of lower incisors resulting from the use of CMA could be controlled using active aligners on the lower arch and applying a lingual radicular torque information on the lower incisors of at least 5 degrees.

Another side effect that can occur using tooth-borne distalization devices is the rotation of the occlusal plane due to the increase of the vertical dimension.

Khosravi et al.[28] in their study about overbite management with Invisalign aligners showed that overbite correction is mostly related to anterior teeth movement without any significant posterior intrusion and/or extrusion.[28] As described by Ravera et al.[3] bite block effect of the aligner causes an intrusive effect on posterior teeth of 0.5 mm[3]. A similar value (0.6 mm) was described by Mantovani et al.[29] Therefore, only the 0.5- to 0.6-mm bite block effect should be considered to counteract the increase of the vertical dimension produced by tooth-borne distalization devices (average increase 2–3 mm).

On the basis of these considerations, tooth-borne distalization devices should be avoided in patients with excessive lower facial height and/or minimal overbite. Clinicians should be aware of the existing evidence related to the limited control of posterior intrusion, overbite correction, and buccolingual inclination provided by CAT.

Two clinical examples will be presented: one in a teen patient and the second in an adult patient.

Case Report 1

DIAGNOSTIC SUMMARY

A 13-year-old female patient presented with molar class II malocclusion, skeletal class II, normal divergence, protrusion of upper and lower incisors, and unerupted upper left canine (Figs. 12.1, 12.2, and 12.3).

The impaction was related to the mesialization of upper left posterior teeth with a consequent absolute lack of space for the canine eruption. Radiographs confirmed the buccal displacement of the impacted upper canine.

The patient's main concern was lack of the upper left canine.

The treatment plan was designed to obtain bodily distal movements of upper molars, premolars, canines, and frontal teeth to achieve a dental molar and canine class I, and recover the proper space for 23 without extractions.

A Pendulum K appliance[30] was bonded on the upper arch to distalize maxillary molars (Fig. 12.4).

Once the class I was overcorrected (8 months treatment), the Pendulum appliance was debonded, and a new intraoral scan was made to start the aligner treatment. The aim of this second phase was to close the remaining spaces in the upper arch, to recover tooth 23 in the arch and to correct lower crowding. The same day temporary thermoformed retainers were provided to the patient.

A set of 49 Invisalign aligners was produced to complete the distalization movements on the upper arch and to correct the lower arch mild crowding. Aligner change was planned every week. During the aligner phase the patient was educated to wear class II elastics (0.25 in, 4.5 oz) bilaterally to reinforce anterior anchorage while distalizing premolars. To anchor class II elastics, buttons were bonded

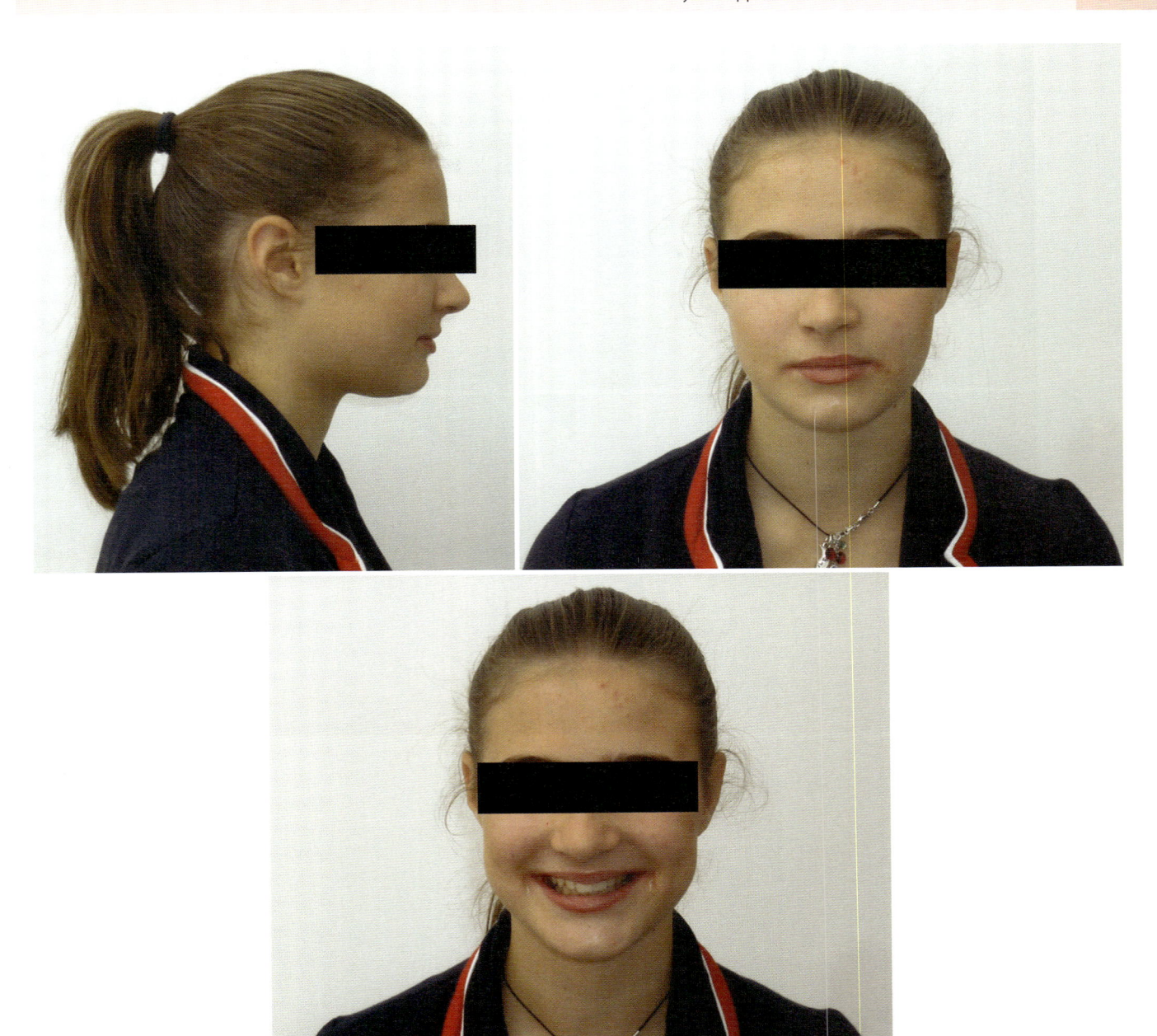

Fig. 12.1 Case 1. Extraoral pictures before treatment.

on the lower first molars, while aligner hooks were used on the upper first premolars region.

Once enough space was obtained, the upper left canine was surgically exposed with a vestibular flap, and a button with stainless steel hook was bonded to the buccal surface of the crown. The tooth was then moved distally first with class II elastics to recover a proper position on the sagittal plane (Fig. 12.5).

When 23 was close enough to the occlusal plane, new intraoral scans were performed to obtain a new set of 15 aligners to finalize the case (Figs. 12.6, 12.7, and 12.8).

The total treatment duration was 22 months.

Fig. 12.2 Case 1. Intraoral pictures before treatment.

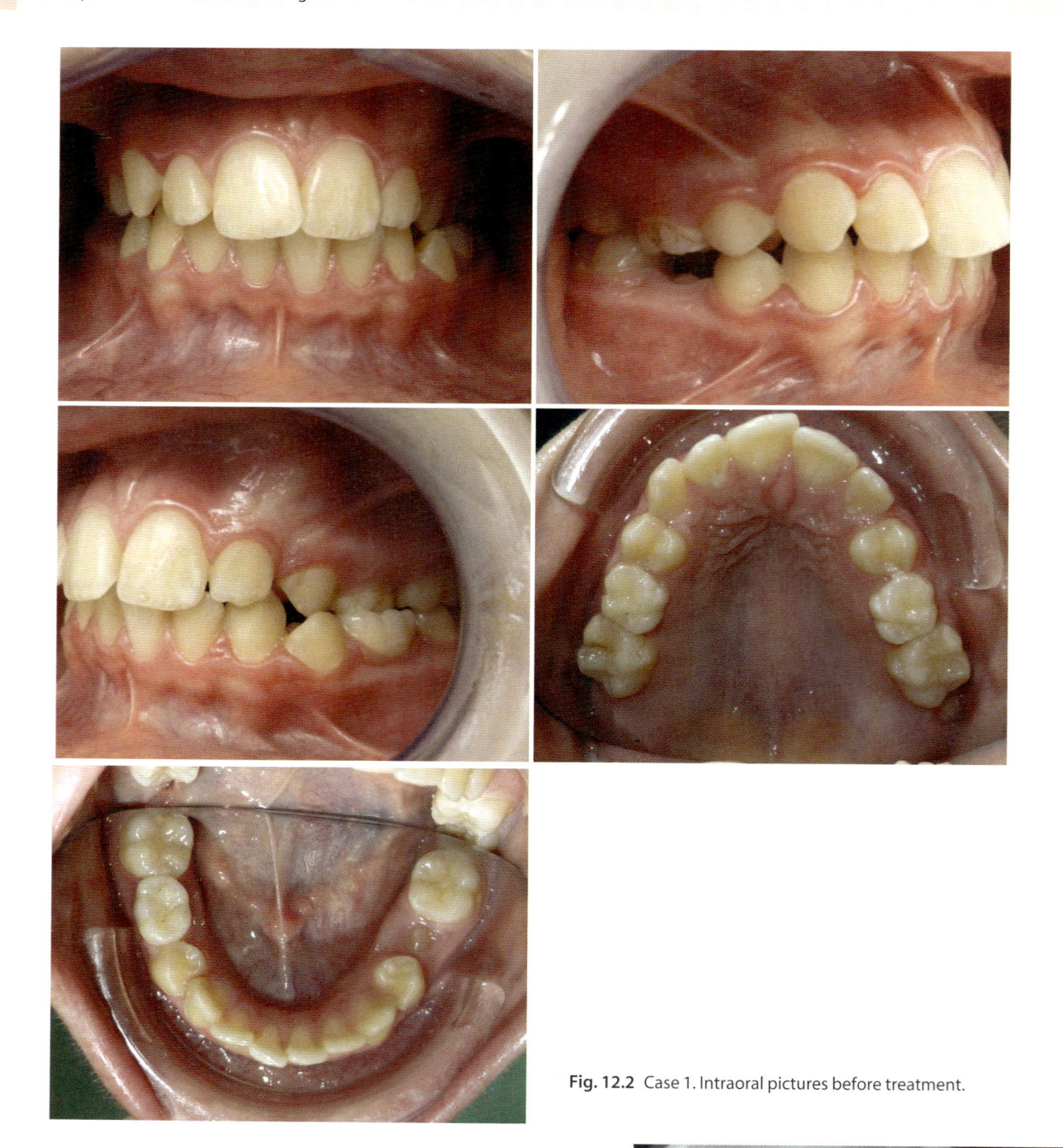

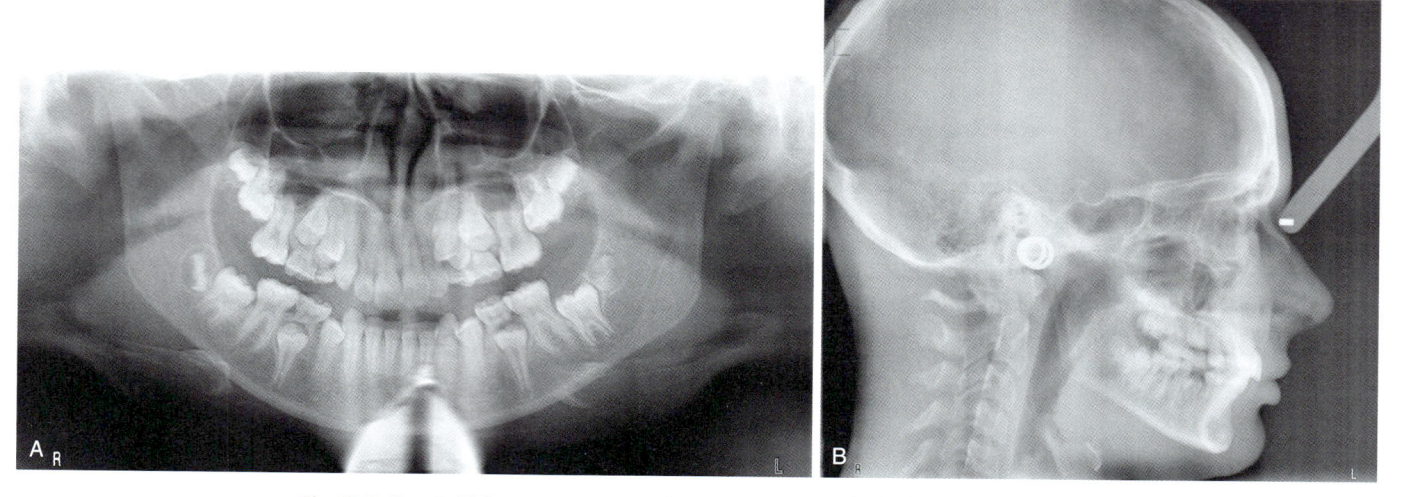

Fig. 12.3 Case 1. (A) Panoramic x-ray before treatment. (B) Lateral x-ray before treatment.

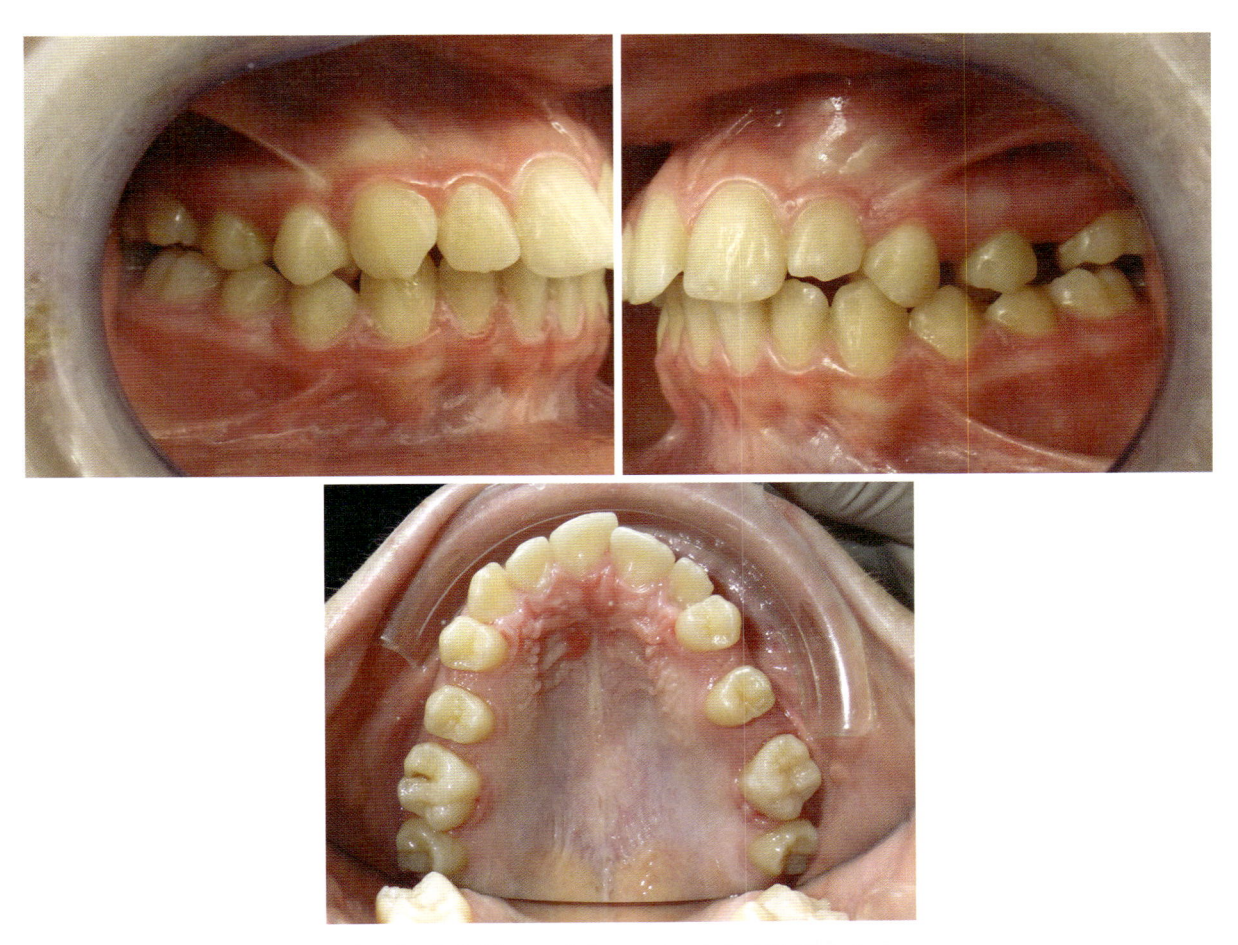

Fig. 12.4 Case 1. Intraoral pictures at end of sagittal first phase.

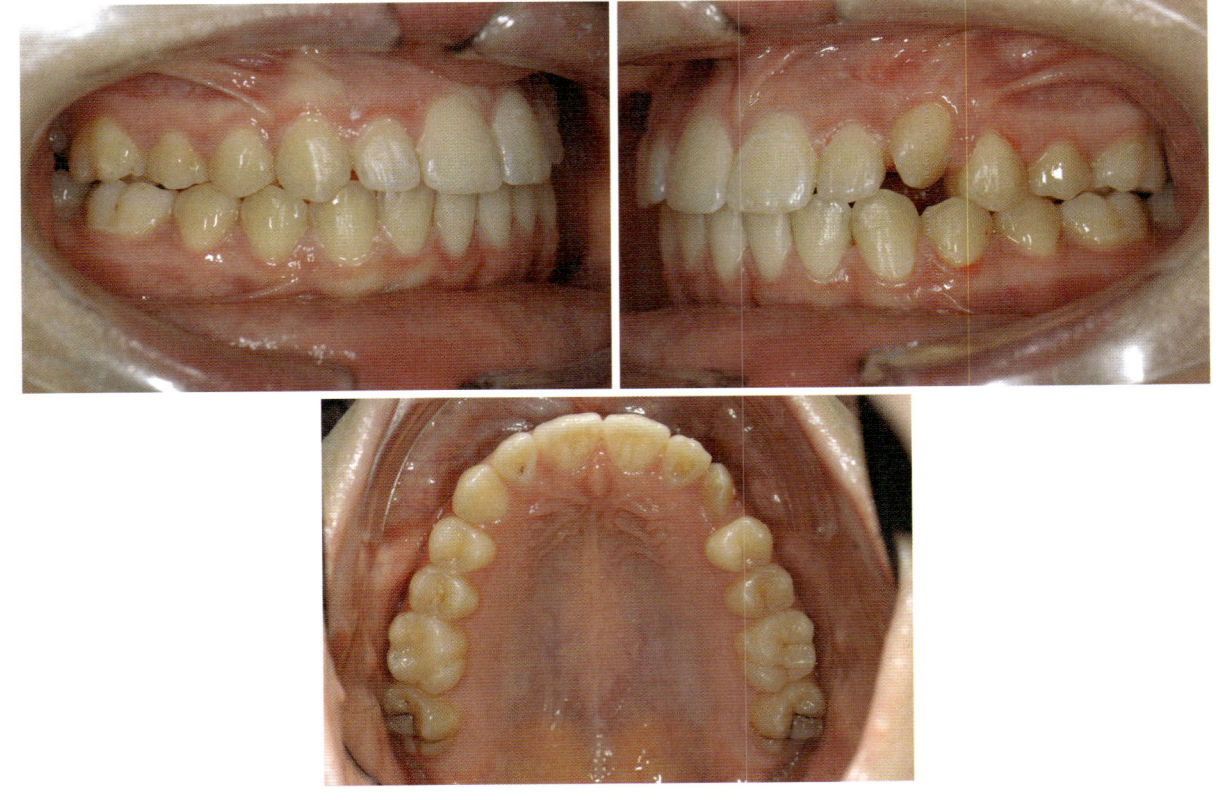

Fig. 12.5 Case 1. Intraoral pictures before additional aligner stage.

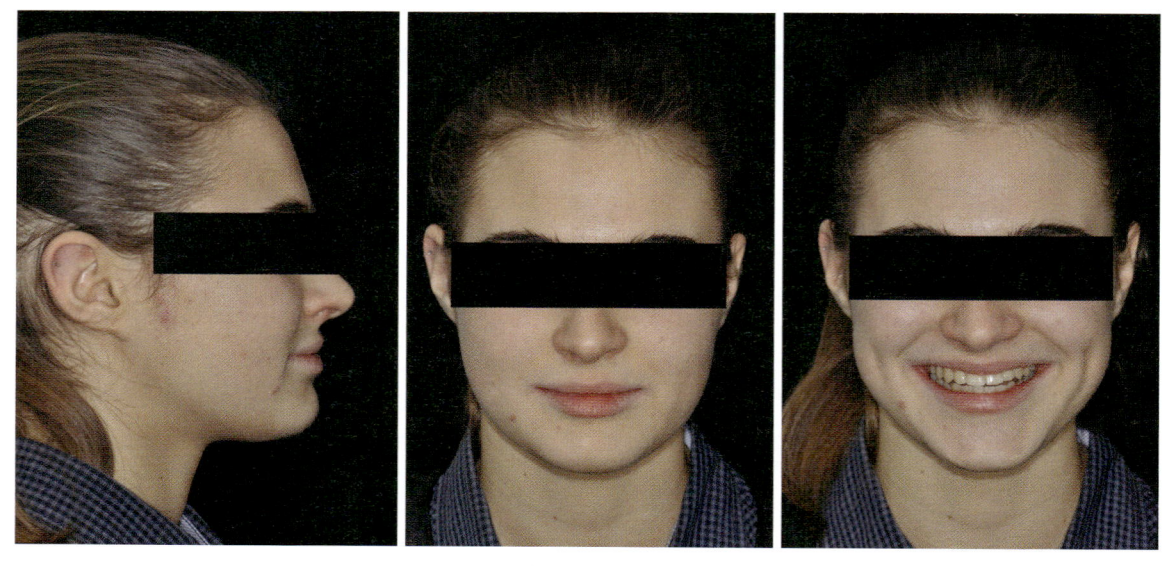

Fig. 12.6 Case 1. Extraoral pictures at end of treatment.

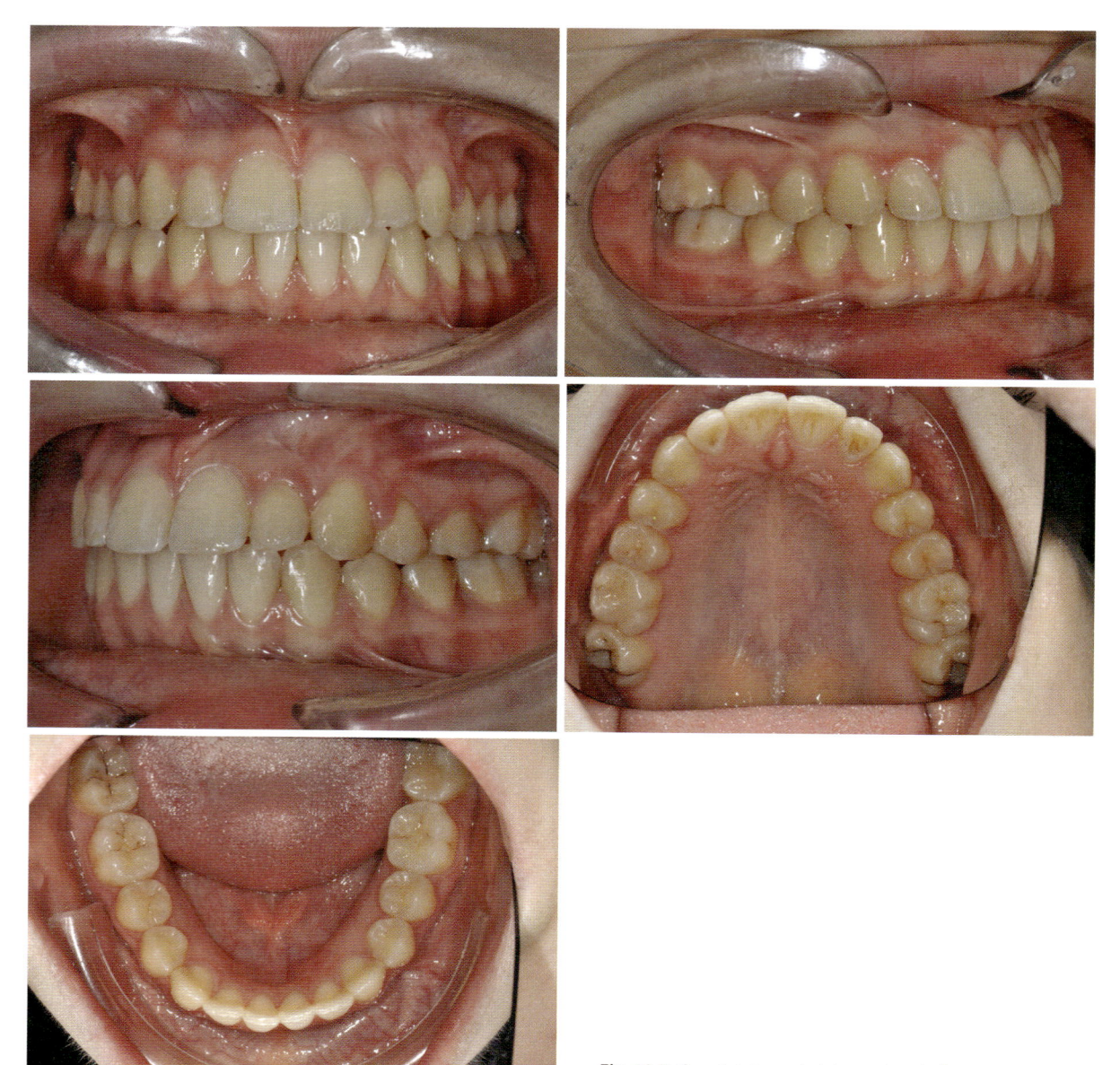

Fig. 12.7 Case 1. Intraoral pictures at end of treatment.

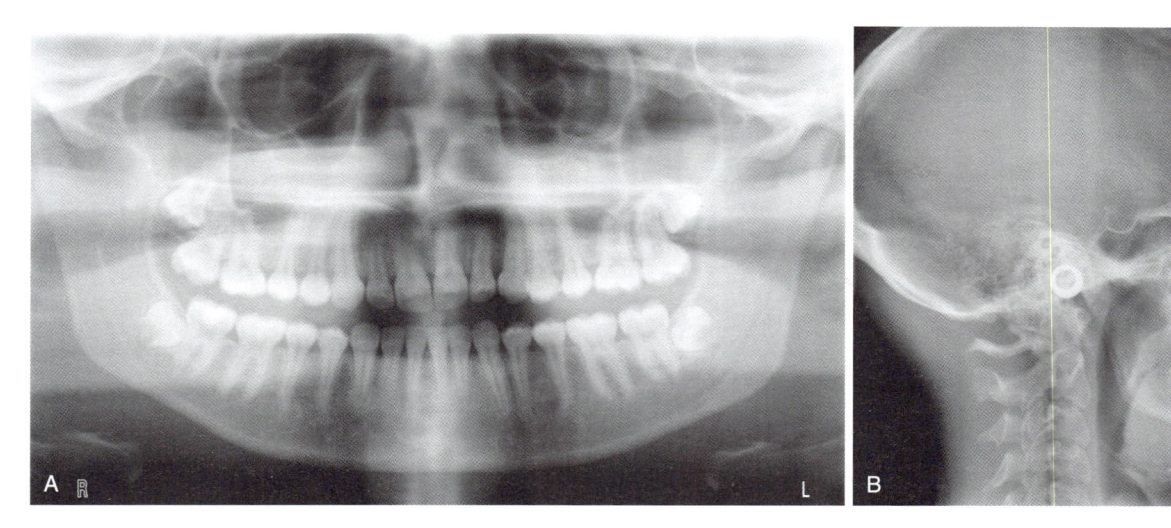

12 • The Hybrid Approach in Class II Malocclusions Treatment   143

Fig. 12.8 Case 1, (A) Panoramic x-ray at end of treatment. (B) Lateral x-ray at end of treatment.

Case Report 2

DIAGNOSTIC SUMMARY

A 25-year-old male patient presented with molar class II malocclusion, skeletal class II, low mandibular plane angle, overbite, and crowding on both upper and lower arches (Figs. 12.9, 12.10, and 12.11).

The patient's main concern was the excessive upper canine buccal displacement and proclination of upper incisors.

The treatment plan was made to obtain bodily distal movements of upper molars, premolars, and canines to achieve a dental molar and canine class I, center midlines, and correct crowding on both arches.

A CMA was bonded in the upper arch on both sides to correct sagittal relationship on molars, bicuspids, and canines (Fig. 12.12).

In the meantime, the lower arch treatment started with a first set of 22 aligners to correct lower crowding. A buccal tube was bonded on lower first molars to allow activation of both CMA through the use, for the first month, of 0.25 in, 6 oz elastic placed from the mesial hook of the CMA to the mesial hook of the lower buccal tubes. From the second month until class I molar and canine resulted, the patient used a 0.19 in, 8 oz elastic with elastic changes three times a day. Aligners were instructed to be changed every 2 weeks at that stage.

Once the class I was obtained on both sides (7 months treatment), the CMA was debonded, and a new intraoral scan was made of the aligner treatment (Fig. 12.13). The aim of this second phase was to close the remaining spaces in the upper arch created during sagittal correction on both sides and to complete crowding correction in the lower arch. Through the same scan and a three-dimensional printing in-office procedure, one temporary thermoformed retainer was provided to the patient who was instructed to wear it day and night.

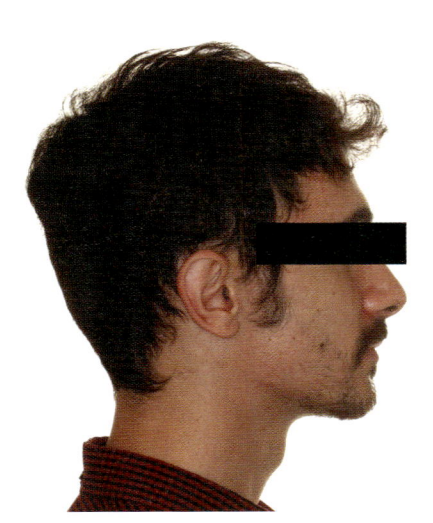

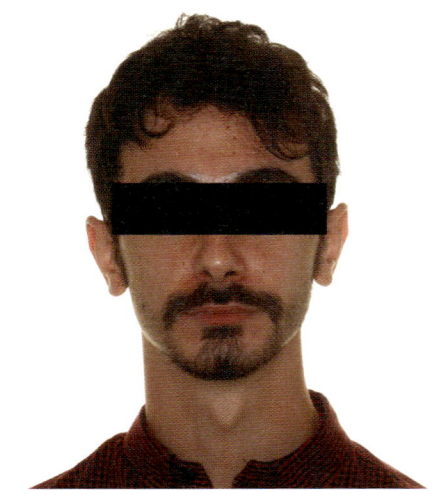

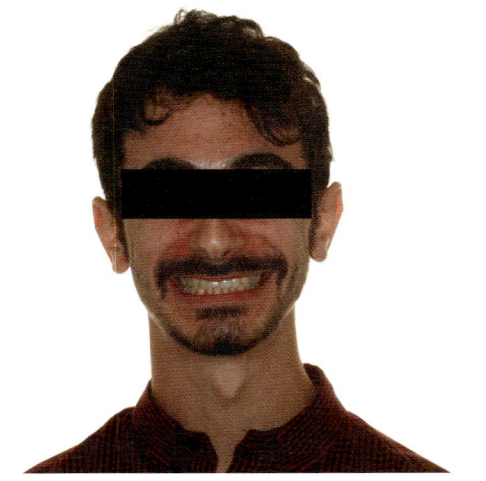

Fig. 12.9 Case 2. Extraoral pictures before treatment.

144 Principles and Biomechanics of Aligner Treatment

Fig. 12.10 Case 2. Intraoral pictures before treatment.

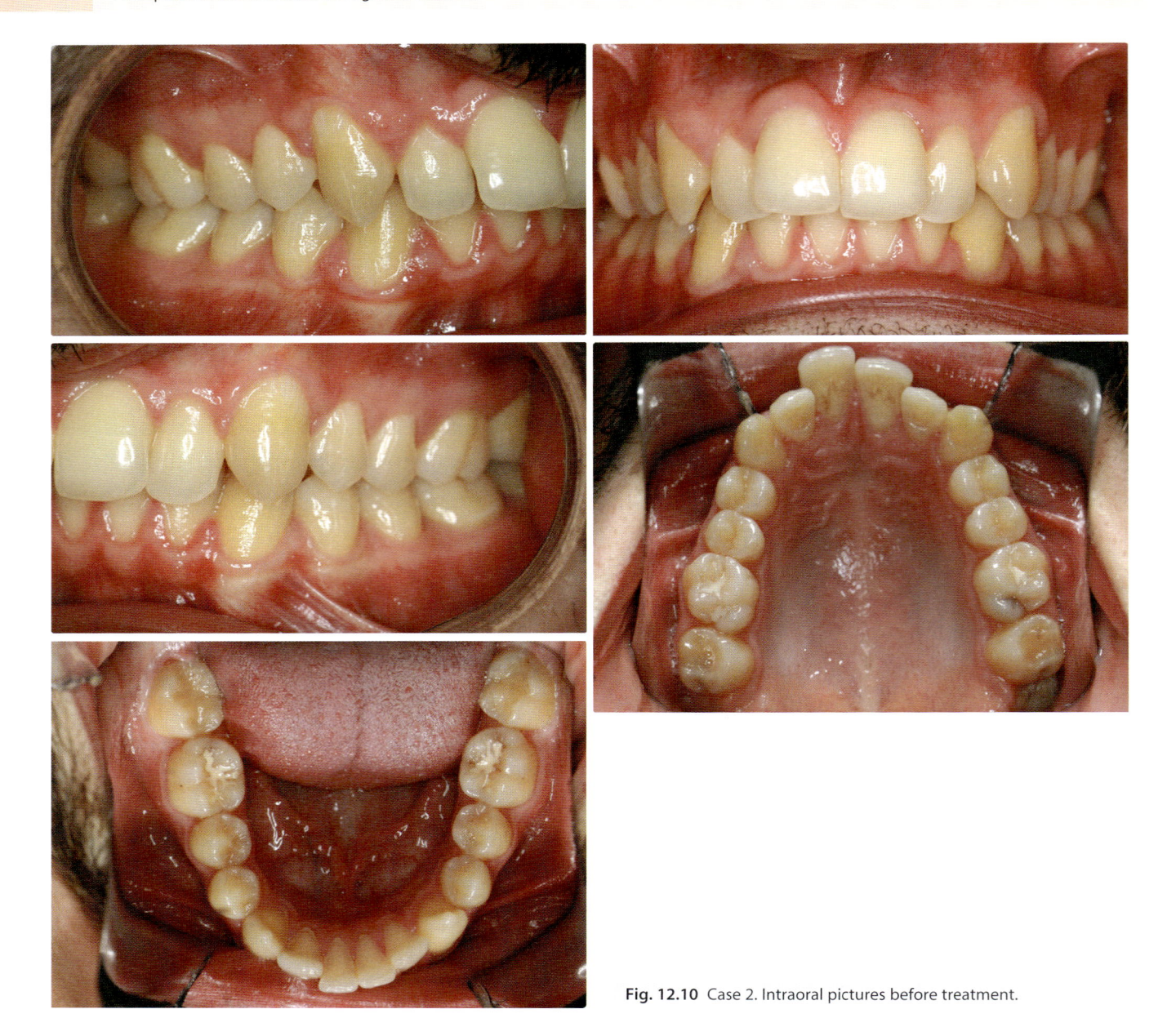

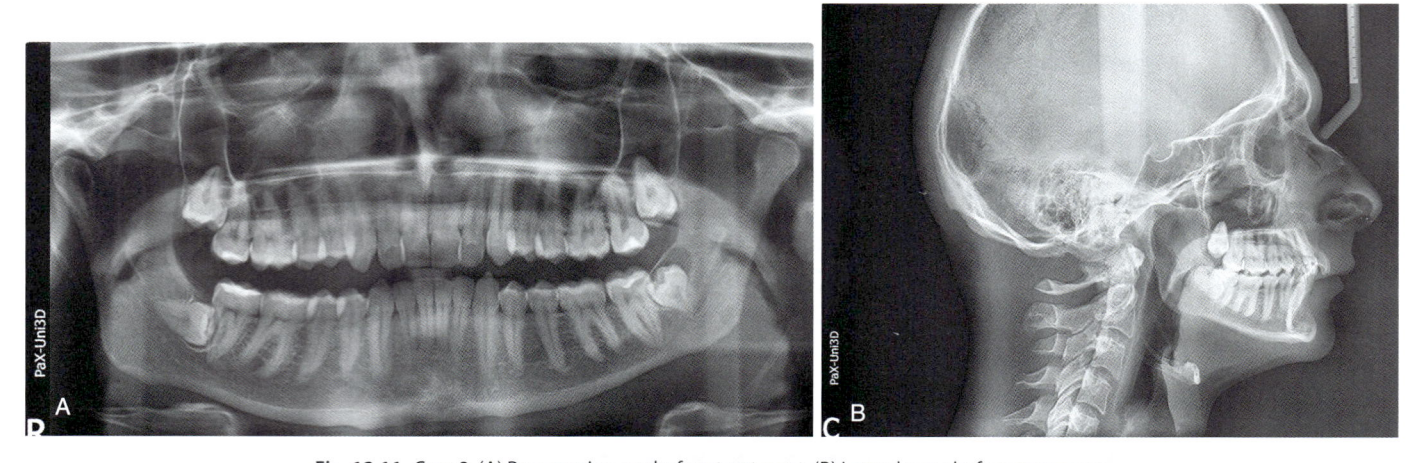

Fig. 12.11 Case 2. (A) Panoramic x-ray before treatment. (B) Lateral x-ray before treatment.

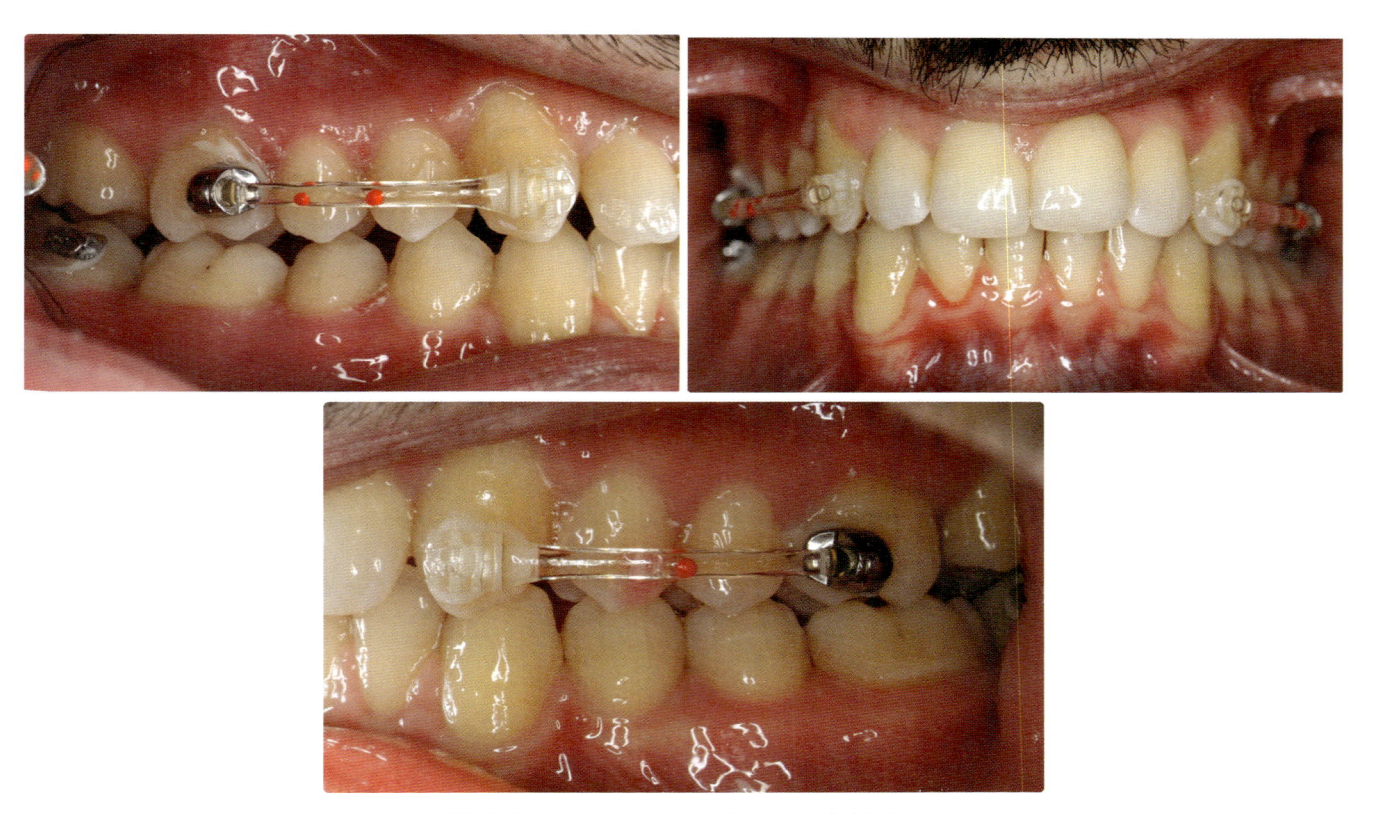

Fig. 12.12 Case 2. Intraoral pictures before sagittal first phase.

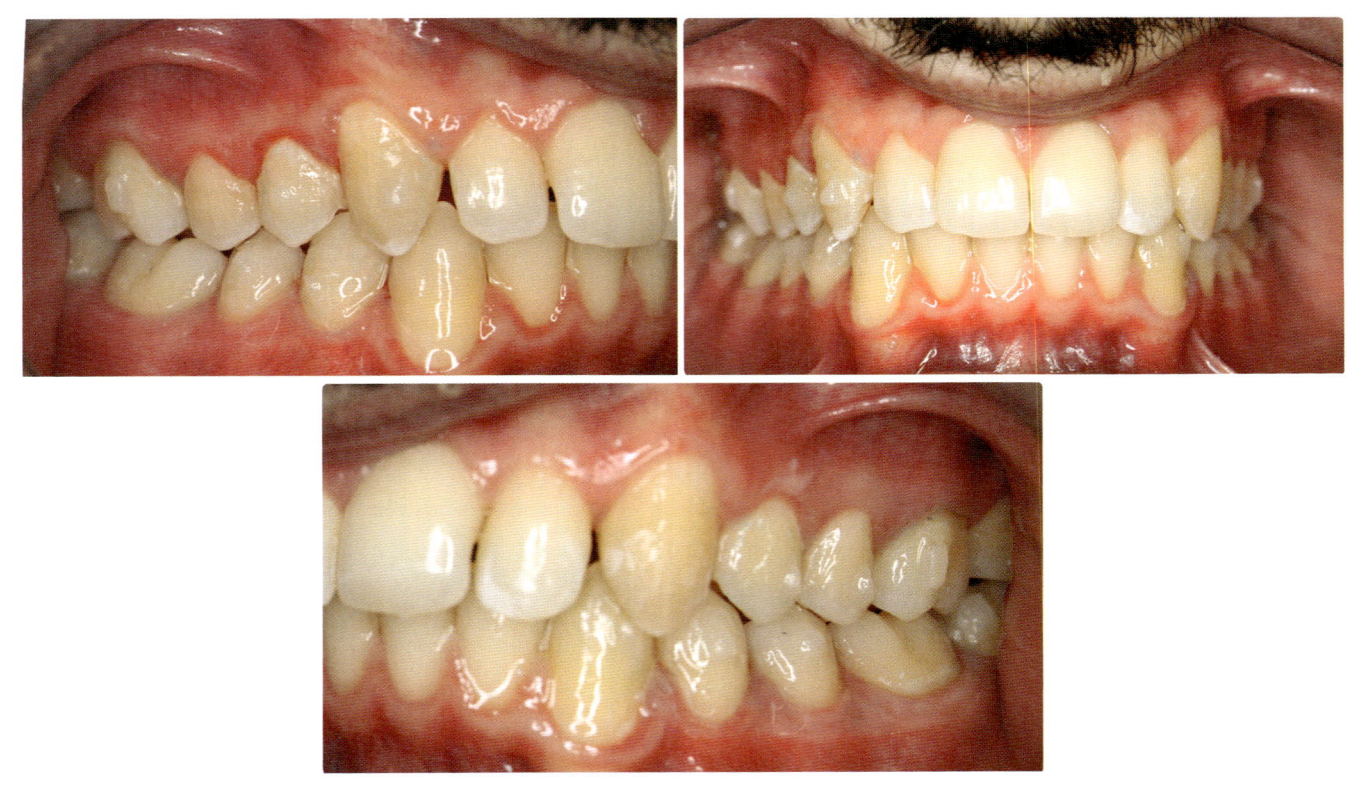

Fig. 12.13 Case 2. Intraoral pictures before additional aligner stage.

A set of 10 Invisalign aligners was produced to perform space closure in the upper arch and to correct the lower arch mild crowding. Aligner change was planned every week.

After 14 months of treatment, class I canine and molar resulted on both sides, midlines centered, and deep bite improved such as upper and lower arch forms. Third molars present, the patient is currently in retention with vacuum-type retainers that are used all nights.

During the retention period, the patient will be followed up to evaluate third molars (Figs. 12.14, 12.15, and 12.16).

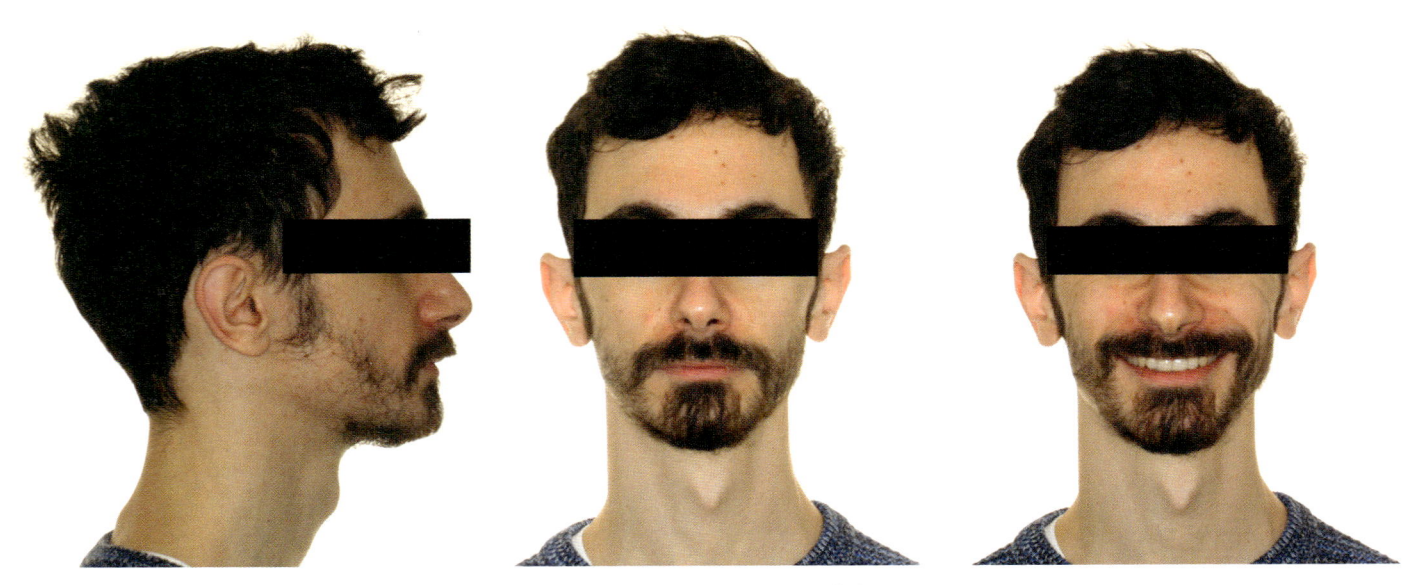

Fig. 12.14 Case 2. Extraoral pictures at end of treatment.

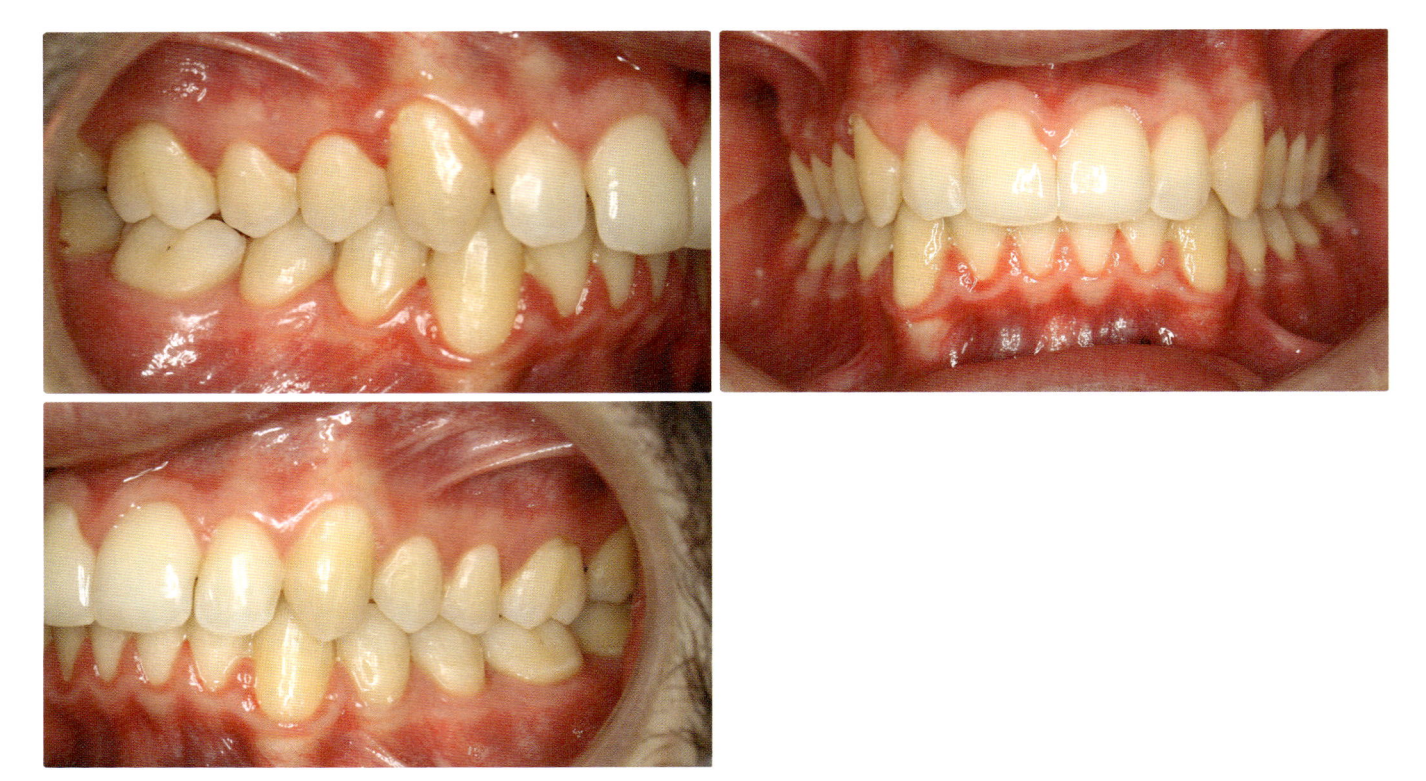

Fig. 12.15 Case 2. Intraoral pictures at end of treatment.

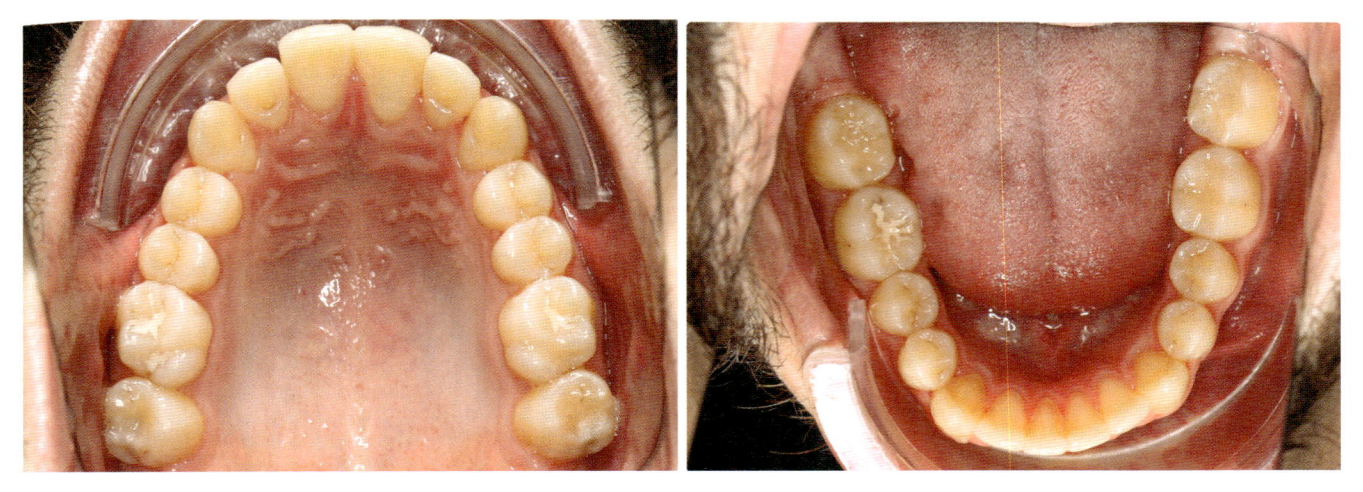

Fig. 12.15, cont'd

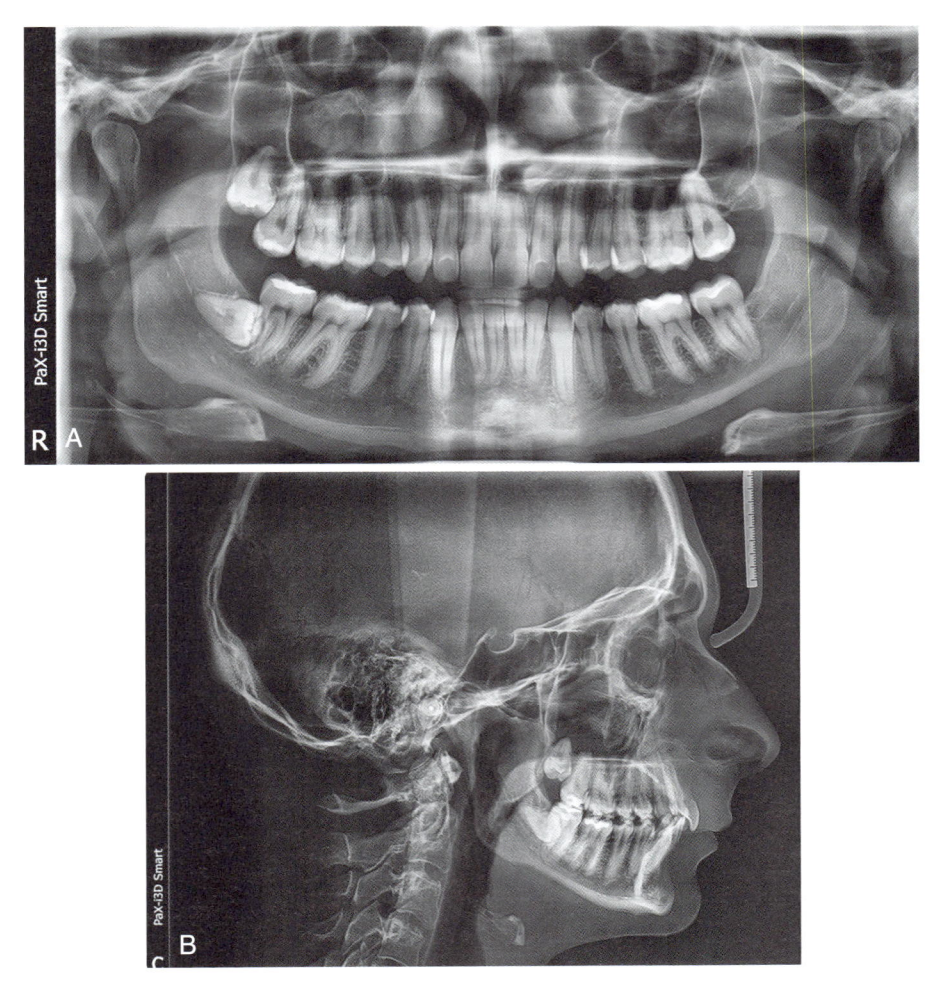

Fig. 12.16 Case 2. (A) Panoramic x-ray at end of treatment. (B) Lateral x-ray at end of treatment.

References

1. Bolla E, Muratore F, Carano A, et al. Evaluation of maxillary molar distalization with the distal jet: a comparison with other contemporary methods. *Angle Orthod.* 2002;72:481-494.
2. Grec RH, Janson G, Branco NC, et al. Intraoral distalizer effects with conventional and skeletal anchorage: a meta-analysis. *Am J Orthod Dentofacial Orthop.* 2013;143:602-615.
3. Ravera S, Castroflorio T, Garino F, et al. Maxillary molar distalization with aligners in adult patients: a multicenter retrospective study. *Prog Orthod.* 2016;17:12.
4. Rossini G, Parrini S, Deregibus A, et al. Controlling orthodontic tooth movement with clear aligners. An updated systematic review regarding efficacy and efficiency. *J Aligner Orthod.* 2017;1:7-20.

5. Garino F, Castroflorio T, Daher S, et al. Effectiveness of composite attachments in controlling upper-molar movement with aligners. *J Clin Orthod.* 2016;50(6):341-347.
6. Richter DD, Nanda RS, Sinha PK, et al. Effect of behavior modification on patient compliance in orthodontics. *Angle Orthod.* 1998;68:123-132.
7. Lombardo L, Colonna A, Carlucci A, et al. Class II subdivision correction with clear aligners using intermaxilary elastics. *Prog Orthod.* 2018;1:19:32.
8. Nedwed V, Miethke RR. Motivation, acceptance and problems of invisalign patients. *J Orofac Orthop.* 2005;66:162-173.
9. Rosvall MD, Fields HW, Ziuchkovski J, et al. Attractiveness, acceptability, and value of orthodontic appliances. *Am J Orthod Dentofacial Orthop.* 2009;135:276.e1-e12.
10. Shah N. Compliance with removable orthodontic appliances. *Evid Based Dent.* 2017;18:105-106.
11. Carano A, Testa M. The distal jet for upper molar distalization. *J Clin Orthod.* 1996;30:374-380.
12. Antonarakis GS, Kiliaridis S. Maxillary molar distalization with noncompliance intramaxillary appliances in class II malocclusion: a systematic review. *Angle Orthod.* 2008;78:1133-1140.
13. Carano A, Testa M, Siciliani G. The lingual distalizer system. *Eur J Orthod.* 1996;18:445-448.
14. Hilgers JJ. The pendulum appliance for class II noncompliance therapy. *J Clin Orthod.* 1992;26:706-714.
15. Proffit W, Fields HW, Sarver DM. *Contemporary Orthodontics.* St. Louis, MO: Mosby Elsevier; 2007.
16. Marure PS, Patil RU, Reddy S, et al. The effectiveness of pendulum, K-loop, and distal jet distalization techniques in growing children and its effects on anchor unit: a comparative study. *J Indian Soc Pedod Prev Dent.* 2016;34:331-340.
17. Byloff FK, Darendeliler MA, Clar E, et al. Distal molar movement using the pendulum appliance. Part 2: the effects of maxillary molar root uprighting bends. *Angle Orthod.* 1997;67:261-270.
18. Chaqués-Asensi J, Kalra V. Effects of the pendulum appliance on the dentofacial complex. *J Clin Orthod.* 2001;35:254-257.
19. Byloff FK, Darendeliler MA. Distal molar movement using the pendulum appliance. Part 1: clinical and radiological evaluation. *Angle Orthod.* 1997;67:249-260.
20. Ghosh J, Nanda RS. Evaluation of an intraoral maxillary molar distalization technique. *Am J Orthod Dentofacial Orthop.* 1996;110:639-646.
21. Carrière L. A new class II distalizer. *J Clinic Orthod.* 2004;38:224-231.
22. Martel D. The Carriere distalizer: simple and efficient. *Int J Orthod Milwaukee.* 2012;23(2):63-66.
23. Rodríguez HL. Unilateral application of the Carriere distalizer. *J Clin Orthod.* 2011;45(3):177-180.
24. Sandifer CL, English JD, Colville CD, Lints JP, et al. Treatment effects of the Carrière distalizer using lingual arch and full fixed appliances. *J World Fed Orthod.* 2014;3(2):e49-e54.
25. Nanda R. *Biomechanics in Clinical Orthodontics.* WB Saunders; 1997.
26. Yin K, Han E, Guo J, et al. Evaluating the treatment effectiveness and efficiency of Carriere distalizer: a cephalometric and study model comparison of class II appliances. *Prog Orthod.* 2019;20(1):24.
27. Kim-Berman H, McNamara Jr JA, Lints JP, et al. Treatment effects of the Carriere Motion 3D Appliance for the correction of class II in adolescents. *Angle Orthod.* 2019;89:839-846.
28. Khosravi R, Cohanim B, Hujoel P, et al. Management of overbite with the Invisalign appliance. *Am J Orthod Dentofacial Orthop.* 2017;151:691-699.
29. Mantovani E, Parrini S, Coda E, et al. Micro computed tomography evaluation of Invisalign aligner thickness homogeneity. *Angle Orthod.* 2021. doi:10.2319/040820-265.1. Epub ahead of print.
30. Kinzinger GS, Wehrbein H, Gross U, et al. Molar distalization with pendulum appliances in the mixed dentition: effects on the position of unerupted canines and premolars. *Am J Orthod Dentofacial Orthop.* 2006;129:407-417.

13 Aligners and Impacted Canines

EDOARDO MANTOVANI, DAVID COUCHAT, TOMMASO CASTROFLORIO

Introduction

Except for the third molars, the impaction of the upper canine is the most common in the permanent dentition, and its recovery is nearly always recommended. The importance of canines, both from a functional and an aesthetic point of view, is crucial to set a proper occlusion. Furthermore, possible adverse sequelae of canine impaction[1] can be as follows:

- Migration of the neighboring teeth and loss of arch length
- External root resorption of the neighboring teeth
- Dentigerous cyst formation
- Infections related to partial eruption

The prevalence of upper canine impaction is ranging between 0.3% and 2.4%, depending on the population, age, sex, and ethnicity.[2-5]

The impacted maxillary canines are more common in white populations[6] and in female patients, with a male to female ratio of approximately 1:3.[7]

Impactions are unilateral in the majority of cases, and the occurrence on the palatal side is three times higher than on the labial side.[8,9]

Some systemic endocrine or infectious diseases are related with failed eruption of one or more teeth (Fig. 13.1).[10] They act as predisposing factors but always in conjunction with a local pathologic condition, such as[11]:

- Supernumerary teeth
- Odontomas
- Dental anomalies
- Cysts
- Previous trauma
- Early extractions
- Ankylosis
- Cleft lip and palate

These factors can be associated with impactions of every tooth and are usually related to incisors or premolars. Therefore, other causes can be identified regarding impacted canines. Since impacted upper canines have been diverted or are angulated aberrantly during development, it has been assumed that eruption of the canine is strongly influenced by environmental factors.[12,13]

The maxillary canine has the longest path of eruption, and a long time period is needed. This could explain the higher percentage of inclusion compared to other teeth.

The upper canine begins its development from the superior part of the maxilla. At age 2 years, the crown is located in correspondence of the apex of deciduous canine, mesially inclined.[14] When the permanent incisors are erupted, the close relationship between the crown of the canine and the distal aspect of the root of lateral incisor is particularly important.[15] Since the upper cuspid is one of the last teeth to reach its position, the lack of space in the arch can have a great influence on the prevalence of impactions, especially regarding the labial ones.[16]

The studies that have investigated palatal impactions pointed out the increased incidence of missing or peg-shaped laterals.[11,17] This leads to the formation of two theories: the genetic theory and the guidance theory.[3,6,18] Both theories share the belief that certain genetic features occur in association with the palatal displacement of maxillary canines. The right side of any patient is genetically identical to the left side. Since many studies indicated 60% to 75% preponderance of unilateral canine impaction, it is reasonable to state that local factors are the prevailing elements.[13]

Zilberman demonstrated that anomalies of the lateral incisors in patients with palatally displaced maxillary canine (PDC) teeth were found to be four times that of the general population.[19] The canine impaction has been related with abnormalities regarding the shape and length of the root of the lateral incisor rather than its agenesis (Fig. 13.2).[20]

However, missing, small, and peg-shaped lateral incisors are three varieties of expression of a single genetic factor. A peg-shaped or small lateral incisor on one side of the mouth and a missing on the other can be frequently seen (Fig. 13.3).

According to the guidance theory of canine impaction, these factors create a genetically determined environment in which the developing canine is deprived of its guidance, thus influencing it to adopt an abnormal eruption path.

Early Diagnosis and Treatment

A tooth is impacted when it fails to erupt into the dental arch within the expected developmental window. Therefore, an early diagnosis is crucial to reduce the consequent issues. Palpation of the labial fornix to assess the crown of the erupting canine is the first clinical attempt needed to identify a possible impaction. In case of a well-marked prominence absence in the late mixed dentition, orthopantomography (OPG) is mandatory (Fig. 13.4).[21]

The early identification signs on radiographs of an abnormal pathway of eruption is needed to prevent canine retention and maxillary incisor root resorption.[22]

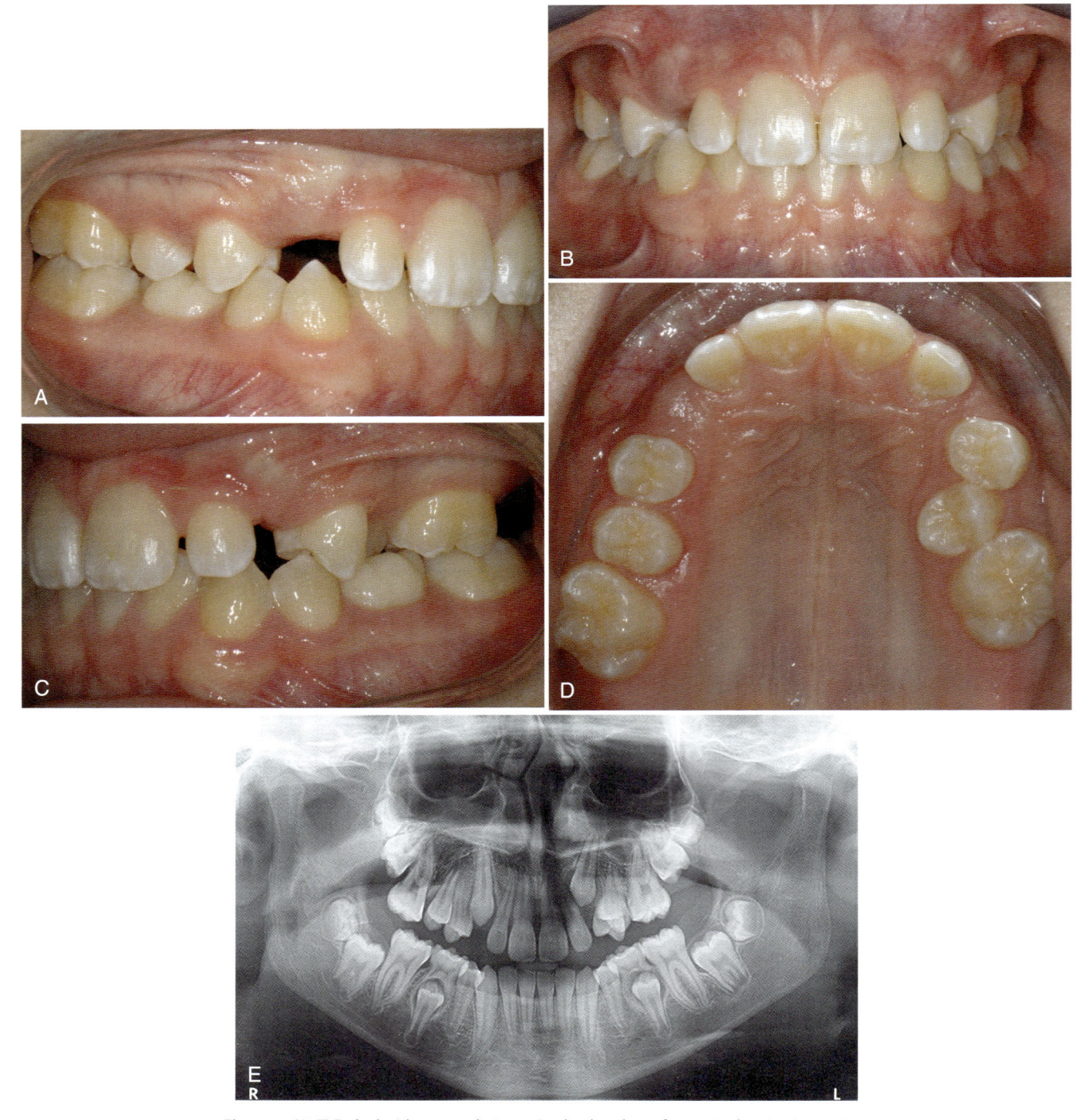

Fig. 13.1 (A–E) Early deciduous teeth extraction leads to loss of space and canine impaction.

The deciduous canine extraction is recommended when limited or absent resorption of its root can be detected, in class I uncrowded malocclusions.[21,23]

Ericson and Kurol,[21] to evaluate the need of primary canine extraction and its corrective effect, determined a method for detection of the permanent canines, based on the following (Fig 13.5):

- The angle of the canine and the midline axis (α)
- The distance from the cusp tip to the occlusal line (d)
- The position sector (s) in the frontal view
  - Between the midline and the axis of the U1
  - Between the axis of U1 and U2
  - Between the axis of U2 and U4

The success rate of early extractions will vary depending on the position of the permanent canine on OPG. If the crown of the permanent canine is distal to lateral incisor root axis, the primary canine extraction normalized the erupting position of the permanent canine in 91% of the cases. In contrast, the success rate decreased to 64% if

13 • Aligners and Impacted Canines   151

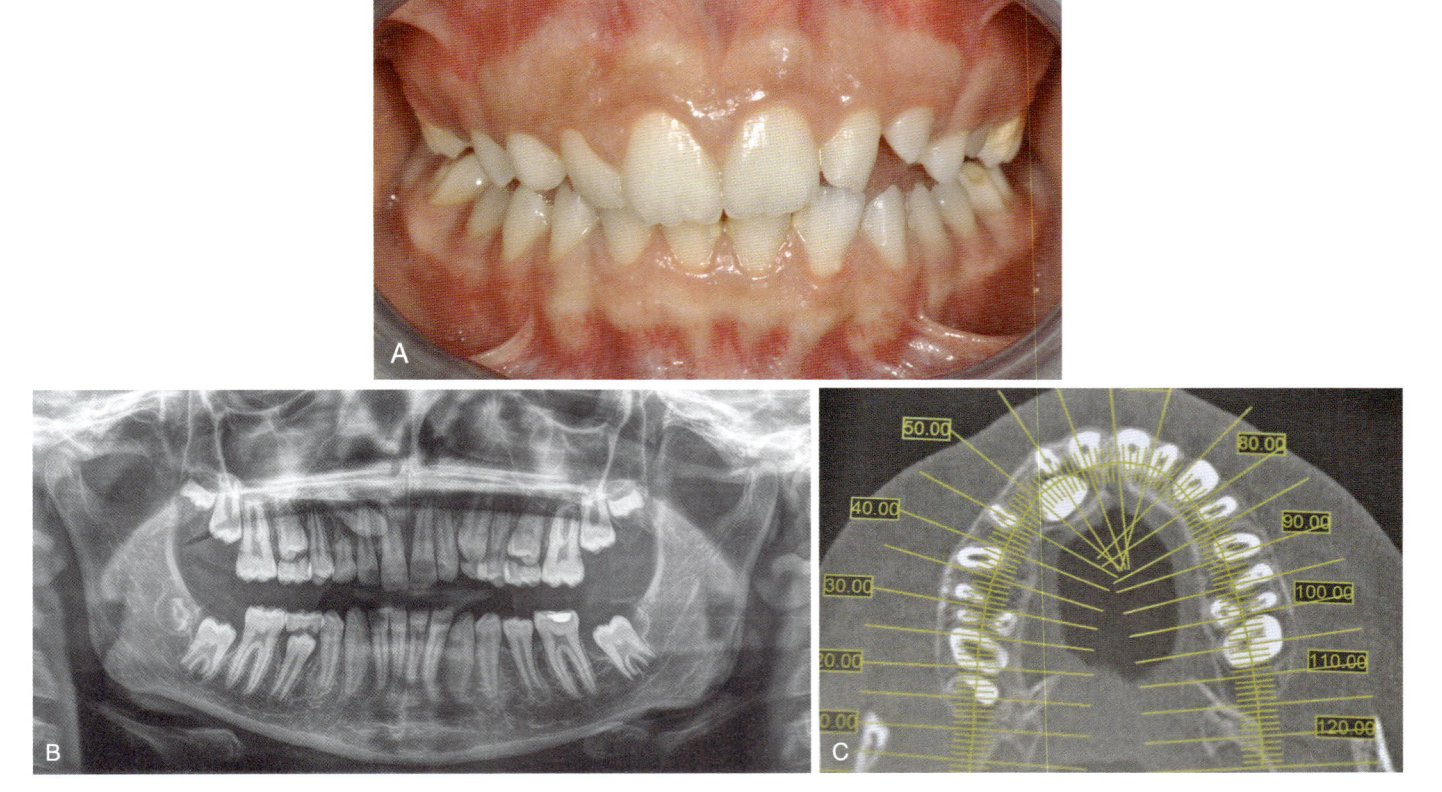

Fig. 13.2 (A–C) Small size lateral incisors and impacted cuspids.

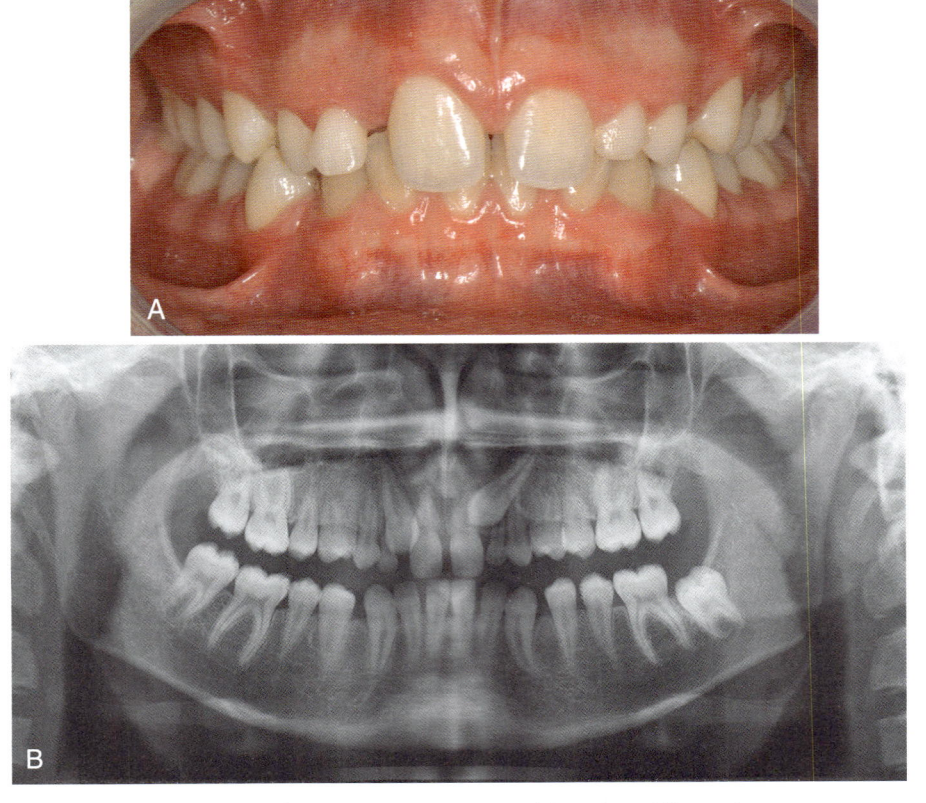

Fig. 13.3 (A) Missing lateral incisors and (B) bilateral cuspid impaction.

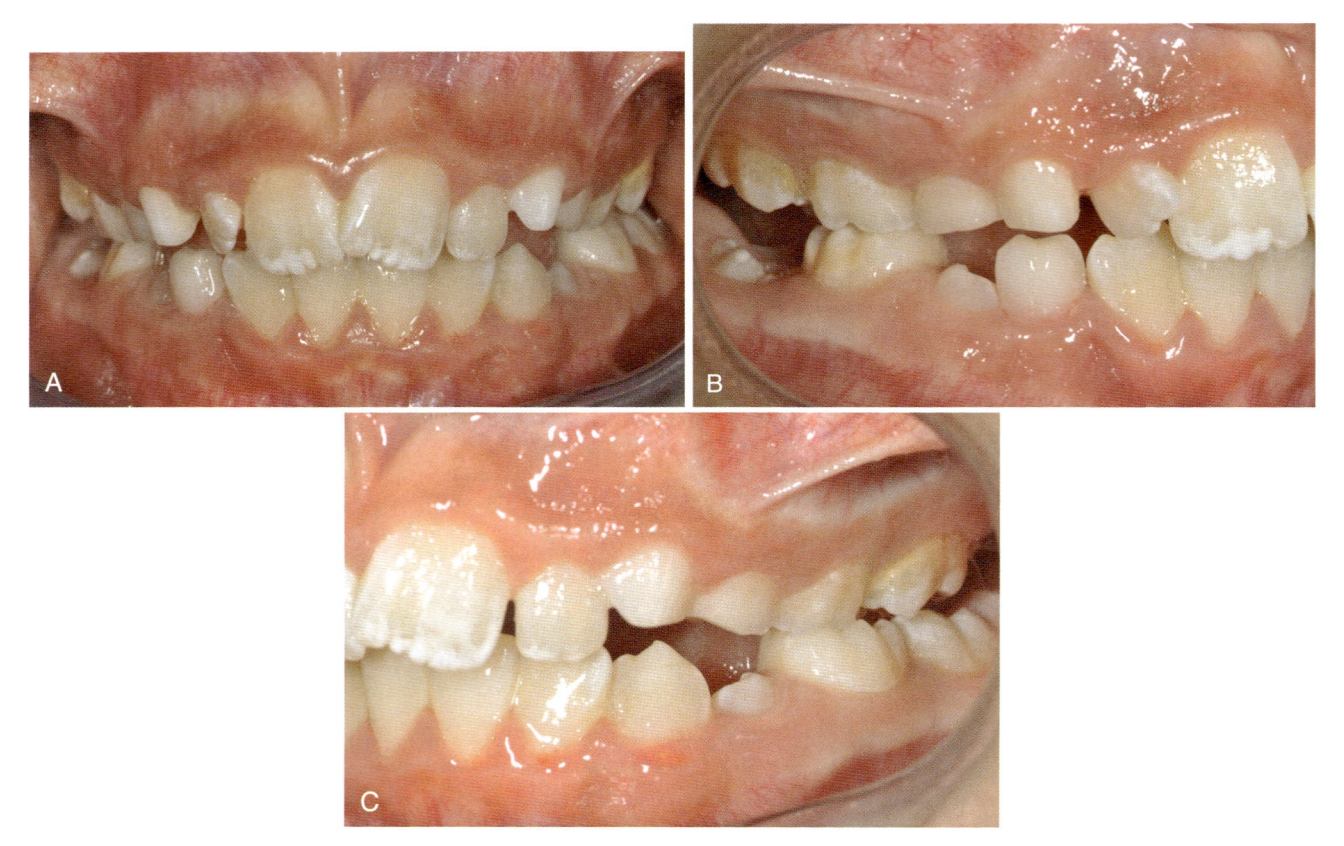

152 Principles and Biomechanics of Aligner Treatment

Fig. 13.4 (A–C) Back of right canine prominence in late mixed-dentition patient.

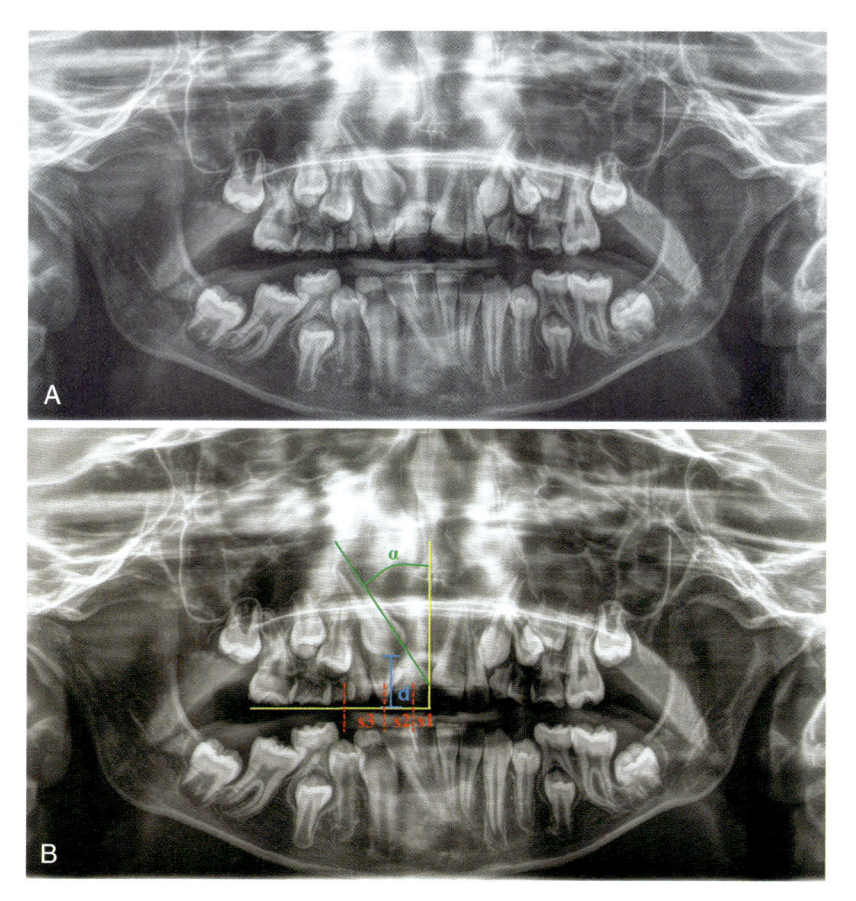

Fig. 13.5 (A, B) The orthopantomography refers to the patient in Fig. 13.4, Ericson and Kurol canine impaction analysis.

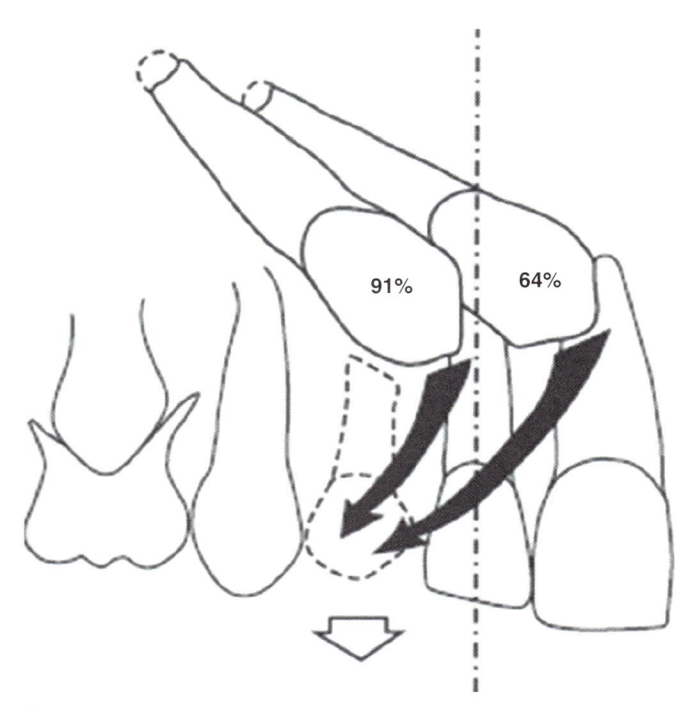

Fig. 13.6 Success rate of early deciduous canine extraction (from Ericson and Kurol).

the permanent canine crown were mesial to the midline of the lateral incisor root (Fig. 13.6).[24]

Bonetti et al. demonstrated that deciduous canine and first molar extractions are more effective as a preventive approach to promote eruption of retained maxillary permanent canines positioned palatally or centrally.[25]

On the lateral cephalometric radiograph the normal inclination of the canine compared to the perpendicular to the Frankfurt plane should be about 10 degrees (Fig. 13.7). Higher values are related with increased need for orthodontic treatment.[26]

Hong et al., using cone-beam computed tomography (CBCT) data, stated that the maxillary transverse dimension had no effect on the occurrence of PDC.[27] Baccetti demonstrated that, in PDC cases not requiring maxillary expansion, the use of a transpalatal arch (TPA) in combination with deciduous canine extraction can be effective for the permanent canine eruption.[28]

On the contrary, there is a strict relationship between the lack of space and the labially impacted canines, in particular a transverse maxillary deficiency located in the anterior portion of the dental arch.[29]

Research using the CBCT approach stated that buccal canine impaction is mostly associated with anterior transverse (dental and skeletal) deficiency.[30]

Subjects with unilateral or bilateral impacted maxillary canines have smaller maxillary transverse dimensions than subjects without impaction.[31]

The effect of rapid palatal expansion as a predictor of automatic eruption has been previously demonstrated.[32,33]

Early treatment of impacted canines is mandatory in case of severely resorbed incisors. When resorption process is halted, the incisors do not suffer from increased mobility or discoloration in the long term.[34]

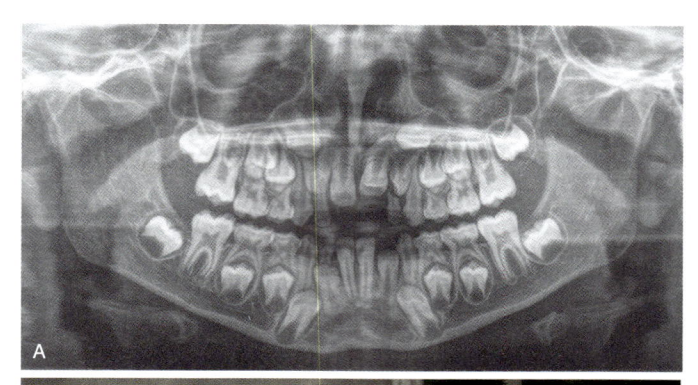

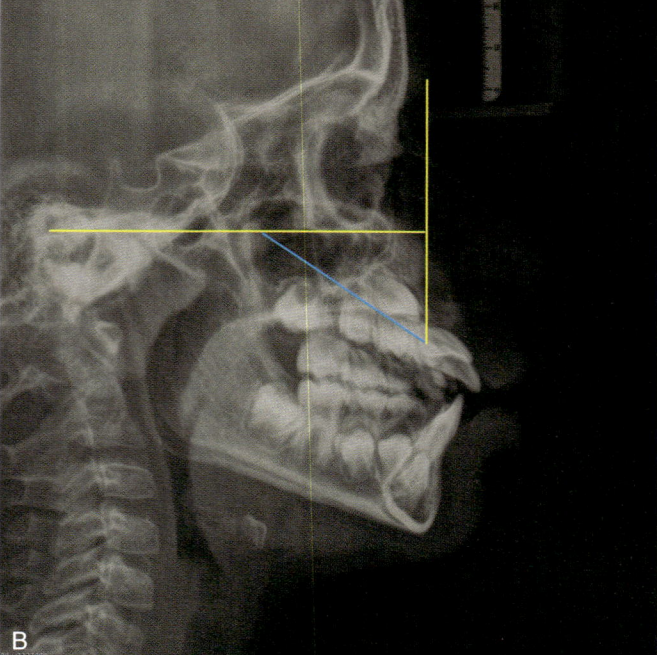

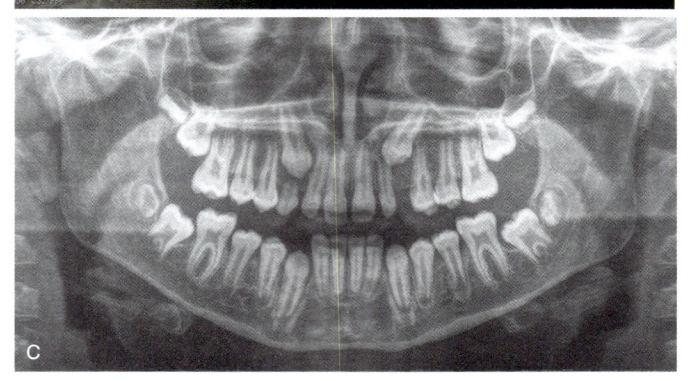

Fig. 13.7 (A–C) Inclination of the canine on lateral cephalometric analysis; parents of this patient refused phase 1 treatment, and upper left canine impaction occurred 3 years later.

Late Diagnosis

Diagnosis of upper canine impaction after the expected age of eruption is primarily clinical, with or without the presence of the corresponding deciduous canine. Ectopic or absent canine prominence is usually detected during the examination. The information provided by OPG gives an overall picture but cannot determine the proper position of the canine. However, when it is possible to identify the cause of failed eruption (e.g., a mechanical obstacle such as odontoma), its removal can allow the tooth to erupt spontaneously.

Lindauer,[35] in his study using panoramic x-ray, found that 22% of PDC had their cusp tip distal to the lateral incisor and remained undetected.

CBCT systems provide three-dimensional (3D) images and useful data for a more accurate locating of impacted teeth.[36]

CT investigations have proven to be superior in detecting root resorption compared with conventional radiographic methods (intraoral and panoramic radiographs). The amount of resorption detected by CT scanning was approximately 50% higher.[37] Root resorption of the maxillary permanent incisors caused by ectopic eruption of the permanent canine has an overall prevalence of 12%, with a prevalence that is four times as high in girls as in boys.[38]

Dental follicles of the ectopically erupting canines are on average wider than those of the normally erupting canines.[39] During eruption, the follicle of the erupting maxillary canine frequently resorbs the periodontal contours of adjacent permanent teeth but not the hard tissues of the roots.

Resorption of neighboring permanent teeth during maxillary canine eruption is most likely an effect of the physical contacts with active pressure during eruption and cellular activities. The resorptive mechanism seems to be confined to the dental follicle and related to metabolic activation.[40] Yan found no significant difference of resorption prevalence between subjects with buccal and palatal impactions. The dominant predictor for resorption was contact relationship less than 1 mm.[41]

Another recent CBCT study found no significant correlation between follicle width and the variables of gender, impaction side, and localization of maxillary impacted canines.[42] Other factors influencing diagnosis and treatment planning, such as ankylosis and root dilaceration, can be identified mostly on CBCT images. Furthermore, CBCT data can provide useful information about shape and size of the impacted canine, especially if further intraarch space is required (Table 13.1).[43]

According to Becker,[44] the major reasons for failure are inadequate anchorage (48.6%), mistaken location and directional traction (40.5%), and ankylosis (32.4%). There is no age limit for orthodontic recovering of impacted canines, but the chance of success decreases with age. A study undertaken in adult patients found 69.5% success rate of impacted maxillary canine treatment among the adults compared with 100% among the younger controls, even though the overall length of orthodontic treatment was similar. All the failed canines were found in the older adult subgroup (>30 years of age).[45]

Table 13.1 Factors Affecting Prognosis

- Depth of impaction
- Lack of space in the dental arch
- Age of the patient
- Cooperation of the patient

Treatment Planning and Orthodontic Management

The main goal of every orthodontic treatment is not only the correction of malocclusion but also a good alignment and healthy periodontal tissues. Regarding impacted canines, the eruption should be in the center of the alveolar ridge.[46]

During physiologic eruption there is a fusion between keratinized gingiva and reduced enamel epithelium with the formation of the junctional epithelium.[47] When this occurs, a proper arrangement of periodontium with an adequate band of keratinized tissue, correct sulcular depth, and connective fibers inserted on cementoenamel junction (CEJ) can be found.[48] If a canine erupts in the alveolar mucosa, lack of junctional epithelium may occur, leading to further mucogingival issues (Fig. 13.8).[49,50]

Teeth erupted in a labial position can promote the thinning of the cortical plate and the formation of bony dehiscence or fenestration. This situation is related to lack of keratinized gingiva and higher prevalence of recessions (Fig. 13.9).[51,52]

The adequate amount of keratinized gingiva has been reported as between 0 and 3 mm[53,54]; however, thinner gingival tissue is at higher risk of gingival recession development during orthodontic movement.[55] When conditions do not allow achievement of the eruption with a good periodontal

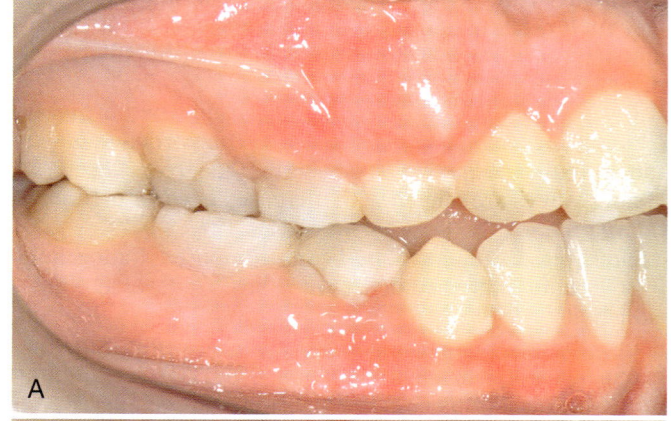

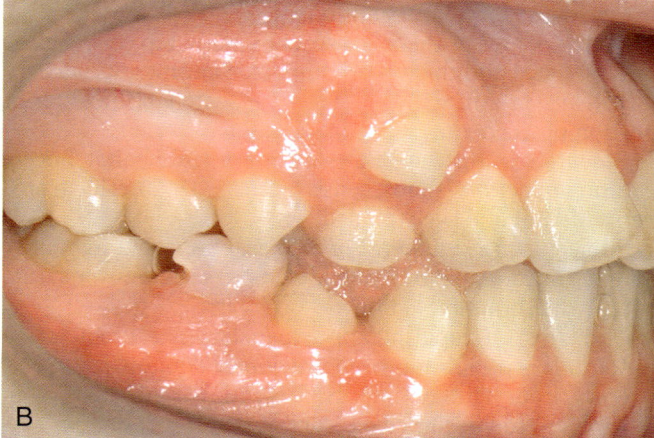

Fig. 13.8 (A, B) Canine eruption in alveolar mucosa.

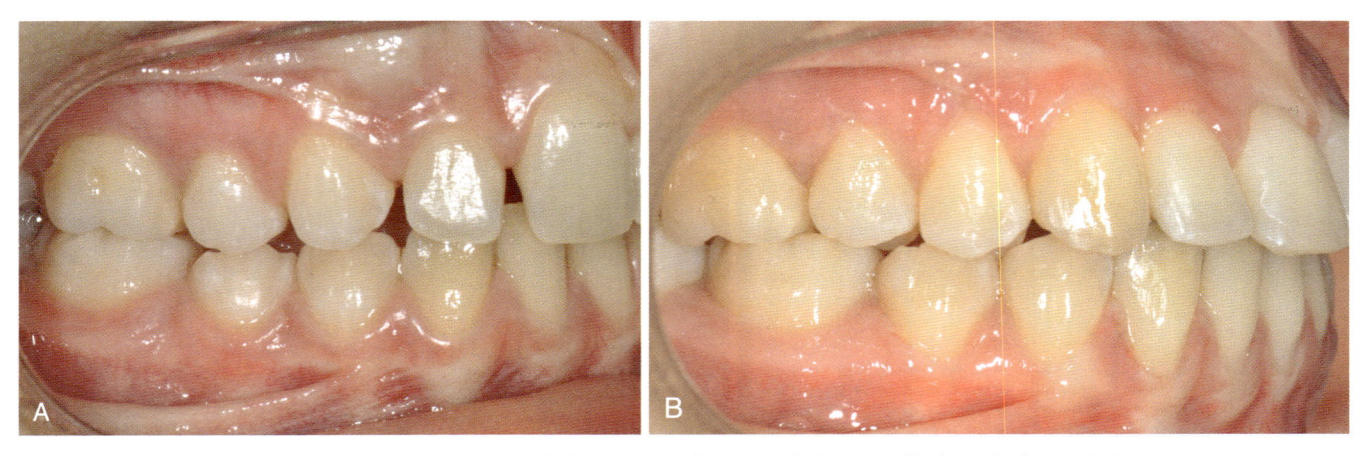

Fig. 13.9 (A, B) Canine erupted labially with lack of keratinized gingiva and higher risk of recession.

support or in a reasonable treatment time, premolar substitution, retention of the primary canine, or prosthetic rehabilitation must be taken into account (Fig. 13.10).

Since a proper diagnosis is mandatory for correct orthodontic and surgical planning, the first issue to deal with is depth of impaction.[56] It can be found as a soft tissue impaction, a partial intraosseous impaction, or a deep full bony impaction. A method of analyzing severity of impactions using CBCT was proposed by Kau.[57] This method utilizes the entire three views (horizontal, vertical, and axial) of a CBCT image. Depending on its anatomic location, the cusp tip and the root tip are each given a number between 0 and 5 in 3D taken from a pretreatment image. The sum of the cusp tip and root tip scores in the three views dictated complexity of treatment.

To obtain the eruption at the center of the alveolar ridge, not only the point of eruption of the cuspid but also the path must be taken into account. Direct traction is provided when relationship with adjacent teeth is favorable. If not, the canine must be moved in a different direction (Fig. 13.11).

A recent classification has been proposed to categorize maxillary impacted canines as type A (high risk) and type B (low risk).[43] Type A teeth represent a high risk of periodontal damage on neighboring teeth, including root resorption. They need early exposure to be pulled away from closer roots. Other teeth must not be moved until they reach a safe position. Type B canines do not require immediate exposure and can be moved directly in their final position. Therefore, combined orthoperiodontal treatment aims to guide the canine at the center of the alveolar ridge in three steps:

1. Initial orthodontic phase
2. Surgical intervention
3. Orthodontic traction and alignment

Usually, before the intervention, a preliminary orthodontic phase is needed to gain space in the arch with aligning and leveling. The initial orthodontic phase should provide a good control of the archform and maintain space for the impacted canine.

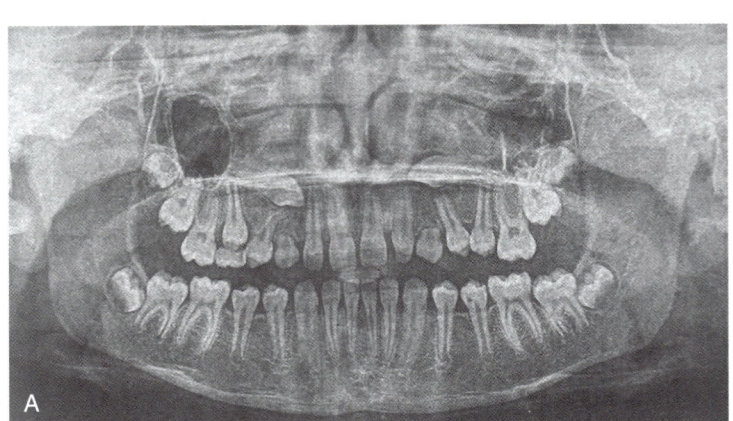

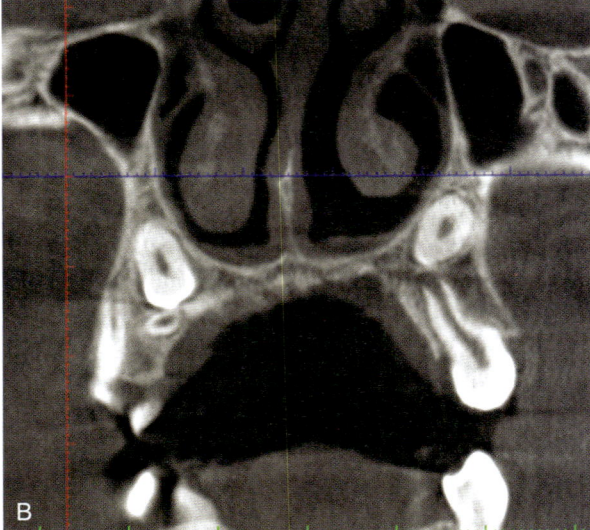

Fig. 13.10 (A–E) Deep horizontal impaction may undermine the eruption with a good periodontal support.

Continued

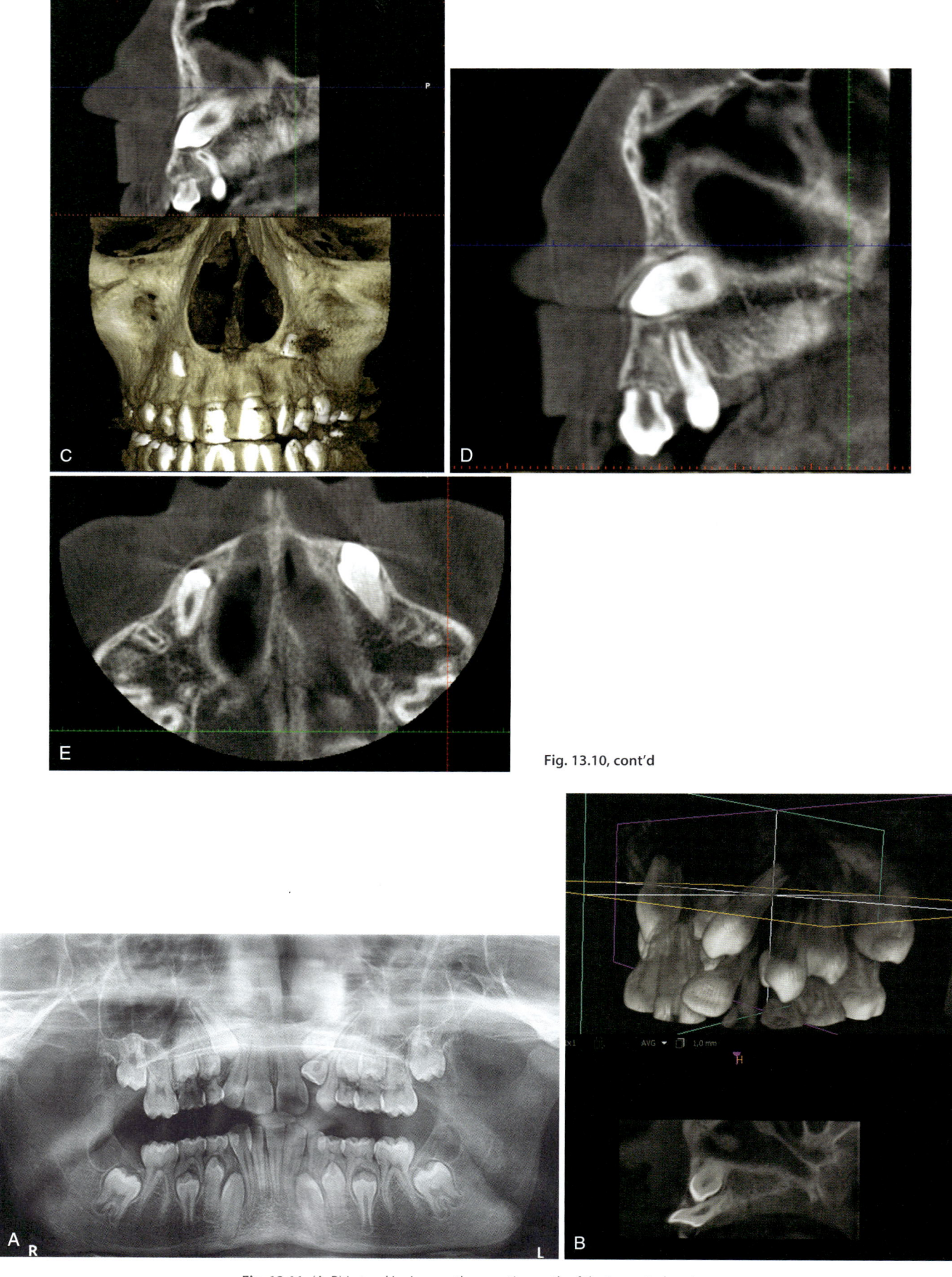

156 Principles and Biomechanics of Aligner Treatment

Fig. 13.10, cont'd

Fig. 13.11 (A, B) Lateral incisor on the eruption path of the impacted canine.

The size of the canine should be calculated automatically using Clincheck software if a contralateral canine is present. Otherwise a digital approximation should be made according to the size of the other teeth. To avoid any risk of interference, roots of incisors and premolars close to the canine should be moved carefully. A proper anchorage is needed before the surgical intervention to support the orthodontic traction; the use of temporary anchorage devices (TADs) can be helpful.

Aim of the surgical exposure is the application of a device for the traction, such as button or a mesh, as close as possible to the cusp tip; the least amount of bone and keratinized tissue removal is desirable. Two methods of surgical-orthodontic traction of impacted teeth can be used: the open flap and closed eruption techniques. The open technique includes surgical exposure of the crown by either complete removal of bone and soft tissue directly overlying the impacted canine[8] or the use of an apically repositioned gingival flap[58] without starting orthodontic traction and waiting on the self-eruption. The closed technique involves elevating a full mucoperiosteal flap, exposing the canine crown to bond an attachment, then suturing. The orthodontic traction is applied until the eruption of the tooth.[59]

Cassina[9] found that open surgical exposure seems to be associated with reduced treatment duration and ankylosis risk over the closed technique. Furthermore the closed technique does not allow direct control of the eruption path, and the detachment of the orthodontic device may require a second surgery. On the other hand, the first intention wound healing can ensure a better postoperative course.

The aim of the postsurgical phase is to bring the impacted tooth into the desired position on the arch. Once the canine has been exposed, continuous light forces (30–50 g) are required using elastics or elastomeric chains. The aligner can be modified with burs or pliers to create proper hooks on which elastics or elastomeric chains can be anchored. Heavy forces may cause loss of anchorage (intrusion) and significant root resorption of the adjacent anchorage teeth. When traction is provided directly by elastomeric chains, if the patient does not wear aligners adequately, unwanted forces can develop and unwanted movement of anchorage teeth can occur. The patient must wear the intraarch elastics for 22 hours a day along with the aligners.

Labial Impactions

Since the amount of attached gingiva after eruption and therefore the final periodontal health is affected by the surgical technique, labial impactions are more challenging to manage. Based on the relationship between the impacted canine height and the mucogingival junction (MGJ), three different surgical techniques are traditionally used to uncover labially impacted canines: gingivectomy, apically positioned flap, and closed eruption.[8]

The gingivectomy is indicated when there is a soft tissue impaction, more than a third of the crown is below the MGJ, and a proper amount of keratinized gingiva (about 3–4 mm) is preserved above the exposed crown.[43]

The apically positioned flap is used in shallow labial impactions when most of the crown is located apically to the MGJ, especially when a little amount of attached gingiva is detected. A minimum of 2 mm of attached gingiva should be embedded in the flap design.

The closed eruption technique is recommended when the position of the crown is coronal to the mucogingival junction, or if the labiolingual position of the impacted canine is toward the center of the alveolar ridge, to avoid massive gingival and bone removal.

Vermette et al.[46] stated that labially impacted teeth mostly need closed eruption technique to reduce unaesthetic sequelae such as increased clinical crown length. In a recent split-mouth study, Lee et al. found that after the closed eruption technique, impacted canines exhibited slight but clinically insignificant periodontal recession compared with the contralateral normal tooth. Occurrence of recession is related to the root developmental stage and pretreatment depth and angle.[60]

Palatal Impactions

According to Becker and Zilberman[61] the ideal treatment approach is from the palatal side. Initial traction should be applied in a lingually downward direction to prevent interference with the neighboring teeth.

A recent review by Parkin[62] stated that when a unilateral PDC is exposed and aligned, there is a small periodontal impact with no clinical relevance in the short term; they found no difference in periodontal health when the open and closed techniques were compared. Before orthodontic treatment, the open technique involves surgical exposure of the canine and the overlying palatal tissue removal. Healing is attained by secondary intention. A large removal of bone and gingival tissue can lead to a significative loss of clinical attachment and gingival recession so that this technique should be avoided in cases of deep impaction.[63] Furthermore, damage of the CEJ can promote an increased risk of ankylosis.[44] The closed technique involves uncovering the canine, attaching an eyelet and gold chain, and then suturing the palatal mucosa back over the tooth.[64,65] In this case, a force is applied on the tooth to speed up the eruption. Criticality of this method is the possible detachment of the orthodontic device. However, the first intention wound healing can lead to better periodontal and aesthetic outcomes with lower morbidity for the patient.

Clinical Case

FIRST VISIT

Date: 8-9-2017
Gender: Male
Age: 16y 5m

ORTHODONTIC DIAGNOSIS

Skeletal
- SKL CL 2, SKL NORMO

Dental
- Molar CL I, canine CL nonassessible, deep bite, increased OVJ, spaces between teeth

158 Principles and Biomechanics of Aligner Treatment

Facial
- Flat profile

Multiple agenesis: 15, 31, 34, 35, 41, 44, 45
Impacted: 13, 23, 33
Figs. 13.12, 13.13, and 13.14 are provided.

TREATMENT PLAN

1. Oral hygiene instructions and motivation
2. Anterior diastemas closure and anchorage preparation
3. Surgical exposure
4. Final alignment

TREATMENT PROGRESS

Figs. 13.15 and 13.16 show details of the treatment progress.

FINAL

Figs. 13.17, 13.18, and 13.19 show final treatment results.

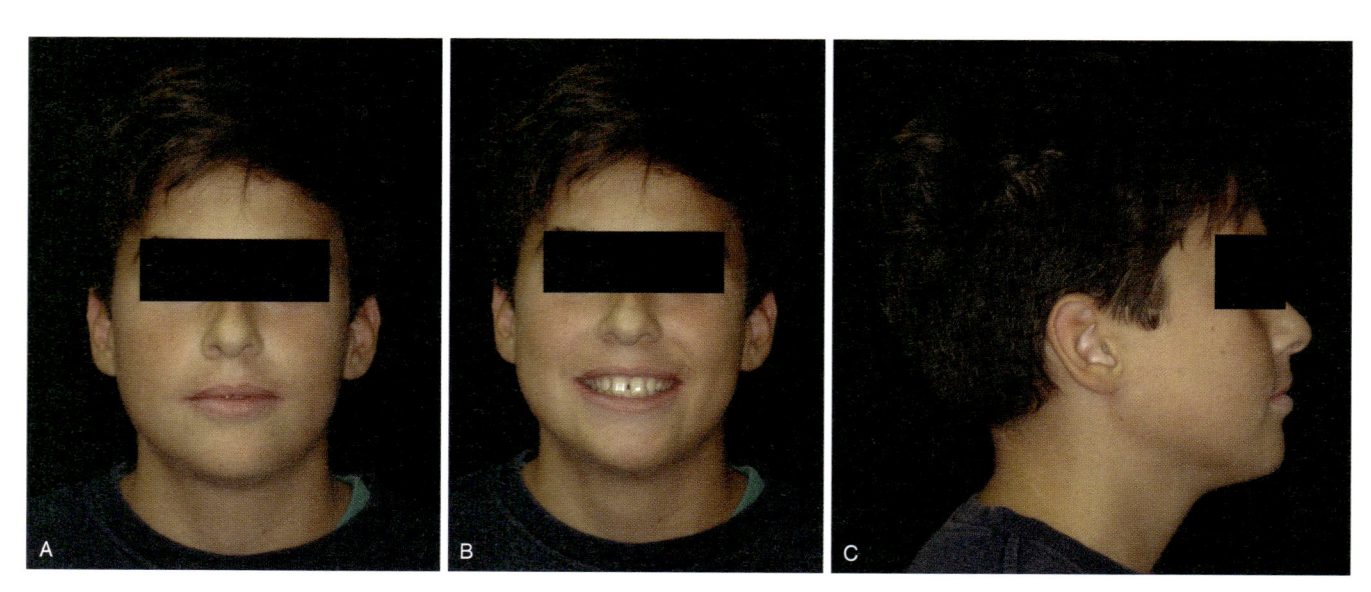

Fig. 13.12 (A–C) Clinical case study baseline extraoral.

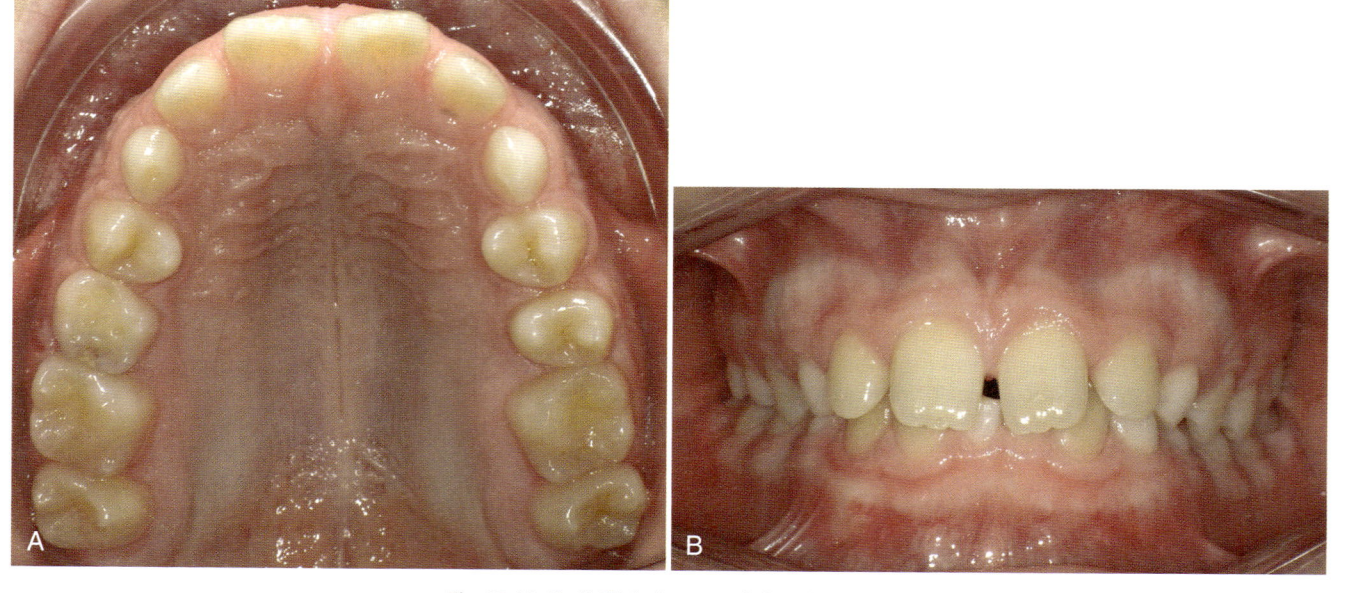

Fig. 13.13 (A–E) Clinical case study baseline intraoral.

13 • Aligners and Impacted Canines 159

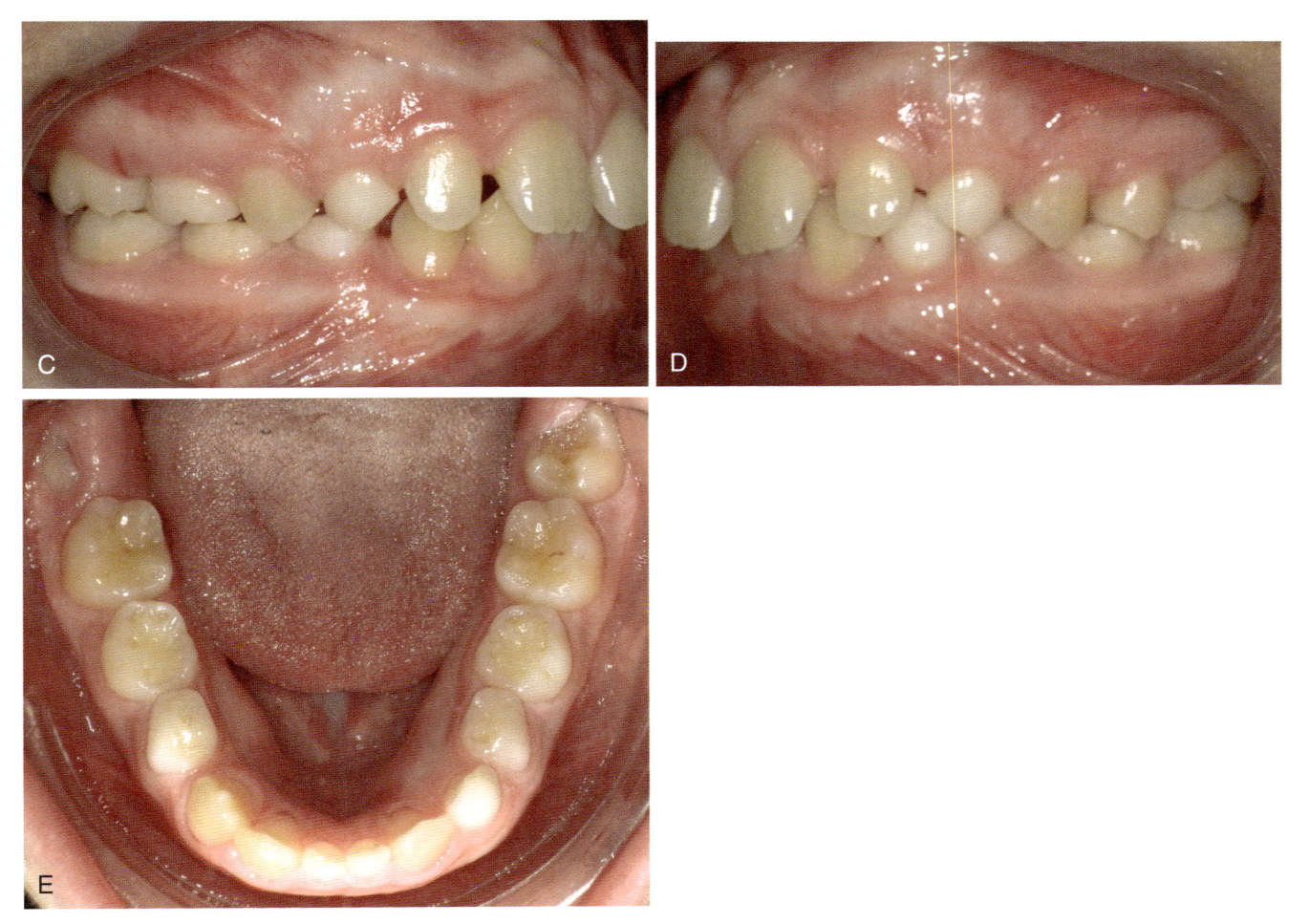

Fig. 13.13, cont'd

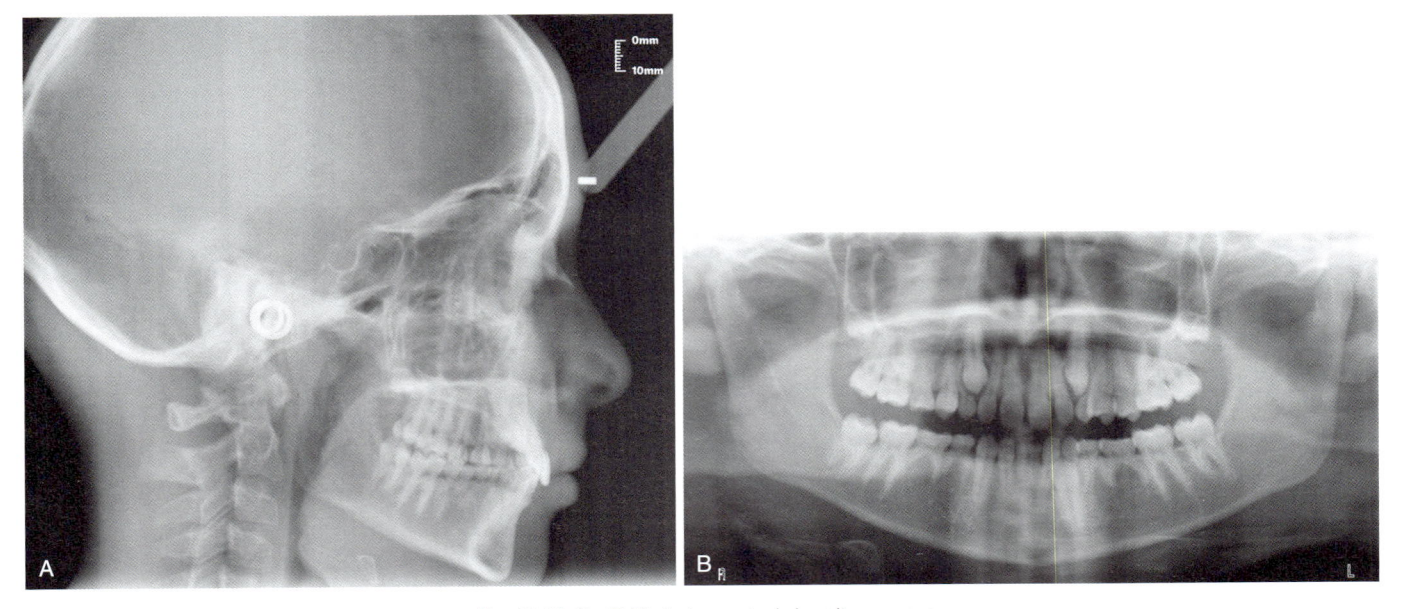

Fig. 13.14 (A–G) Clinical case study baseline x-rays.

Continued

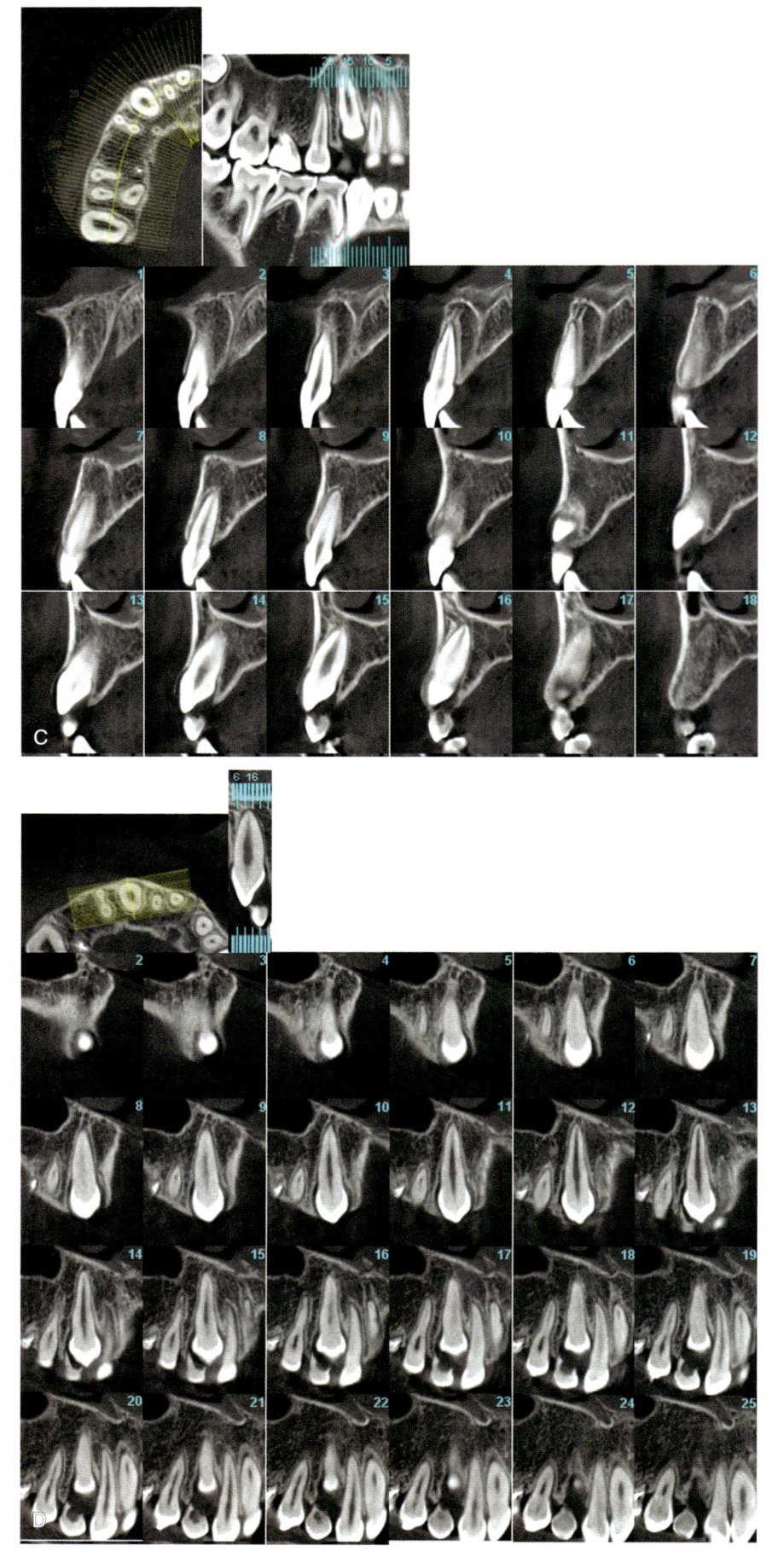

160 Principles and Biomechanics of Aligner Treatment

Fig. 13.14, cont'd

13 • Aligners and Impacted Canines 161

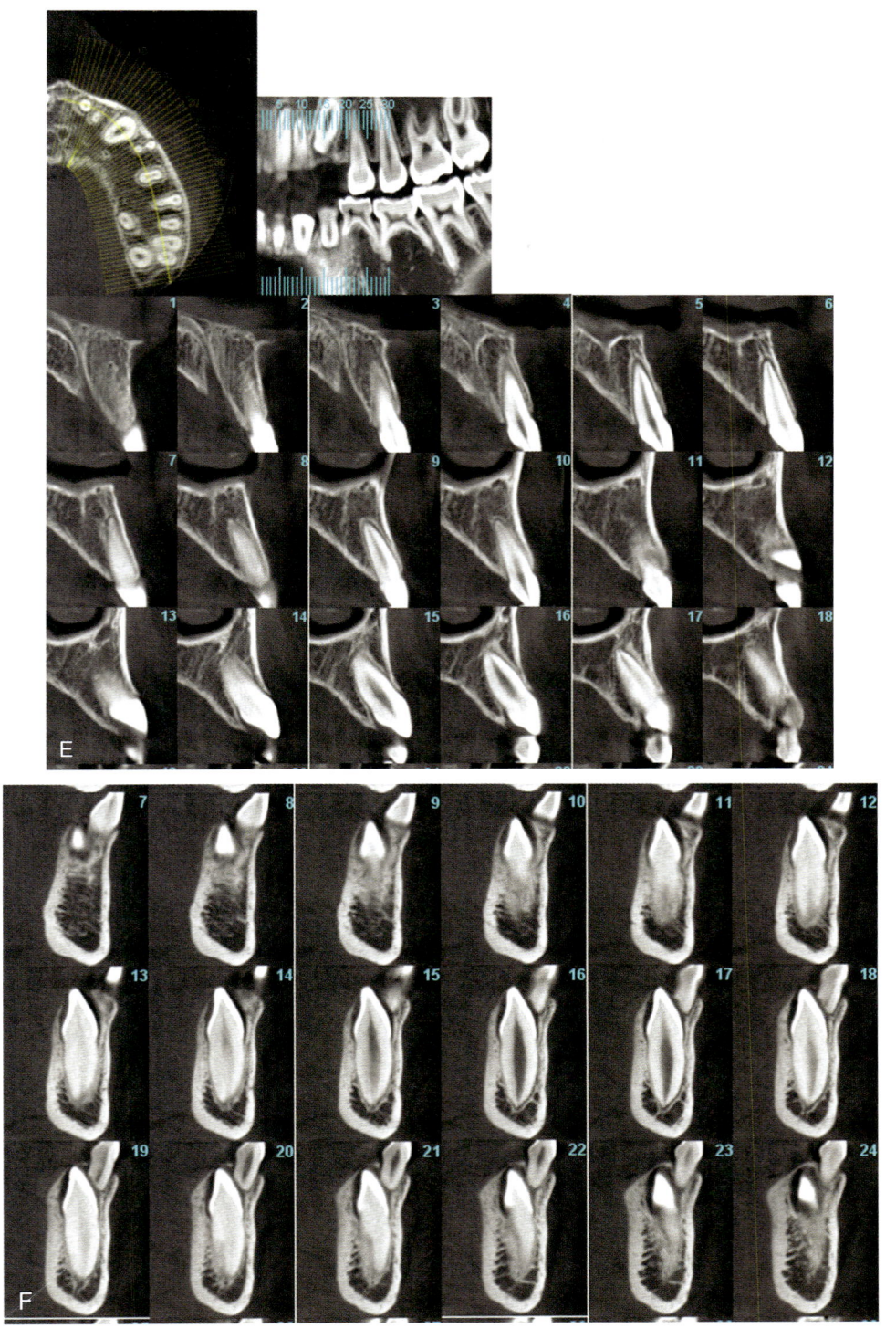

Fig. 13.14, cont'd

Continued

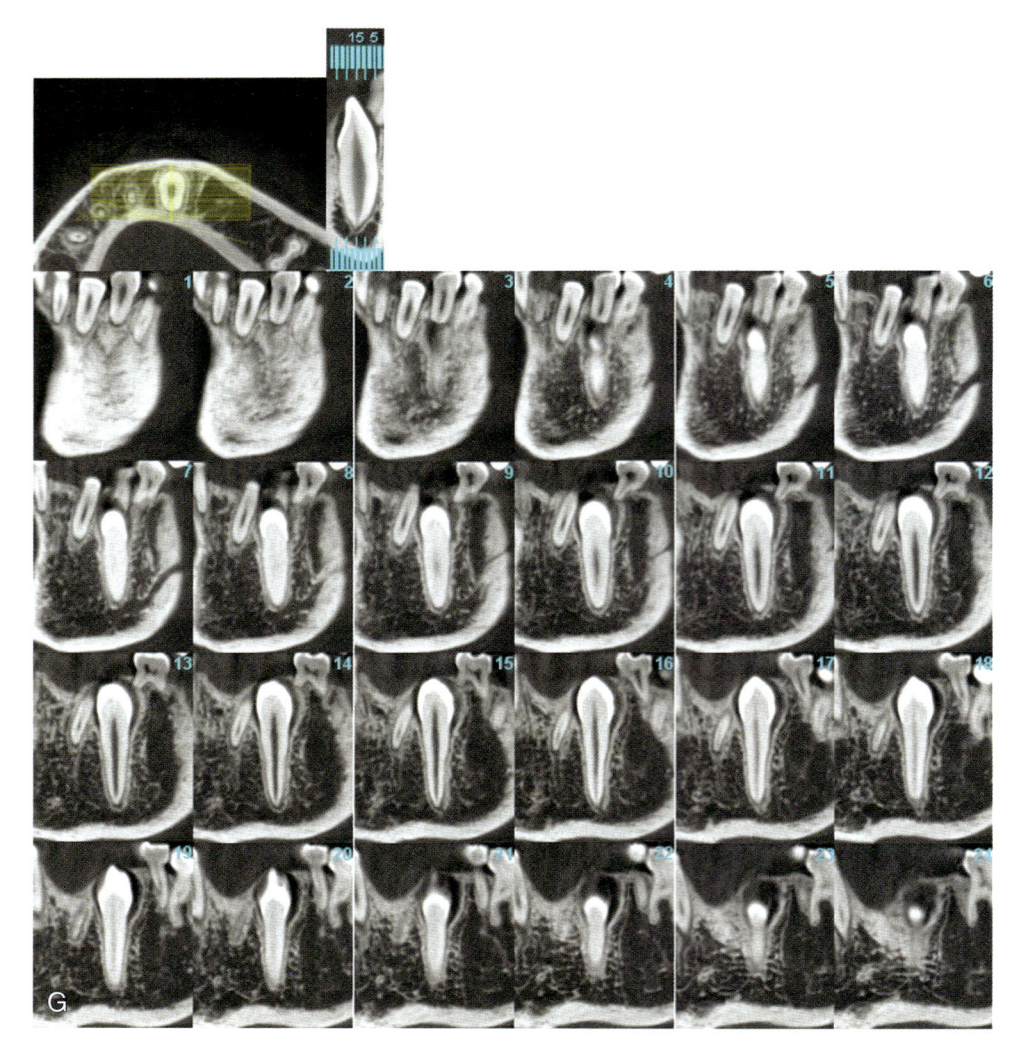

162 Principles and Biomechanics of Aligner Treatment

Fig. 13.14, cont'd

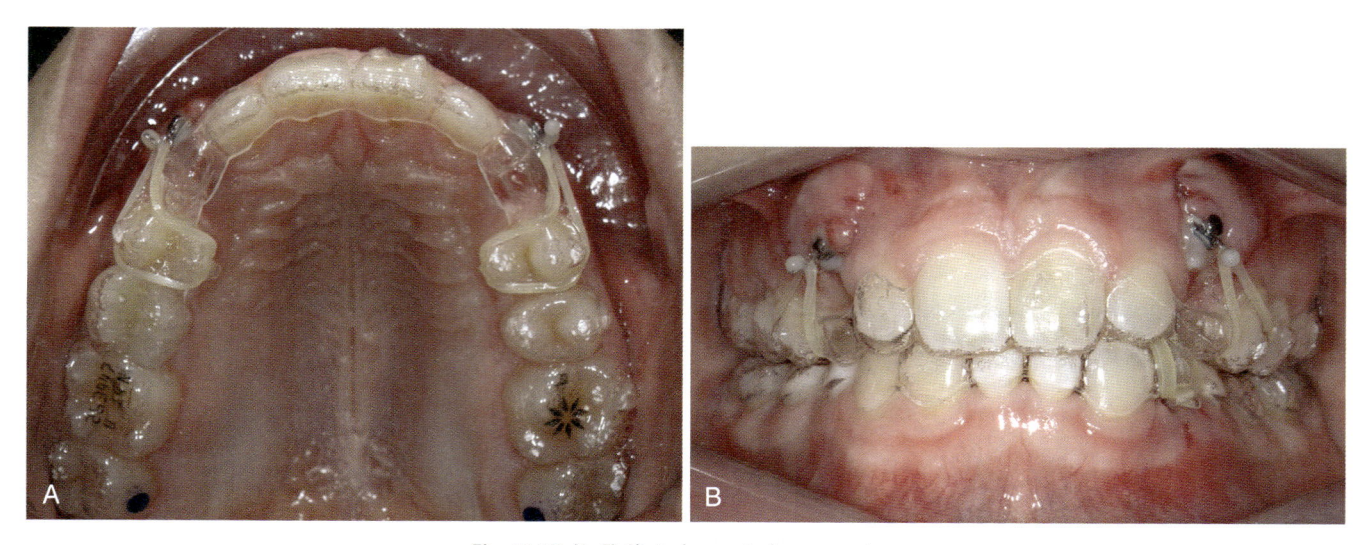

Fig. 13.15 (A–E) Clinical case study progression.

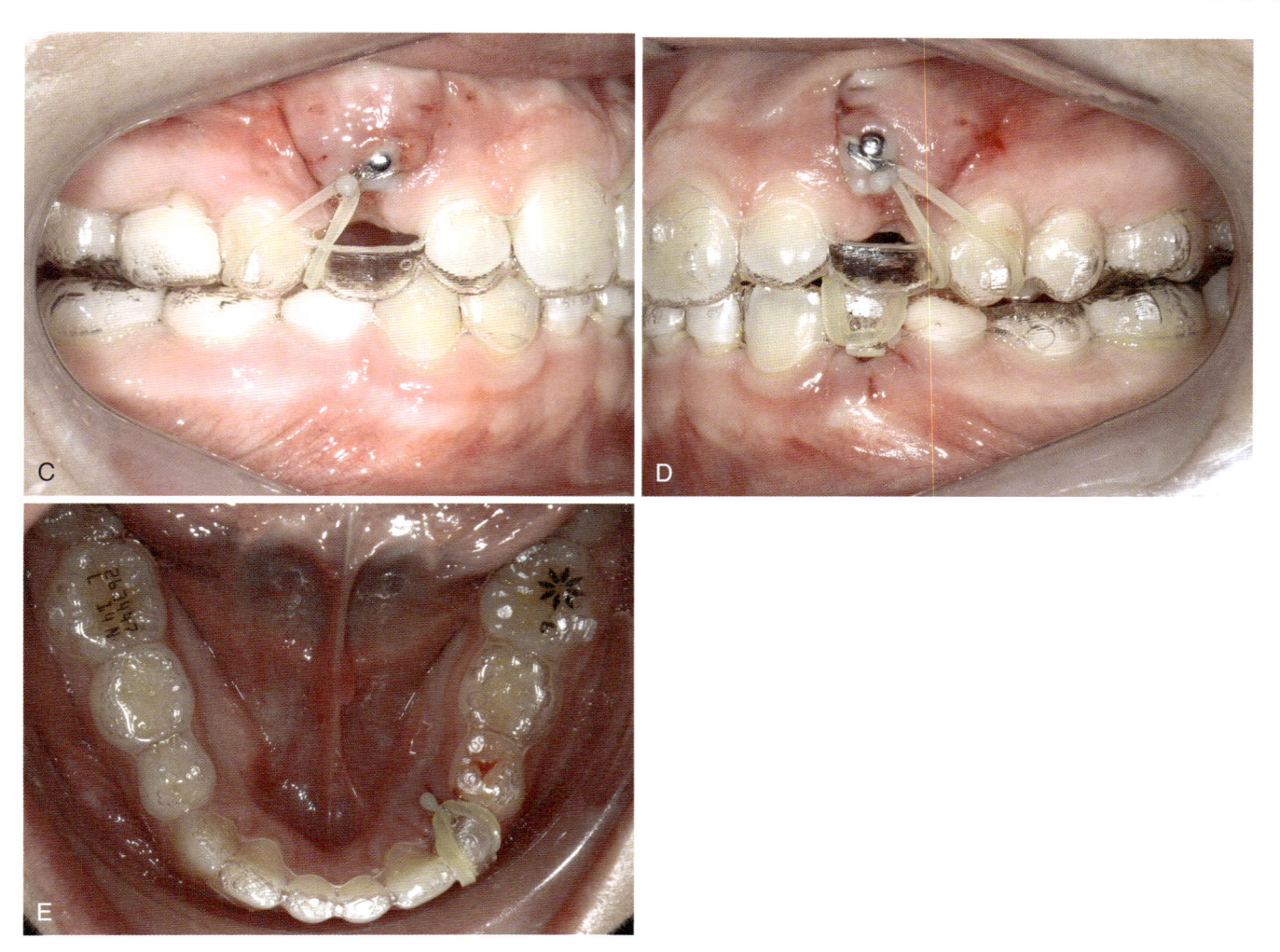

13 • Aligners and Impacted Canines

Fig. 13.15, cont'd

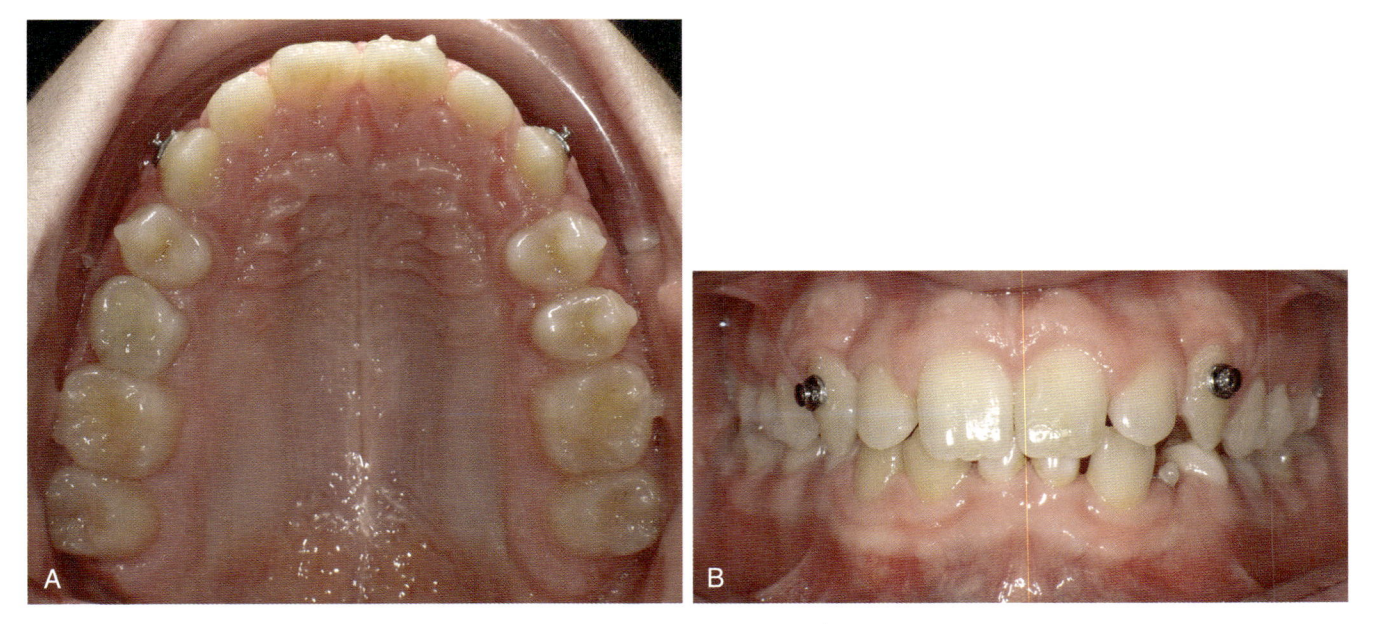

Fig. 13.16 (A–F) Clinical case study progression.

Continued

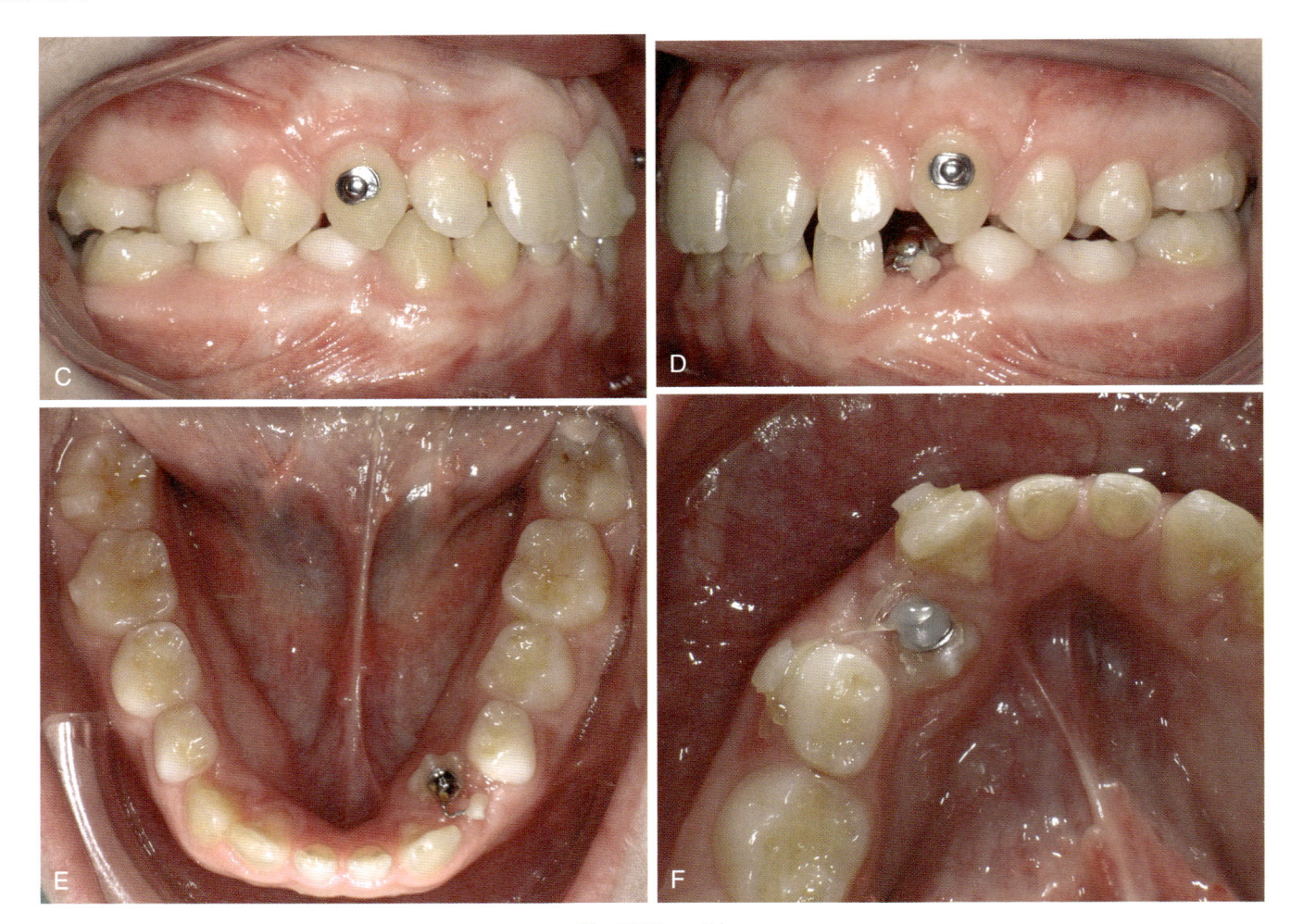

164 Principles and Biomechanics of Aligner Treatment

Fig. 13.16, cont'd

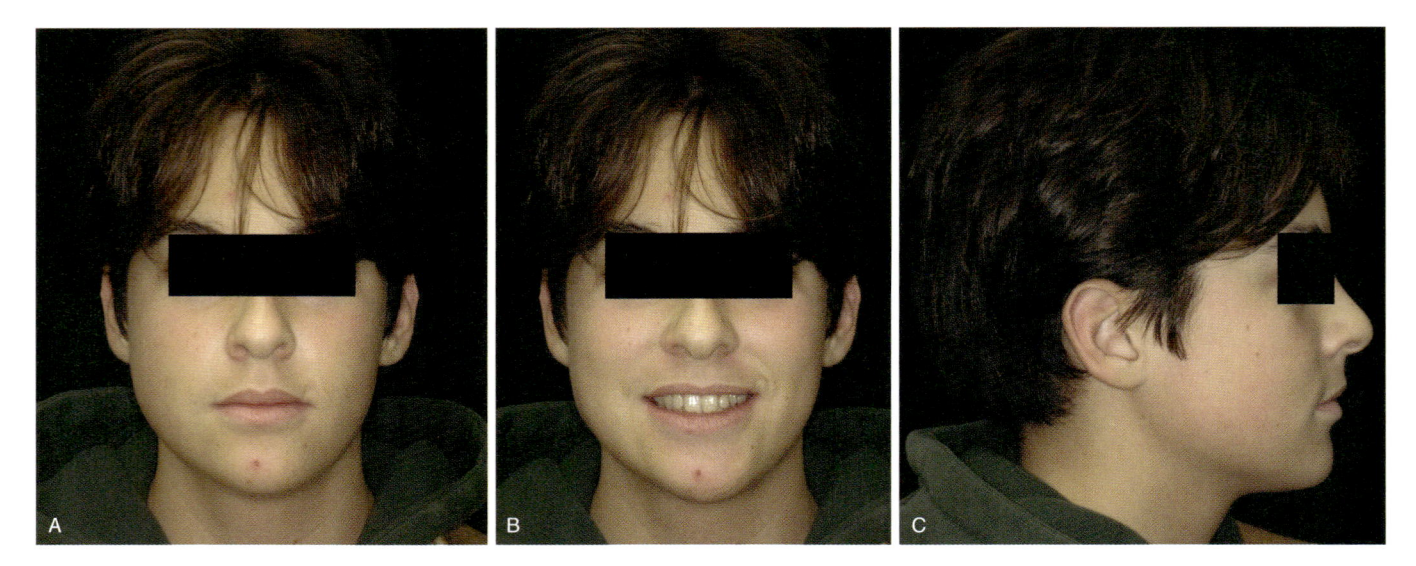

Fig. 13.17 (A–C) Clinical case study extraoral final.

13 • Aligners and Impacted Canines 165

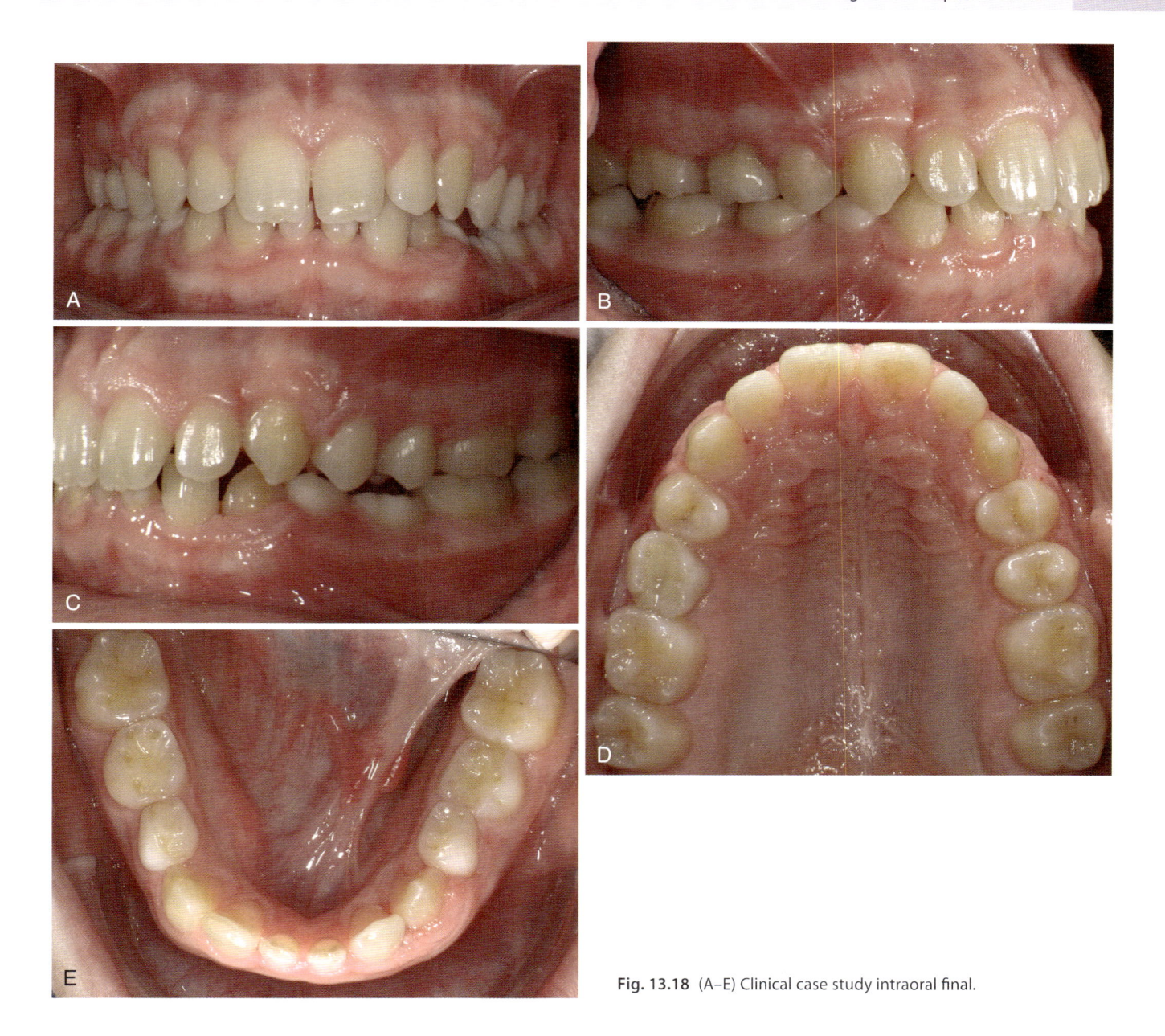

Fig. 13.18 (A–E) Clinical case study intraoral final.

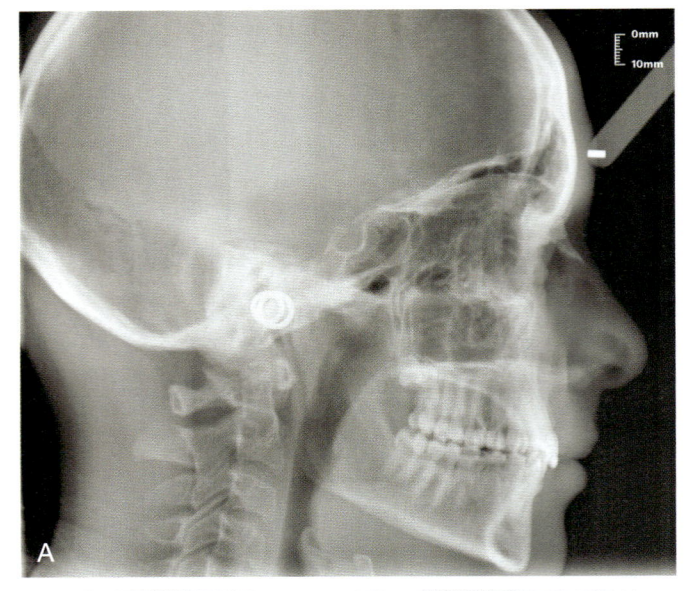

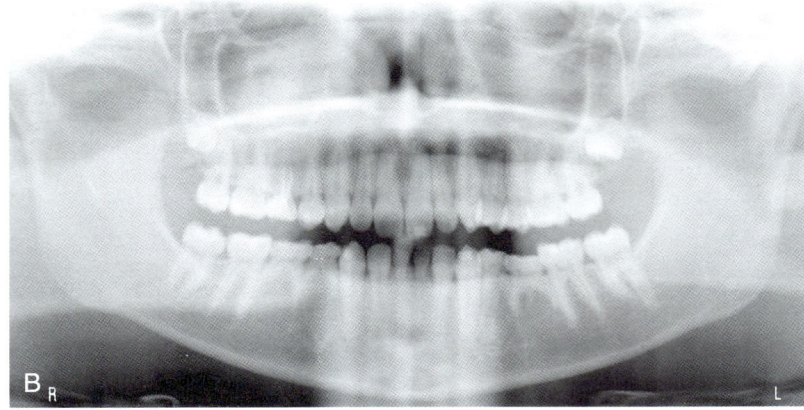

Fig. 13.19 (A, B) Clinical case study final x-rays.

References

1. Shafer WG, Hine MK, Levy BM. *A Textbook of Oral Pathology.* 2nd ed. Philadelphia: WB Saunders; 1963.
2. Dachi SF, Howell FV. A survey of 3874 routine full mouth radiographs. II. A study of impacted teeth. *Oral Surg Oral Med Oral Pathol.* 1961;14:1165-1169.
3. Sacerdoti R, Baccetti T. Dentoskeletal features associated with unilateral or bilateral palatal displacement of maxillary canines. *Angle Orthod.* 2004;74:725-732.
4. Ericson S, Kurol J. Radiographic assessment of maxillary canine eruption in children with clinical signs of eruption disturbance. *Eur J Orthod.* 1986;8(3):133-140.
5. Wang H, Li T, Lv C, Huang L, Zhang C, Tao G, Li X, Zou S, Duan P. Risk factors for maxillary impacted canine-linked severe lateral incisor root resorption: A cone-beam computed tomography study. *Am J Orthod Dentofacial Orthop.* 2020 Sep;158(3):410-419.
6. McDonald F, Yap WL. The surgical exposure and application of direct traction of unerupted teeth. *Am J Orthod.* 1986;89(4):331-340.
7. Peck S, Peck L, Kataja M. The palatally displaced canine as a dental anomaly of genetic origin. *Angle Orthod.* 1994;64(4):249-256.
8. Cooke J, Wang HL. Canine impactions: incidence and management. *Int J Periodontics Restorative Dent.* 2006;26(5):483-491.
9. Kokich VG. Surgical and orthodontic management of impacted maxillary canines. Am J Orthod Dentofacial Orthop. 2004;126(3):278-283.
10. Cassina C, Papageorgiou SN, Eliades T. Open versus closed surgical exposure for permanent impacted canines: a systematic review and meta-analyses. *Eur J Orthod.* 2018;40(1):1-10.
11. Bishara SE, Kommer DD, McNeil MH, et al. Management of impacted canines. *Am J Orthod.* 1976;69(4):371-387.
12. Becker A, Smith P, Behar R: The incidence of anomalous maxillary lateral incisors in relation to palatally-displaced cuspids. *Angle Orthod* 51(1):24-9, 1981.
13. Kokich VG, Mathews DP. Surgical and orthodontic management of impacted teeth. *Dent Clin North Am.* 19934;37(2):181-204.
14. Becker A, Chaushu S. Etiology of maxillary canine impaction: a review. *Am J Orthod Dentofacial Orthop.* 2015;148(4):557-567.
15. Dewel BF. Clinical observations on the axial inclination of teeth. *Am J Orthod.* 1949;35(2):98-115.
16. van der Linden F. *Development of the Human Dentition.* Quintessence; 2016.
17. Jacoby H. The etiology of maxillary canine impactions. *Am J Orthod.* 1983;84(2):125-132.
18. Liuk IW, Olive RJ, Griffin M, et al. Maxillary lateral incisor morphology and palatally displaced canines: a case-controlled cone-beam volumetric tomography study. *Am J Orthod Dentofacial Orthop.* 2013;143(4):522-526.
19. Peck S, Peck L, Kataja M. Concomitant occurrence of canine malposition and tooth agenesis: evidence of orofacial genetic fields. *Am J Orthod Dentofacial Orthop.* 2002;122(6):657-660.
20. Zilberman Y, Cohen B, Becker A. Familial trends in palatal canines, anomalous lateral incisors, and related phenomena. *Eur J Orthod.* 1990;12(2):135-139.
21. Brin I, Becker A, Shalhav M. Position of the maxillary permanent canine in relation to anomalous or missing lateral incisors: a population study. *Eur J Orthod.* 1986;8(1):12-16.

22. Ericson S, Kurol J. Radiographic assessment of maxillary canine eruption in children with clinical signs of eruption disturbance. *Eur J Orthod*. 1986;8(3):133-140.
23. Garib DG, Janson G, Baldo Tde O, et al. Complications of misdiagnosis of maxillary canine ectopic eruption. *Am J Orthod Dentofacial Orthop*. 2012;142(2):256-263.
24. Williams BH. Diagnosis and prevention of maxillary cuspid impaction. *Angle Orthod*. 1981;51(1):30-40.
25. Ericson S, Kurol J. Early treatment of palatally erupting maxillary canines by extraction of the primary canines. *Eur J Orthod*. 1988;10(4):283-295.
26. Alessandri Bonetti G, Zanarini M, Incerti Parenti S, et al. Preventive treatment of ectopically erupting maxillary permanent canines by extraction of deciduous canines and first molars: a randomized clinical trial. *Am J Orthod Dentofacial Orthop*. 2011;139(3):316-323.
27. Crescini A. *Trattamento Chirurgico-Ortodontico dei Canini Inclusi*. Bologna: Ed Martina; 2010.
28. Hong WH, Radfar R, Chung CH. Relationship between the maxillary transverse dimension and palatally displaced canines: a cone-beam computed tomographic study. Angle *Orthod*. 2015;85(3):440-445.
29. Baccetti T, Sigler LM, McNamara Jr JA. An RCT on treatment of palatally displaced canines with RME and/or a transpalatal arch. *Eur J Orthod*. 2011;33(6):601-607.
30. McConnell TL, Hoffman DL, Forbes DP, et al. Maxillary canine impaction in patients with transverse maxillary deficiency. *ASDC J Dent Child*. 1996;63(3):190-195.
31. Yan B, Sun Z, Fields H, et al. Etiologic factors for buccal and palatal maxillary canine impaction: a perspective based on cone-beam computed tomography analyses. *Am J Orthod Dentofacial Orthop*. 2013;143(4):527-534.
32. Arboleda-Ariza N, Schilling J, Arriola-Guillén LE, et al. Maxillary transverse dimensions in subjects with and without impacted canines: a comparative cone-beam computed tomography study. *Am J Orthod Dentofacial Orthop*. 2018;154(4):495-503.
33. Geran RG, McNamara Jr JA, Baccetti T, et al. A prospective long-term study on the effects of rapid maxillary expansion in the early mixed dentition. *Am J Orthod Dentofacial Orthop*. 2006;129(5):631-640.
34. Koutzoglou SI, Kostaki A. Effect of surgical exposure technique, age, and grade of impaction on ankylosis of an impacted canine, and the effect of rapid palatal expansion on eruption: a prospective clinical study. *Am J Orthod Dentofacial Orthop*. 2013;143(3):342-352.
35. Becker A, Chaushu S. Long-term follow-up of severely resorbed maxillary incisors after resolution of an etiologically associated impacted canine. *Am J Orthod Dentofacial Orthop*. 2005;127(6):650-654.
36. Lindauer SJ, Rubenstein LK, Hang WM, et al. Canine impaction identified early with panoramic radiographs. *J Am Dent Assoc*. 1992;123(3):91-92, 95-97.
37. Botticelli S, Verna C, Cattaneo PM, et al. Two- versus three-dimensional imaging in subjects with unerupted maxillary canines. *Eur J Orthod*. 2011;33(4):344-349.
38. Bjerklin K, Ericson S. How a computerized tomography examination changed the treatment plans of 80 children with retained and ectopically positioned maxillary canines. *Angle Orthod*. 2006;76(1):43-51.
39. Ericson S, Kurol J. Radiographic examination of ectopically erupting maxillary canines. *Am J Orthod Dentofacial Orthop*. 1987;91(6):483-492.
40. Ericson S, Bjerklin K. The dental follicle in normally and ectopically erupting maxillary canines: a computed tomography study. *Angle Orthod*. 2001;71(5):333-342.
41. Ericson S, Bjerklin K, Falahat B. Does the canine dental follicle cause resorption of permanent incisor roots? A computed tomography study of erupting maxillary canines. *Angle Orthod*. 2002;72(2):95-104.
42. Yan B, Sun Z, Fields H, et al. Maxillary canine impaction increases root resorption risk of adjacent teeth: a problem of physical proximity. *Am J Orthod Dentofacial Orthop*. 2012;142(6):750-757.
43. Dağsuyu İM, Kahraman F, Okşayan R. Three-dimensional evaluation of angular, linear, and resorption features of maxillary impacted canines on cone-beam computed tomography. *Oral Radiol*. 2018;34(1):66-72.
44. Evans M. Management of impacted maxillary canines. In: Eliades T, Katsaros C. *The Ortho-Perio Patient, Clinical Evidence & Therapeutic Guidelines*. 1st ed. Quintessence; 2019.
45. Becker A, Chaushu G, Chaushu S. Analysis of failure in the treatment of impacted maxillary canines. *Am J Orthod Dentofacial Orthop*. 2010;37(6):743-754.
46. Becker A, Chaushu S. Success rate and duration of orthodontic treatment for adult patients with palatally impacted maxillary canines. *Am J Orthod Dentofacial Orthop*. 2003;124(5):509-514.
47. Vermette ME, Kokich VG, Kennedy DB. Uncovering labially impacted teeth: apically positioned flap and closed-eruption techniques. *Angle Orthod*. 1995;65(1):23-32.
48. Orban B. *Orban's Oral Histology and Embryology*. 5th ed. St Louis, MO: The C; 1962.
49. Maynard Jr JG, Ochsenbein C. Mucogingival problems, prevalence and therapy in children. *J Periodontol*. 1975;46(9):543-552.
50. Lang NP, Löe H. The relationship between the width of keratinized gingiva and gingival health. *J Periodontol*. 1972;43(10):623-627.
51. Ochsenbein C, Maynard JG. The problem of attached gingiva in children. *ASDC J Dent Child*. 1974;41(4):263-272.
52. Gorman WJ. Prevalence and etiology of gingival recession. *J Periodontol*. 1967;38(4):316-322.
53. Sperry TP, Speidel TM, Isaacson RJ, et al. The role of dental compensations in the orthodontic treatment of mandibular prognathism. *Angle Orthod*. 1977;47(4):293-299.
54. Miyasato M, Crigger M, Egelberg J. Gingival condition in areas of minimal and appreciable width of keratinized gingiva. *J Clin Periodontol*. 1977;4(3):200-209.
55. Wennström J, Lindhe J, Nyman S. Role of keratinized gingiva for gingival health. Clinical and histologic study of normal and regenerated gingival tissue in dogs. *J Clin Periodontol*. 1981;8(4):311-328.
56. Wennström JL, Lindhe J, Sinclair F, et al. Some periodontal tissue reactions to orthodontic tooth movement in monkeys. *J Clin Periodontol*. 1987;14(3):121-129.
57. Crescini A, Nieri M, Buti J, et al. Orthodontic and periodontal outcomes of treated impacted maxillary canines. *Angle Orthod*. 2007;77(4):571-577.
58. Kau CH, Pan P, Gallerano RL, et al. A novel 3D classification system for canine impactions—the KPG index. *Int J Med Robot*. 2009;5(3):291-296.
59. Levin MP, D'Amico R. Flap design in exposing unerupted teeth. *Am J Orthod*. 1974;65:419-422.
60. Becker A, Shpack N, Shteyer A. Attachment bonding to impacted teeth at the time of surgical exposure. *Eur J Orthod*. 1996;18:457-463.
61. Lee JY, Choi YJ, Choi SH, et al. Labially impacted maxillary canines after the closed eruption technique and orthodontic traction: a split-mouth comparison of periodontal recession. *J Periodontol*. 2019;90(1):35-43.
62. Becker A, Zilberman Y. The palatally impacted canine: a new approach to treatment. *Am J Orthod*. 1978;74(4):422-429.
63. Parkin N, Benson PE, Thind B, et al. Open versus closed surgical exposure of canine teeth that are displaced in the roof of the mouth. *Cochrane Database Syst Rev*. 2017;21:8.
64. Kohavi D, Becker A, Zilberman Y. Surgical exposure, orthodontic movement, and final tooth position as factors in periodontal breakdown of treated palatally impacted canines. *Am J Orthod*. 1984;85(1):72-77.
65. Crescini A, Nieri M, Buti J, et al. Short- and long-term periodontal evaluation of impacted canines treated with a closed surgical-orthodontic approach. *J Clin Periodontol*. 2007;34(3):232-242.

14 Aligner Orthodontics in Prerestorative Patients

KENJI OJIMA, CHISATO DAN, and TOMMASO CASTROFLORIO

Introduction

According to a recent American Association of Orthodontists statement, today one in four orthodontic patients is an adult.[1] In this specific category of patients, orthodontics can be called on to treat either primary malocclusions that have not been treated before or secondary malocclusions due to orthodontic relapse or pathologic tooth migration related to periodontal disease (see Chapter 16). Advances in orthodontics have also made treatment more comfortable and less noticeable than ever for individuals of all ages. Many of today's treatment options are designed to minimize the appearance of the appliance to better fit any lifestyle. Apart from the innovations in the field, the increasing demand of orthodontic treatment from adult patients is due to an increased awareness by patients of the need for good oral health, enabling the patient to reach adulthood with a greater number of teeth in the mouth.[2] It also happens by the increase on esthetic requirement from society.[3,4] Despite possible functional problems, many of those seeking orthodontic treatment are keen to improve dental esthetics and, potentially, their quality of life regarding both functional aspects and appearance. The relative importance of esthetics in current society is understood when analyzing the positive attributes associated with physical attractiveness.[5]

Many of the adults looking for orthodontic treatment have worn or abraded teeth, previous restorations, missing teeth, supraeruption and occlusal plane discrepancies, malformed teeth, collapse of the vertical dimension due to the loss of posterior teeth, and many other problems requiring an interaction between orthodontics and restorative dentistry.[6] However, the connection between the two specialties is required for young patients when agenesis spaces should be managed or when the recovery of a proper smile esthetics requires crown shape modifications.

Orthodontic diagnosis aims, among others, to determine the degree of harmonization required to correct dental or dentomaxillary disorders and to indicate whether prosthetic or restorative compensation is needed and what form it should take.[7] Dental professionals should always carefully consider tooth position in prosthodontic treatment to determine whether orthodontic treatment can improve prosthodontic treatment outcomes. Controlling tooth position with orthodontics can help the prosthodontist in creating restorations that are more stable, functional, and esthetic.

Space Management in the Anterior Region

Space management represents the field in which the cooperation between orthodontist and prosthodontists is very common. The most frequent reason is represented by agenesis, especially of the upper lateral incisor, because of its relative high prevalence and impact on a high esthetic value area.

Patients with congenitally missing maxillary lateral incisors often need a challenging interdisciplinary treatment, whether canine substitution, single implants, or tooth-supported restorations are chosen. Currently, it would be inappropriate to remove enamel and dentin to place crowns on adjacent teeth in patients with dental agenesis, mainly if these individuals have no restorations or wear of their existing teeth.[8] In case of unilateral agenesis of the maxillary lateral incisor, space closure should not be used, except in exceptional cases, because of subsequent esthetical and functional problems.[7]

If the treatment plan calls for opening of the edentulous spaces, implants would be an ideal alternative for replacing the missing teeth. Research has shown that the success rate of implants is very high. However, maxillary lateral incisor implants are challenging aesthetically. The amount of space is often small, the alveolar ridge may be deficient, the papillae are occasionally short, the adjacent roots could be too close, the gingival levels may be uneven, and the patient could be too young. Any of these issues could compromise the aesthetic outcome of even the finest surgical implant placement.[9]

In this approach, orthodontic treatment combines:

1. Functional placement of the canine
2. Creation of sufficient space to accommodate a cosmetic replacement for the missing lateral incisor

Working with aligners, the functional placement of the canine requires the use of attachments to properly control the movement of the root in the three dimensions. A good option to obtain predictable movements is always represented by their sequentialization. If the canine requires distalization, mesiodistal root tipping, and torque control, then a good suggestion is to plan distalization steps of 2 mm, application of mesial root tipping of at least 2 degrees every 2 mm of distalization, and (only once distalization and mesiodistal root tipping have been completed) planning the root torque information.[10] The control of all those movements can be achieved with the use of rectangular and vertical attachments.

If a patient is congenitally missing one maxillary lateral incisor, the amount of space to accommodate a cosmetic replacement is determined by opposite lateral incisor. However, in some patients the contralateral incisor could be peg shaped. If this is the case, management of spaces should be performed on the basis of surrounding teeth and tissue esthetics and function. The same approach should be used when both lateral incisors are congenitally missing.

The fundamental criteria for esthetic analysis should include facial, dentogingival, and dental esthetics.[11] In recent years, several computer software programs for digital smile design (DSD) have been introduced to clinical practice and research. They are multiuse conceptual tools that can strengthen diagnostic vision, improve communication, and enhance treatment predictability by permitting careful analysis of the patient's facial and dental characteristics that may have been overlooked by clinical, photographic, or diagnostic cast-based evaluation procedures.[12]

With today's implant technology, assuming a 3.25-mm lateral incisor implant, most surgeons would probably be comfortable placing a maxillary lateral incisor implant in a patient with an interradicular space greater than 5.5 mm, leaving at least 1 mm of alveolar bone on either side of the implant. If the interradicular space were less than 4 mm, many surgeons would suggest orthodontic retreatment. Therefore, speaking specifically to minimizing the risk of root movement during retention that would impede implant placement, Olsen and Kokich[13] recommend leaving extra space for the surgeon (i.e., a minimum of 6.3 mm between the crowns and 5.7 mm between the roots). This correlates well with the space traditionally suggested for implant placement of 1 mm on either side of the implant.

Case Study

A 27-year-old female presented with the chief complaint of an unaesthetic lateral profile due to protruded upper teeth, in addition to lower dental crowding. She had a short face, an acute nasolabial angle, a mildly convex profile, and lip incompetence, with class I canine and molar relationships and significant overjet and overbite (Fig. 14.1). Furthermore multiple restorations were present. The panoramic radiograph confirmed that 1.2 was missing (Fig. 14.2).

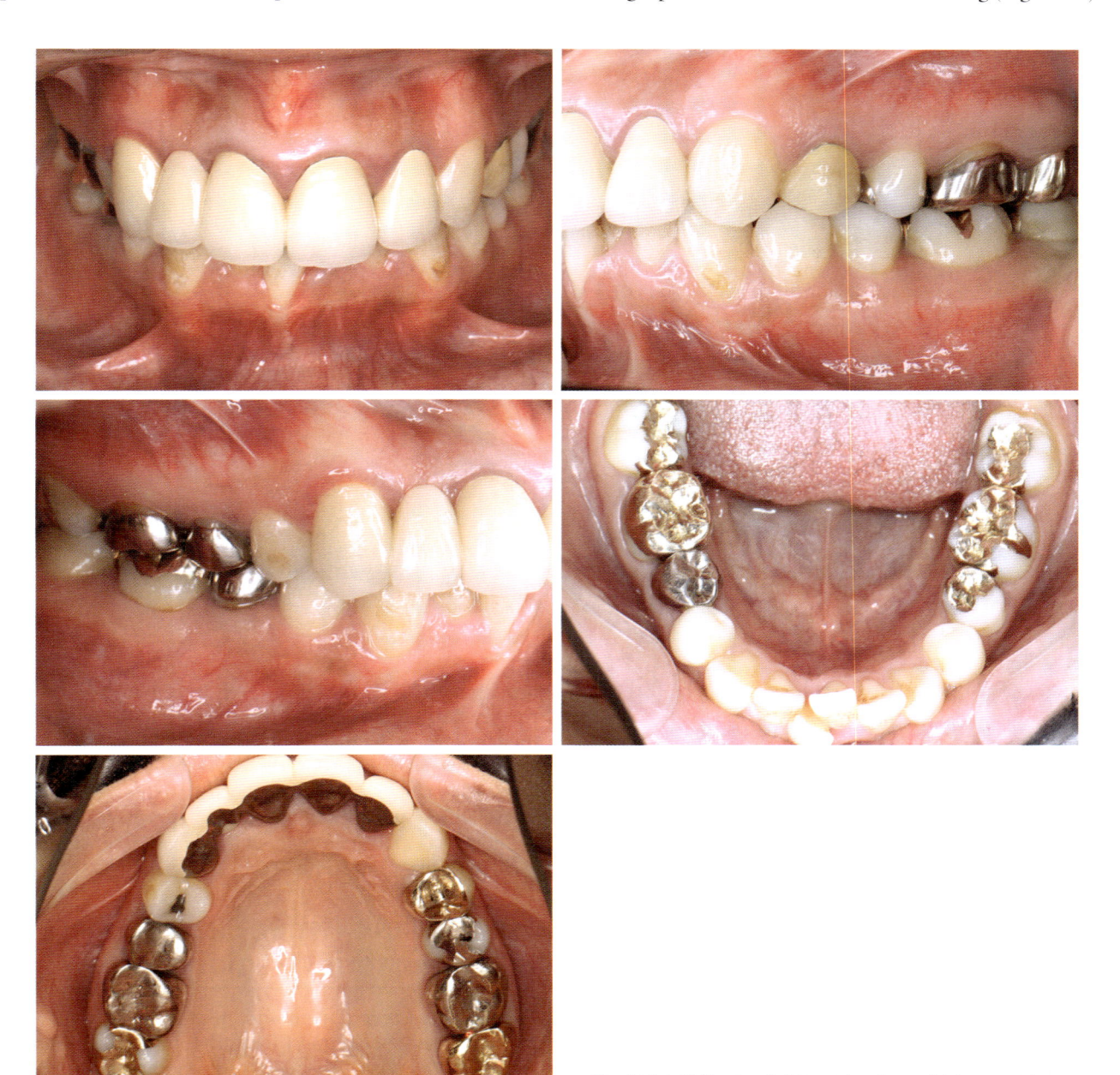

Fig. 14.1 Initial intraoral pictures showing multiple restorations.

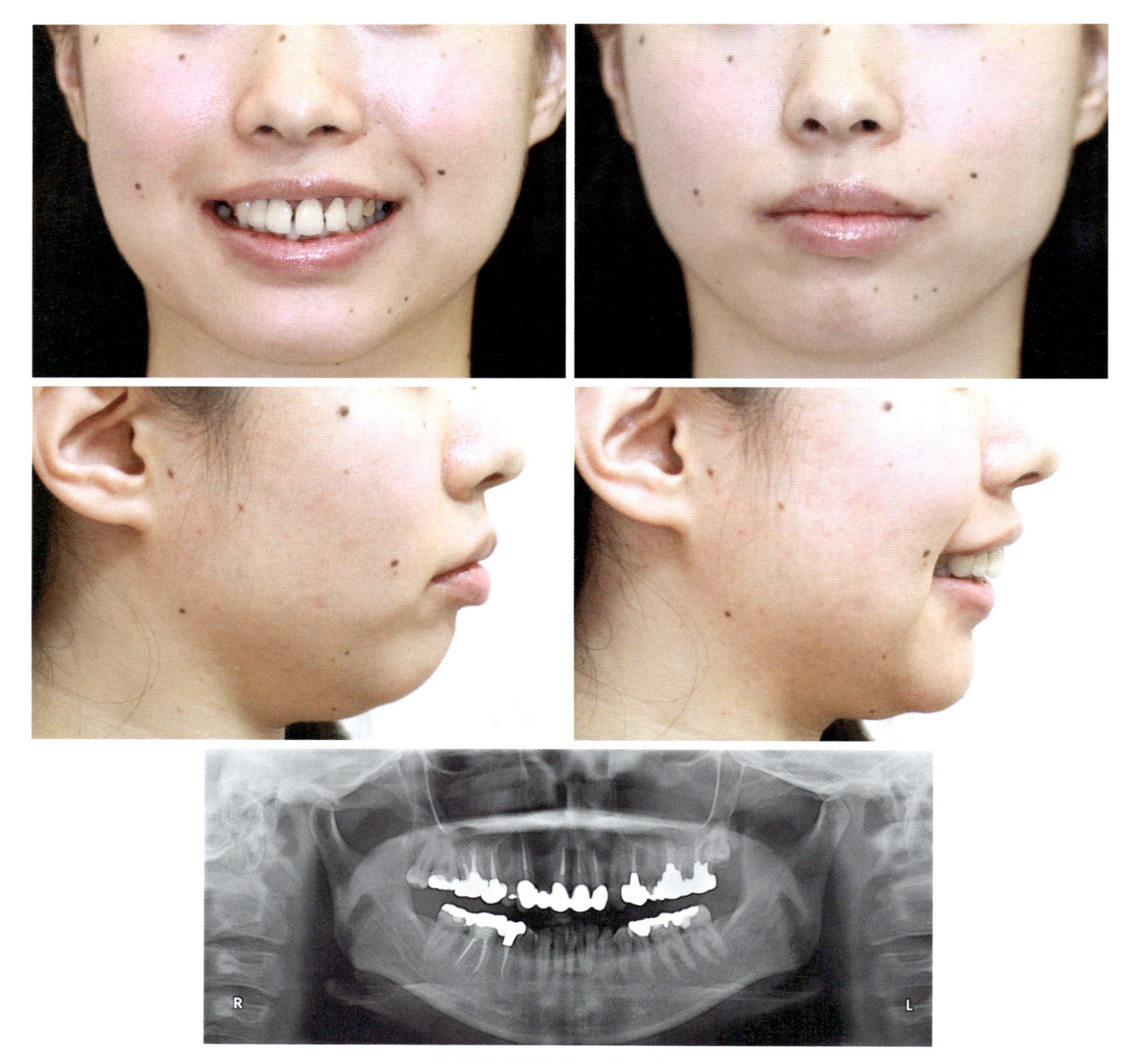

Fig. 14.2 Initial orthopantomograms.

This patient did not wish to change her facial esthetics but to merely improve the appearance of her anterior teeth. Therefore the goals of esthetic interdisciplinary treatment were to reduce the protrusive profile and obtain a class I canine occlusion, with normal overjet and overbite, by means of orthodontic treatment; enhance dental esthetics and the smile line with orthodontics and prosthetic restorations; and replace the upper right lateral incisor with an implant.

Prior to clear aligner treatment, the dental bridge from the upper right canine to the upper left lateral incisor was sectioned and polyvinyl siloxane (PVS) impressions were taken. Clear aligner treatment in the upper arch was designed to intrude and retract the anterior teeth, supported by class II elastics to bonded buttons on the upper canines and lower first molars. In the lower arch, intrusion and proclination of the anterior teeth were planned. A temporary resin pontic replaced the missing upper right lateral incisor during aligner treatment (Figs. 14.3, 14.4, and 14.5). At the conclusion of 19 months of aligner treatment, the severe overjet and overbite were improved, and the original vertical dimension was unaltered. An upper right lateral incisor implant was placed, followed by final esthetic restorations (Figs. 14.6, 14.7, and 14.8).

Space Management in the Posterior Region

The mesial tipping of mandibular second molars is a frequent source of request for orthodontic intervention by restorative dentists. Inadequate mandibular arch length,

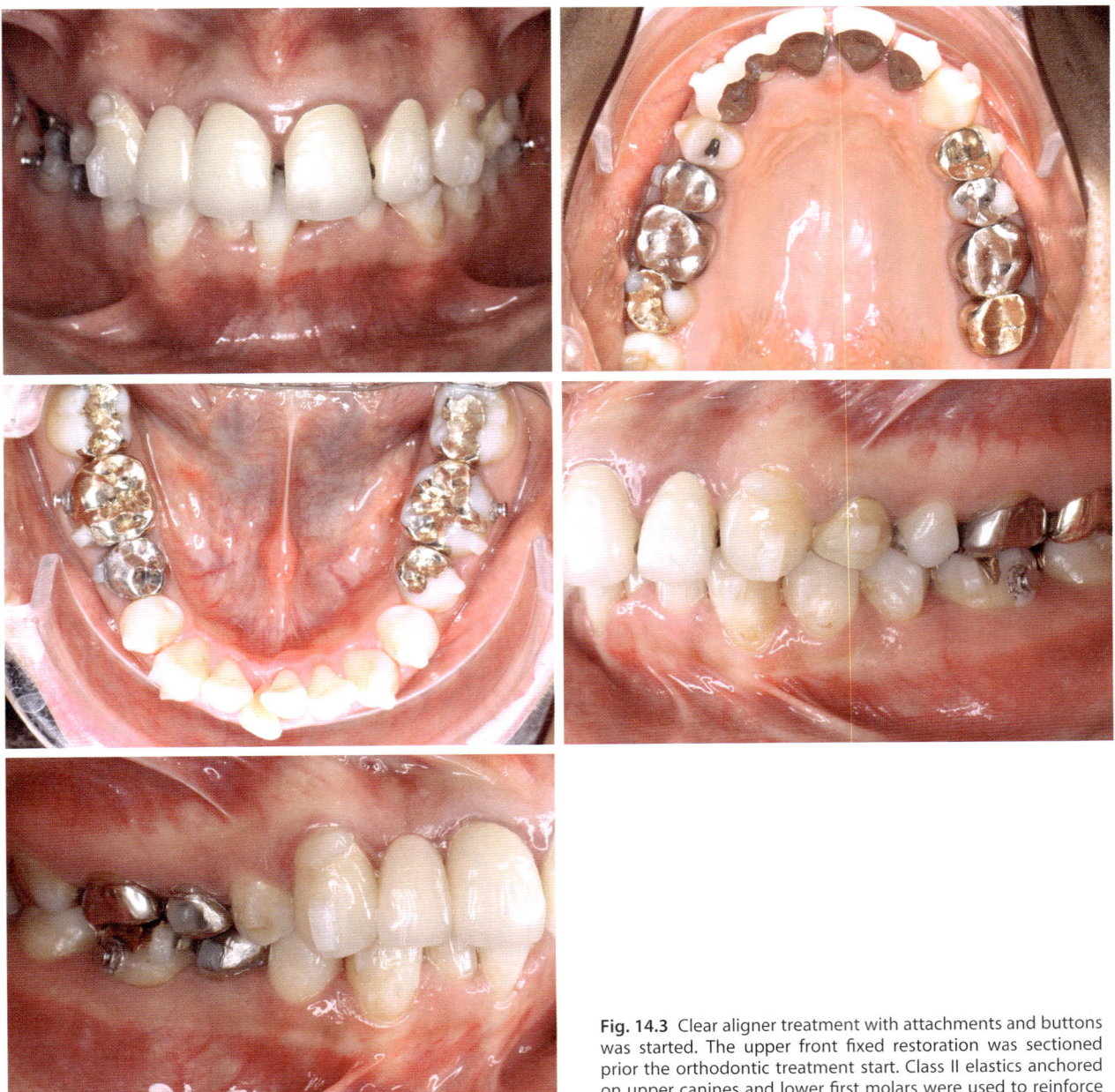

14 • Aligner Orthodontics in Prerestorative Patients 171

Fig. 14.3 Clear aligner treatment with attachments and buttons was started. The upper front fixed restoration was sectioned prior the orthodontic treatment start. Class II elastics anchored on upper canines and lower first molars were used to reinforce canine class I relationship.

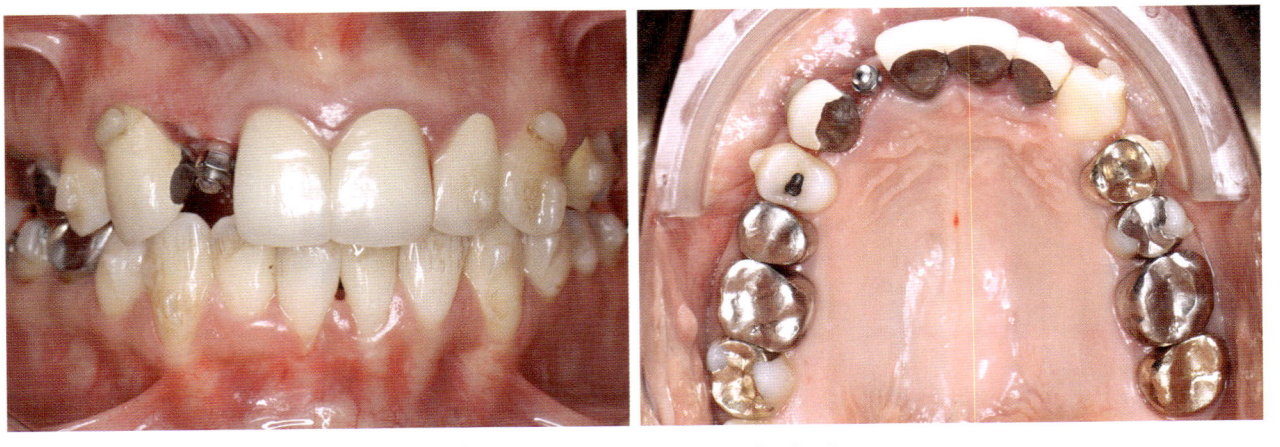

Fig. 14.4 An implant was placed in 1.2 area.

Continued

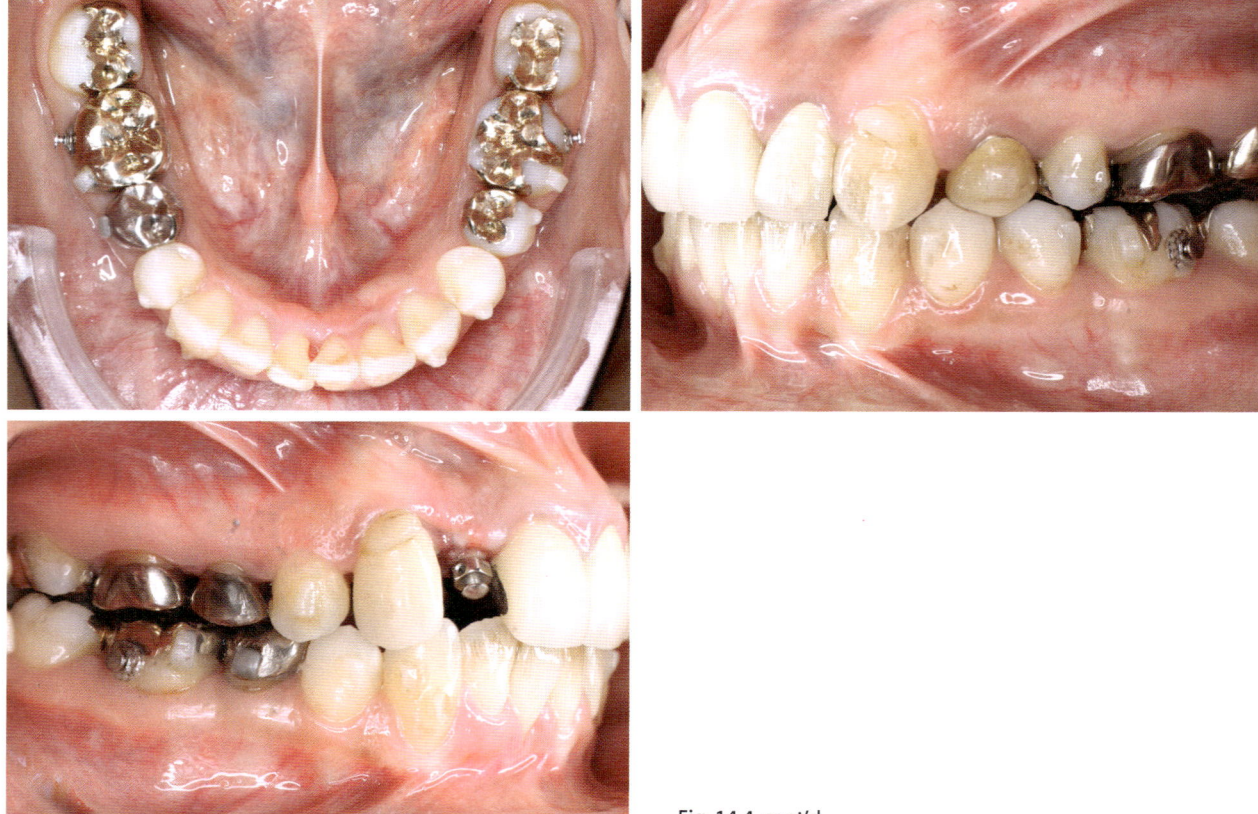

Fig. 14.4, cont'd

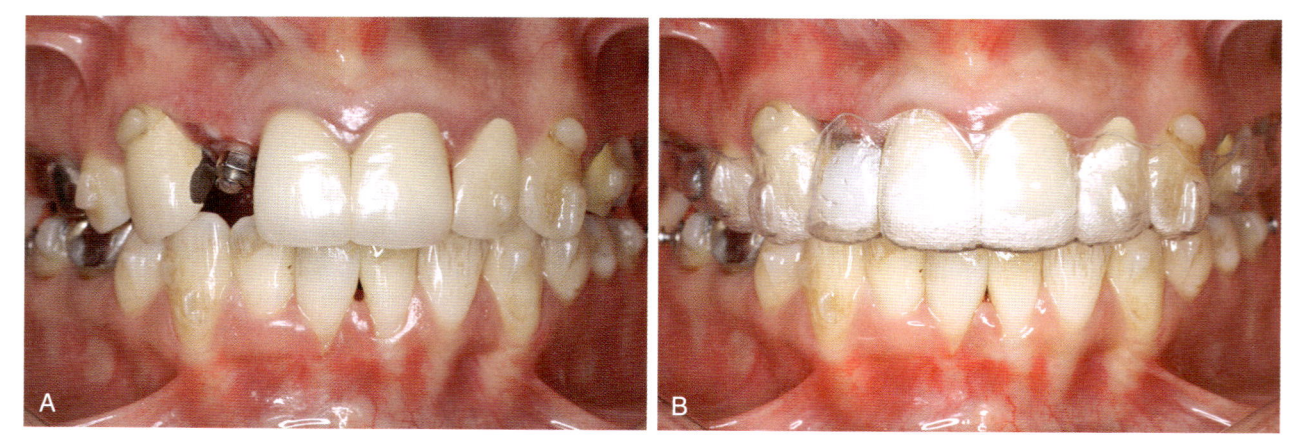

Fig. 14.5 Frontal view of 1.2 implant with (A) and without (B) aligner.

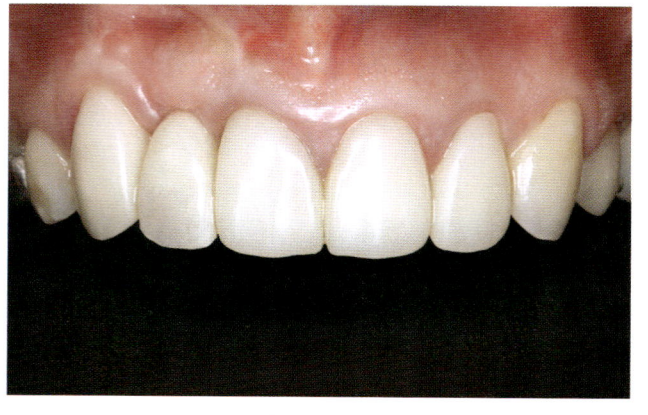

Fig. 14.6 Frontal view of the final upper anterior restoration.

14 • Aligner Orthodontics in Prerestorative Patients

Fig. 14.7 Final intraoral pictures.

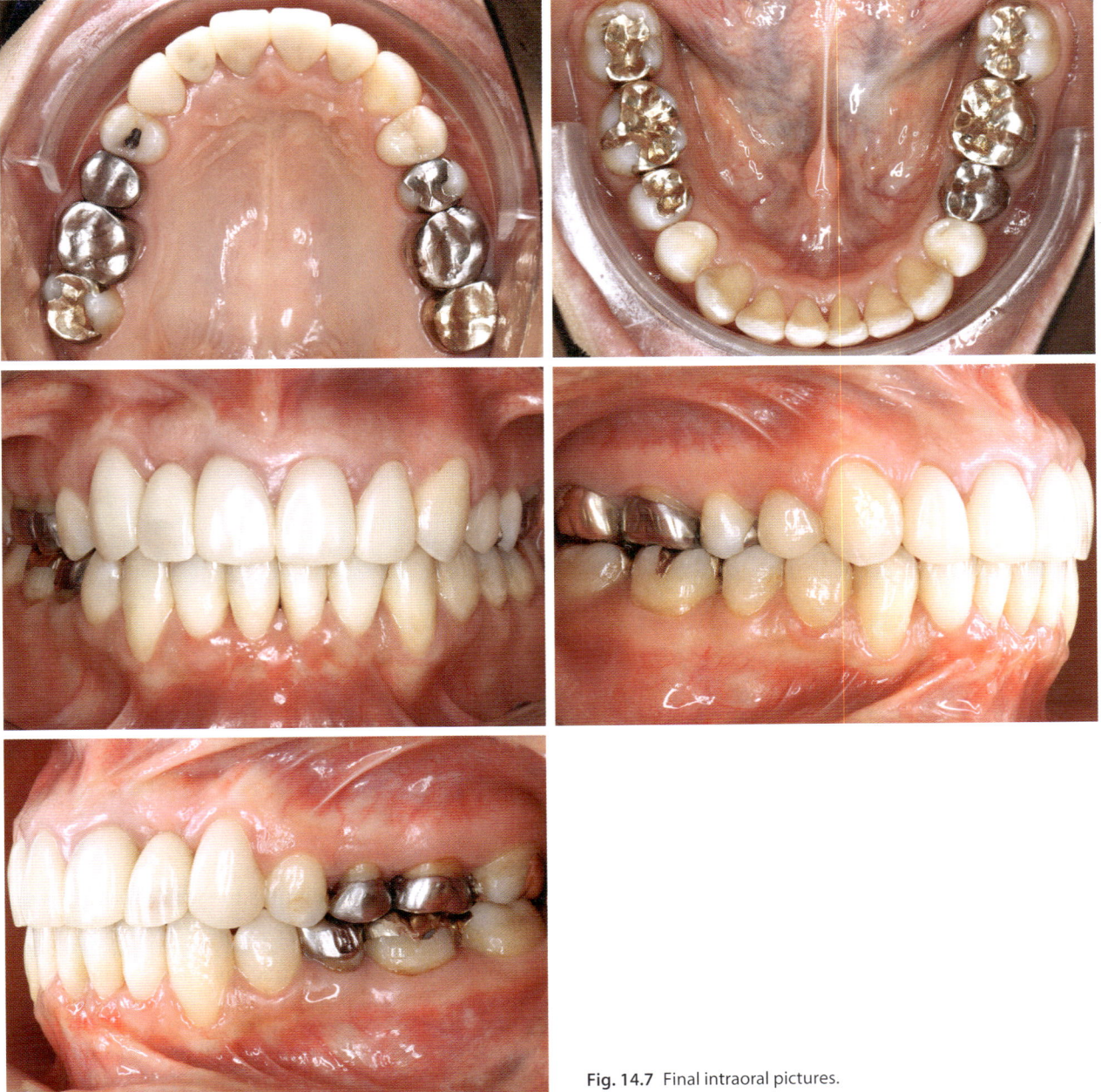

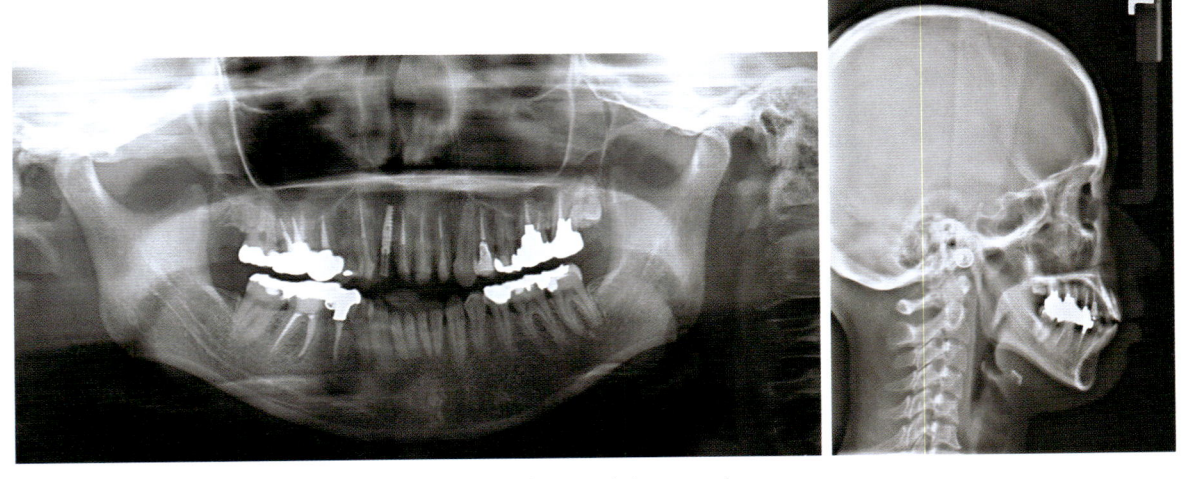

Fig. 14.8 Final extraoral pictures and x-rays.

Continued

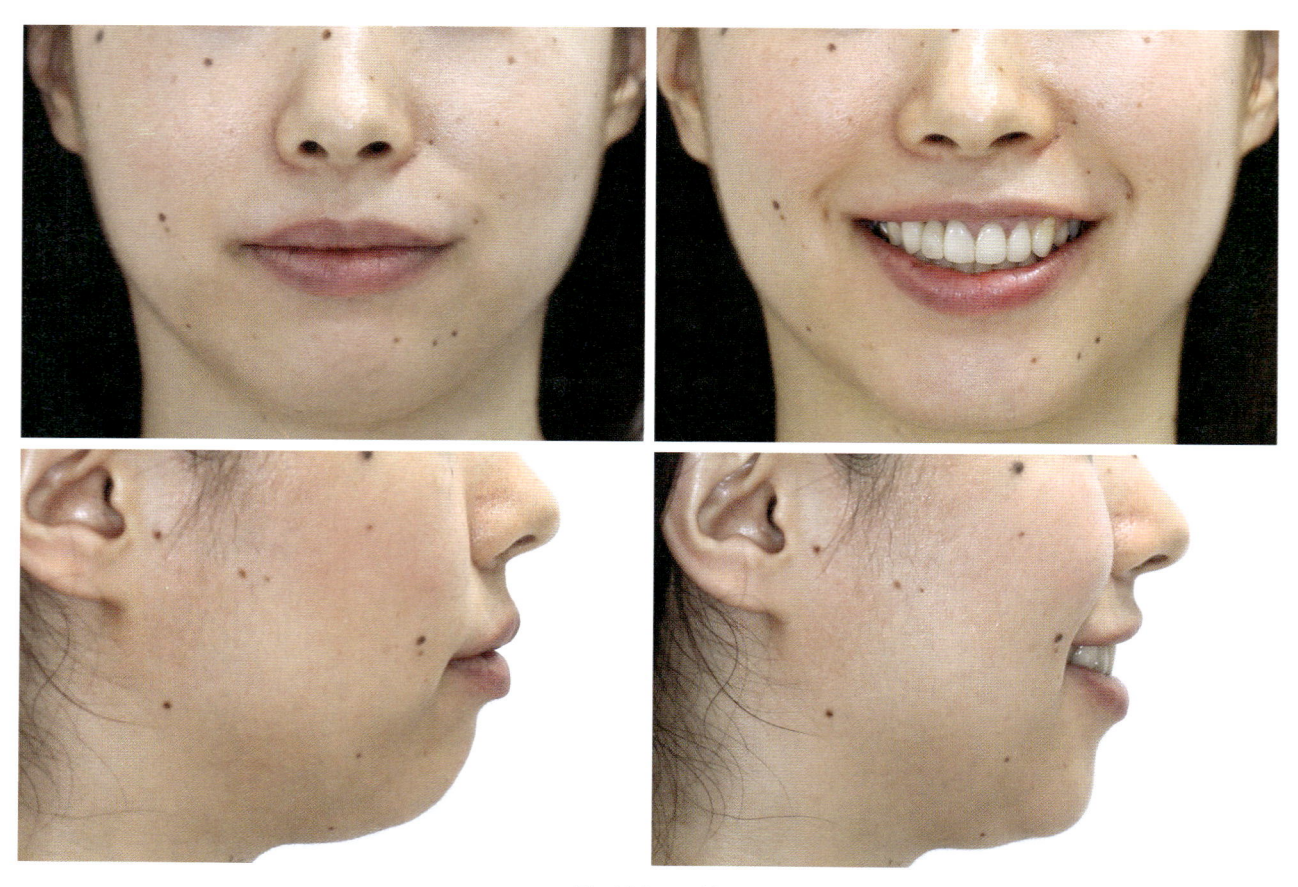

Fig. 14.8, cont'd

excessive teeth size, loss of the adjacent first molar, premature eruption of the mandibular third molar, and unusually mesial eruption pathway of the second molar can also cause its partial or total impaction.[14] Zachrisson[15] stated that in case of severe mesial tipping of lower second molars, periodontal status can be aggravated, with angular bone loss, and an apparent pocket at the mesial surface of a tipped mandibular molar. In excessive inclination cases, overeruption of the antagonist molar with subsequent premature contacts and occlusal interferences hamper prosthetic intervention.

Repositioning of the second molar eliminates pathologic condition and facilitates the placement of a prosthetic restoration. Among the limitations of aligners, severely tipped teeth (>45 degrees) were included.[16] Uprighting a severe mesial tipped molar using aligners could be quite risky since the fitting loss could produce a worsening of the mesial tipping. As well described by Brezniak,[17] if the tooth is not performing the desired movement, the aligner will surrender to the stiffer teeth and become distorted. Its gingival edges move away from the teeth, and no force can be exerted in the gingival area while the force is concentrated only in the occlusal part. This distortion prevents any possible couple to be developed, and no bodily movement of the tooth is possible. This occlusal force encourages intrusion that, for a severe mesial tipped molar, means worsening of its tipping. Therefore when planning, uprighting of molars with aligners is preferable to reduce the velocity of the angular movement and to accurately control the fitting of aligners at every appointment (Figs. 14.9 through 14.20). The intrusion effect and thus the worsening of the mesial tipping could be accelerated if a large attachment has been displaced on the buccal surface of the molar and if the aligner is losing fitting. Attachments are helpful especially in those cases with rounded shape teeth but close controls in the office are required. To increase the efficiency of the uprighting mechanics and to increase the stiffness of the aligner, pontics mesially to the tipped teeth should be avoided. Pontics are equivalent to loops bent on an archwire. They increase elasticity and then a potential undesired distortion of the aligner if it is going to lose fitting.

The use of temporary anchorage devices (TADs) can support the uprighting of severe mesially tipped molars. For this instance, cutouts should be planned on the aligner portion covering the tipped teeth to permit the placement of bonded buttons or brackets or tubes on the tooth crown, which can be connected with sectional mechanics or elastic moduli to TADs. A systematic review indicated mandibular molar uprighting as a frequent and complicated procedure, which requires good anchorage control.[14] Even a small amount of anchorage loss can result in aligner distortion with adverse effects, not only on the moving tooth but also on other tooth units. The introduction of TADs as anchorage control auxiliaries was a "game changer" in orthodontics, making, among others as discussed in other chapters of this book, molar uprighting easier and reliable with aligner orthodontics.

14 • Aligner Orthodontics in Prerestorative Patients   175

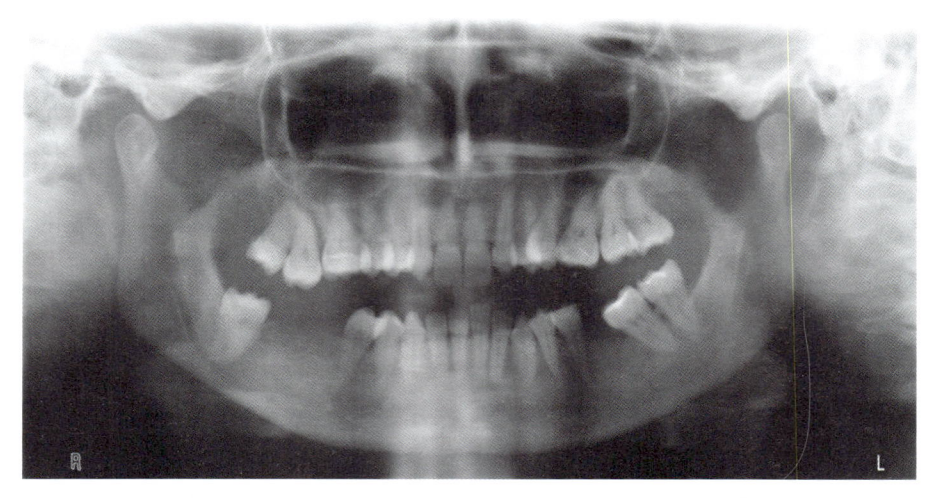

Fig. 14.9 Initial orthopantomogram of a patient for which a prerestorative orthodontic treatment was required. 12.2 and 2.2 were congenitally missing. The interdisciplinary treatment plan was designed to recover a proper interarch relationship and preparing the case for future restorations on upper front teeth and in the lower arch after the uprighting of 3.7 and intrusion of overerupted 1.7.

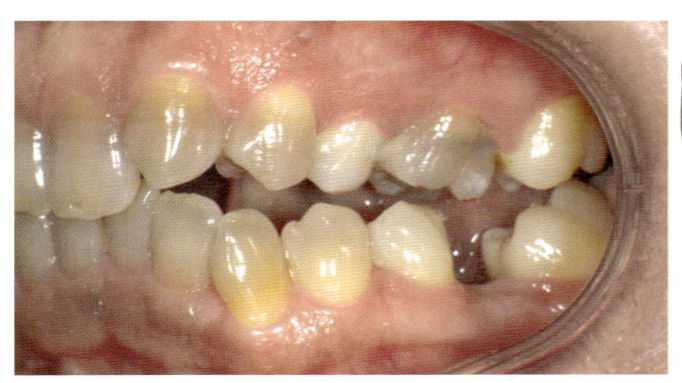

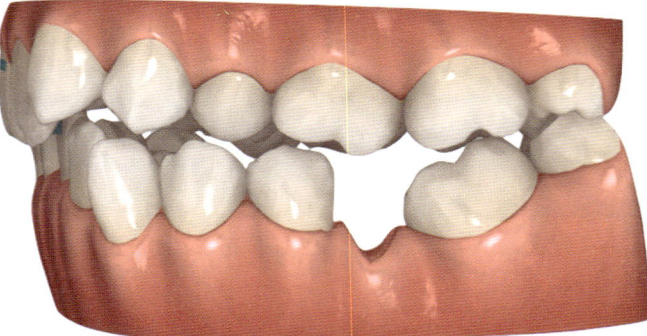

Fig. 14.10 Initial intraoral and ClinCheck lateral views in relation to the mesial tipping of 3.7, caused by the premature loss of 3.6.

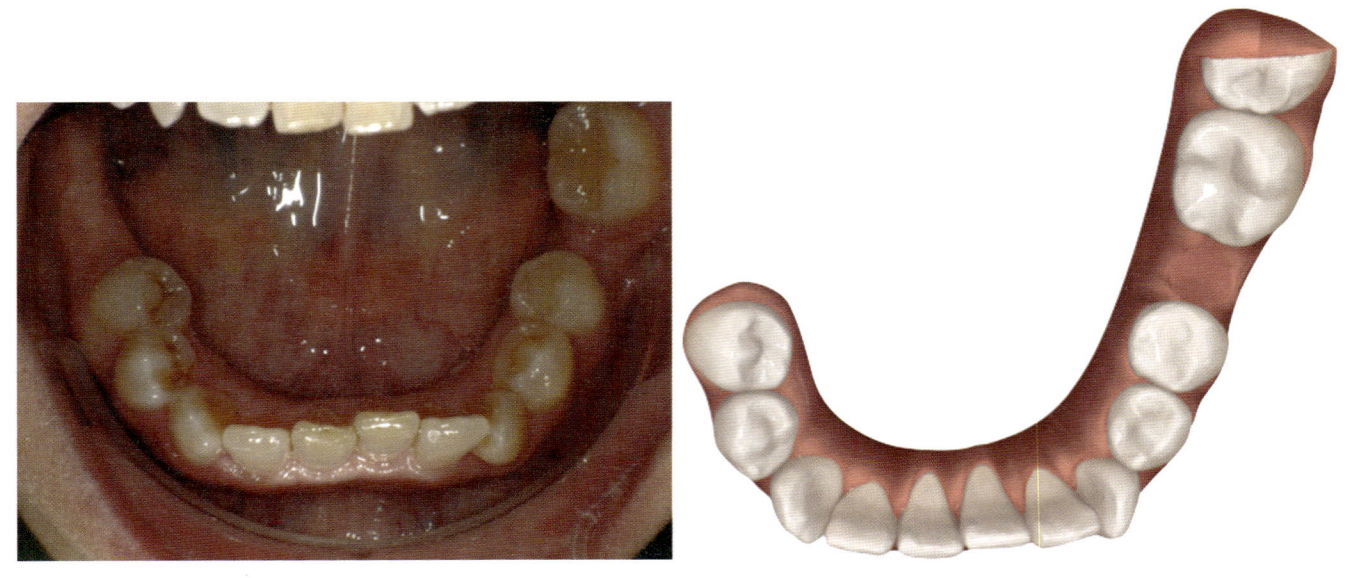

Fig. 14.11 Initial intraoral and ClinCheck occlusal views in relation to the mesial tipping of 3.7.

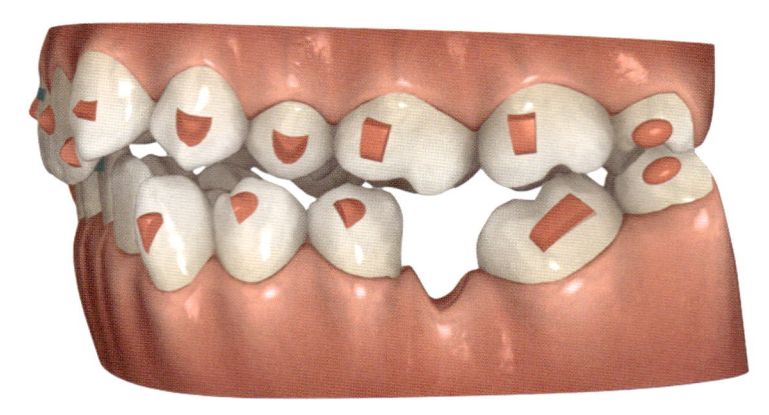

176 Principles and Biomechanics of Aligner Treatment

Fig. 14.12 Attachment configuration used to recover a proper alignment and leveling of the arches and the uprighting of 3.7. Pontic was not prescribed in 3.6 area to increase the stiffness of the aligner.

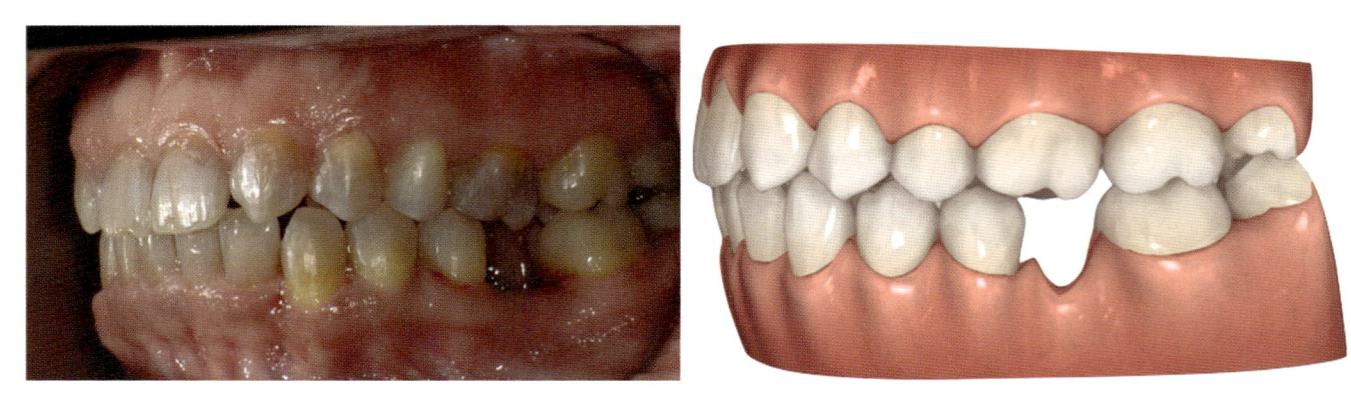

Fig. 14.13 Final intraoral and ClinCheck lateral views with successful uprighting of 3.7.

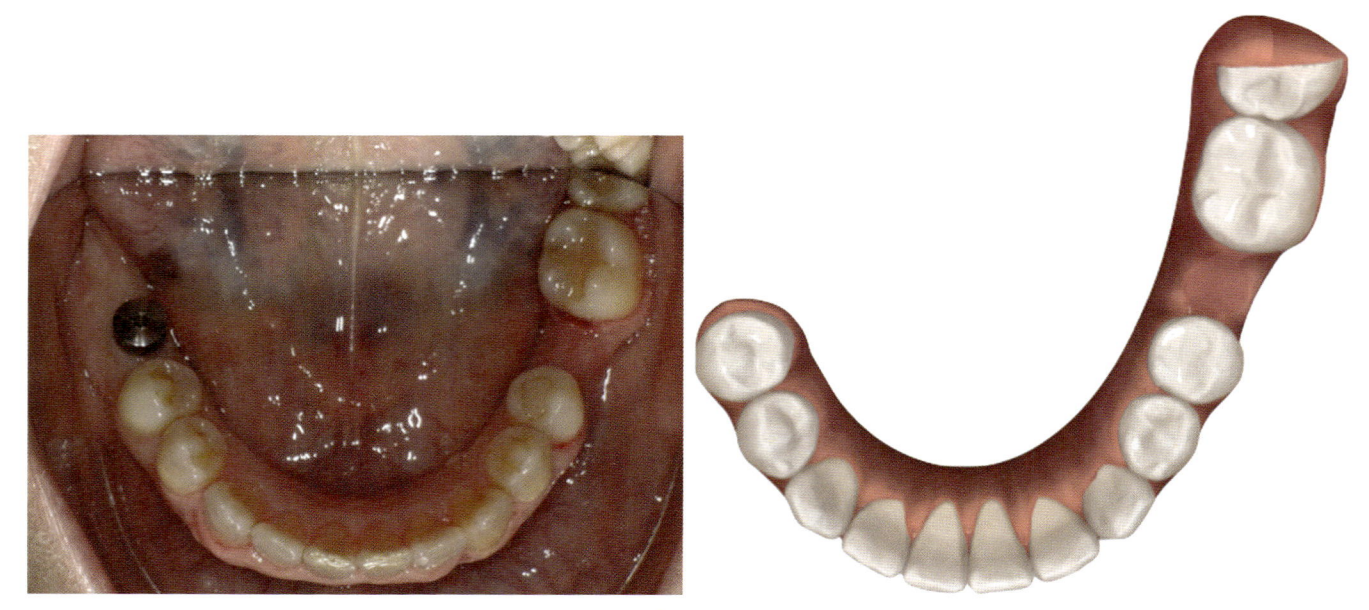

Fig. 14.14 Final intraoral and ClinCheck occlusal views with successful uprighting of 3.7.

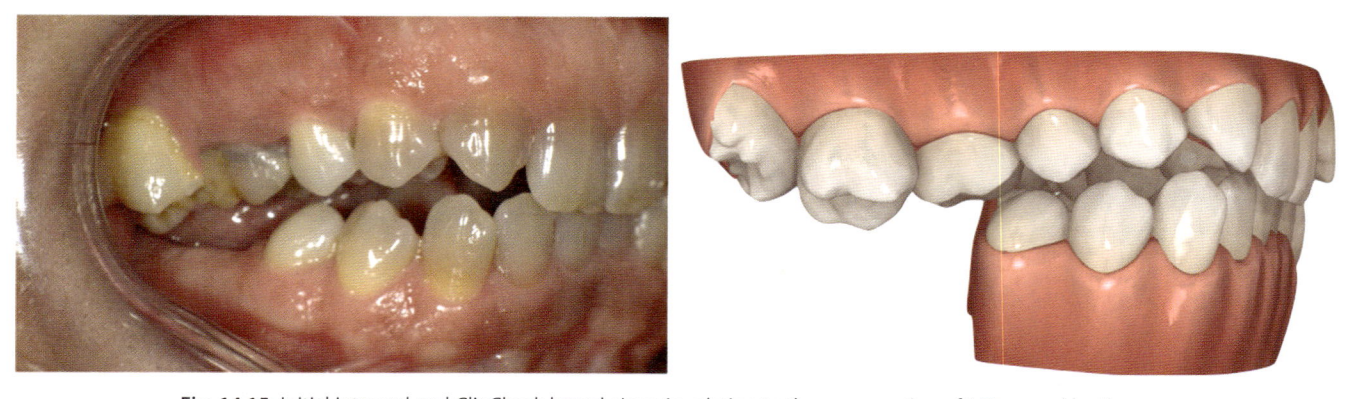

Fig. 14.15 Initial intraoral and ClinCheck lateral views in relation to the overeruption of 1.7, caused by the premature loss of 4.6.

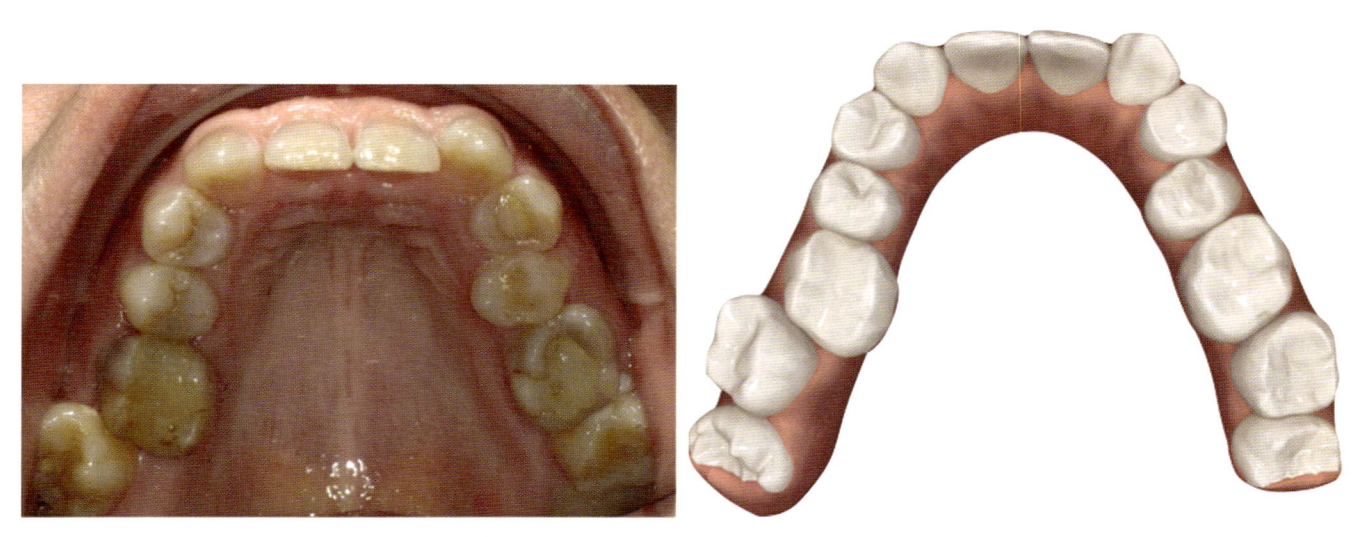

Fig. 14.16 Initial intraoral and ClinCheck occlusal views of the upper arch.

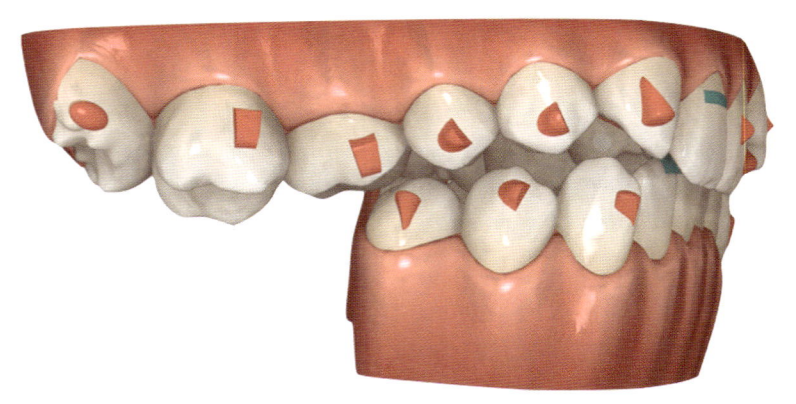

Fig. 14.17 Attachment configuration used to recover a proper alignment and leveling of the arches.

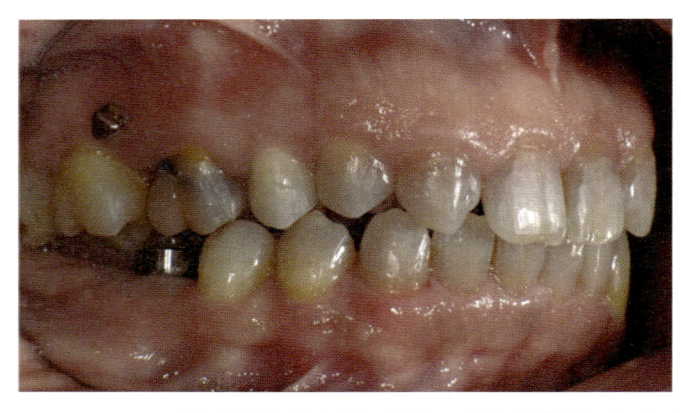

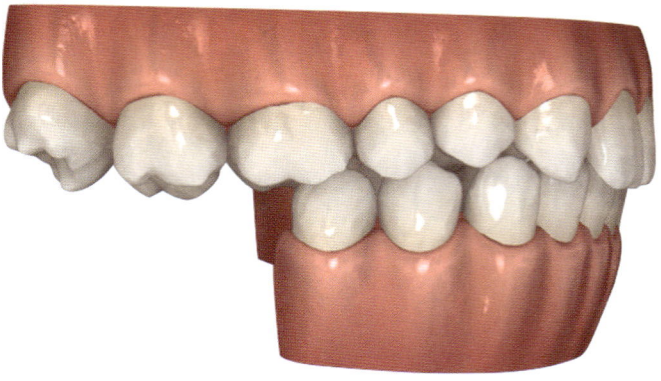

Fig. 14.18 Final lateral intraoral and ClinCheck views of the right side showing intrusion and leveling of 1.7 obtained with the aid of a buccal miniscrew and a segmented auxiliary arch bonded on 1.8 and 1.6 after proper modification of the aligners.[30] Intrusion of 1.4 was planned to level gingival edge to the 2.4 one. An implant was placed in 4.6 area during the final stages of the orthodontic treatment.

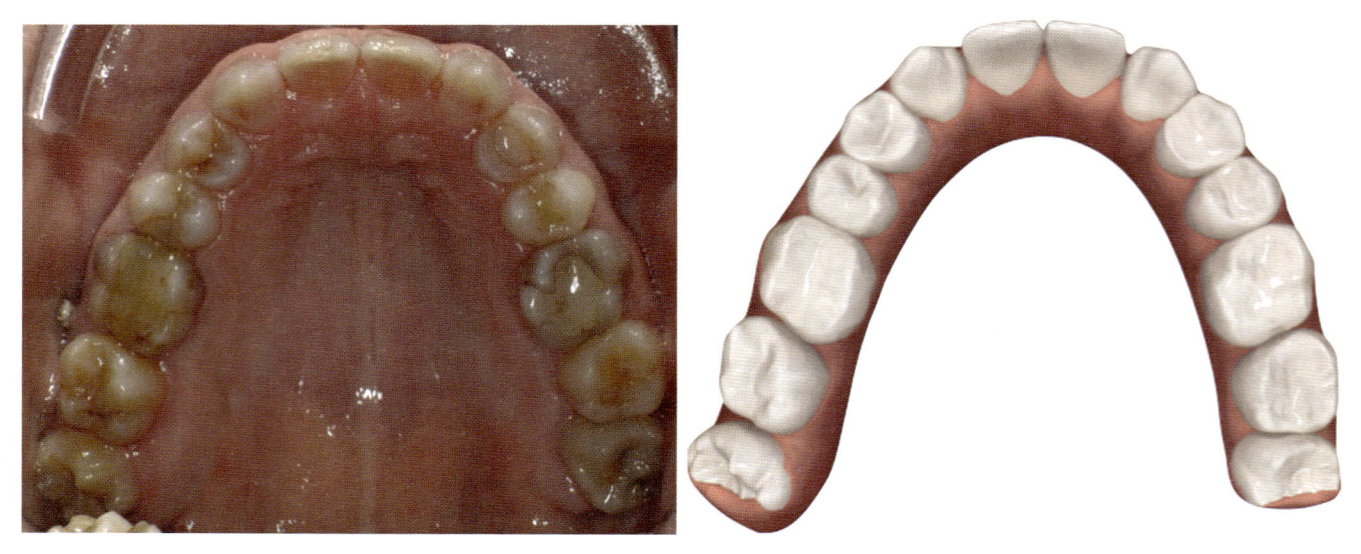

Fig. 14.19 Final intraoral and ClinCheck occlusal views of the upper arch.

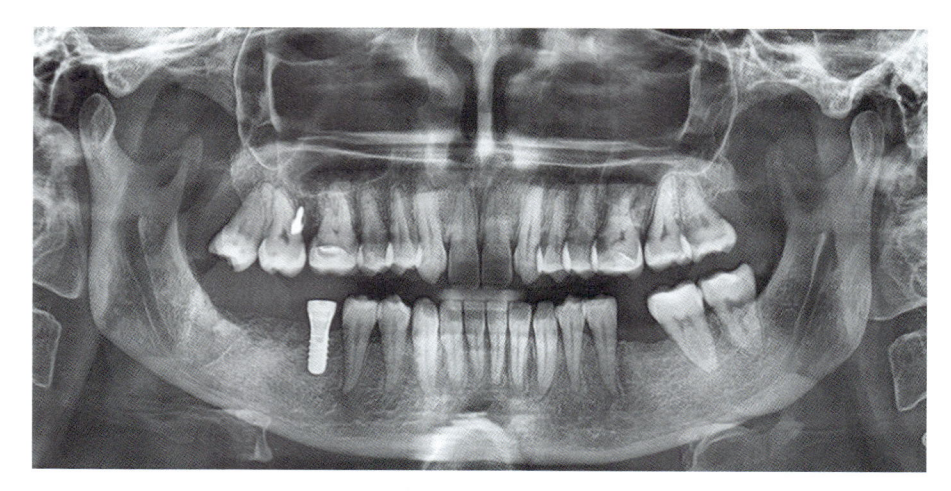

Fig. 14.20 Final orthopantomogram.

Management of Posterior Overerupted Molars

It is common for adult patients with dental loss, particularly of molars and premolars, to have an extrusion of the antagonist. An early loss of any molar is bound to cause supraeruption of the opposing molar into the available space. Overeruption of such a molar can lead to occlusal interference and functional disturbances and cause great difficulty during prosthetic reconstruction.[18]

Orthodontic treatment of overerupted molars has always been considered challenging by orthodontists, even more when considering aligner treatment. This is primary due to the great volume of these teeth and to the need for excellent anchorage control to have the required forces directed through the center of resistance of the tooth. Furthermore molar intrusion is one of the less predictable movements to be performed with aligners. According to a recent paper, posterior intrusion could be taken into account with aligners if a maximum 0.5- to 1-mm molar intrusion has been planned.[19]

In these cases, the use of TADs along with orthodontic biomechanics incorporated into the aligner treatment plan is used to obtain better case control while minimizing unwanted side effects. To avoid tipping of the molar that should be intruded, forces need to be applied both buccally and lingually, and interproximal spaces are required to obtain intrusion.

Therefore, when planning the mechanics required to obtain intrusion of an overerupted molar with aligners, it is important to have interproximal spaces open to permit the intrusion movement, planning interproximal reduction and controlling that at every stage of movement the tooth has no interproximal friction. Attachments should be prescribed on adjacent teeth to provide anchorage (rectangular and horizontal attachments) but not on the tooth requiring intrusion. However, if the tooth requiring intrusion is the most distal one, then a buccal attachment should be placed.

TADs can be of help in increasing the amount of molar intrusion over the maximum value of predictability with aligners only (see Figs. 14.9 through 14.20). Two mini-implants can be installed on each side, one buccally and another palatally, to have more controlled movement and to make it less complex for the professional, with more predictable results.[18] For pure intrusion, a total of three mini-implants could be used in a tooth, in agreement with Paccini et al.[20] The skeletal anchorage can be used connecting it to buttons bonded on the tooth crown with elastic chains or NiTi coils, and, in this case, cutouts should be planned on the aligner. Another option could be represented by the use of elastic chains or other elastic modulus connecting the palatal and buccal miniscrews, passing over the occlusal surface of the aligner.

A finite element study investigating the use of TADs for molar intrusion showed that unilateral force unleashed higher stress in root apex and higher evidence for dental tipping directed to mini-implant sites; the bilateral force promoted a more homogeneous stress distribution without evidence of dental tipping. Bilateral intrusion technique suggested a vertical movement of intrusion and lower probability of root apex resorption.[21]

Management of Patients With a History of Temporomandibular Disorders

Temporomandibular disorders (TMDs) are a group of musculoskeletal and neuromuscular conditions involving the temporomandibular joints (TMJs), the masticatory muscles, and associated tissues. Current understanding and evidence-based literature failed to demonstrate a relationship between various occlusal factors and TMD signs and symptoms. TMD has moved from a dental and mechanical-based model to a biopsychosocial and medical model that integrates a host of biologic, behavioral, and social factors to the onset, maintenance, and progression of TMD. Management of TMD is typically symptomatic, aimed at decreasing pain, decreasing loading on the muscles and joints, and facilitating the restoration of function and quality of life of patients.[22] Orthodontics is generally described as neutral in that it neither causes, cures, nor mitigates TMD.[23]

Some early case reports showed for some patients treated with aligners, jaw muscle tenderness and wear facets on their aligners.[24] Several clinicians speculated about the wear facets concluding that aligners may have acted as occlusal splints.[25] A more credible hypothesis is related to an adaptation mechanism involving repetitive tooth clenching. Perhaps it is possible that patients are triggered to clench on the aligners to alleviate orthodontic pain.[26] As previously reported, orthodontic pain can be reduced by repetitive chewing of gum or plastic wafers during the first 8 hours after the appliance is activated. Aligner chewing and clenching can result in wear facets and muscle tenderness in some patients treated with aligners. Therefore it is a possibility that patients undergoing clear aligner treatment may have transient symptoms of facial muscular pain and TMD as a result of repetitive clenching to relieve orthodontic pain.[26,27] This is the reason why aligners should not be used in patients with active TMDs. As a general rule, TMD needs to be managed before starting any orthodontic treatment. Treatment should address not only the physical diagnosis but also the psychologic distress and the psychosocial dysfunction.[28] The first stage in TMD treatment is symptom focused and behavioral, and it includes (as determined by the problem list) patient education, physiotherapy, pharmacotherapy, psychologic therapy (e.g., cognitive behavioral therapy, stress management, and self-regulatory skills), control of overuse behaviors, and intraoral TMD appliances.[29] Only once symptoms have been controlled and with the awareness that TMDs are cyclic in nature (therefore with a proper informed consent available), an orthodontic treatment can be planned. The following case is helpful in explaining a possible aligner orthodontics approach to a TMD patient after a first conservative phase and pain relief.

DIAGNOSIS AND TREATMENT PLAN

The reasons why aligners could be used to move teeth orthodontically in a patient with a history of TMD are represented by the possibility of accurately planning the sequence of movements, thus reducing and preventing phases in which premature contacts can trigger the occlusal hypervigilance of some patients and by the possibility of using the aligners as physical pro memoria to help the patient to avoid clenching and gnashing of the teeth at least during the awake part of the day. Since the possibility of involuntary clenching or gnashing to alleviate orthodontic pain has been described, the orthodontic treatment plan should consider small amounts of movement from the very early stages of treatment to reduce orthodontic pain as much as possible.

Case Study

A 28-year-old female patient presented with anterior open bite, shift of the lower midline and of the mandible toward the left side, canine class II on the left side, and canine class I on the right side. Furthermore diastemas were present in the lower arch, and posterior fixed prosthodontic restorations were present (Fig. 14.21). The patient had a history of TMD with headaches in the temple region, neck pain, and back. All these symptoms were controlled with physiotherapy, cognitive behavioral therapy, and pharmacotherapy; only once the pain was relieved was the treatment plan designed.

The panoramic x-ray highlighted the presence of interproximal spaces in the lower arch and the missing of both lower first molars with consequent installation of bridges (Fig. 14.22). A TMJ cone-beam computed tomography (CBCT) scan highlighted a protruded position of the right condyle (Fig. 14.23).

The first step of the interdisciplinary treatment consisted in the substitution of the old prosthetic restorations with provisional ones built in a stabilized mandible position thanks to a repositioning splint[25] built by the prosthodontist in centric relation (Figs. 14.24, 14.25, and 14.26).

Once the provisional bridges were fixed, an intraoral scan was performed to start aligner treatment. The virtual treatment plan is illustrated in Figs. 14.27 and 14.28.

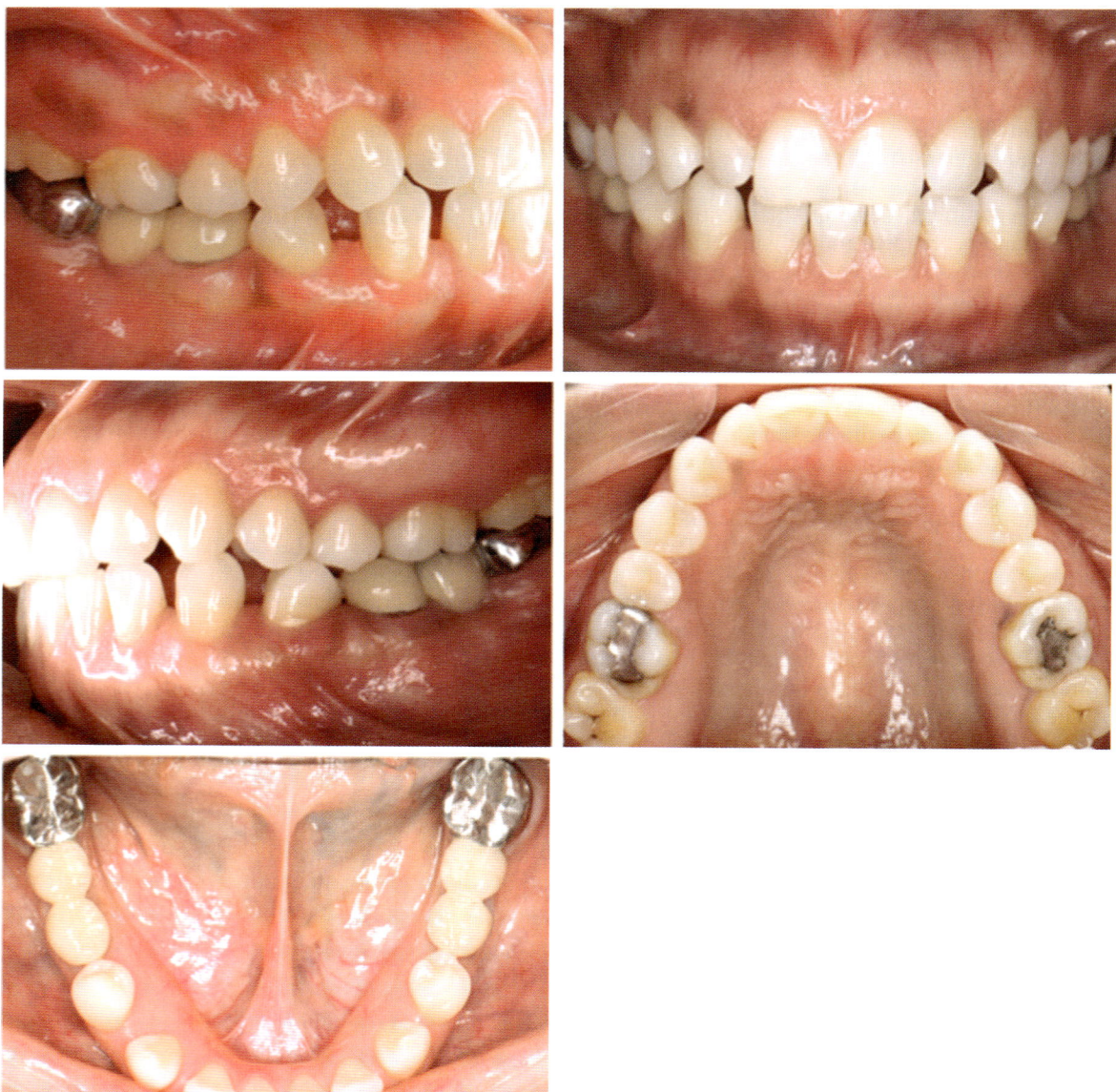

Fig. 14.21 Initial intraoral pictures.

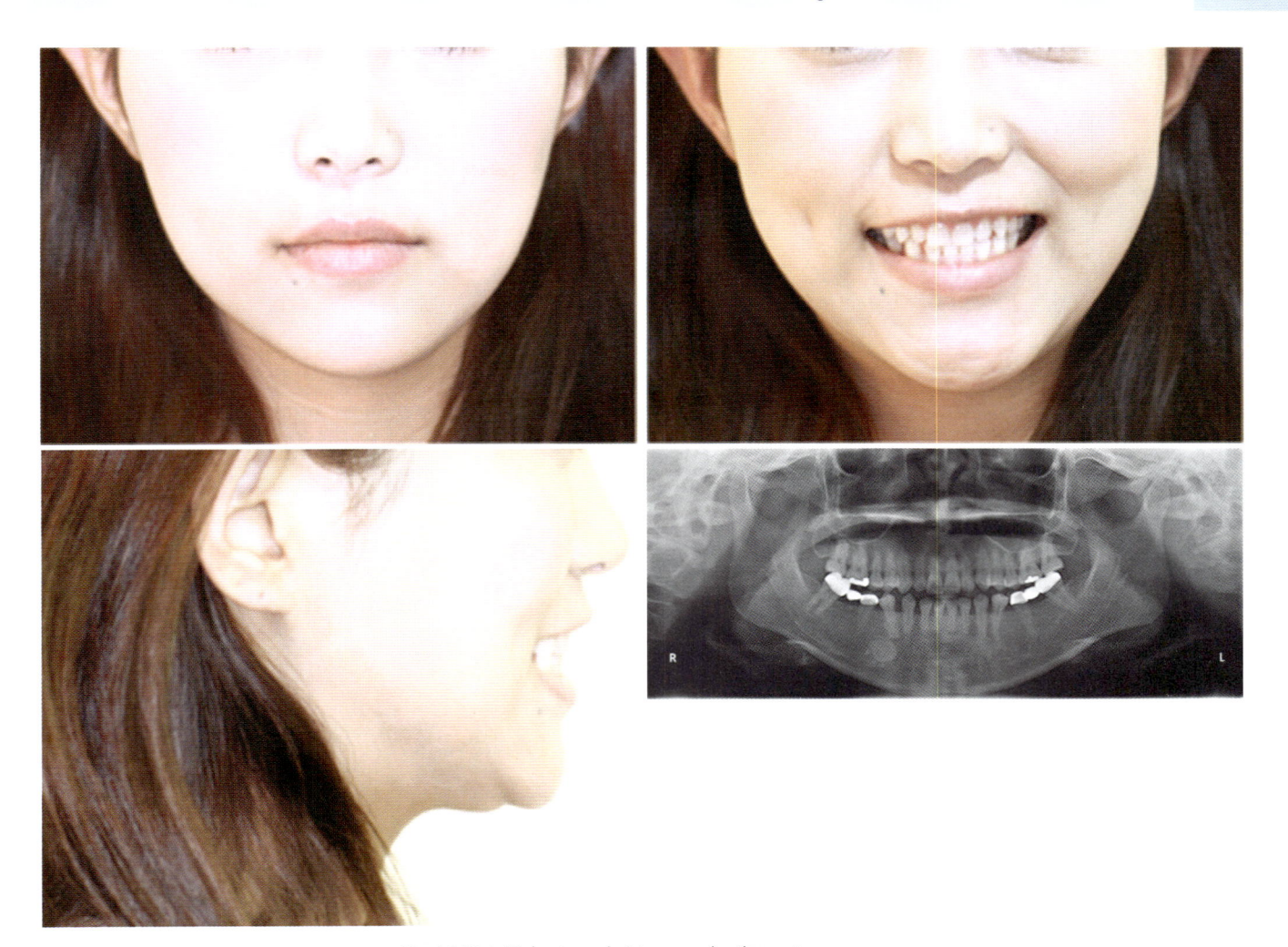

14 • Aligner Orthodontics in Prerestorative Patients

Fig. 14.22 Initial extraoral pictures and orthopantomogram.

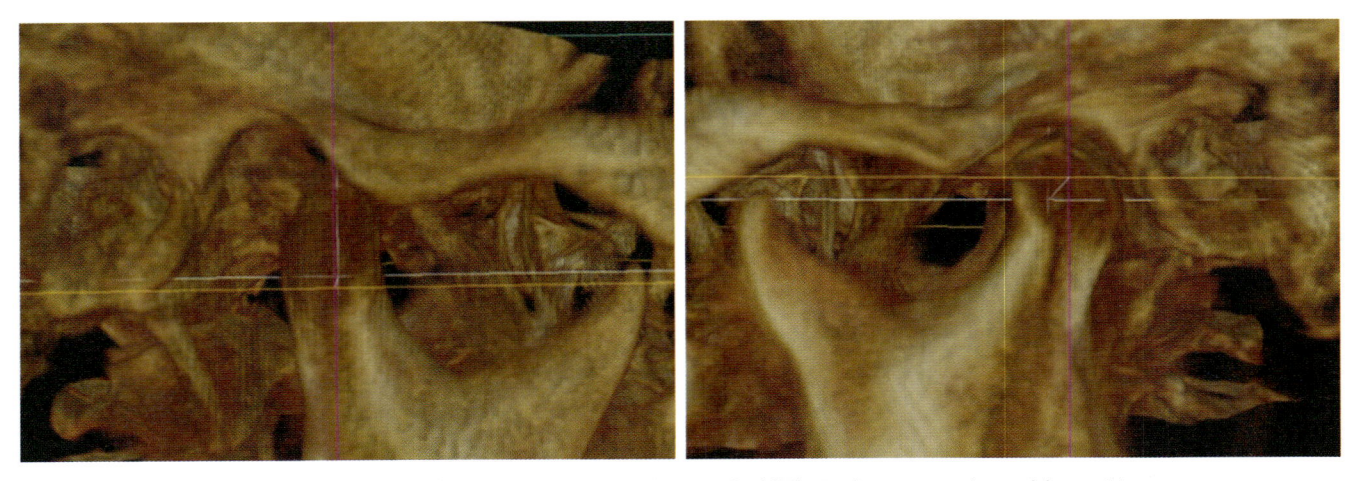

Fig. 14.23 Initial cone-beam computed tomography scans highlighting the asymmetric condyles position.

182 Principles and Biomechanics of Aligner Treatment

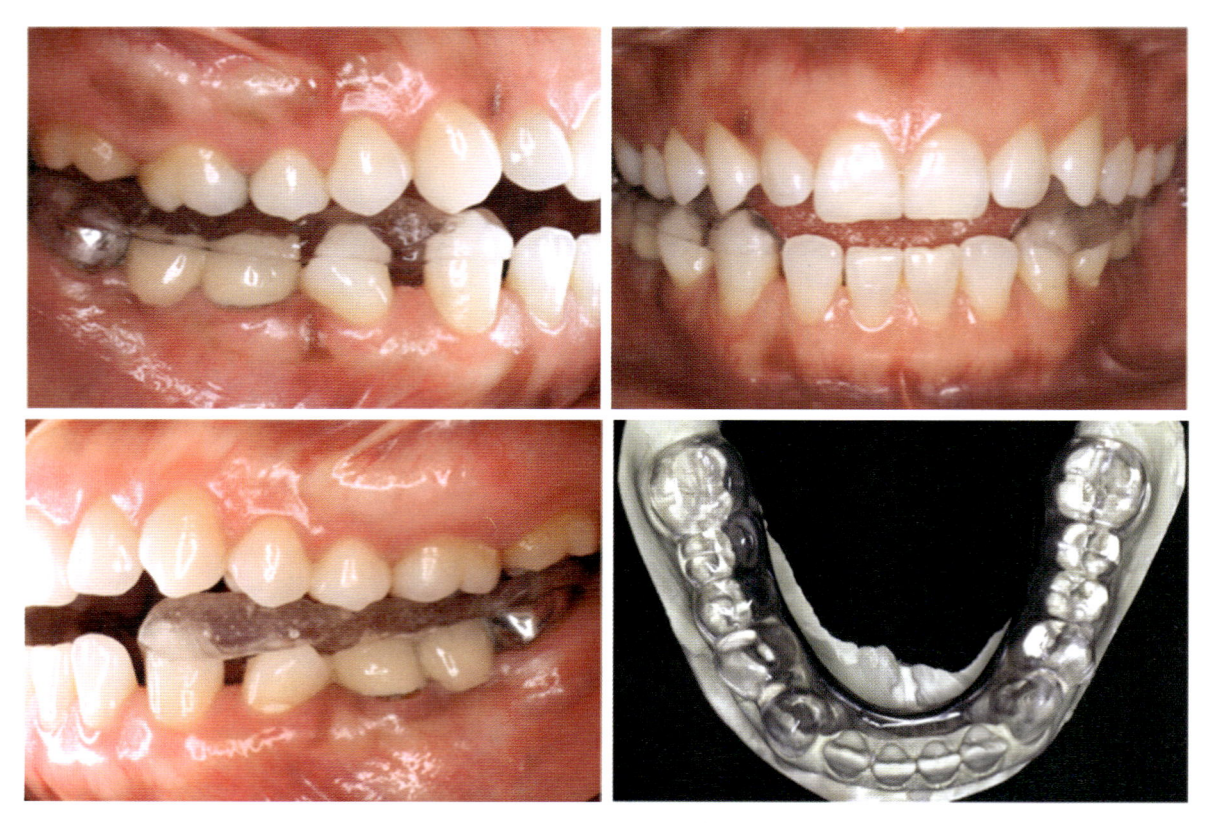

Fig. 14.24 Lower occlusal splint.

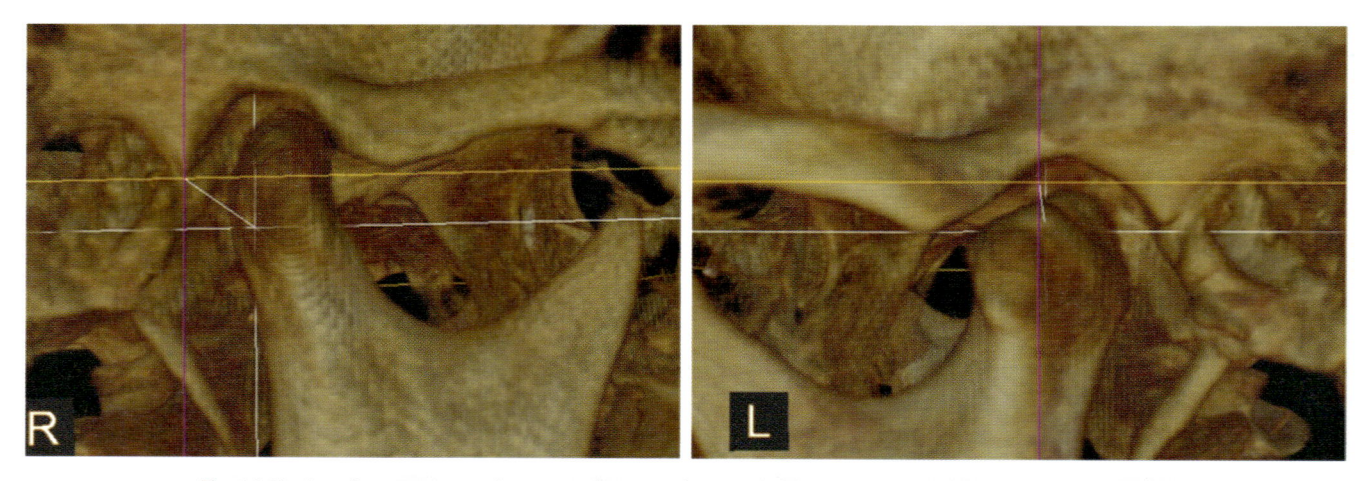

Fig. 14.25 Cone-beam computed tomography scans showing condyle repositioning due to the splint effect.

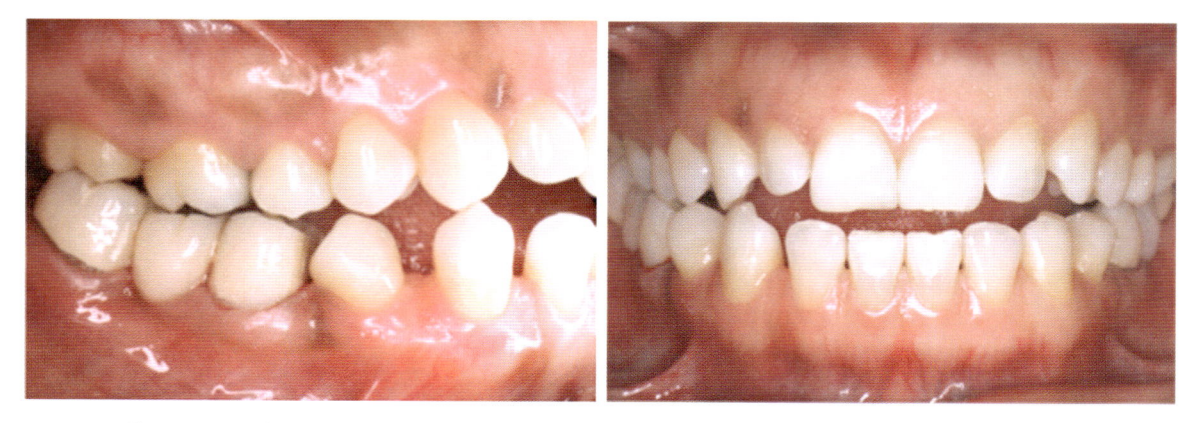

Fig. 14.26 Acrylic provisionals used to keep the new mandible position during the orthodontic treatment.

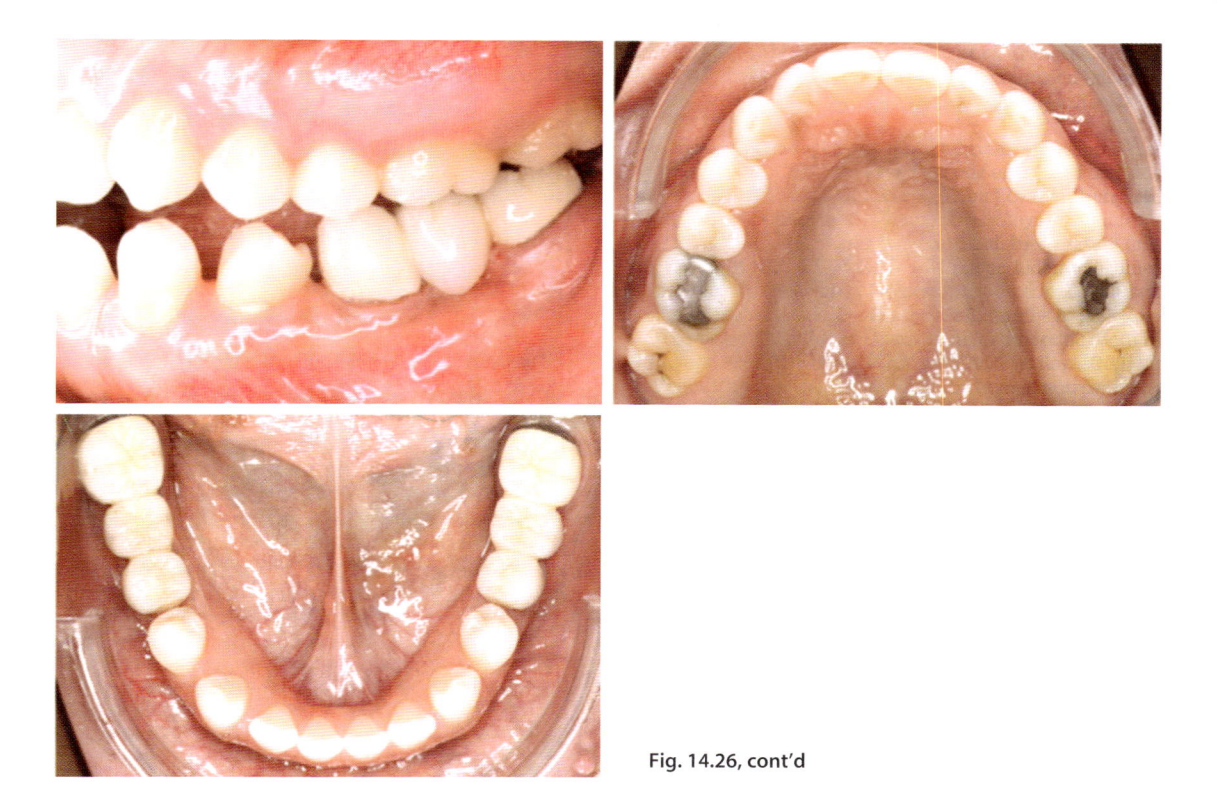

14 • Aligner Orthodontics in Prerestorative Patients 183

Fig. 14.26, cont'd

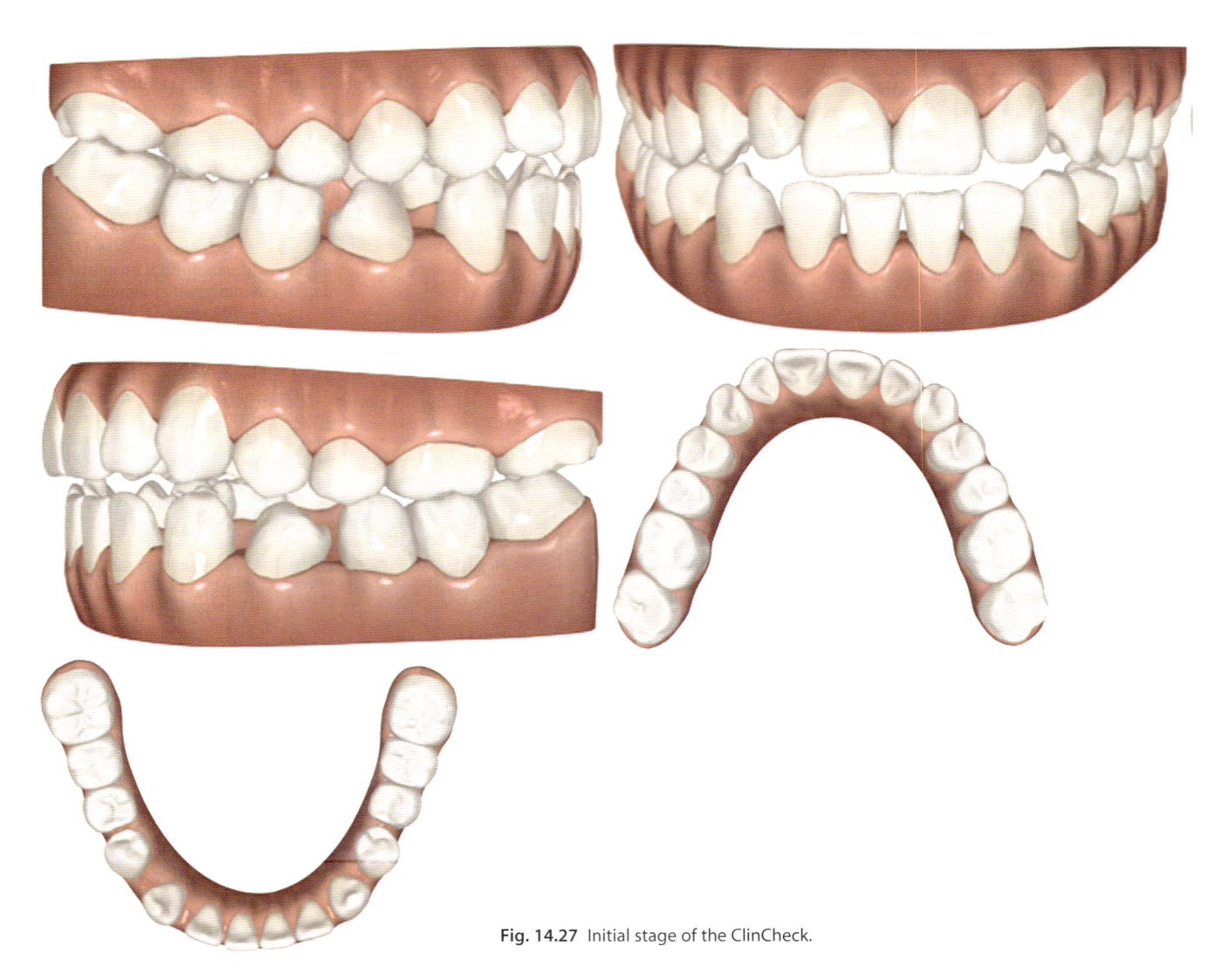

Fig. 14.27 Initial stage of the ClinCheck.

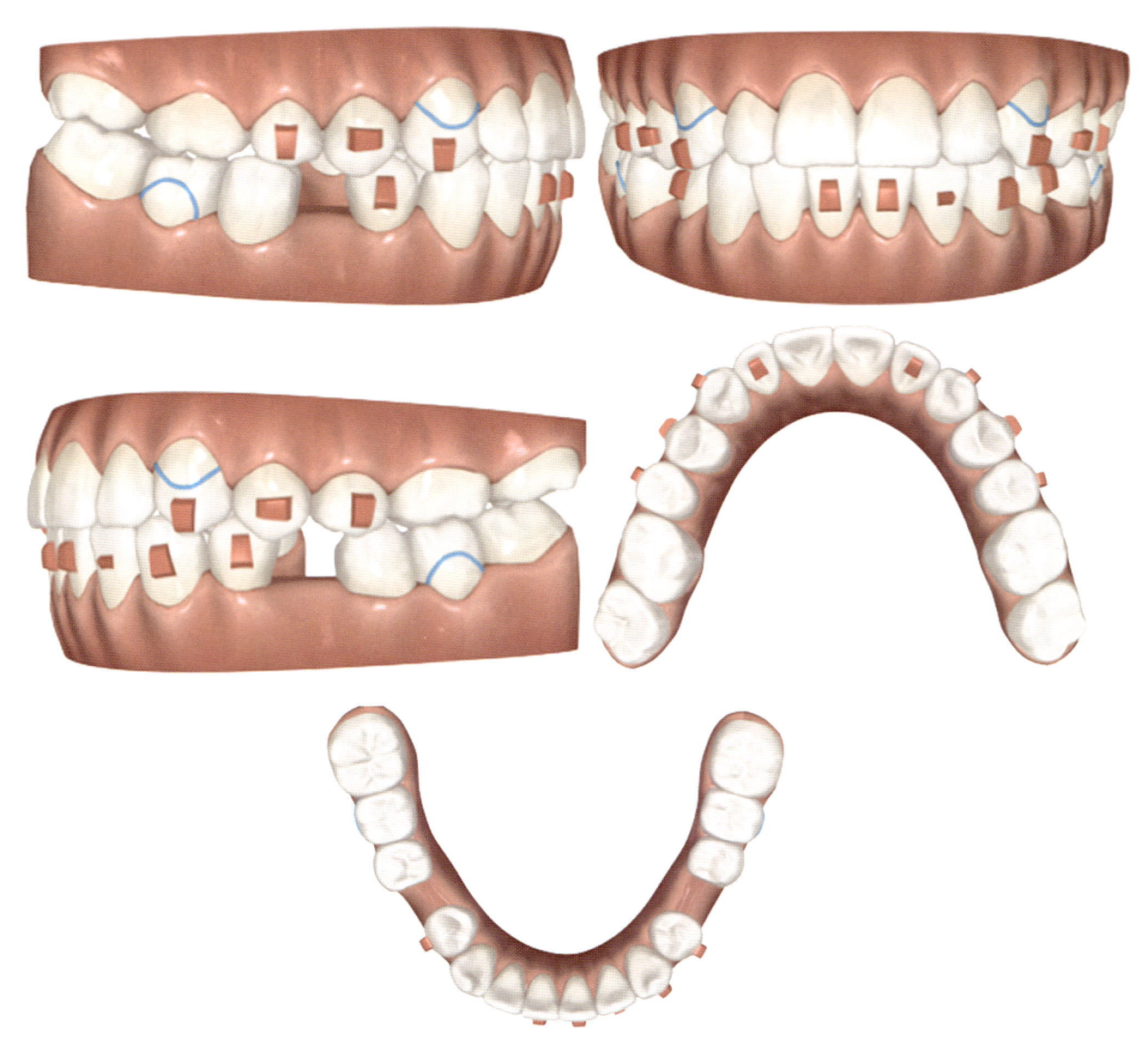

Fig. 14.28 Final stage of the first ClinCheck.

A phase I treatment was planned with 28 aligners and concluded in 6 months with a 5-day aligner change regimen (supported by additional vibrational forces with AcceleDent Aura, OrthoAccel Inc., Bellair, TX, USA). Fig. 14.29 illustrates the intraoral situation at the end of phase I. To complete the orthodontic treatment, the pontic sections of the lower left and right bridges were cut and a new intraoral scan was performed to design the biomechanics required for the final phase of the orthodontic treatment. Then 44 aligners were planned and a 5- to 7-day aligner change regimen was applied to close the treatment in 14 months. Additional vibrational forces were used in this phase, too (Figs. 14.30 and 14.31).

Space for the installation of a first molar implant was secured (Figs. 14.32 and 14.33).

Final pictures show the alignment of the midlines and the set of a functional occlusion with good esthetic results (Figs. 14.34 and 14.35).

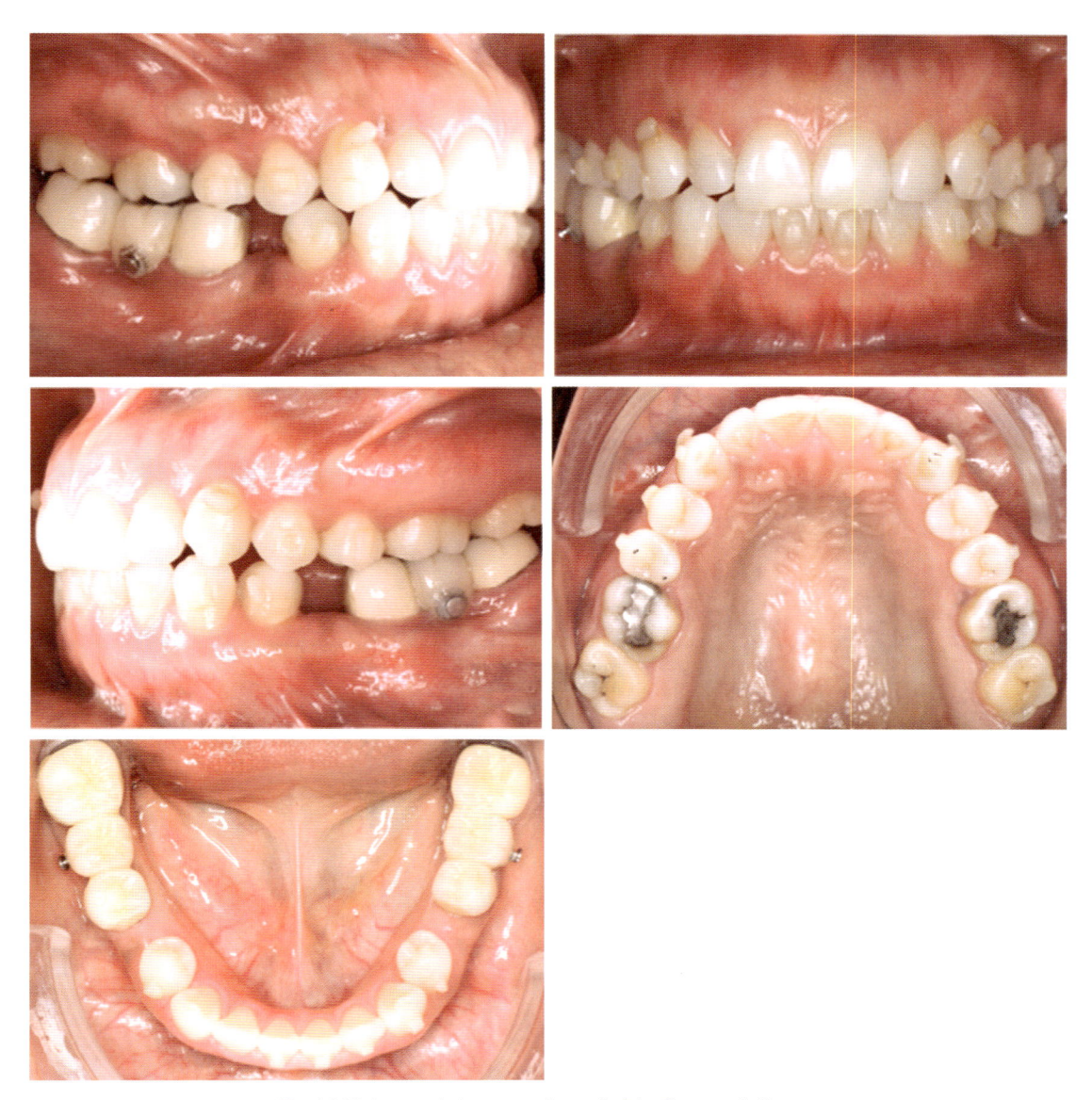

14 • Aligner Orthodontics in Prerestorative Patients 185

Fig. 14.29 Intraoral pictures at the end of the first set of aligners.

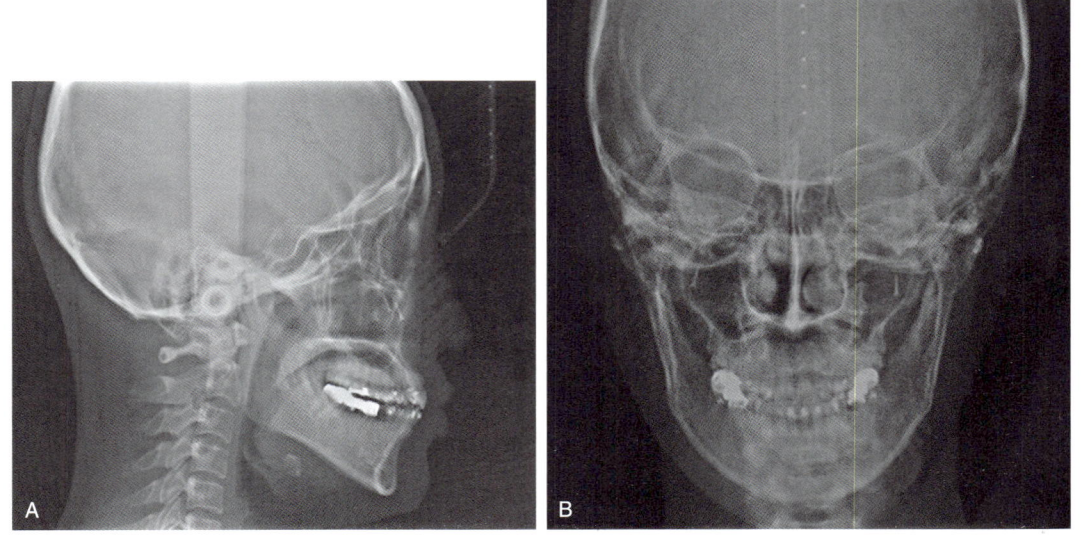

Fig. 14.30 (A) Lateral and (B) posteroanterior x-rays at the end of the first set of aligners.

186 Principles and Biomechanics of Aligner Treatment

Fig. 14.31 Intraoral pictures at the end of the second set of aligners.

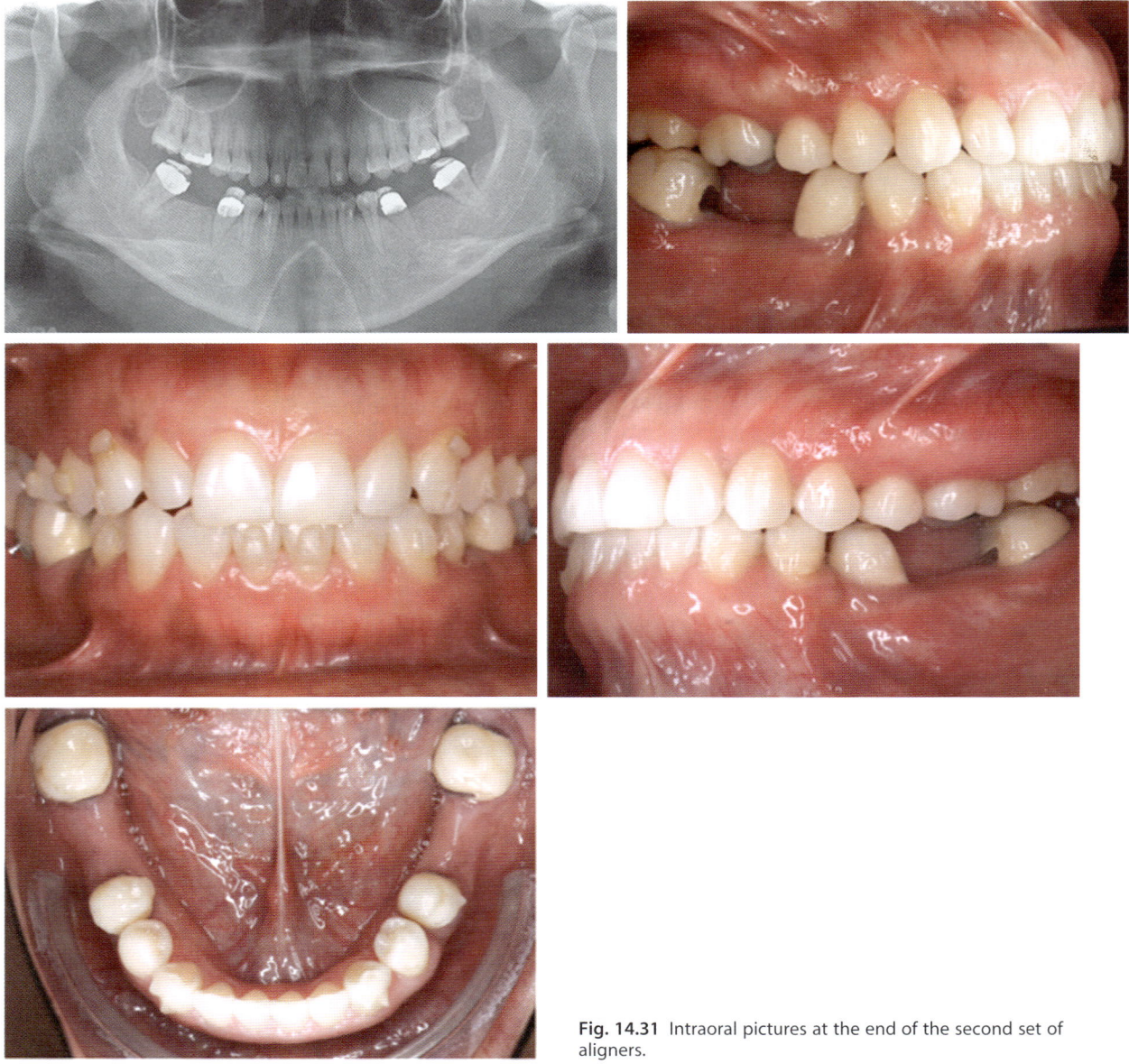

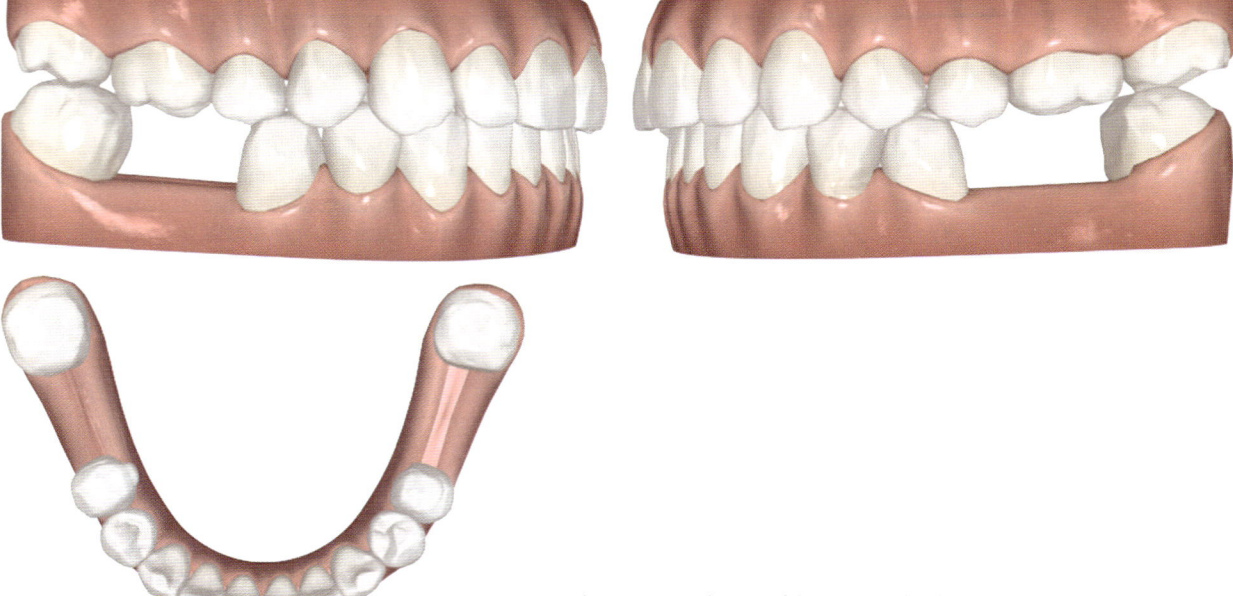

Fig. 14.32 Final stage of the second ClinCheck.

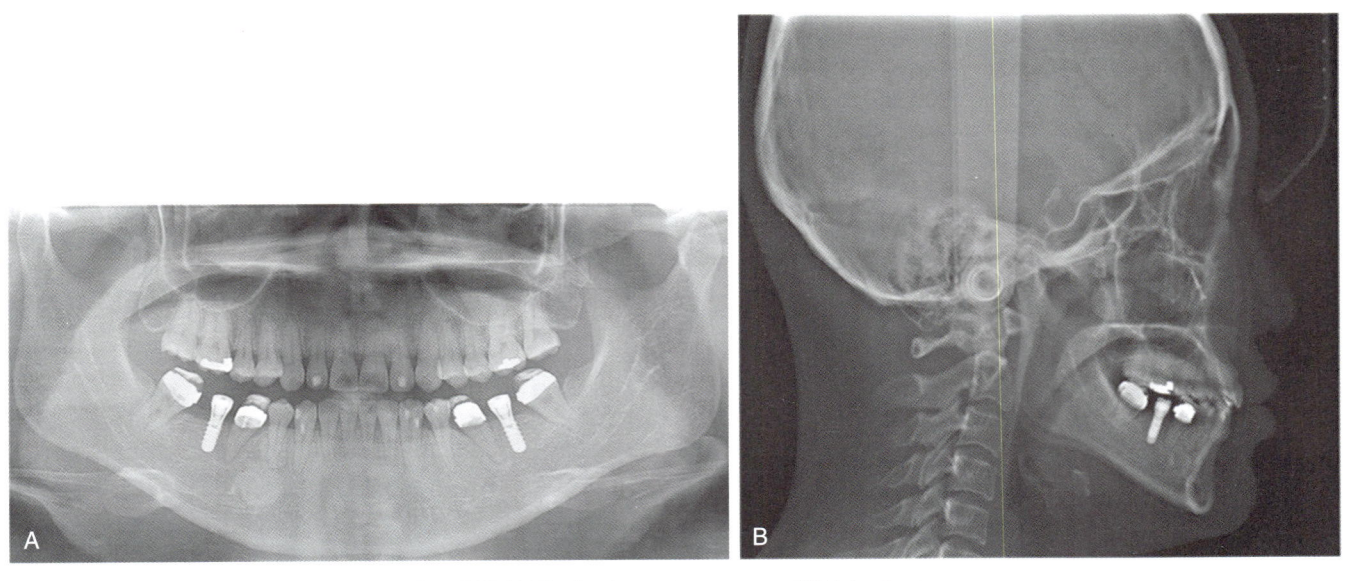

14 • Aligner Orthodontics in Prerestorative Patients   187

Fig. 14.33 (A) Final orthopantomogram and (B) lateral x-ray.

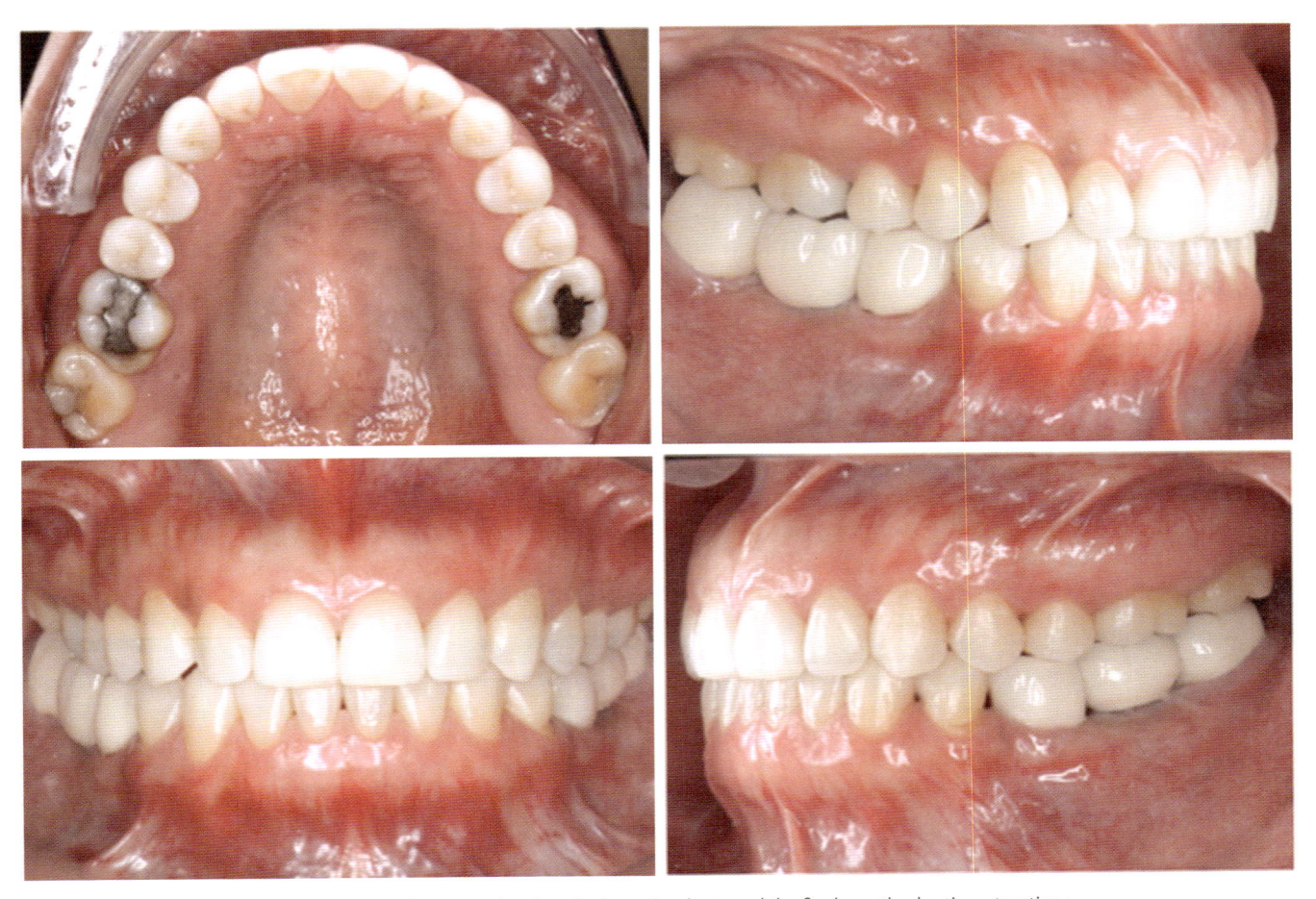

Fig. 14.34 Intraoral pictures showing the lower implants and the final prosthodontic restorations.

Continued

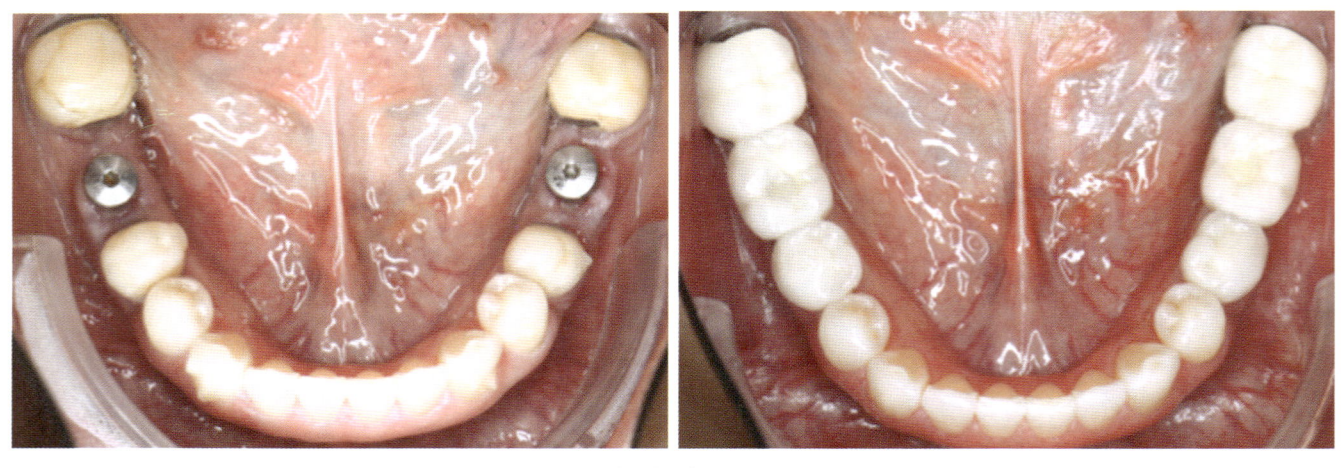

188 Principles and Biomechanics of Aligner Treatment

Fig. 14.34, cont'd

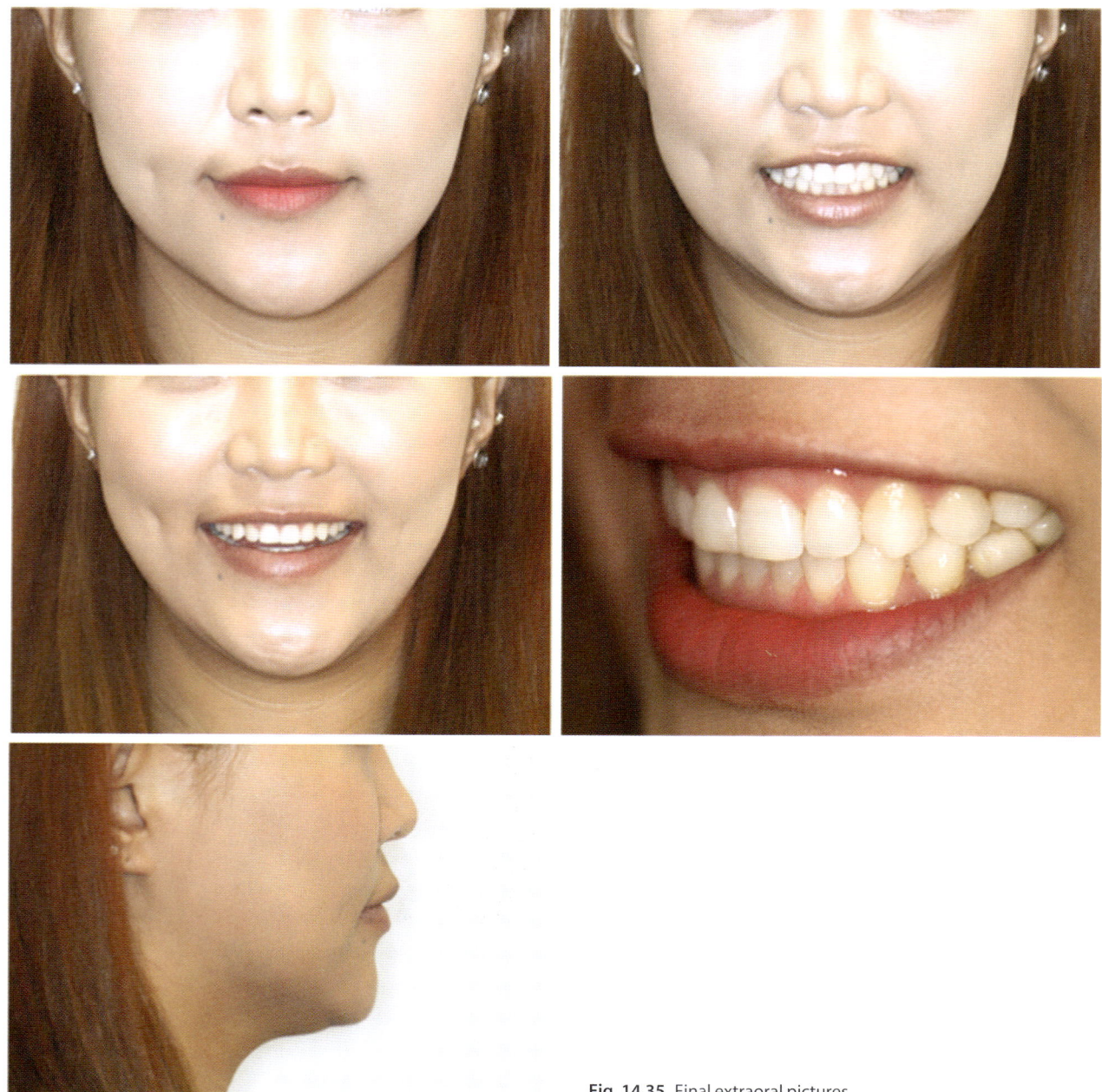

Fig. 14.35 Final extraoral pictures.

References

1. American Association of Orthodontists. Adult orthodontics. https://www.aaoinfo.org/_/adult-orthodontics. Accessed February 27, 2021.
2. Nattrass C, Sandy JR. Adult orthodontics: a review. *Br J Orthod.* 1995;22:331-337.
3. Hamdan AM. The relationship between patient, parent and clinician perceived need and normative orthodontic treatment need. *Eur J Orthod.* 2004;26:265-271.
4. Gosney MB. An investigation some of the factors influencing the desire for orthodontic treatment. *Br J Orthod.* 1986;13:87-94.
5. Parrini S, Rossini G, Castroflorio T, et al. Laypeople's perceptions of frontal smile esthetics: a systematic review. *Am J Orthod Dentofacial Orthop.* 2016;150:740-750.
6. Kokich VG, Spear FM. Guidelines for managing the orthodontic-restorative patient. *Semin Orthod.* 1997;3:3-20.
7. Sanama Y. The link between orthodontics and prosthetics. In: Melsen B, ed. *Adult Orthodontics.* Chichester, UK: Blackwell Pub Ltd; 2012.
8. de Avila ÉD, de Molon RS, de Assis Mollo Jr F, et al. Multidisciplinary approach for the aesthetic treatment of maxillary lateral incisors agenesis: thinking about implants? *Oral Surg Oral Med Oral Pathol Oral Radiol.* 2012;114(5):e22-e28.
9. Kokich VG. Maxillary lateral incisor implants: planning with the aid of orthodontics. *Tex Dent J.* 2007;124:388-398.
10. Samoto H, Vlaskalic V. A customized staging procedure to improve the predictability of space closure with sequential aligners. *J Clin Orthod.* 2014;48:359-367.
11. Magne P, Belser U. Natural oral esthetics. In: *Bonded Porcelain Restorations in the Anterior Dentition: A Biomimetic Approach.* 1st ed. Qunitessence Pub; 2010:57-98.
12. Coachman C, Calamita M. Digital smile design: a tool for treatment planning and communication in esthetic dentistry. *Quintessence Dent Technol.* 2012;35:103-111.
13. Olsen TM, Kokich Sr VG. Postorthodontic root approximation after opening space for maxillary lateral incisor implants. *Am J Orthod Dentofacial Orthop.* 2010;137:158.e1; discussion 158-159.
14. Magkavali-Trikka P, Emmanouilidis G, Papadopoulos MA. Mandibular molar uprighting using orthodontic miniscrew implants: a systematic review. *Prog Orthod.* 2018;19:1.
15. Zachrisson BU, Bantleon HP. Optimal mechanics for mandibular molar uprighting. *World J Orthod.* 2005;6:80-87.
16. Phan X, Ling PH. Clinical limitations of Invisalign. *J Can Dent Assoc.* 2007;73:263-266.
17. Brezniak N. The clear plastic appliance: a biomechanical point of view. *Angle Orthod.* 2008;78:381-382.
18. Taffarel IP, Meira TM, Guimarães LK, et al. Biomechanics for orthodontic intrusion of severely extruded maxillary molars for functional prosthetic rehabilitation. *Case Rep Dent.* 2019;15:8246129.
19. Weir T. Clear aligners in orthodontic treatment. *Aust Dent J.* 2017;62(suppl 1):58-62.
20. Paccini JV, Cotrim-Ferreira FA, Ferreira FV, et al. Efficiency of two protocols for maxillary molar intrusion with mini-implants. *Dental Press J Orthod.* 2016;21:56-66.
21. Sugii MM, Barreto BC, Francisco Vieira-Júnior W, et al. Extruded upper first molar intrusion: comparison between unilateral and bilateral miniscrew anchorage. *Dental Press J Orthod.* 2018;23:63-70.
22. Kandasamy S, Rinchuse DJ. Orthodontics and TMD. In: Kandasamy S, Greene CS, Rinchuse DJ, et al., eds. *TMD and Orthodontics. A Clinical Guide for the Orthodontist.* Springer Pub; 2015:81-95.
23. Manfredini D, Stellini E, Gracco A, et al. Orthodontics is temporomandibular disorder-neutral. *Angle Orthod.* 2016;86:649-654.
24. Boyd RL. Esthetic orthodontic treatment using the Invisalign appliance for moderate to complex malocclusions. *J Dent Educ.* 2008;72:948-967.
25. Schupp W, Haubrich J, Neumann I. Invisalign treatment of patients with craniomandibular disorders. *Int Orthod.* 2010;8:253-267.
26. Tran J, Lou T, Nebiolo B, et al. Impact of clear aligner therapy on tooth pain and masticatory muscle soreness. *J Oral Rehabil.* 2020;47:1521-1529.
27. Lou T, Tran J, Castroflorio T, et al. Evaluation of masticatory muscle response to clear aligner therapy using ambulatory electromyographic recording. *Am J Orthod Dentofacial Orthop.* 2021;159:e25-e33.
28. Ohrbach R. Disability assessment in temporomandibular disorders and masticatory system rehabilitation. *J Oral Rehabil.* 2010;37:452-480.
29. Greene CS, Rinchuse DJ, Kandasamy S, et al. Management of TMD signs and symptoms in the orthodontic practice. In: Kandasamy S, Greene CS, Rinchuse DJ, et al., eds. *TMD and Orthodontics. A Clinical Guide for the Orthodontist.* Springer Pub; 2015:119-124.
30. Giancotti A, Germano F, Muzzi F, et al. A miniscrew-supported intrusion auxiliary for open-bite treatment with Invisalign. *J Clin Orthod.* 2014;48:348-358.

15 Noncompliance Upper Molar Distalization and Aligner Treatment for Correction of Class II Malocclusions

BENEDICT WILMES and JÖRG SCHWARZE

Upper Molar Distalization in Aligner Treatment

The distalization of the upper molars may be considered as a treatment option for patients with an angle class II malocclusion characterized with an increased overjet and/or anterior crowding. There has been an increasing trend in the clinical use of purely intraoral appliances, which require minimal need for patient cooperation. Unfortunately, most tooth-borne appliances for upper molar distalization produce an unwanted side effect of anchorage loss resulting in maxillary incisor proclination, reported to be 24% to 55% of observed tooth movement.[1] Pure bodily tooth movement with sequential plastic aligner therapy is challenging to achieve to a high degree of predictability. As a consequence, molar distalization is limited when relying on aligner movement alone. While there are limited reports of successful upper molar distalization of up to 2.5 mm in the literature,[2] a very long treatment time and high level of patient compliance are expected with requirement for intermaxillary class II elastics to be worn during the long period of the sequential upper molar distalization.[3] Moreover, the potential side effects of class II elastics must be considered in terms of mesial shift of the lower anchorage teeth.

To minimize anchorage loss and need for class II elastics, mini-implants have been incorporated into the design of maxillary distalization appliances.[4,5] Mini-implants can be positioned intraorally with minimal degrees of surgical invasiveness, are readily integrated with concomitant biomechanical initiatives, and are relatively cost effective.[6-8] Various designs of implant supported distalization appliances have been published. The retromolar region is an unsuitable area for mini-implant insertion due to the unfavorable anatomic conditions (poor bone quality and thick soft tissue).[9] Additionally, the alveolar process has also been shown to be inappropriate in cases of a desired molar distalization since the mini-implants are in the direct path of the moving teeth resulting in a failure rate that is much higher as compared to the anterior palate.[10] Therefore, the palatal area posterior from the rugae (T zone[11]) seems to be the preferred insertion site for mini-implants where the treatment objective is for distal movement of the maxillary molars without associated anchorage loss and maxillary incisor displacement. Furthermore, good bone quality with thin attached mucosa implies minimal risk of tooth-root injuries and a very high success rate in the anterior palatal region.[9] In contrast to treatment strategies involving the interradicular positioning of mini-implants, the molar teeth can be distalized, and the premolars are free to move distally due to the stretch of the interdental fibers without any interference since the palatally positioned mini-implants are not in the path of moving teeth. Within the T zone, the mini-implants can be inserted in a median or paramedian orientation,[11] with both insertion sites showing a similar stability.[12]

Clinical Procedure and Rational of the Beneslider

The Beneslider[13-15] is a maxillary molar tooth distalization appliance, principally designed on the use of one or two mini-implants coupled in a median or paramedian orientation in the anterior palate (Fig. 15.1). By modifying the angulation of the 1.1-mm stainless steel wire, it is possible to achieve a simultaneous intrusion or extrusion of the molars.[16-18] The distalization forces are transferred to the molars by the use of bonded tubes. The advantages of a bonded tube are esthetics, and the adaptability and fit of the aligners is not undermined by the presence of stainless steel molar bands. The aligner material could cover this bonded connection (Fig. 15.2) or the aligner could be cut out in this connection area ("button cutout") (Fig. 15.3).

It seems advantageous that the Beneslider appliance can be fitted directly without the requirement for adjunctive laboratory work in terms of welding or soldering, or the need to record an intraoral impression. Alternatively, the clinician has the choice to record an intraoral impression and transfer the clinical setup to a plaster cast model using an impression cap and laboratory analogue from the Benefit system.

Following distalization of the maxillary molar teeth, steel ligatures can be used (see Fig. 15.2) or springs removed (see Fig. 15.3) to modify the Beneslider from an active distalization device to a passive molar anchorage device. The primary objective is to stabilize the maxillary molar teeth during the retraction of the maxillary anterior teeth. Our experience in using the Beneslider appliance in conjunction with aligners commenced with a two-phase approach[16]:

15 • Noncompliance Upper Molar Distalization and Aligner Treatment for Correction of Class II Malocclusions

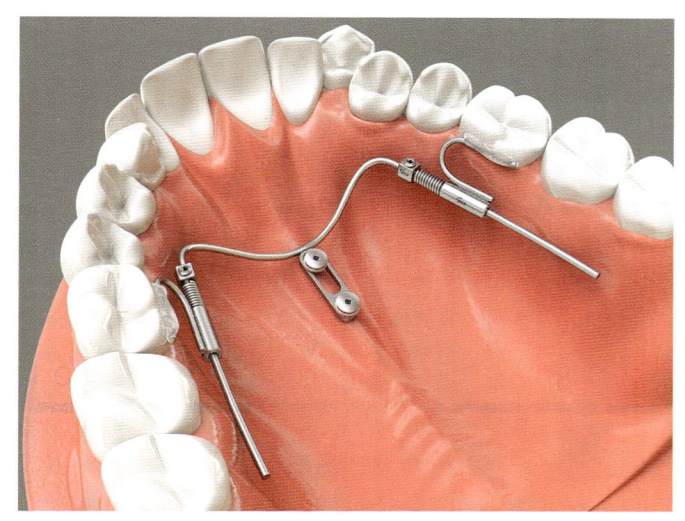

Fig. 15.1 The Beneslider appliance is based on one or two mini-implants with exchangeable abutments.

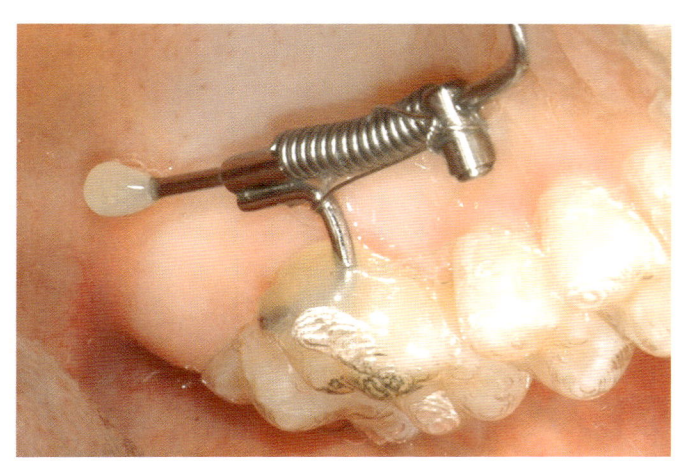

Fig. 15.2 The aligners can cover the bonded connection like a big attachment. After distalization, steel ligatures are to modify the active Beneslider into a passive anchorage device.

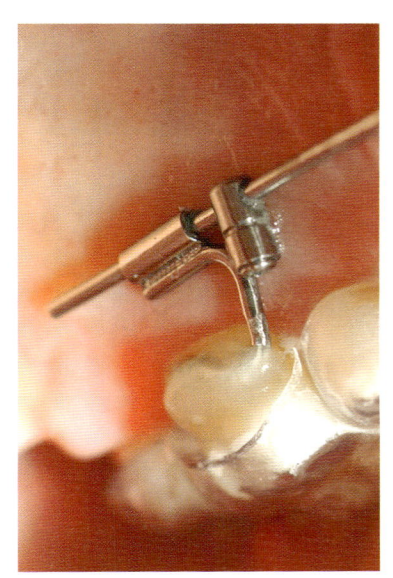

Fig. 15.3 The aligners can be cut out in this connection area ("button cutout"). Springs are removed in this case to modify the active Beneslider into a passive anchorage device.

the initial phase involving molar distalization and the secondary phase for the final detailing of the occlusion with sequential thermoplastic aligners. With a two-phase approach, an impression (or scan) is recorded *after* distalization. To reduce the total treatment time, we now recommend simultaneous distalization with the Beneslider and alignment with sequential aligners. With a single-phase approach, the impressions for aligners are taken *prior to* distalization of the maxillary molars, and the anticipated tooth movement to be produced by the Beneslider appliance is programmed in the digital software platform. For distalization, either a sequential step-by-step distalization or an entire maxillary arch can be chosen since the stretch of the interdental fibers supports the simultaneous distal drift of maxillary anterior teeth.

If the aligner material should cover the connection area with the molars (see Fig. 15.2), the impressions for aligners should be done after the insertion of the Beneslider appliance. The Beneslider should be not activated prior to the delivery of the aligners. If the aligners have a cutout area (see Fig. 15.3), the impressions for aligners are able to be recorded either before or after insertion of the Beneslider appliance. Distalization forces can be applied to the first or second maxillary molar teeth. Our clinical experiences have shown that force application to the first molar is a superior approach, as direct force application to the second molar teeth is associated with precocious distalization of the second molars, leading to improper tracking and fitting of the sequential plastic aligners, a risk that is reduced if the maxillary first molar teeth are connected to the Beneslider.

Clinical Case

A 39-year-old female patient presented with anterior crowding class II malocclusion (Fig. 15.4; Table 15.1). The maxillary teeth were migrated mesially, especially on the left side. Due to the absence of the second lower right molar, the upper second right molar was elongated.

The patient was very unhappy with the protrusion of the upper front teeth and specifically requested an invisible orthodontic treatment option to be performed on a nonextraction basis. Following the insertion of two Benefit mini-implants in the anterior palate (Fig. 15.5A), the Beneslider appliance was passively installed (see Fig. 15.5B; note springs are not activated). With the goal to distalize and intrude the upper right second molar simultaneously, the guiding wire of the Beneslider was angulated apically (see Fig. 15.5B).[17] Secondly, intraoral scans were recorded for fabrication of clear aligners (Invisalign, Align Technology, Inc.).

Using the aligner planning software (e.g., ClinCheck), the molar movements have to be planned parallel to the guiding wires of the Beneslider, including the intrusive vertical component in the first quadrant. During the distalization period, molar derotations and uprighting movements were not allowed (see Fig. 15.5C). In this patient, a sequential distalization was chosen. The aligner material should cover the connection area (Fig. 15.6). After delivery and insertion of the aligners, the Beneslider was activated by pushing the 240-g NiTi springs distally using the activation lock (see Fig. 15.6). The maxillary molars were to be distalized

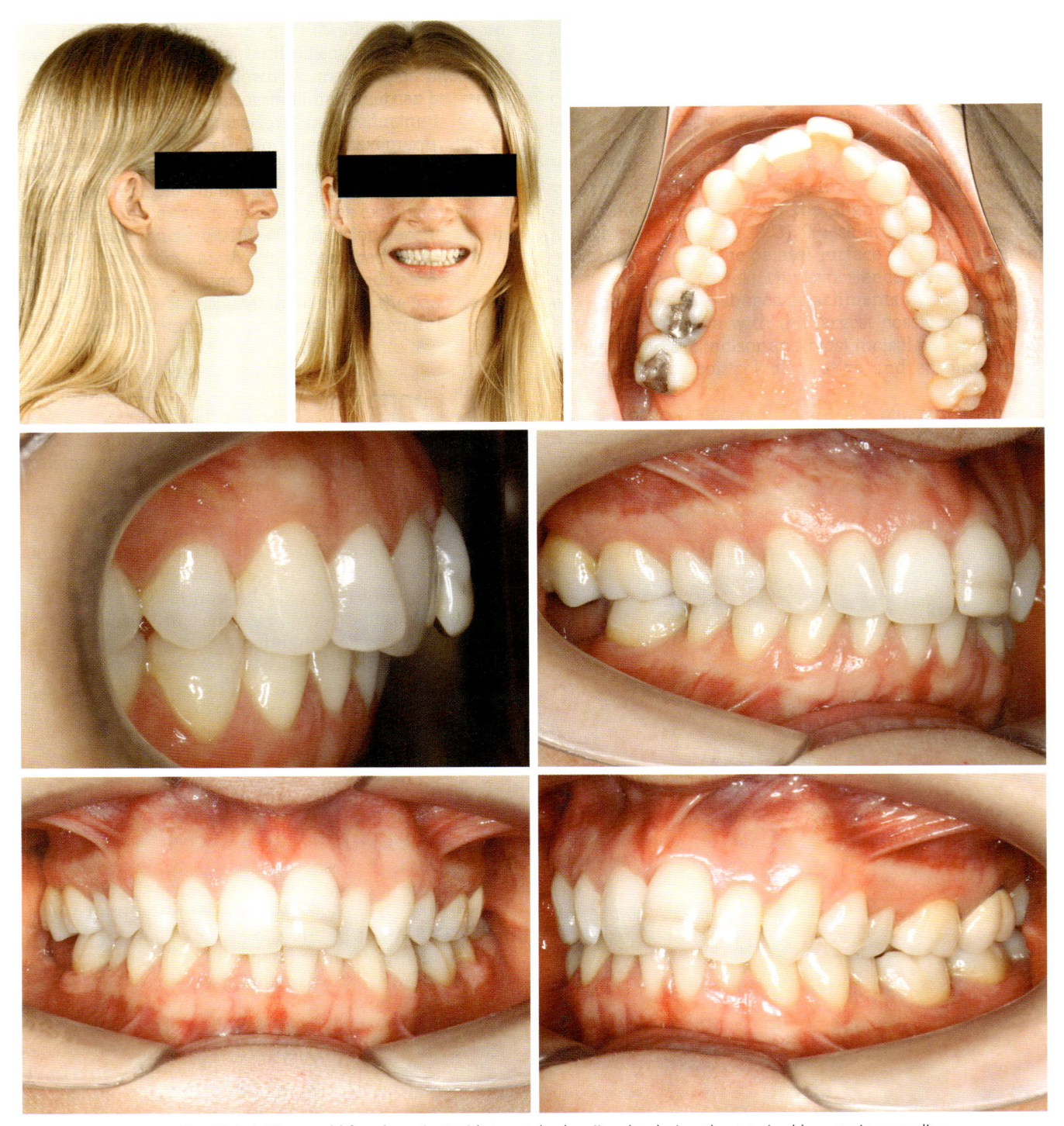

Fig. 15.4 A 37-year-old female patient with an angle class II malocclusion characterized by anterior crowding and a deep bite.

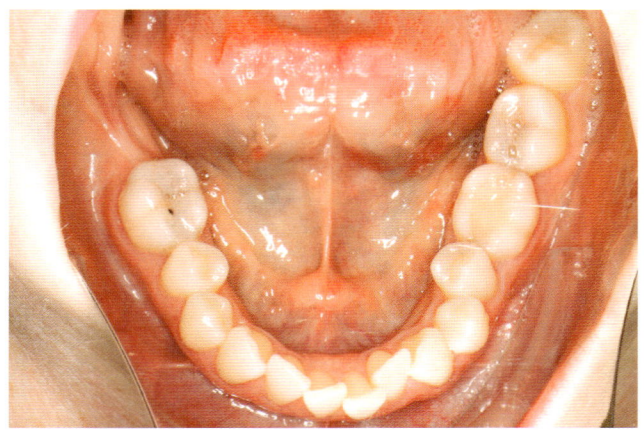

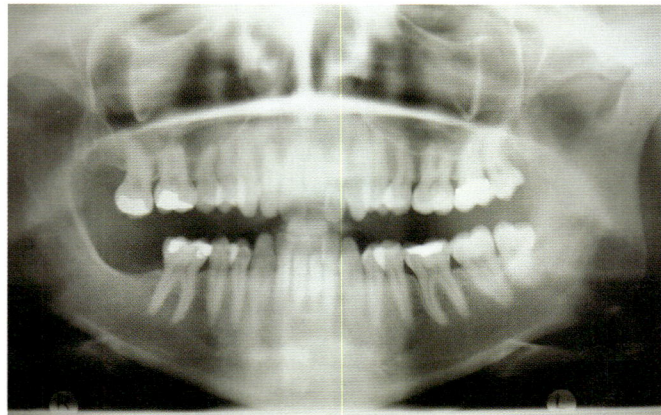

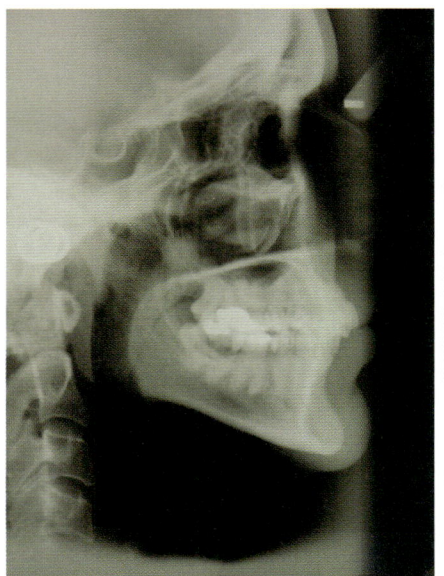

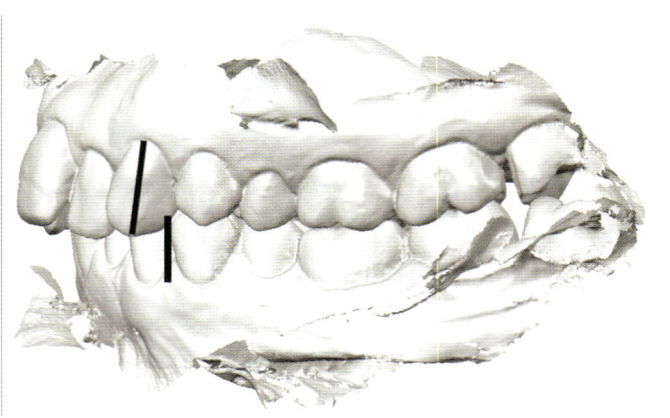

Fig. 15.4, cont'd

Table 15.1 Cephalometric Summary

	Pretreatment	Posttreatment
NSBa	123.9°	124.5°
NL-NSL	7.9°	6.3°
ML-NSL	35.0°	38.3°
ML-NL	27.2°	32.1°
SNA	80.5°	78.5°
SNB	76.2°	74.0°
ANB	4.3°	4.6°
Wits	3.7 mm	2.6 mm
U1-NL	117.6°	106.6°
L1-ML	93.3°	94.5°
U1-L1	121.9°	126.8°
Overjet	6.1 mm	3.9 mm
Overbite	2.0 mm	1.6 mm

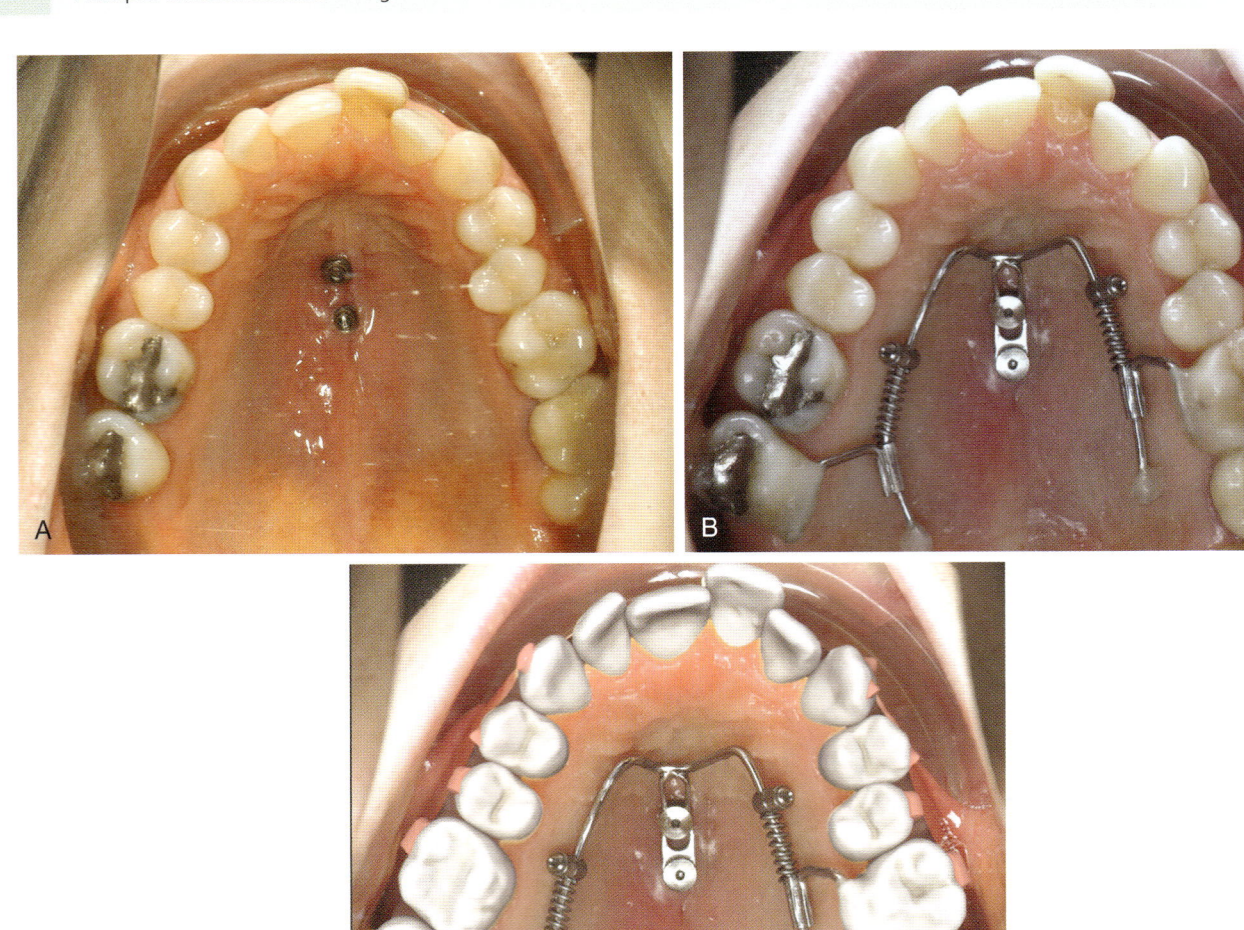

Fig. 15.5 After insertion of two Benefit mini-implants in the anterior palate (A) and installation of the Beneslider mechanics (B). Superimposition of an intraoral picture of the maxillary arch and the ClinCheck to demonstrate desired tooth movement directions (C).

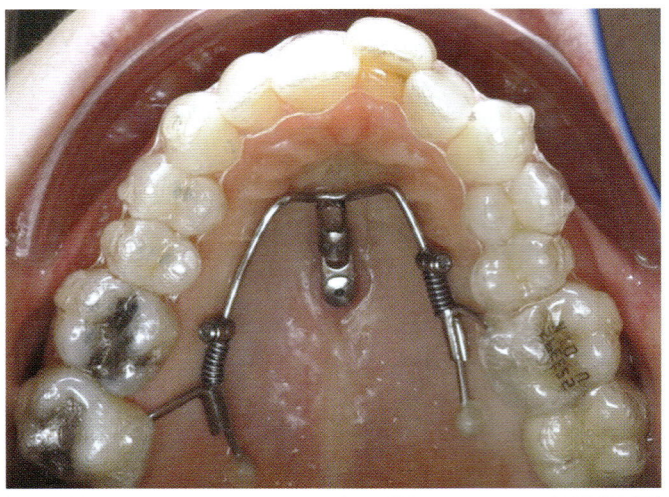

Fig. 15.6 Beneslider was activated by pushing open springs distally after delivery of the aligners. Connection areas of the Beneslider with the molars are covered by the aligner ("big attachment").

approximately 4 to 5 mm. The patient reportedly adapted to the appliance without issue. The panoramic radiograph denotes bodily distalization of all maxillary posterior teeth after 5 months (Fig. 15.7).

During the follow-up controls, molar distalization is visible with small spaces between molars and bicuspids (Figs. 15.8, 15.9, 15.10, and 15.11; note sequential distalization). As soon as the maxillary molar teeth were distalized into an angle class I occlusion, steel ligatures were used between the bonded tube and the activation lock to deactivate the Beneslider (Fig. 15.12; see Figs. 15.10 and 15.11). The Beneslider was converted from a distalization device to a molar anchorage device. After all spaces were closed to the distal, the Beneslider was removed and scans for a refinement and molar derotation were recorded. Comprehensive treatment was completed after 19 months, and the palatal mini-implants were removed without the adjunctive use of local anesthesia (Fig. 15.13). Upper incisors were reclined significantly (U1-NL has changed from 117.6 to

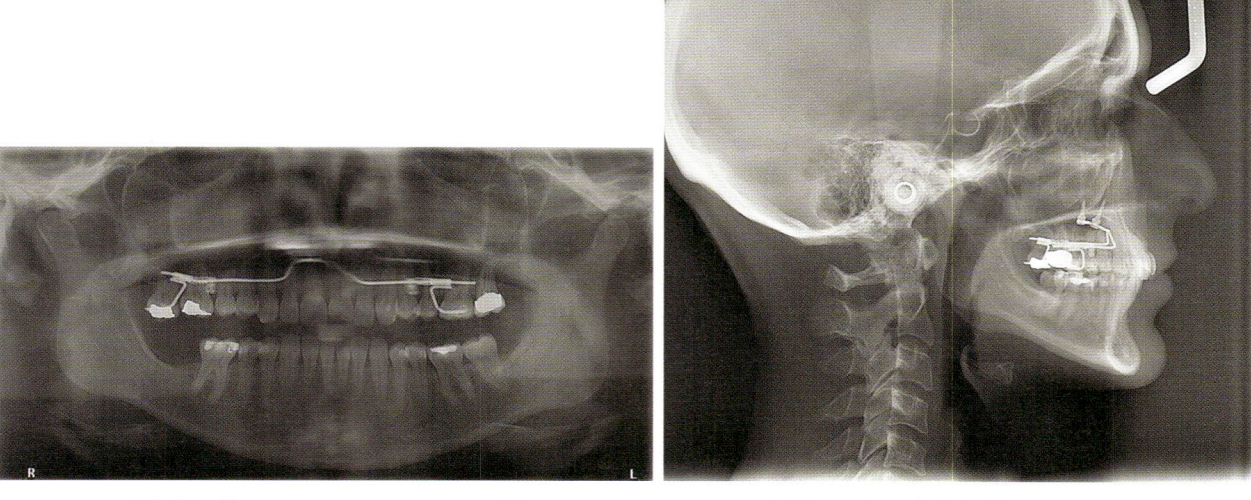

Fig. 15.7 Radiographs after 5 months of treatment. Ortopantomography and lateral x-ray after 5 months of treatment.

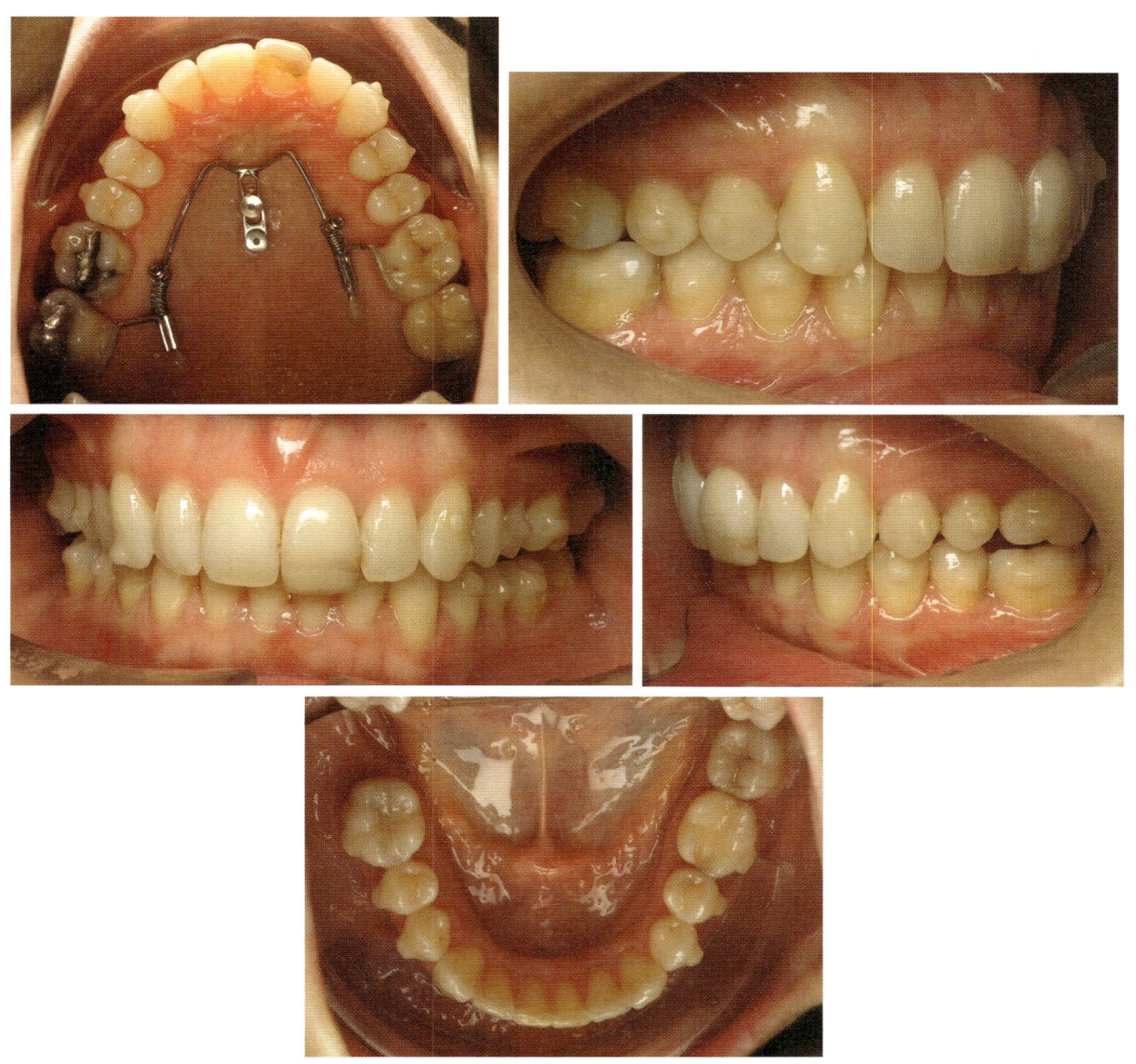

Fig. 15.8 Intraoral pictures after 8 months.

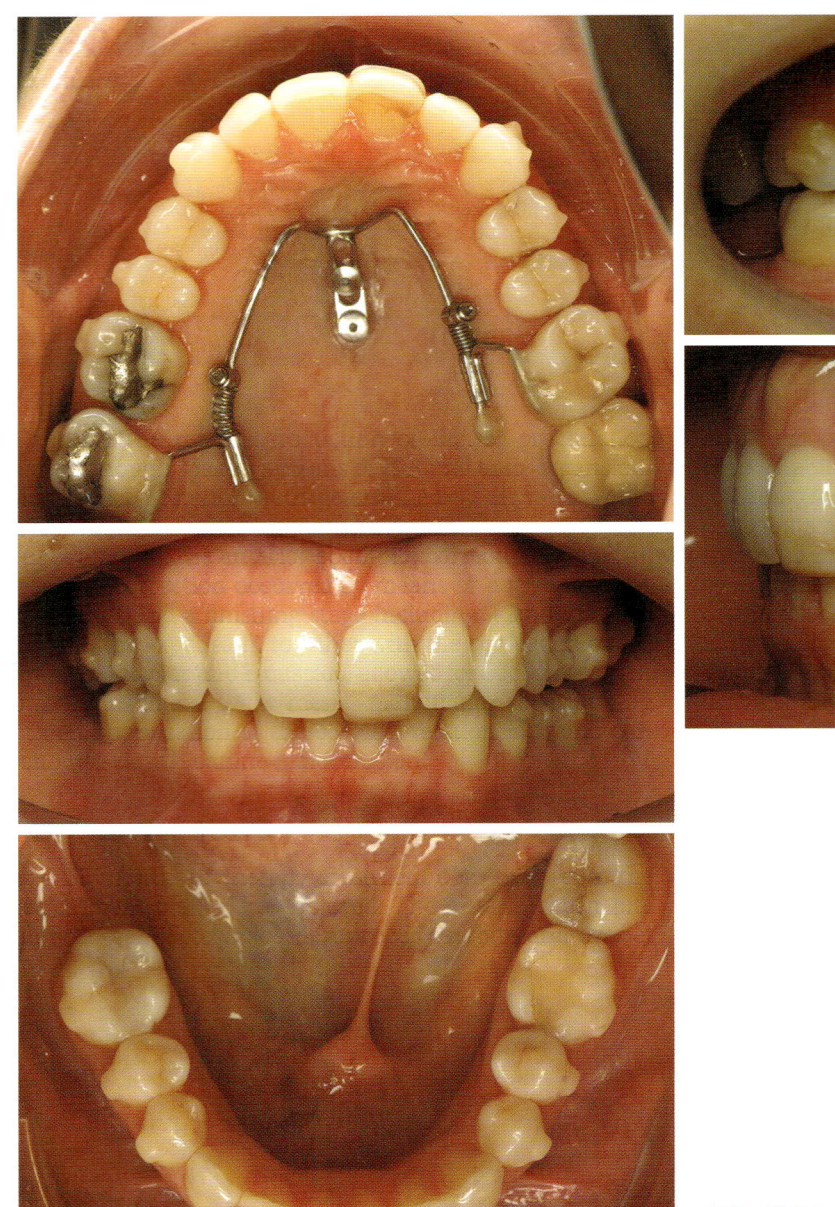

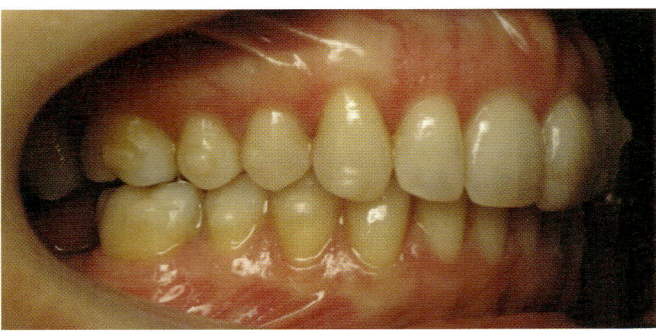

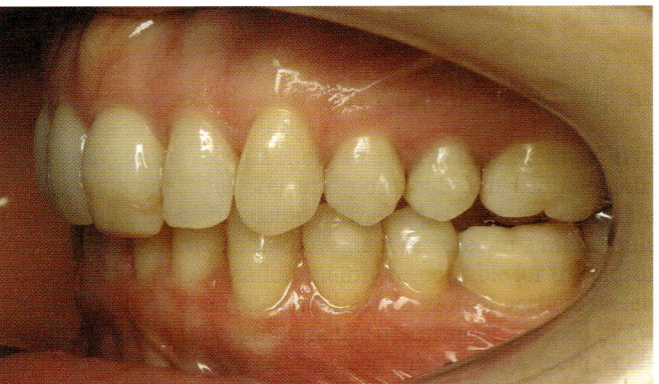

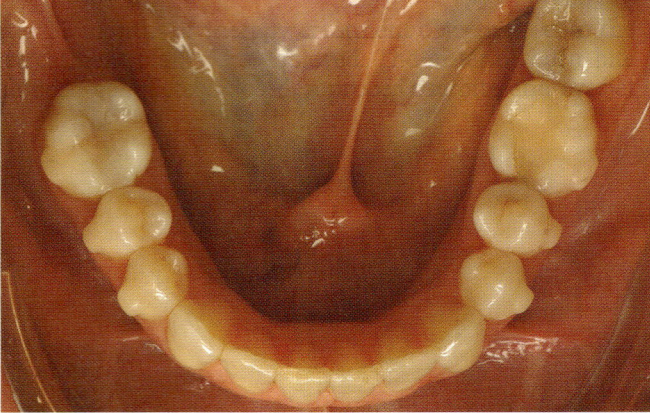

Fig. 15.9 Intraoral pictures after 10 months showing many small spaces due to the semisequential distalization.

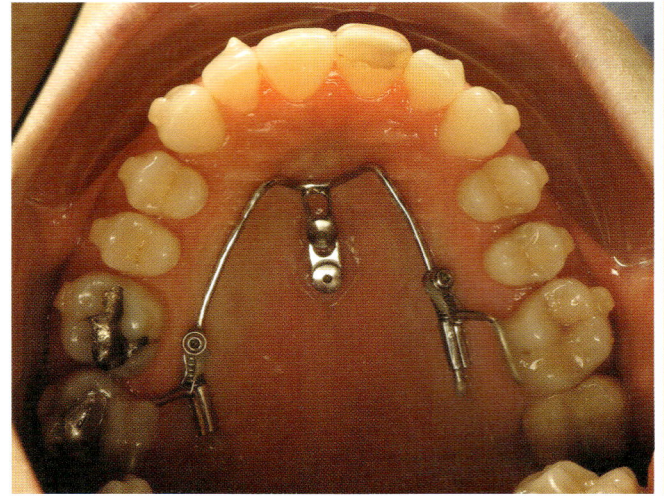

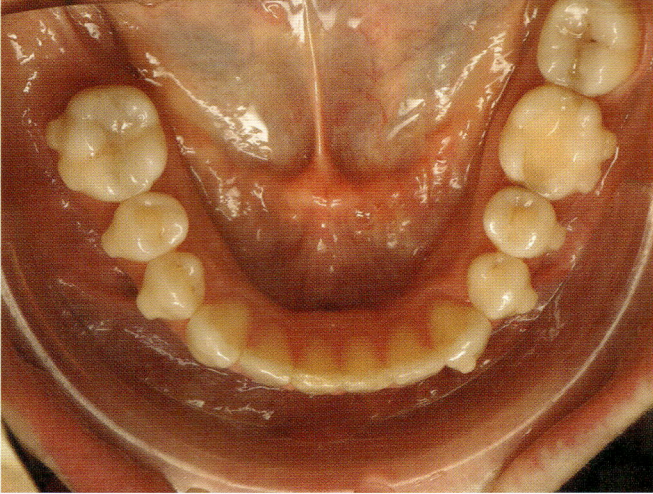

Fig. 15.10 Intraoral pictures after 12 months. Molars are distalized in a Class I occlusion The Beneslider is modified into a molar anchorage device by two steel ligatures, which are deactivating the Beneslider. From this moment, bicuspid, canine, and incisor retractions are following.

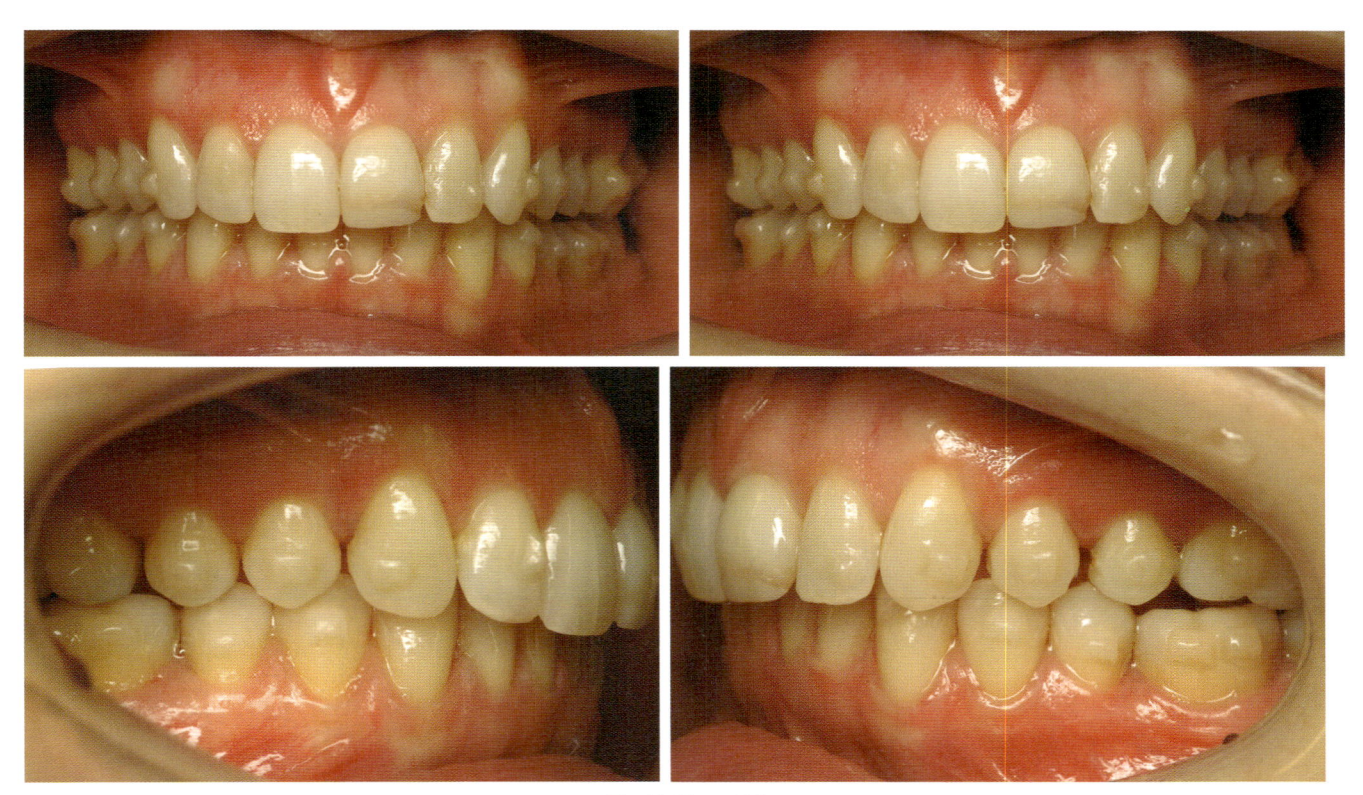

15 • Noncompliance Upper Molar Distalization and Aligner Treatment for Correction of Class II Malocclusions 197

Fig. 15.10, cont'd

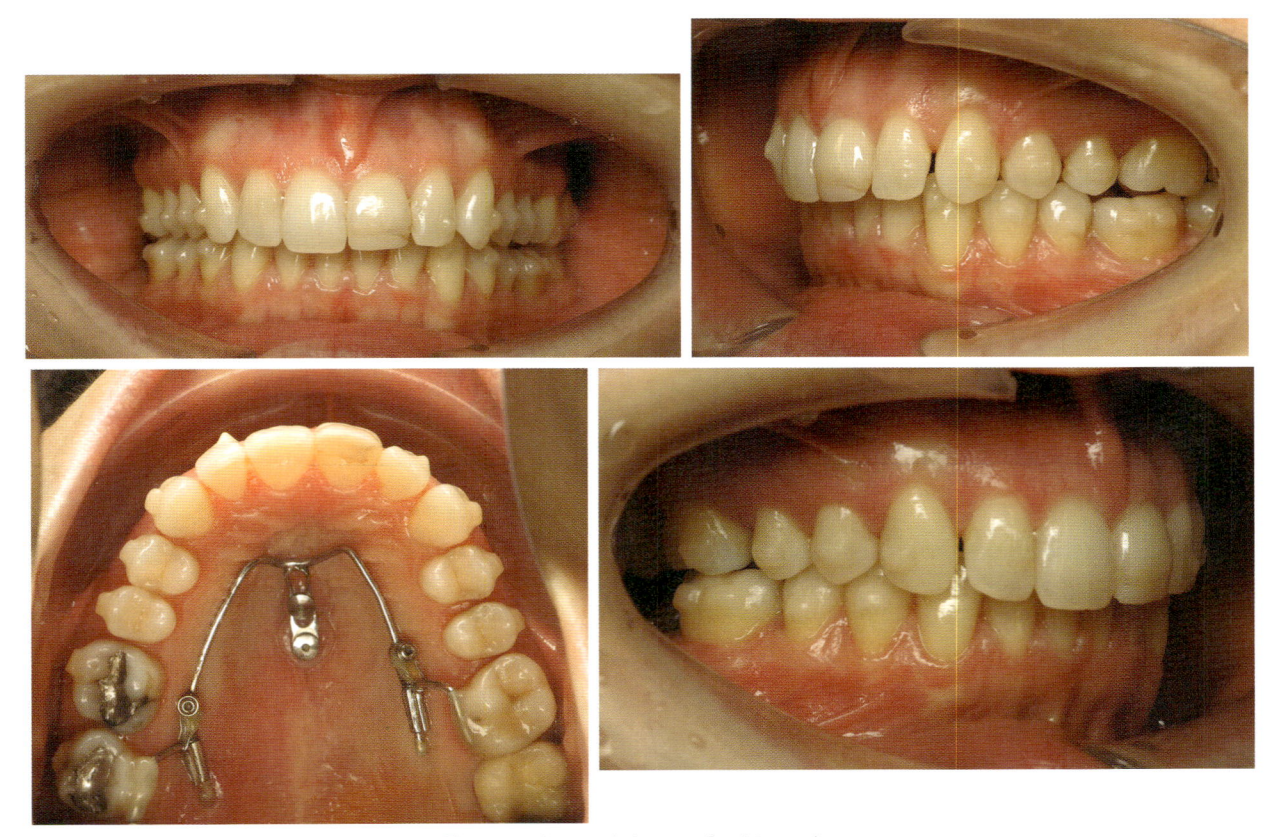

Fig. 15.11 Intraoral pictures after 14 months.

Continued

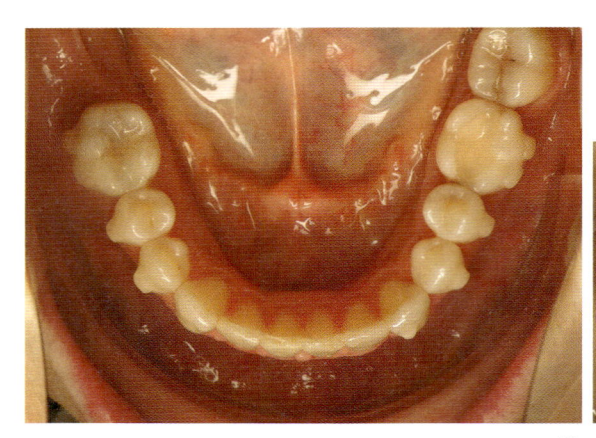

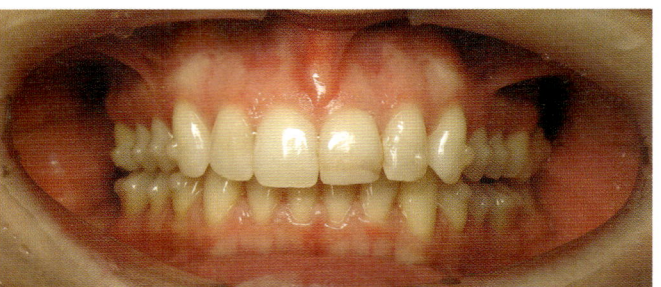

198 Principles and Biomechanics of Aligner Treatment

Fig. 15.11, cont'd

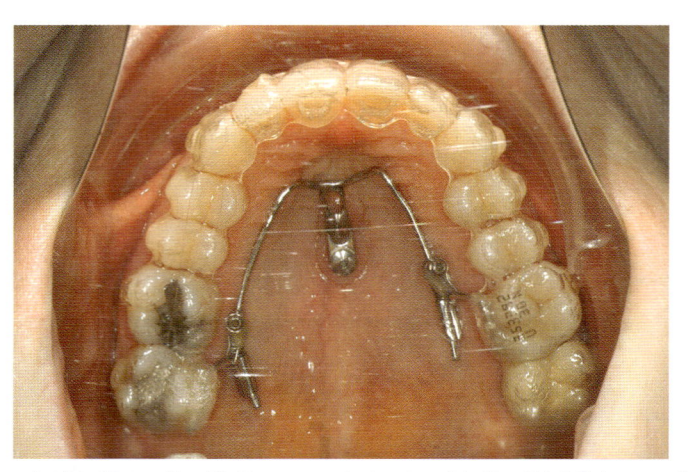

Fig. 15.12 Upper arch after 15 months. All spaces were to be closed to the distal. Subsequently, the Beneslider was removed for refinement.

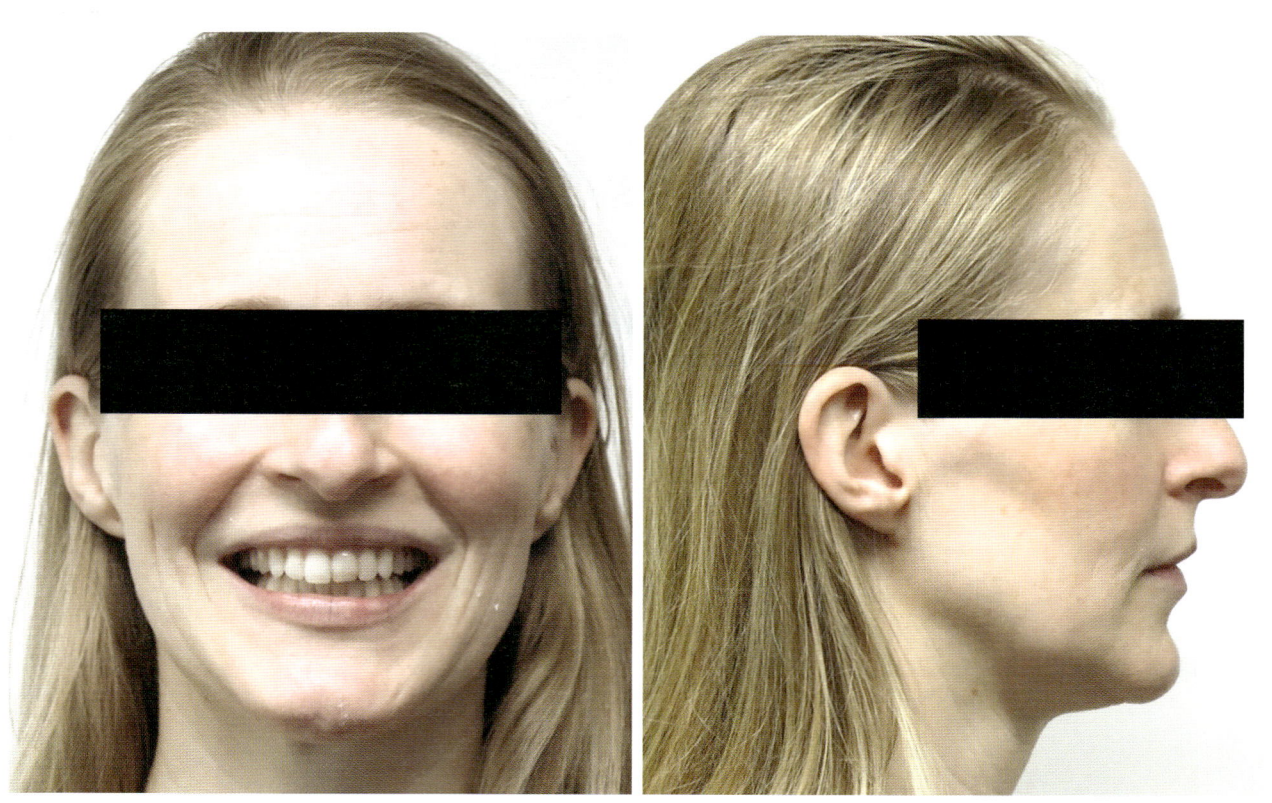

Fig. 15.13 Treatment result after 19 months.

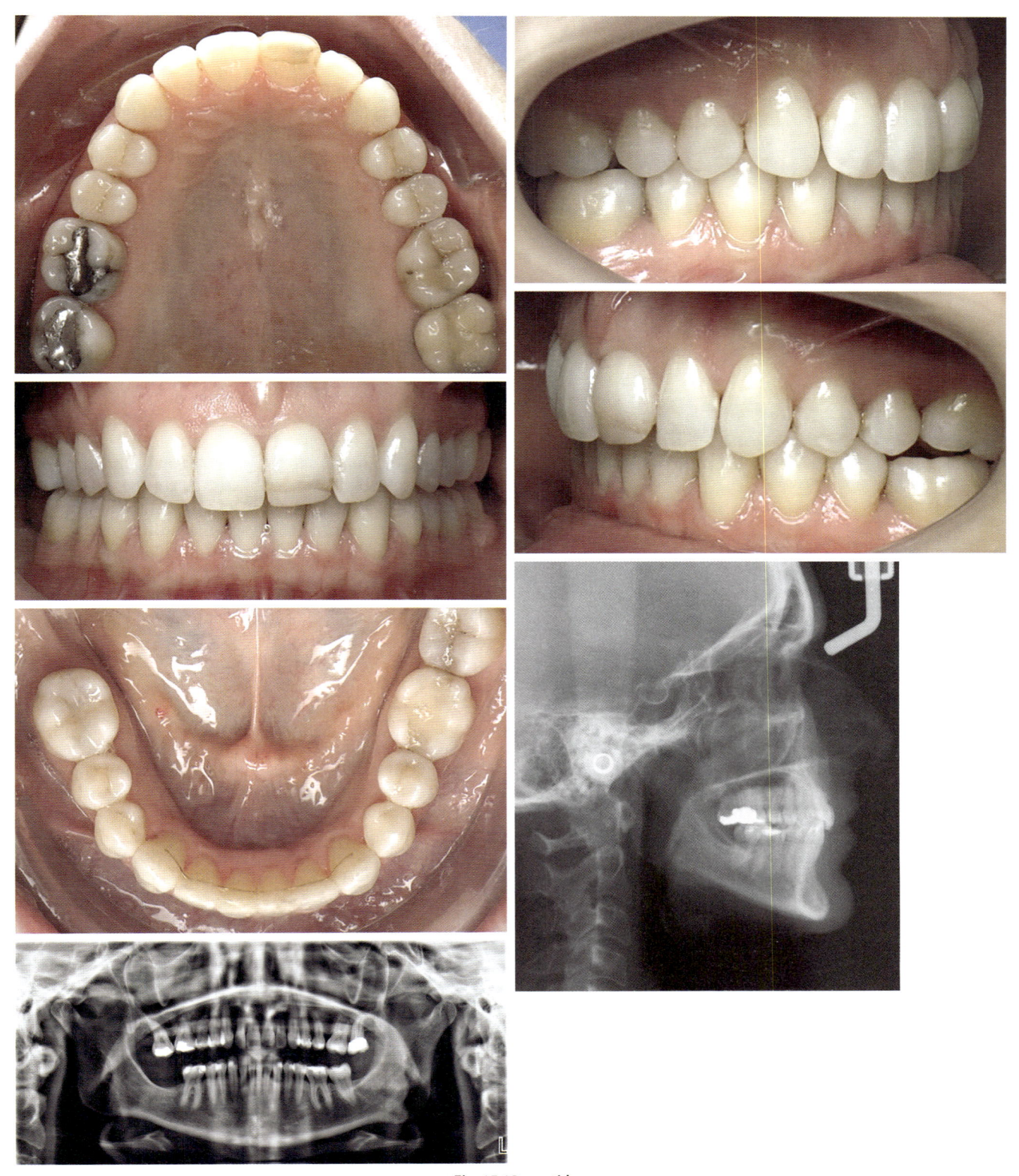

Fig. 15.13, cont'd

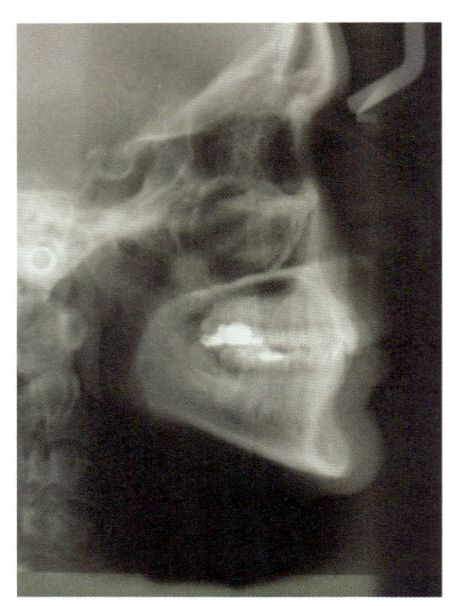

Fig. 15.14 Superimposition of before and after cephalograms (S-N). Upper incisor retraction is significant.

106.6 degrees) (Fig. 15.14), and the patient was very happy with the achieved result.

Clinical Considerations

For distalization, either a sequential step-by-step distalization or an entire maxillary arch can be chosen. In this case, a sequential distalization was chosen. The advantage of sequential distalization is the aligner fitting is probably better because all teeth are enclosed by aligner material, and therefore bodily retractions of bicuspids and canines can be achieved easier. Disadvantage is the longer treatment time, which is visible in the case shown in this chapter.

Our initial approach to combine aligner therapy and the Beneslider appliance involved a two-phase protocol: (1) distalization, and after distalization of the maxillary molar, (2) impression/scan and finishing with aligners.[17]

Advantages of this two-phase procedure are as follows:

- No need for coordination of tooth movement with Beneslider and aligners
- An expected requirement for fewer aligners to achieve treatment objectives

A disadvantage of the two-phase procedure is:

- An expected increased treatment time

The potential drawback of the one-phase method is the coordination between the Beneslider appliance and planned aligner tooth movements. If the distalization force and/or the rate of distal molar movement are excessive compared to the aligner staging, the fit and accuracy of the aligner may be undermined with the appearance of maxillary interdental spacing. A second factor to be considered is the possibility of insufficient aligner wear by the patient. If this is recognized during active treatment, the rate of distalization may be reduced or the wear time of on aligner may be prolonged (e.g., wearing each aligner for 2 weeks instead of one). The rate of the maxillary molar distal movement associated with the use of a Beneslider appliance is approximately 0.6 mm per month[19]; this rate of molar distalization speed should be kept in mind when determining the appropriate aligner staging (ClinCheck).

The distalization force can be directly applied to the first or second molar teeth. To achieve a maximum retention with the teeth that are to be moved distally, we recommend bonding the Beneslider to the first molar teeth instead of the second molars. If the distalization forces are applied to the second molars and the aligner fitting at the second molars is not perfect, small unexpected spaces can develop in between the upper first and second molar teeth. In this situation, the distalization force must be reduced to regain aligner fitting.

The anterior palate has proven to be the most convenient region of the maxilla for insertion of mini-implants.[10,11] Since there are no roots, blood vessels, or nerves, the risk of a complication associated with the placement of a mini-implant is minimal. Even the penetration of the nasal cavity does not result in any problems. Recently, a CAD/CAM-manufactured insertion guide was introduced (Easy Driver, Parma, Italy), which facilitates safe and precise insertion of mini-implants in the anterior hard palate, availing the opportunity for the use of palatal implants to the less experienced clinician. Secondly, these insertion guides allow for the insertion of mini-implants and installation of the appliance in a single office visit.[20]

Conclusions

- By using palatal mini-implants and a Beneslider device, unilateral or bilateral distal tooth movement can be realized without anchorage loss and need for class II elastics.
- The Beneslider can be easily integrated in aligner therapy by using bonded tubes on the palatal surfaces.
- A combined, single-phase treatment approach with simultaneous distalization and alignment is possible.

References

1. Fortini A, Lupoli M, Giuntoli F, et al. Dentoskeletal effects induced by rapid molar distalization with the first class appliance. *Am J Orthod Dentofacial Orthop.* 2004;125:697-704; discussion 704-695.
2. Simon M, Keilig L, Schwarze J, et al. Forces and moments generated by removable thermoplastic aligners: incisor torque, premolar derotation, and molar distalization. *Am J Orthod Dentofacial Orthop.* 2014;145:728-736.
3. Simon M, Keilig L, Schwarze J, et al. Treatment outcome and efficacy of an aligner technique—regarding incisor torque, premolar derotation and molar distalization. *BMC Oral Health.* 2014;14:68.
4. Kinzinger G, Gulden N, Yildizhan F, et al. Anchorage efficacy of palatally-inserted miniscrews in molar distalization with a periodontally/miniscrew-anchored distal jet. *J Orofac Orthop.* 2008;69:110-120.
5. Aaboud M, Aad G, Abbott B, et al. Search for dark matter at [Formula: see text] in final states containing an energetic photon and large missing transverse momentum with the ATLAS detector. *Eur Phys J C Part Fields.* 2017;77:393.
6. Costa A, Raffaini M, Melsen B. Miniscrews as orthodontic anchorage: a preliminary report. *Int J Adult Orthodon Orthognath Surg.* 1998;13: 201-209.
7. Kanomi R. Mini-implant for orthodontic anchorage. *J Clin Orthod.* 1997;31:763-767.

8. Melsen B, Costa A. Immediate loading of implants used for orthodontic anchorage. *Clin Orthod Res.* 2000;3:23-28.
9. Ludwig B, Glasl B, Bowman SJ, et al. Anatomical guidelines for miniscrew insertion: palatal sites. *J Clin Orthod.* 2011;45:433-441.
10. Hourfar J, Bister D, Kanavakis G, et al. Influence of interradicular and palatal placement of orthodontic mini-implants on the success (survival) rate. *Head Face Med.* 2017;13:14.
11. Wilmes B, Ludwig B, Vasudavan S, et al. The T-zone: median vs. paramedian insertion of palatal mini-implants. *J Clin Orthod.* 2016;50:543-551.
12. Nienkemper M, Pauls A, Ludwig B, et al. Stability of paramedian inserted palatal mini-implants at the initial healing period: a controlled clinical study. *Clin Oral Implants Res.* 2015;26:870-875.
13. Wilmes B, Drescher D. A miniscrew system with interchangeable abutments. *J Clin Orthod.* 2008;42:574-580; quiz 595.
14. Wilmes B, Drescher D, Nienkemper M. A miniplate system for improved stability of skeletal anchorage. *J Clin Orthod.* 2009;43:494-501.
15. Wilmes B, Drescher D. Application and effectiveness of the Beneslider molar distalization device. *World J Orthod.* 2010;11:331-340.
16. Wilmes B, Nienkemper M, Ludwig B, et al. Esthetic class II treatment with the Beneslider and aligners. *J Clin Orthod.* 2012;46:390-398.
17. Wilmes B, Neuschulz J, Safar M, et al. Protocols for combining the Beneslider with lingual appliances in class II treatment. *J Clin Orthod.* 2014;48:744-752.
18. Wilmes B, Katyal V, Willmann J, et al. Mini-implant-anchored Mesialslider for simultaneous mesialisation and intrusion of upper molars in an anterior open bite case: a three-year follow-up. *Aust Orthod J.* 2015;31:87-97.
19. Nienkemper M, Wilmes B, Pauls A, et al. Treatment efficiency of mini-implant-borne distalization depending on age and second-molar eruption. *J Orofac Orthop.* 2014;75:118-132.
20. De Gabriele O, Dallatana G, Riva R, et al. The easy driver for placement of palatal mini-implants and a maxillary expander in a single appointment. *J Clin Orthod.* 2017;51:728-737.

16 Clear Aligner Orthodontic Treatment of Patients with Periodontitis

TOMMASO CASTROFLORIO, EDOARDO MANTOVANI, and KAMY MALEKIAN

Malocclusions Related to Periodontal Disease

There is no direct influence between malocclusion and periodontal breakdown; however, quicker progression of periodontal disease is associated with occlusal discrepancies and is reduced by occlusal treatment.[1,2] It has been demonstrated that in crowded areas plaque accumulation increases[3] and, with respect to noncrowded areas, an increased number of periopathogenic species can be found.[4] Furthermore, an altered topography of the gingiva and the alveolar bone is commonly found when teeth are crowded.[5]

There is a strict relationship between crowding and periodontitis because anterior teeth migration is enhanced by periodontal disease, leading to a further crowding in lower arch, which then hinders a proper periodontal health.[6] Sanavi demonstrated that deep bite is directly related to periodontal breakdown due to soft tissue impingement on the upper and lower incisors (Fig. 16.1).[7] Furthermore, multiple types of occlusal contacts have been associated with deeper probing depths: premature contacts in centric relation, posterior protrusive contacts, balancing contacts, combined working and balancing contacts, and length of slide between centric relation and centric occlusion.[8] Another correlation was found in mesially inclined molars where the periodontal destruction was 10% greater than that found in normally inclined teeth.[9]

Orthodontic Treatment in Patients With Periodontal Disease

Orthodontics is needed in combination with periodontal and prosthodontic treatment to treat patients with a secondary malocclusion or in whom there is aggravation of an existing malocclusion related to periodontal disease.[2] Despite the high number of published articles, there is still a lack of good evidence about many of the treatments, including orthodontics and periodontal therapy.[10]

The prevalence of pathologic tooth migration (PTM) among periodontal patients has been reported to range from 30.03% to 55.8%; periodontal bone loss appears to be the major factor in the etiology of PTM.[11] In a recent study, Khorshidi et al. found that pathologic migration prevalence was 11.4% (35/314 patients); however, there was no pathologic migration in patients with mild chronic periodontitis. PTM prevalence is increased by the severity of periodontal disease, and no statistically significant difference between males and females was found.[12]

In early stages of PTM, spontaneous correction of migrated teeth sometimes occurs after periodontal therapy. When only a light degree of pathologic migration is considered, it has been hypothesized that this is due to wound contraction during healing (Fig. 16.2).[13] Soft tissue forces of the tongue, cheeks, and lips are known to cause tooth movement and in some situations can cause PTM. The transseptal fibers play a key role in PTM by forming a chain from tooth to tooth and helping maintain contacts between teeth. If the continuity of the chain is weakened by periodontal disease, the balance of forces is upset, and displacement of the teeth can occur (Fig. 16.3).

Occlusal factors such as posterior bite collapse, shortened dental arches, occlusal interferences, and bruxism are connected to the etiology of PTM.

Patients with periodontal issues are commonly characterized by general flaring with spacing between the upper incisors, deepening of the bite (sometimes extrusion of a single tooth can occur), increased overjet, and crowding in the lower incisor region.[14] Interposition of the lower lip behind the flared incisors can worsen the situation. An orthodontic treatment provided without a proper oral hygiene can result in iatrogenic damages: Moving a tooth into an infected infrabony defect can enhance the destruction of connective tissue.[15] However, a combined ortho-perio treatment is efficient in the treatment of periodontitis and could effectively decrease the levels of inflammatory cytokines.[16] Furthermore, the treatment should aim for the patient's expectations and aesthetic goals.

Orthodontic treatment can allow the optimization of clinical situations[17] such as:

- Leveling of bone peaks
- Bringing a tooth back to the alveolar ridge
- Implant site preparation

Orthodontic treatment is indicated when the worsening of periodontal status can be promoted by tooth malposition such as:

- Severe tooth crowding
- Premature contacts
- Severe deep bite associated with direct trauma on periodontal tissues
- Mesial inclination of molars associated with angular bony defect

Orthodontic treatment is mandatory when:

- The periodontal disease has caused PTM and abnormal tooth mobility.
- A previous orthodontic therapy made with unskillfulness has created further periodontal tissue damage.

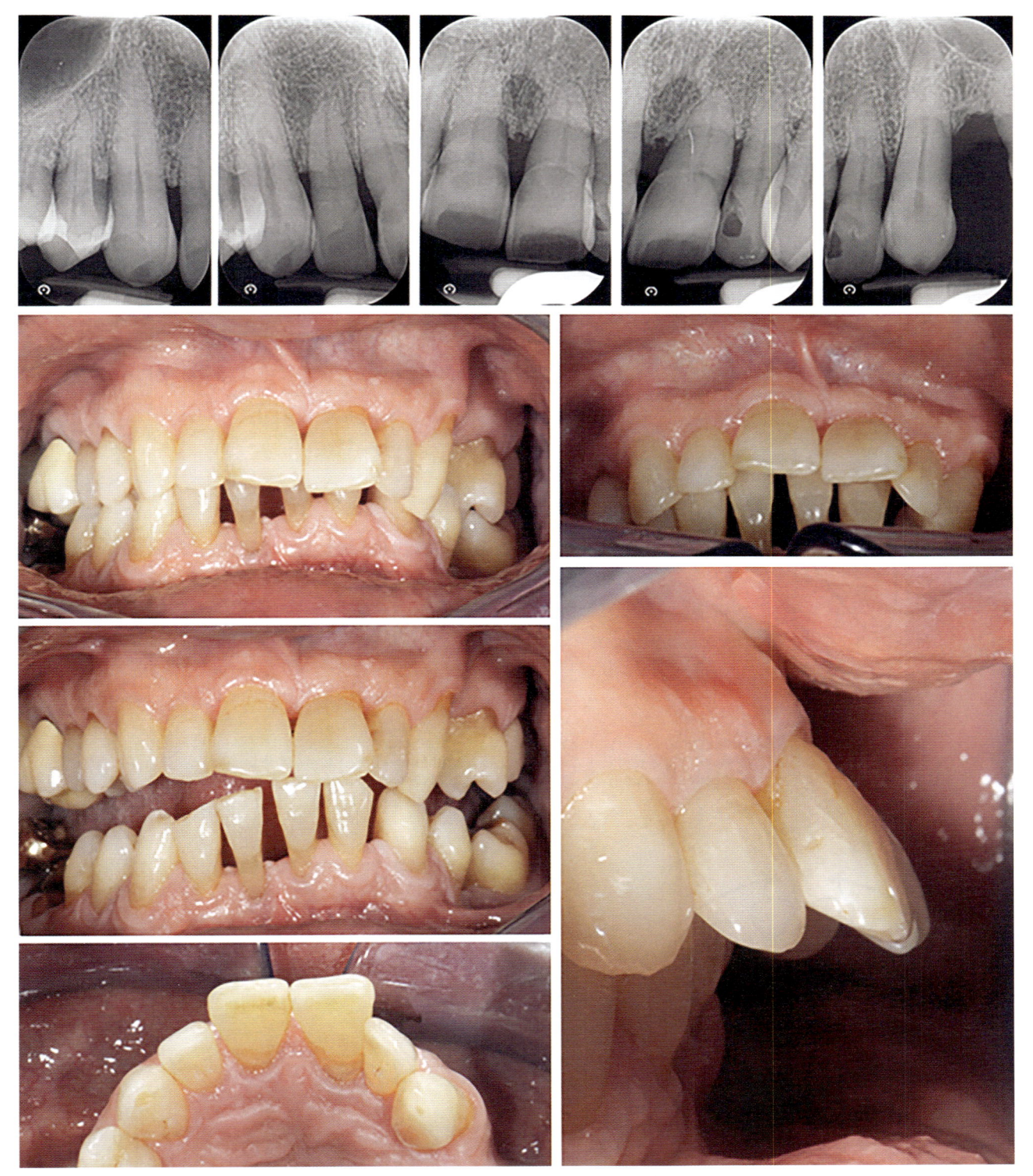

Fig. 16.1 Pathologic tooth migration in an old man.

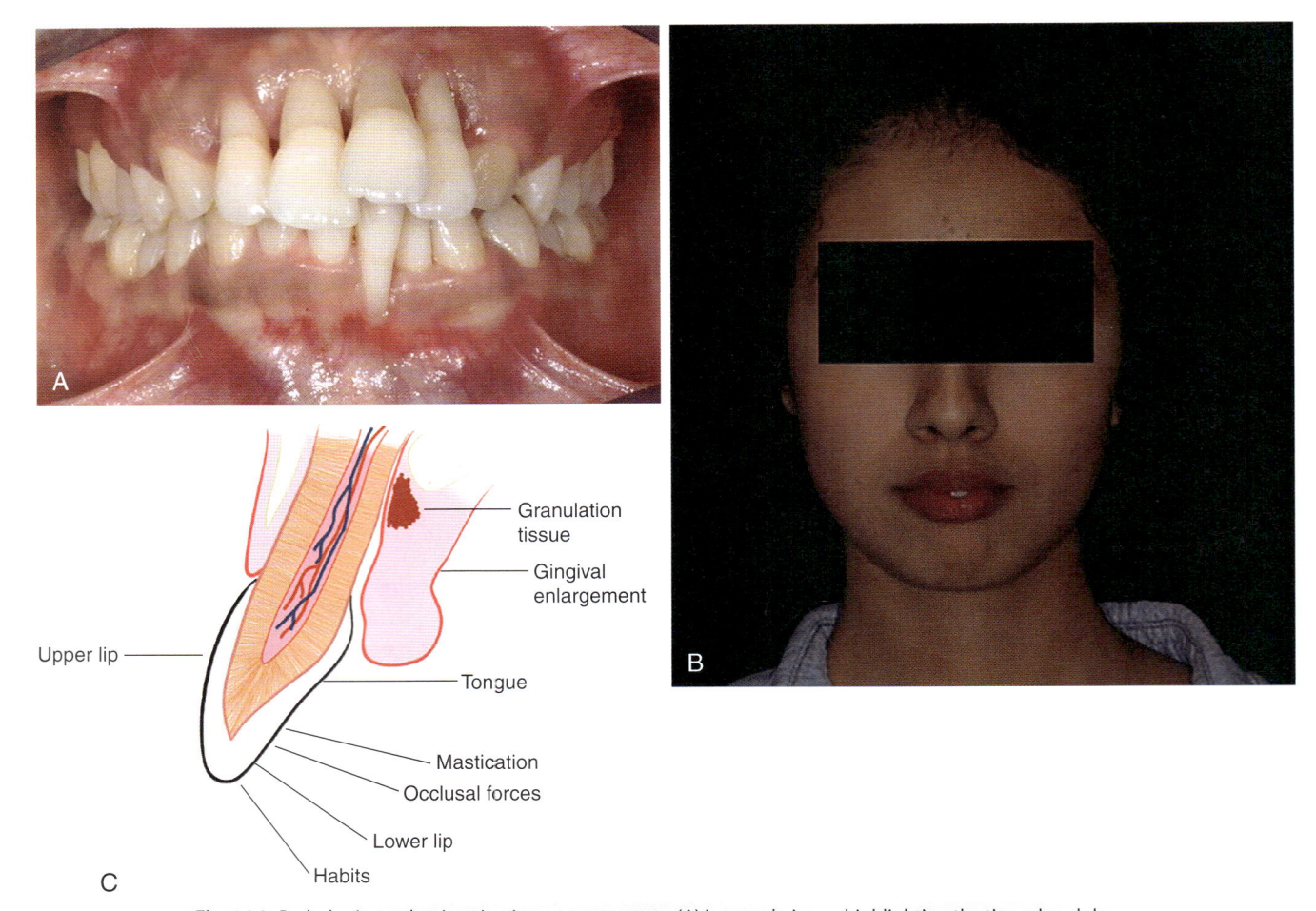

204 Principles and Biomechanics of Aligner Treatment

Fig. 16.2 Pathologic tooth migration in a young woman. (A) Intraoral picture highlighting the tissue breakdown. (B) Extraoral picture (please note the position of element 2.1). (C) Scheme representing tissue breakdown. (From Brunsvold MA. Pathologic tooth migration. J Periodontol. 2005;76[6]:859-866. doi:10.1902/jop.2005.76.6.859.)

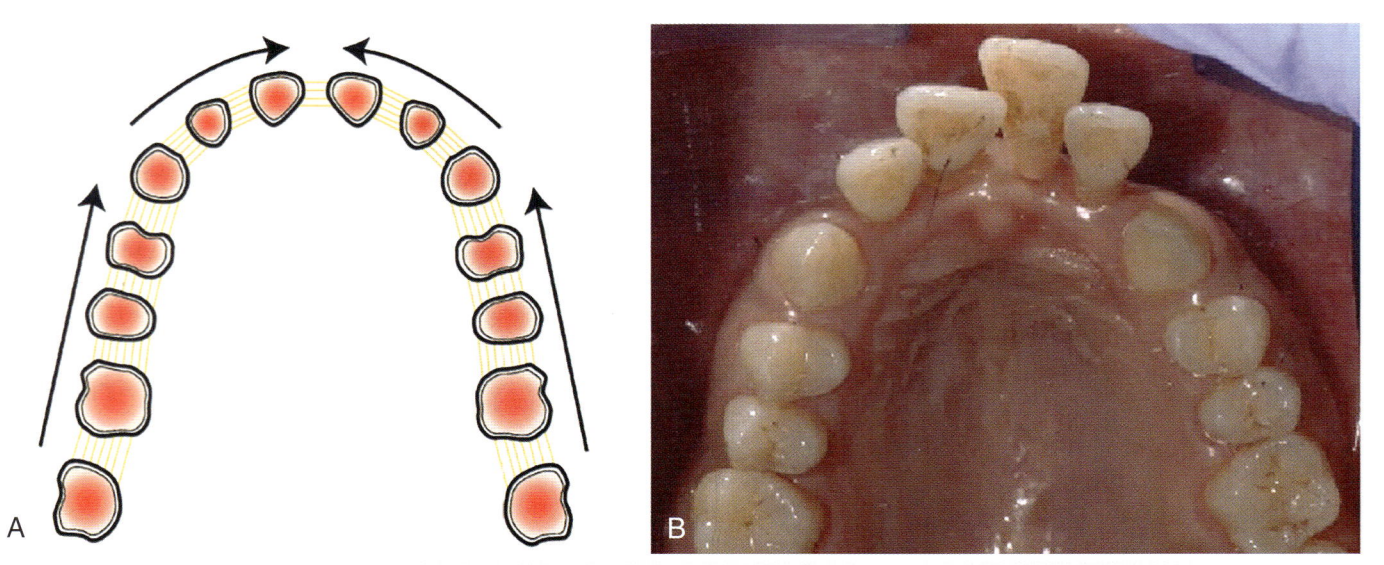

Fig. 16.3 Transseptal fibers balance loss and pathologic tooth migration. (A) Scheme from Brunsvold MA. Pathologic tooth migration. (B) Occlusal view of the patient of figure 16.2. *J Periodontol*. 2005;76[6]:859-866. doi:10.1902/jop.2005.76.6.859.)

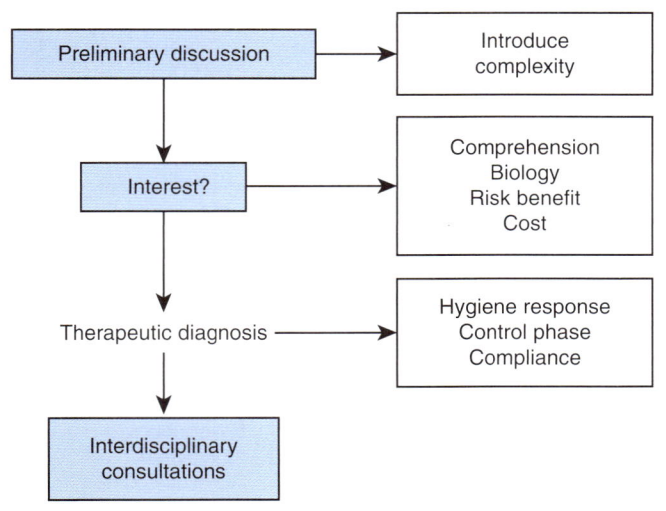

Fig. 16.4 Preliminary evaluation of an ortho-perio patient. (From Nanda R. *Esthetics and Biomechanics in Orthodontics*. 2nd ed. St. Louis, MO: Elsevier; 2015:500.)

Diagnosis and Treatment Planning

PATIENT EXPECTATIONS

A very careful consideration of the patient's chief complaint is due in order to clearly determine the patient's needs and plan realistic treatment goals.[18] These objectives generally should be economically, occlusally, periodontally, and restoratively realistic.[17] The preliminary periodontal assessment is a fundamental screening process during which adherence to issues of home oral hygiene and regular appointment attendance is determined (Fig. 16.4).[19]

MULTIDISCIPLINARY TEAM

Since several skills and knowledge are needed to provide full treatment planning, in addition to a periodontist and an orthodontist, a restorative dentist, prosthodontist, and oral or maxillofacial surgeon can be involved. The importance of the team approach in achieving the best possible results in the management of adult orthodontic patients with bone loss cannot be overstated.[20] In this phase, good communication between specialists is mandatory, and roundtable discussion is required to discuss complicated cases.[21]

PERIODONTAL ASSESSMENT

Main concept: orthodontic tooth movement without preexisting inflammation.

Periodontitis is characterized by microbially associated, host-mediated inflammation that results in loss of periodontal attachment. The bacterial biofilm formation initiates gingival inflammation and promotes tissue breakdown (Tables 16.1 and 16.2).[22]

The primary goal is to eliminate periodontal disease and stabilize the dentition. The clinical and radiologic assessments of the periodontal situation are mandatory before treatment planning. Assessment also enables the identification of recessions, horizontal bone loss, and lesions such as crater defects (one-, two-, and three-wall defects and furcation defects).

Limiting factors are:

- Periodontal pockets >4 mm
- Plaque index and bleeding on probing >10%
- Thin-scalloped gingival biotype
- Diabetes out of control
- Smoking >10/day
- Severe tooth mobility

Prior to orthodontic treatment, the following can be performed:

- Oral hygiene motivation
- Prophylaxis or therapy to control inflammation
- Surgery to eliminate deep pockets
- Augmentation of attached gingiva
- Frenectomy
- Elimination of gingival clefts

It is mandatory that the orthodontist and periodontist discuss the management of periodontal issues and plan the correction.[23]

Patients with a malocclusion may present with preexisting mucogingival problems or fragile periodontal support that is susceptible to attachment loss during or after orthodontic treatment (Fig. 16.5).[24] A proper amount of attached gingiva is needed to dissipate the mechanical trauma induced by mastication and tooth brushing. If teeth are inside the alveolar ridge, predictable soft tissue grafting

Table 16.1 Framework for Staging and Grading of Periodontitis

		DISEASE SEVERITY AND COMPLEXITY OF MANAGEMENT			
		Stage I: Initial Periodontitis	Stage II: Moderate Periodontitis	Stage III: Severe Periodontitis With Potential for Additional Tooth Loss	Stage IV: Advanced Periodontitis With Extensive Tooth Loss and Potential for Loss of Dentition
Evidence or risk of rapid progression, anticipated treatment response, and effects on systemic health	Grade A				
	Grade B		Individual Stage and Grade Assignment		
	Grade C				

Table 16.2 Periodontitis Stage

PERIODONTITIS STAGE		Stage I	Stage II	Stage III	Stage IV
Severity	Interdental CAL at site of greatest loss	1–2 mm	3–4 mm	≥5 mm	≥5 mm
	Radiographic bone loss	Coronal third (<15%)	Coronal third (15%–33%)	Extending to mid-third of root and beyond	Extending to mid-third of root and beyond
	Tooth loss	No tooth loss due to periodontitis		Tooth loss due to periodontitis ≤4 teeth	Tooth loss due to periodontitis of ≥5 teeth
Complexity	Local	Maximum probing ≤4 mm Mostly horizontal bone loss	Maximum probing depth ≤5 mm Mostly horizontal bone loss	In addition to stage II complexity: Probing depth ≥6 mm Vertical bone loss ≥3 mm Furcation involvement class II and III Moderate ridge defect	In addition to stage III complexity: Need for complex rehabilitation due to: Masticatory dysfunction Secondary occlusal trauma (tooth mobility ≥2) Severe ridge defect Bite collapse, drifting, flaring <20 remaining teeth (10 opposing pairs)
Extent and Distribution	Add to stage as descriptor	For each stage, describe extent as localized (<30% of teeth involved), generalized, or molar/incisor patter			

CAL, Clinical attachment level.

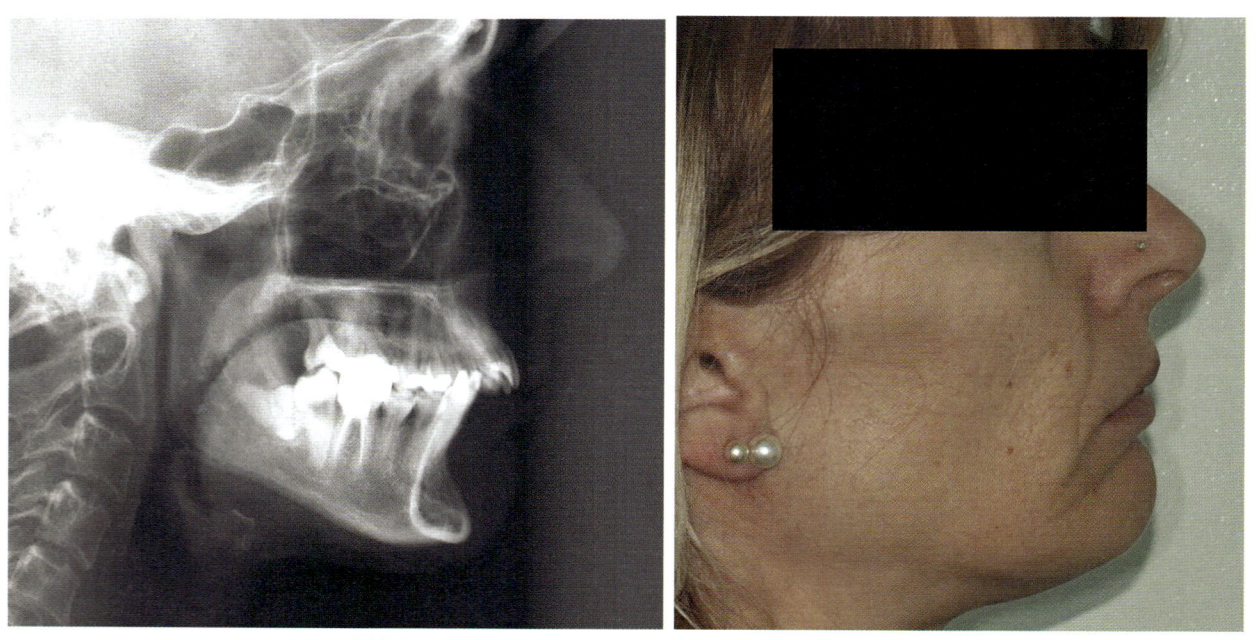

Fig. 16.5 In this class II adult patient, incisors are crowded, extruded, and proclined. Soft and hard tissue grafting can be helpful before orthodontic treatment to prevent the development of recessions.

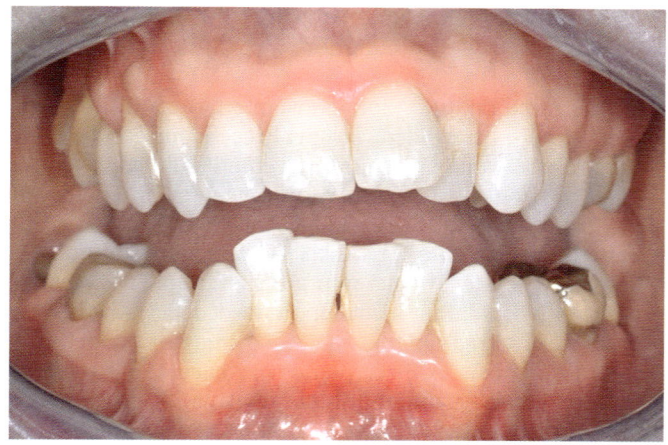

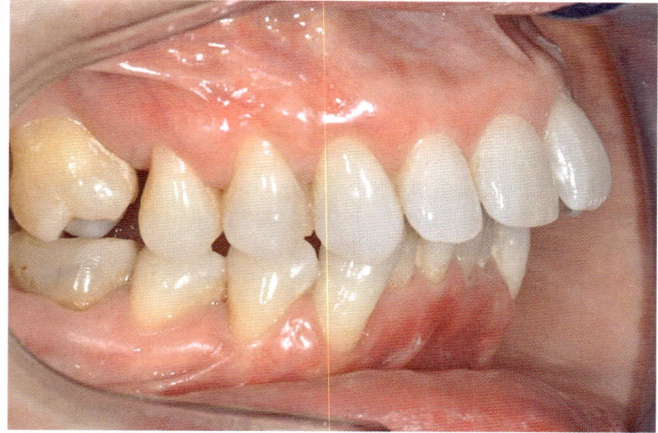

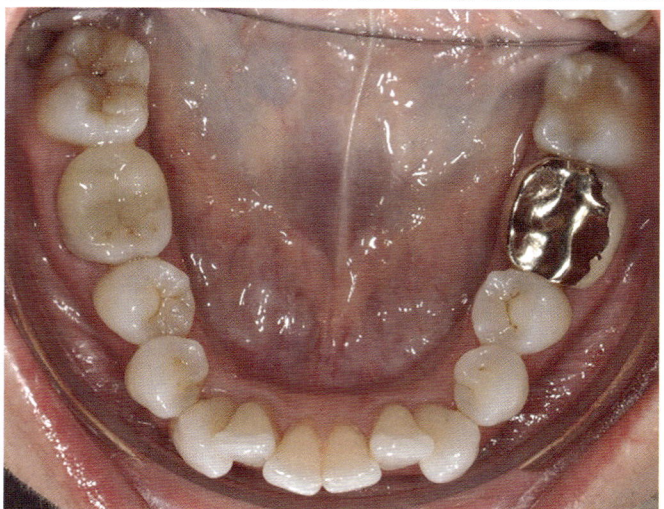

Fig. 16.5, cont'd

procedures such as the subepithelial connective tissue graft (SCTG) and the free gingival graft (FGG) may be performed prior to tooth movement to prevent gingival recession.[25]

In a systematic review, Kloukos et al. investigated the indication and timing of soft tissue augmentation in orthodontic patients. No randomized controlled trial was identified, and only limited data were available.[26] Furthermore, osseous defects cannot allow many adult patients to clean teeth adequately and require correction prior to or during orthodontic therapy. These osseous defects include interproximal craters; one-, two-, and three-wall defects; furcation defects; and horizontal defects. Interproximal craters are two-wall defects, where attachment loss occurs on the mesial and distal surfaces of the adjacent roots and the remaining walls are the buccal and lingual ones. Orthodontic movement cannot improve interproximal craters; if the crater is mild to moderate, then resective surgery and bone recontouring should be executed.

In one-wall defects, there has been destruction of three of the four interproximal walls, leaving one wall remaining. These defects are difficult for a periodontist to manage because resection could be too destructive and regeneration is inappropriate. Orthodontic eruption of the tooth can eliminate the defect associated with occlusal reduction.[27]

Three-wall defects must be treated prior to orthodontics with regenerative therapy.[28] A provisional splinting of the teeth undergoing periodontal surgery is needed to provide stabilization. Roccuzzo et al. demonstrated that the enamel matrix derivative (EMD) alone and in association with various grafts give the best results for the treatment of intrabony defects, with improvements in terms of clinical attachment level (CAL) gain and pocket depth (PD) reduction. In this study, the orthodontic treatment was initiated 8 to 12 months after guided tissue regeneration (GTR) procedures and aimed at correcting malposition, creating contact points, and providing nontraumatic occlusion.[29]

Since the fibroblastic and osteoblastic turnover is necessary to heal the defect before moving the adjacent teeth, the timing of orthodontic treatment after regenerative therapy is still debated.[30-32] Sanz et al. recommended waiting to begin orthodontic therapy until at least 6 months after the completion of periodontal regenerative therapy to carry out the movement in fully healed sites.[33]

Furcation defects are typically divided into three classifications: class 1, 2, or 3. Class 1 furcation defects are usually monitored during orthodontic therapy. Class 2 and 3 furcation defects should be treated by the periodontist before the orthodontic treatment to allow a proper hygiene.

Sometimes, if the periodontal health of adjacent teeth can be maintained, hopeless teeth are used during orthodontic treatment to provide anchorage and occlusal function for the patient.

The orthodontist must evaluate the horizontal bone loss because there is an alteration of crown/root ratios. If horizontal bone loss has occurred in only one area, reduction of crown length will avoid the creation of bony defects between adjacent teeth after leveling.

During orthodontic treatment, the following can be performed:

- Prophylaxis and plaque removal every month to control inflammation
- Surgical exposure of impacted teeth according to periodontal concepts
- Fibrotomy every 10 days during forced eruption

After orthodontic treatment, the following can be performed:

- Supportive therapy
- Clinical crown lengthening
- Gingivoplasty
- Root coverage

ORTHODONTIC ASSESSMENT: DETERMINATION OF FINAL OCCLUSION

Dental history in adult patients should not be overlooked and, along with restorative requirements, is a key factor in determining the final occlusion. A specific evaluation of parafunctional habits, temporomandibular disorders, cracked teeth, and wear facets is mandatory (Table 16.3). Particular focus is on the following:

- Tooth movements within bone limits
- Oval-shaped roots (buccolingual dimension wider than the mesiodistal dimension)
- Presence of fremitus
- Evaluation of tongue pressure

CONSIDERATIONS

- Evaluate teeth with intact or reduced periodontal support.
- Prevent plaque buildup (avoid fixed appliances).

Table 16.3 Orthodontic Movements And Malocclusion Features

Issues	Goals
Crowding	Alignment
Flaring	Closure of diastemas and retraction, intrusion
Black triangles	Reshaping by interproximal reduction, retraction, intrusion
Bone peaks and gingival margins need leveling	Intrusion/extrusion
Removal of occlusal interference	Retraction and intrusion, selective grinding
Worn/lost teeth	Prosthetic rehabilitation/space closure
Prevention of relapse	Retention

- Avoid excessive ridge expansion.
- Avoid excessive proclination.

Every orthodontic tooth movement beyond the cortical plate should be avoided. Gingival recessions can be related to excessive expansions and movements outside the alveolar bone housing (i.e., when an alveolar bone dehiscence has been created) (Fig. 16.6).[34] Vanarsdall suggested that patients with a transverse skeletal maxillomandibular discrepancy greater than 5 mm are susceptible to recessions, especially if palatal expansion is needed.[35] With the introduction of three-dimensional (3D) imaging in orthodontics, a diagnosis in three planes of space can be obtained with relative ease and minimal radiation.[36]

In a recent study on adolescent patients, an evaluation using cone-beam computed tomography (CBCT) scans before and after orthodontic alignment stated that bone thickness (BT) decreased and height from the cementoenamel junction to the alveolar crest (BH) increased significantly for the incisors and mesiobuccal root of the first molars. Arch dimensions generally increased together with tipping, and expansion related to alignment resulted in horizontal and vertical bone loss at the incisors and mesiobuccal root of the first molars. Thinner BTs and more severe crowding before treatment increased the risk for buccal bone loss.[37] As extraction may worsen the soft tissue profile, especially in adult patients, protraction of the lower incisors is an alternative dealing with cases of lower crowding or increased overjet. A beneficial effect on the soft tissue profile through smoothing of the mentolabial sulcus can be achieved, but the optimal position of the lower incisors is still not clear.

No association between proclination and gingival recession has been found by Artun and Grobéty,[38] while others consider lower incisor proclination a risk.[39] Diedrich[40] stated that the specific anatomy must be taken into consideration, such as the gingival health and the force system.

The morphology of mandibular anterior alveolus differs in hypodivergent, hyperdivergent, and norm divergent patients, but the evaluation of symphysis morphology on cephalometric radiographs might not be a solid method aimed at predicting gingival recession in the anterior region of the mandible. The relationship between periodontal status of mandibular incisors and selected cephalometric parameters has recently been investigated: the width of keratinized gingiva (WKT) was found to correlate with ANB, WITS, and symphysis length, while gingival thickness (GT) was associated with WITS and symphysis length. Both WKT and GT are regarded as significant risk factors for gingival recession.

In a recent study, no higher occurrence of gingival recession in cases of pronounced proclination of lower incisors without violating the osseous envelope of the alveolar process has been found. It can be speculated that if the gingiva maintains appropriate thickness, it is more resistant and less affected by tension from large proclination.[41] In a retrospective study, Melsen found that gingival recession on mandibular incisors was not significantly increased during orthodontic treatment. Thin gingival biotype, visual plaque, and inflammation are useful predictors of gingival recession.[42]

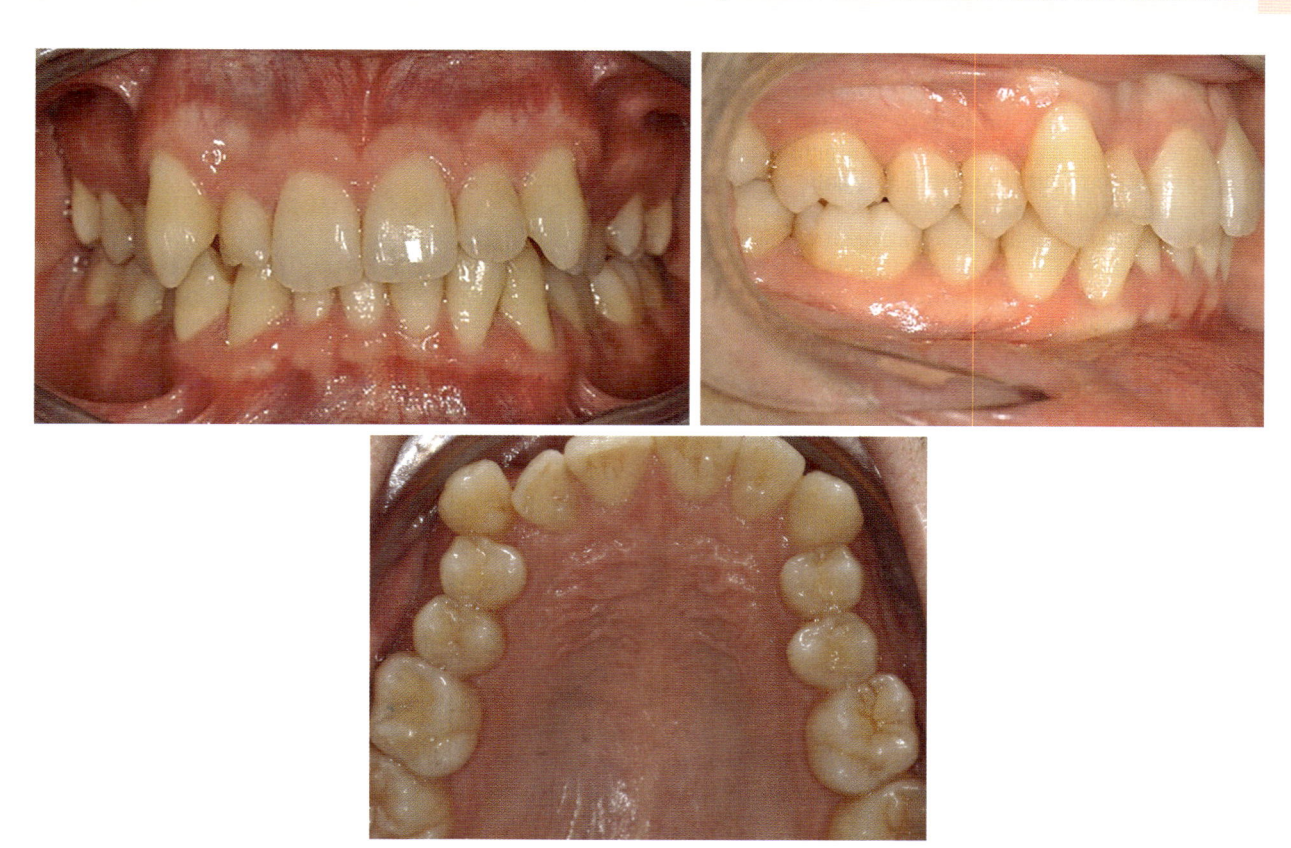

Fig. 16.6 In this adult patient, a previous excessive orthodontic expansion promoted a gingival recession on teeth 13 and 23. The occlusal instability has led to orthodontic relapse.

Teeth can be moved with their surrounding periodontium when careful attention is paid to local anatomy and periodontal health. Furthermore, tooth movement with or through bone can be provided using different force systems.[43] When an optimal oral hygiene has been achieved, it is possible to apply orthodontic forces, even if the periodontal tissue has reduced connective tissue attachment and alveolar bone height.[44,45] Traditional fixed orthodontic appliances induce microbial changes toward periodontopathogenic anaerobic bacteria because of the increased plaque accumulation.[46] These effects are normalized after removal of orthodontic appliances without lasting detrimental effects, but in some patients there is a significant risk for irreversible periodontal destruction.[47] Thus the use of clear aligners that promote a better periodontal health when compared to fixed appliances[48-50] may be the optimal choice in patients with periodontal involvement. With clear aligners, it is possible for good control of oral hygiene throughout treatment, while the first months with fixed appliances are always difficult to manage.[51]

The forces and moments generated by aligners of the Invisalign system are always within the range of orthodontic forces.[52] The forces and couples delivered by aligners are determined by the shape of the crown and the type and amount of displacement of the particular tooth and therefore the contacts between tooth and the inner surface of the appliance. Tipping movement is predictable with thermoplastic appliances, but difficulties about root control have been reported.[53]

Since the gingival margin of the aligner is elastic, it is not surprising that an aligner would have difficulty controlling the forces applied in this region. The introduction of Power Ridges demonstrates that when a torque correction of about 10 degrees is required, torque loss is negligible. The force couple generated by a thermoplastic aligner torquing an upper incisor consists of a tipping force near the gingival margin and a resulting force produced by movement of the tooth against the opposite inner surface of the appliance, near the incisal edge.[54] The undesirable mesial movement of first molar compensation requires programmed forward mesial root rotation, in effect producing crown tipback rotation.[55]

In an in vitro study, Simon et al.[56] investigated the influence of auxiliaries, such as attachments and Power Ridges, on performing root movements of upper central incisor torque. A loss of torque up to 50% must be considered; however, it must be noted that the efficacy of fixed orthodontic appliances does not reach 100% either. Conventional orthodontic brackets and wires do not completely fill the bracket slots so that the wire is able to twist, leading to a loss of moment known as torque play. The loss of torque between an arch of 0.019 × 0.025 in. section (usual size for the final stages of orthodontic treatment) and a 0.022 × 0.028 in. slot is about 10 degrees.

A more recent study stated that Invisalign is able to achieve predicted tooth positions with high accuracy in nonextraction cases.[57] Lombardo et al.[58] stated that some tooth movements can be achieved with aligners more easily than others. In particular, vestibulolingual tipping and rotation reached 72.9% and 66.8% of the prescribed movement, respectively. In a retrospective study, Sfondrini et al.[59] found no differences between aligners and brackets about buccolingual inclination control on upper incisors. These studies led to different conclusions probably because of the development and improvements in materials, technologies, and treatment protocols. Several factors are involved in determining successful tooth movement: the attachment's shape and position, the aligner's material and thickness, the amount of activation present in each aligner, and the techniques used for the production of the aligners.[60]

Treatment outcomes depend also on the patient's characteristics, bone density and morphology, crown and root morphology of teeth, as well as on factors related to the clinician such as the accuracy in performing the requested amount of interproximal reduction (IPR), which is usually underestimated.

The plastic foil used for the fabrication is thinned out by thermoforming at the gingival edge of the aligners, thus representing the area where they are less rigid. Furthermore, to avoid loss of anchorage, simultaneous movement of multiple teeth should not be performed.

Planning clear aligner therapy (CAT) with virtual setup software facilitates choosing an appropriate number of anchor teeth and the proper sequence of tooth movement to minimize the risk of anchorage loss.[61] However, an aligner alone cannot provide proper anchorage control, especially in situations in which tooth morphology is not favorable (i.e., small clinical crowns, reduced undercuts). To overcome clear aligner limitations, the development of effective attachments (rectangular and vertical), for both anchorage management and better root control, is increasing. The use of conventional bulk-fill resins for the attachment creation leads to a higher precision.[62]

The 3D planning, especially when associated with CBCT data, can allow a proper control; moreover, the velocity of movements can be selectively slow (0.12 mm/20 g/14 days). A CBCT examination is useful to evaluate the spatial position of the teeth within bone. They may be positioned off-axis and present radiographically with fenestrations and dehiscences.[24] Anticipated orthodontic treatment can improve tooth position in the bone so that mucogingival deficiencies can be subsequently reevaluated (Fig. 16.7).[63]

In periodontal patients there is interproximal bone loss, and the periodontal objectives are more valuable than the occlusal ones. The role of the orthodontist should be leveling the bone peaks. The marginal ridges are not always helpful for positioning the posterior teeth. If they are worn or abraded, it is more important to find the best position to facilitate restoration.

Tooth shape is another factor with great importance in treatment planning. In the majority of patients, we find three main tooth shapes: rectangular, triangular, and barrel-shaped teeth. Especially when the crown has a triangular shape, the distance between the bone crest and the contact point is relatively large, and the interproximal papilla tends to be absent. Tarnow demonstrated that the papilla is present in 100% of cases when the distance from the contact point to the interdental bone crest is 5 mm or less.[64] Since adults have narrower pulp chambers, IPR can be performed and black triangles closed (Fig. 16.8).

Orthodontic Movements

With a healthy periodontal tissue, the supracrestal fibers control the extrusive component of forces applied horizontally to teeth. When the bone support is reduced, forces are distributed over a smaller area, and the resistance to extrusion is lower.[65] Furthermore, the center of resistance of a periodontally involved tooth is shifted apically because of the bone resorption. That is why occlusal forces induce tipping and extrusion of the incisors. When planning the orthodontic treatment, the apical displacement of the center of resistance should be taken into account, and the moment-to-force ratio therefore must be adapted to the individual situation (Figs. 16.9 and 16.10).

To provide a uniform loading on periodontal ligament, translation and controlled tipping movements should be preferred.[66] The orthodontic treatment with clear aligners in periodontal patients should be similar to the segmented arch approach. The active and reactive units should be identified and force delivery planned 3D.

OPTIMAL CONTROL OF BIOMECHANICS

- Use of light forces
- Center of resistance
- Avoid roundtrip
- Slow movements
- Selective movements
- Need for further anchorage (implants, temporary anchorage devices [TADs]) (free anchorage lost teeth)

Taking the tooth long axis as a reference, three kinds of movement can be performed.

Mesiodistal Movements

Mesiodistal movements are mainly used to close diastemas and eliminate the black triangles, after providing IPR and the creation of a surface of contact.[66] Space opening for implant placement is a predictable movement that can be carried out both in anterior and posterior regions.[67] Surgical bone augmentation could be needed at the end of orthodontics due to high interindividual variability of neoformed bone thickness.[68]

A mesially inclined molar is not a cause of periodontal disease itself[69]; however, molars uprighting alone can be performed to achieve root parallelism before implant placement. In presence of an infraosseous defect, GTR should be executed prior to orthodontics. A strict control of oral hygiene on the distal side of an uprighting tooth is mandatory to avoid subgingival plaque formation. Additional anchorage using miniscrews may be needed in case of tricky malpositions. The mesialization of molars is a translation movement that can be performed using light forces (Fig. 16.11); however, considering the high risk of complications such as bone fenestration, bone loss, and radicular resorption, it should be managed carefully.[70]

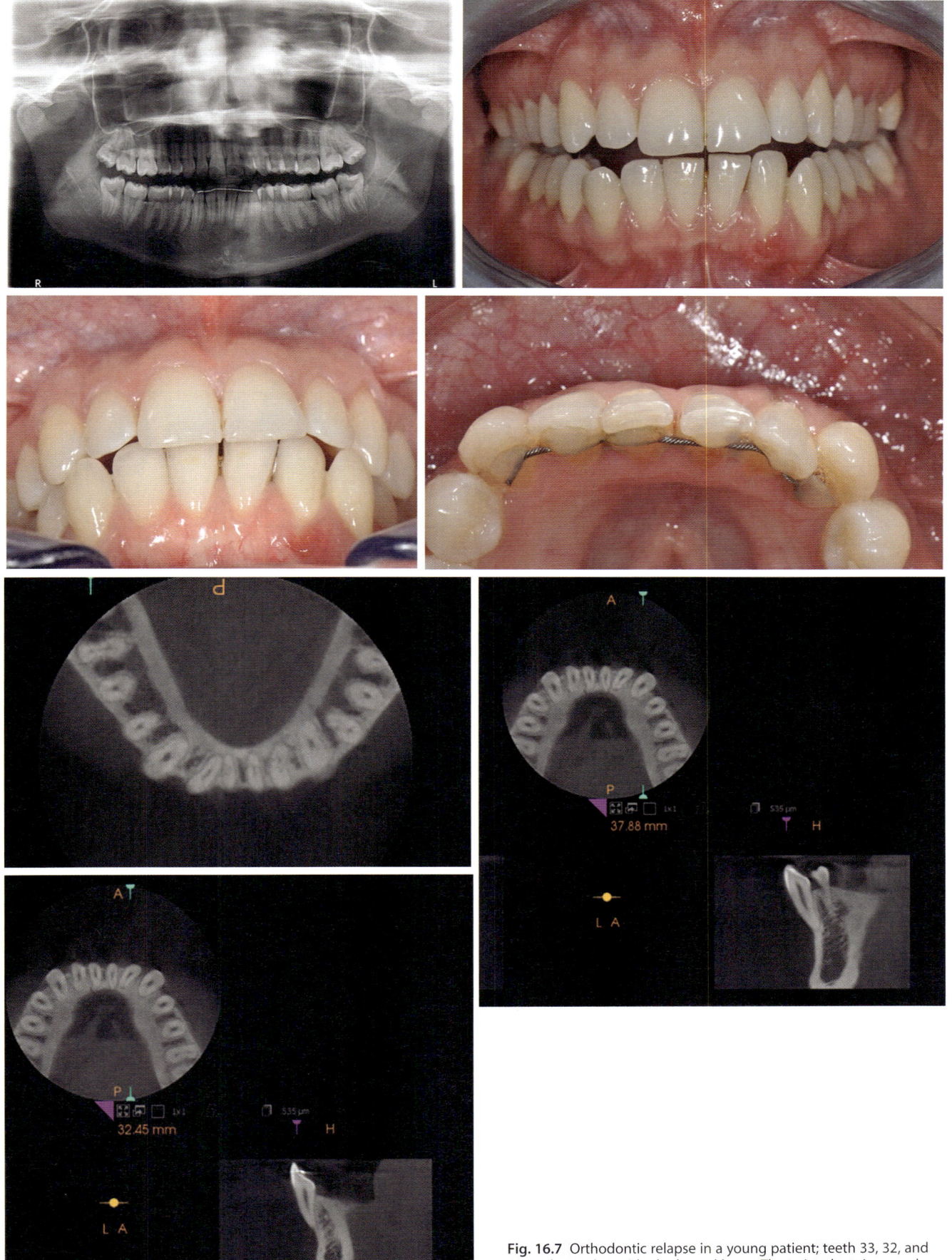

Fig. 16.7 Orthodontic relapse in a young patient; teeth 33, 32, and 43 are located outside the buccal bone. The twisted retainer, probably not passive, allowed a radicular torque movement[48] on tooth 32 that promoted a gingival recession with lack of adherent gingiva.

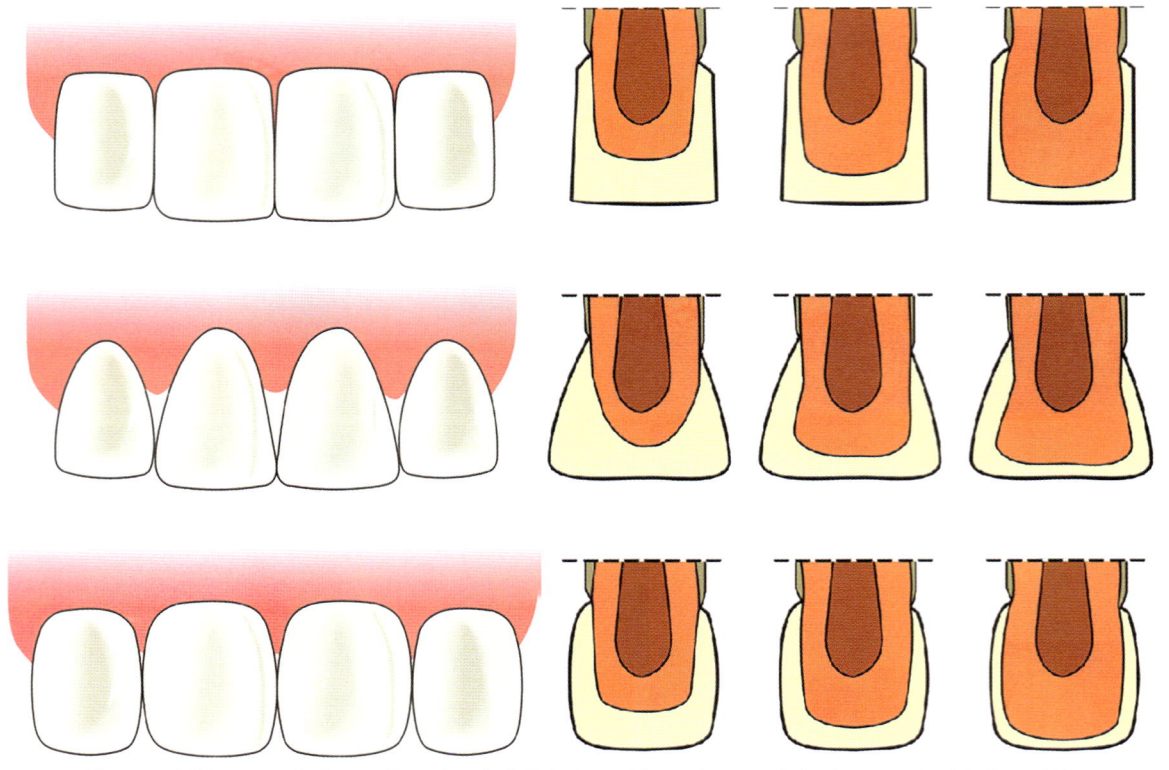

212 Principles and Biomechanics of Aligner Treatment

Fig. 16.8 Different tooth shapes. (From Nanda R. *Esthetics and Biomechanics in Orthodontics*. 2nd ed. St. Louis, MO: Elsevier; 2015:500.)

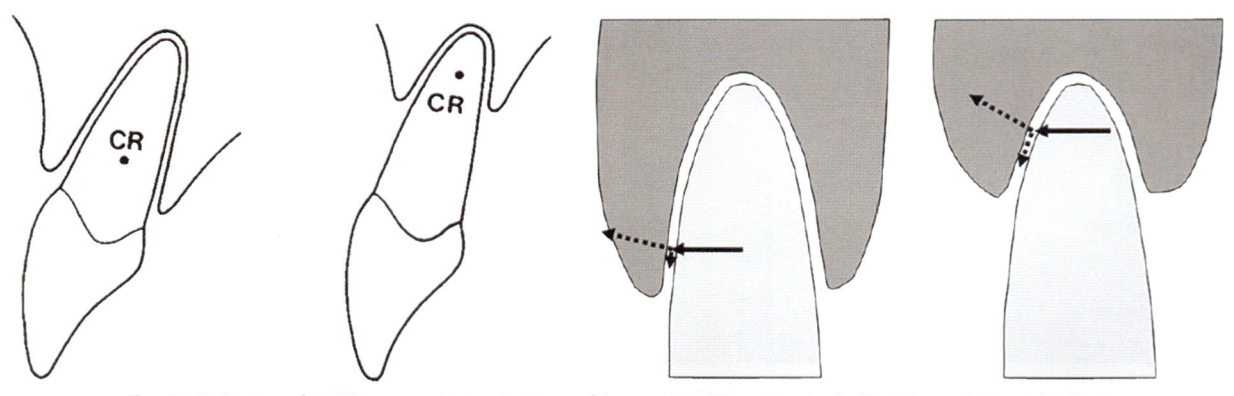

Fig. 16.9 Center of resistance variation in case of bone loss. (From Nanda R. *Esthetics and Biomechanics in Orthodontics*. 2nd ed. St. Louis, MO: Elsevier; 2015:500.)

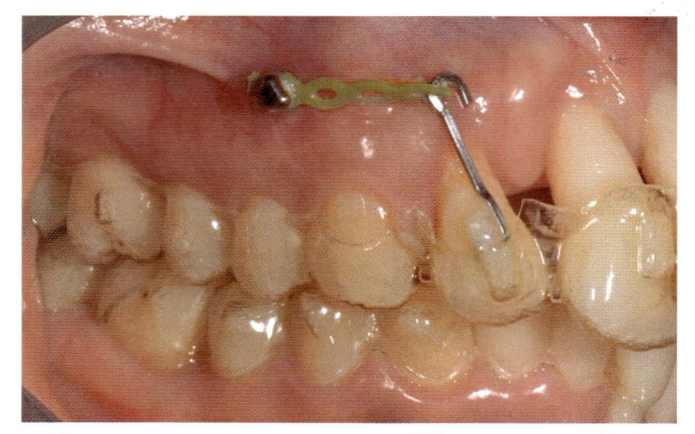

Fig. 16.10 In this patient, a stainless steel power-arm has been bonded to tooth 12, and retraction has been performed using maximum anchorage.

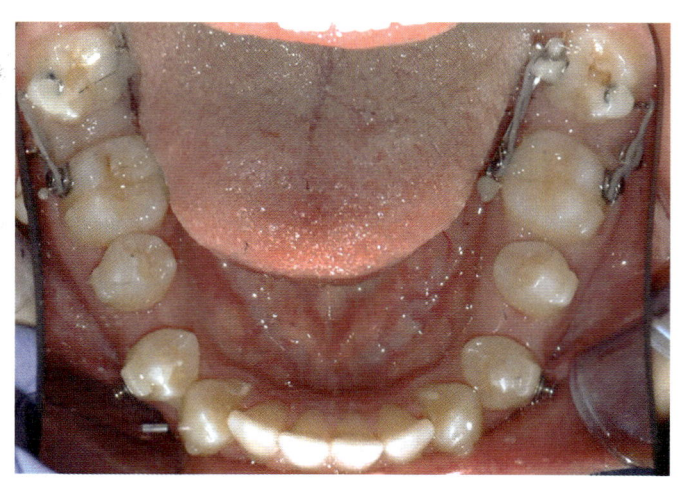

Fig. 16.11 Mesialization of lower third molars.

Vestibulolingual Movements

Vestibulolingual movements are needed to position teeth inside the alveolar bone. After a proper evaluation of bone thickness, typical localized recessions on incisors can be improved through retraction of teeth within the alveolar walls.[71]

The most effective movements, translation and lingual root torque, must be carried out on lower incisors only after a previous evaluation of mandibular symphyseal dimensions (height, depth, and angle). Orthodontics can be subsequently followed by mucogingival surgery for complete root covering.

In selected cases, bodily movements can be associated with corticotomies and bone tissue grafting to prevent further periodontal damage.[72] An efficient torque control is also needed, in combination with intrusion, during retraction of flared incisors after pathologic tooth migration.

Vertical Movements

The vertical movements are the main issue in periodontal patients since they are used to restore the correct alveolar bone and gingival margin levels. Moving a tooth with a vertical defect can increase the risk of further attachment loss. If intrusion is needed, the probing depth has to be reduced before orthodontics. Three-wall defects can be successfully treated with regenerative surgery followed by orthodontic intrusion.[73]

Intrusion is indicated when vital teeth are extruded, in both anterior and posterior regions. In an animal study, Melsen[74] demonstrated that intrusion can improve the quantity of new attachment if carried out under healthy conditions. A proper intrusive force should be 5 to 20 g per tooth and is affected by the periodontal support. Before providing vertical movements, a correct diagnosis should take into account the presence of recession and the labial sulcular depth of the maxillary incisors. If no recession has occurred, the gingival margins are used as a guide in tooth positioning.

If the sulcular depth is uniformly 1 mm, the discrepancy in gingival margins may be due to uneven wear or trauma of the incisal edges (Fig. 16.12). Treatment for this problem is the intrusion. When the gingival margins are aligned, the discrepancy in the incisal edges presents itself, and restoration of the short teeth can be provided.

Orthodontic intrusion should be planned to also properly treat lower incisors with incisal edge abrasion. These teeth typically are overerupted to maintain contact, and no space for restoration is left. Endodontic treatment and periodontal crown lengthening with bone removal are avoided by orthodontics that provides the correct restorative space.

Periodontal patients are usually characterized by flared and extruded upper incisors and horizontal bone loss.[11] A combination of retraction and intrusion is needed, while a simple retroclination would deepen the bite.[2] The available molars and premolars are used as anchorage units. Additional scaling and root planning every 2 weeks are mandatory during active intrusion.

Despite contrasting evidence about intrusion in patients with reduced periodontal support, Melsen[75] found creation of new attachment with a consequent reduction of root to crown ratio and Cardaropoli et al.[76,77] demonstrated the reduction of probing pocket depth and the gain of clinical attachment after combined ortho-perio treatment of extruded teeth with infrabony defects. The use of light (15–50 g) and continuous forces together with proper

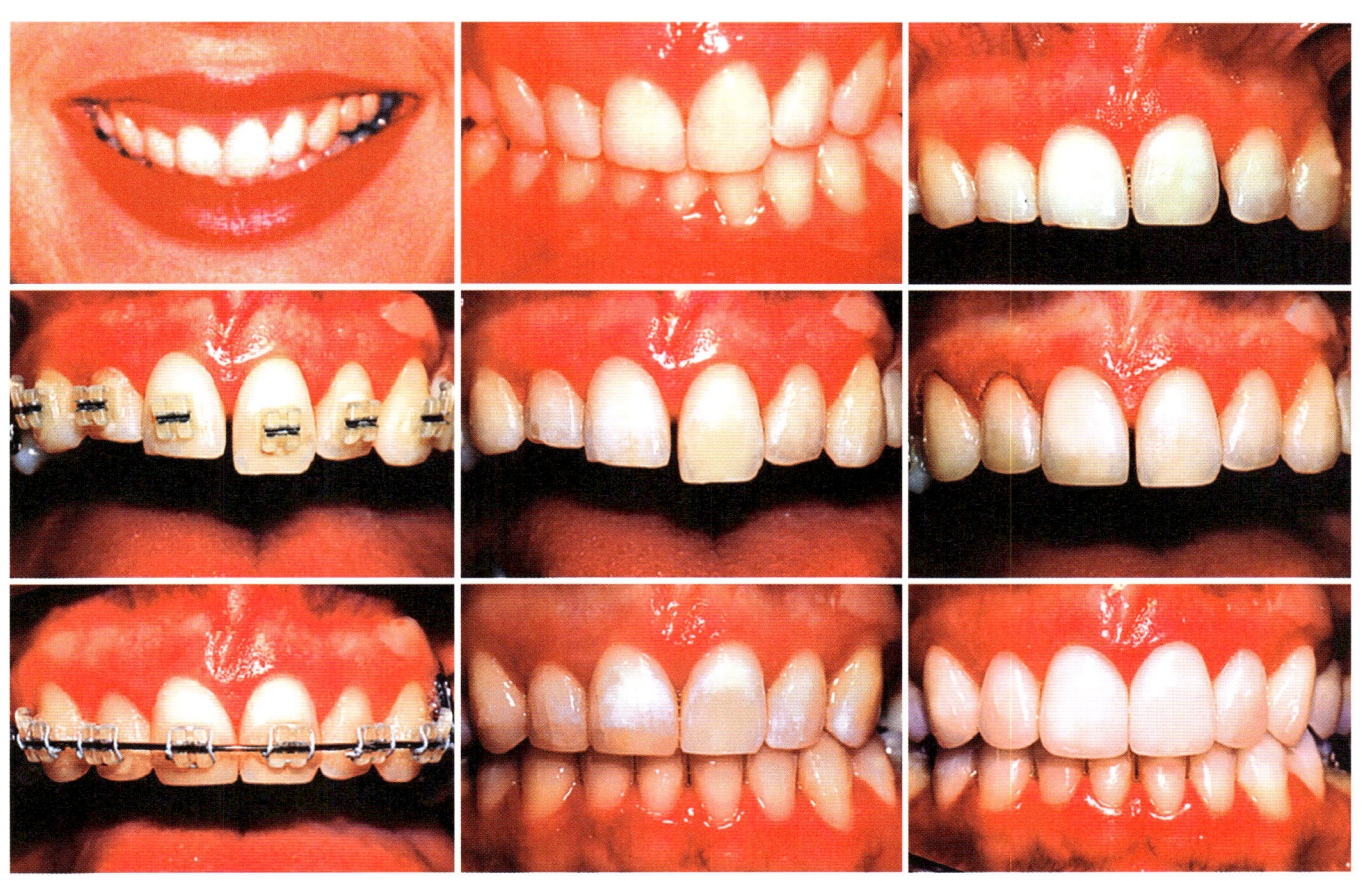

Fig. 16.12 Selective intrusion of worn teeth. (From Nanda R. *Esthetics and Biomechanics in Orthodontics*. 2nd ed. St. Louis, MO: Elsevier; 2015:500.)

torque control seems to be relevant.[78-81] Nevertheless, there can be transformation of supragingival plaque in subgingival and risk of angular defect formation.[82] Moreover, attention must be paid to root morphology, since there is a higher risk of resorption of short and pipette-shaped roots.[83]

When a periodontally involved tooth needs prosthetic rehabilitation or the gingival margin is more apical than the others, orthodontic extrusion has a beneficial effect on the bone level. Extrusion movements can be executed to level gingival margins, recover the interdental papilla, and reduce probing depth.[84] Extrusion can be performed either with light or heavy forces. Fundamentals are direction of movement and torque control because uncontrolled tipping can lead to vestibularization of the root. A constant occlusal grinding is due to avoid premature contacts. At the end of the movement, a fixed retention should be performed for at least 3 months to prevent relapse.

In case of healthy periodontium, when the crown is lost because of decay or trauma, extrusion is performed associated with fibrotomy every 10 days (or followed by surgical crown lengthening).[85] In case of attachment loss, extrusion is executed to level gingival margins and reduce angular defects. Allow 3 to 8 months for connective fibers to heal after regenerative therapy. A single compromised tooth can be extruded for leveling of gingival margins, providing hard and soft tissue augmentation before the implant placement. In this case, the use of light forces (1 mm/month) is recommended.

If a patient is missing multiple teeth, treatment plans can eventually include placement of dental implants to have a further anchorage for the orthodontics.[86] Before the orthodontic loading, a proper amount of time is needed for the osteointegration. TADs such as microscrews and bone plates are also effective in enhancing tooth movements without the biomechanical side effects.

FINAL FLOWCHART

- Reestablish periodontal health
- Periodontal reassessment
- If possible, regenerative and/or mucogingival surgery and implant placement
- Orthodontic treatment
- Periodontal maintenance/supportive therapy
- Orthodontic retention
- Prosthodontic finalization

Retention

Reduced periodontal tissues are a risk factor for orthodontic relapse.[87] In addition, the periodontally involved teeth could be significantly mobile. The purpose of retention is to stabilize them and reduce mobility. Every action that intends to prevent relapse should be performed immediately after the completion of orthodontic movement.[88]

Since the presence of retainers bonded to all anterior teeth can increase plaque accumulation and gingivitis, the use of removable retainers should be recommended when excessive mobility is not an issue.[89] Moreover, fixed retainers can produce inadvertent tooth movement, and regular observation is needed.[90] Parafunctional habits, such as onychophagia, might be involved.

The orthodontic patient with periodontal involvement may be missing one or more teeth. Since pathologic tooth migration is worsened by lack of posterior occlusal support, a final prosthetic rehabilitation should always be planned. A fixed or removable prosthesis can help stabilize the remaining teeth in the arch and provide an occlusal stop for teeth in the opposing arch.

Occlusal splint, can be eventually used as orthodontic retention in patients with parafunctional habits, including:

- Removable retainers
- When mobility is excessive:
  - Lower fixed retainer (3-3, 4-4 in case of deep bite)
  - Intra- or extracoronal fixed retainer in other sextant
- Prosthetic rehabilitation of edentulous sellae
- Occlusal night guard

Conclusions

Clear aligners are safer than conventional orthodontics for stable periodontal patients. Aligners allow patients to have excellent hygiene control, especially during long treatments. ClinCheck software is a diagnostic tool that provides a virtual setup both for orthodontics and prosthodontics. It offers a precise 3D plan control of each movement and the possibility of selective anchorage. The keys to success are based on both lifelong supportive periodontal treatment and orthodontic retention. Patient adhesion to the supportive periodontal treatment is mandatory to maintain stable long-term results.[91-93]

Clinical Case

FIRST VISIT

Date: 19-09-2016
Gender: Male
Age: 49y
Profession: Employed
Chief complaint: Bleeding gums and drifting of front teeth
Attitude: Patient is concerned about his dentition and is positive about keeping his teeth
Expectations: Patient has realistic expectations and wants to restore his dentition in health
Medical anamnesis
　　General appraisal of patient: Fit and healthy
　　Family medical anamnesis:
　　Past pathologic anamnesis: Hypertensive
　　Recent pathologic anamnesis: None
Drug therapy
Allergies or sensitivities: None
Habits: Former smoker who quit 6 months back
Occupation and stress level: Employed in a multinational company; medium stress level
Last physical examination: 6 months back, nothing significant
Dental anamnesis (Figs. 16.13 and 16.14)
Date and reason for the last dental visit: 6 months back for bleeding gums
Major dental treatments: No
Missing teeth (reason): 1.5 (caries)
Adverse dental experiences: None
History of periodontal disease: Yes
Previous periodontal treatments: Only supragingival scaling
Oral habits: None
Oral hygiene practices: Brushes twice daily with a manual toothbrush
Prophylaxis frequency: Once every year
TMJ and muscles of mastication: Both unremarkable

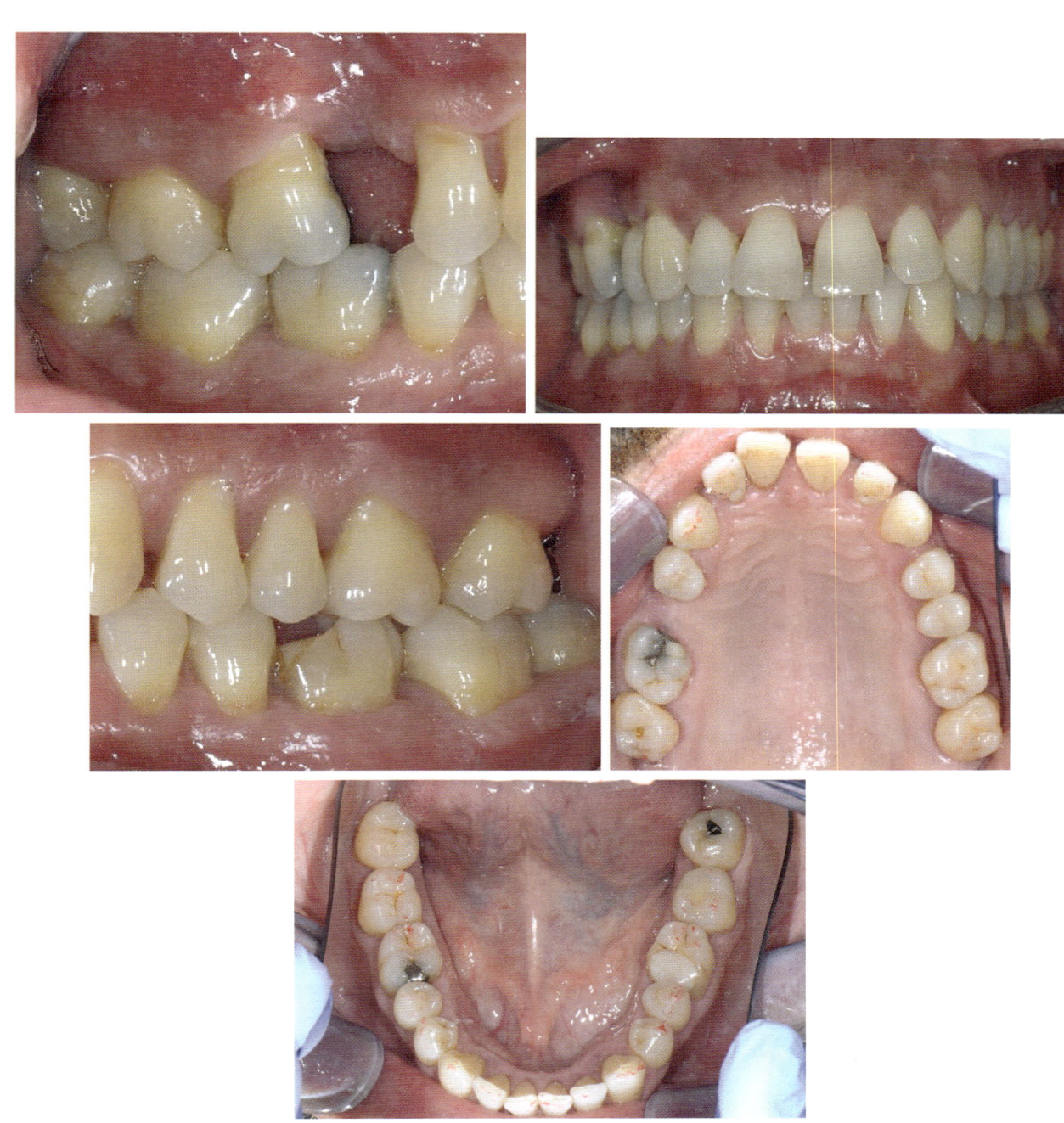

Fig. 16.13 Baseline intraoral view.

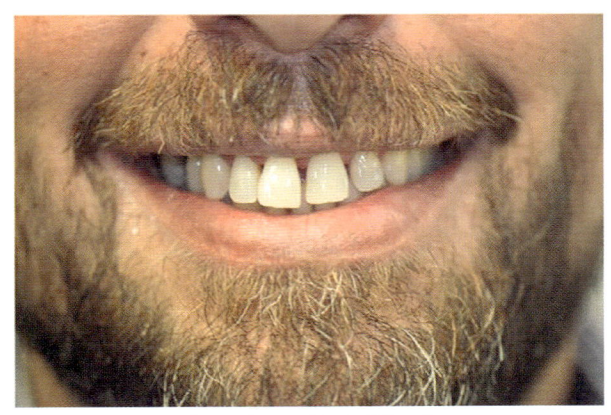

Fig. 16.14 Baseline smile.

INTRAORAL CLINICAL EXAM

Dental analysis
- Angle class: Molar and canine class 1
- Missing teeth: 1.5
- Dental malpositions: 1.1 extruded and proclined
- Decays: None
- Inadequate restorations: 3.6 premature contacts in centric occlusion: None
- Occlusal trauma: None
- Occlusal wear: None

Working contacts on right side: 1.3 (canine guided) (Fig. 16.15)
- Balancing contacts on left side: None

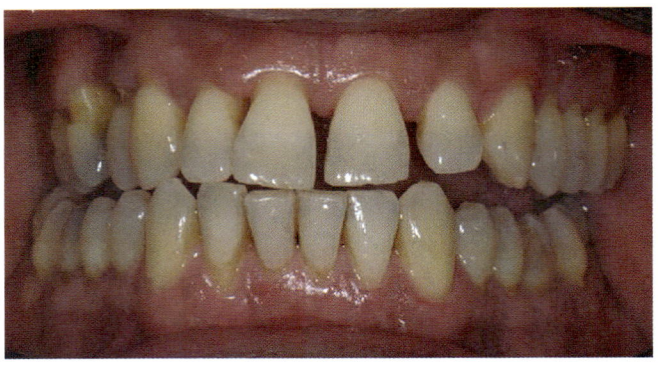

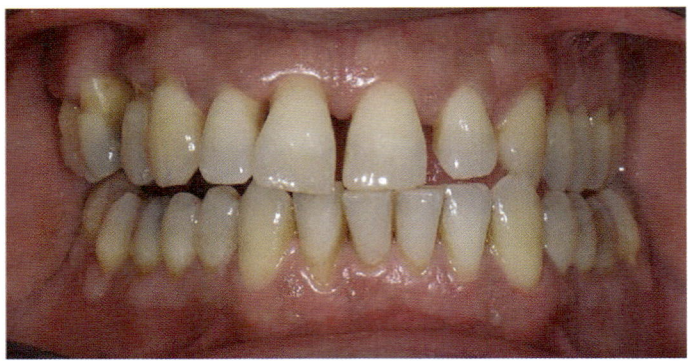

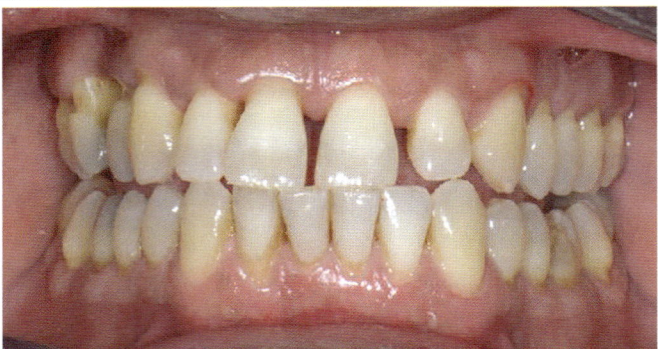

Fig. 16.15 Working contacts.

Working contacts on left side: 2.3 (canine guided)
- Balancing contacts on right side: None

Protrusive contacts: 1.1, 1.2
- Posterior interferences: 3.8, 4.8

X-RAY STATUS

- Amount of bone resorption: 60% bone loss (vertical and horizontal) (Fig. 16.16)
- Interradicular translucencies: None
- Lamina dura and periodontal ligament enlargements: None
- Periapical pathologies: None
- Retained teeth: None
- Root fragments/foreign bodies: None
- Decays: None
- Devitalized teeth: None

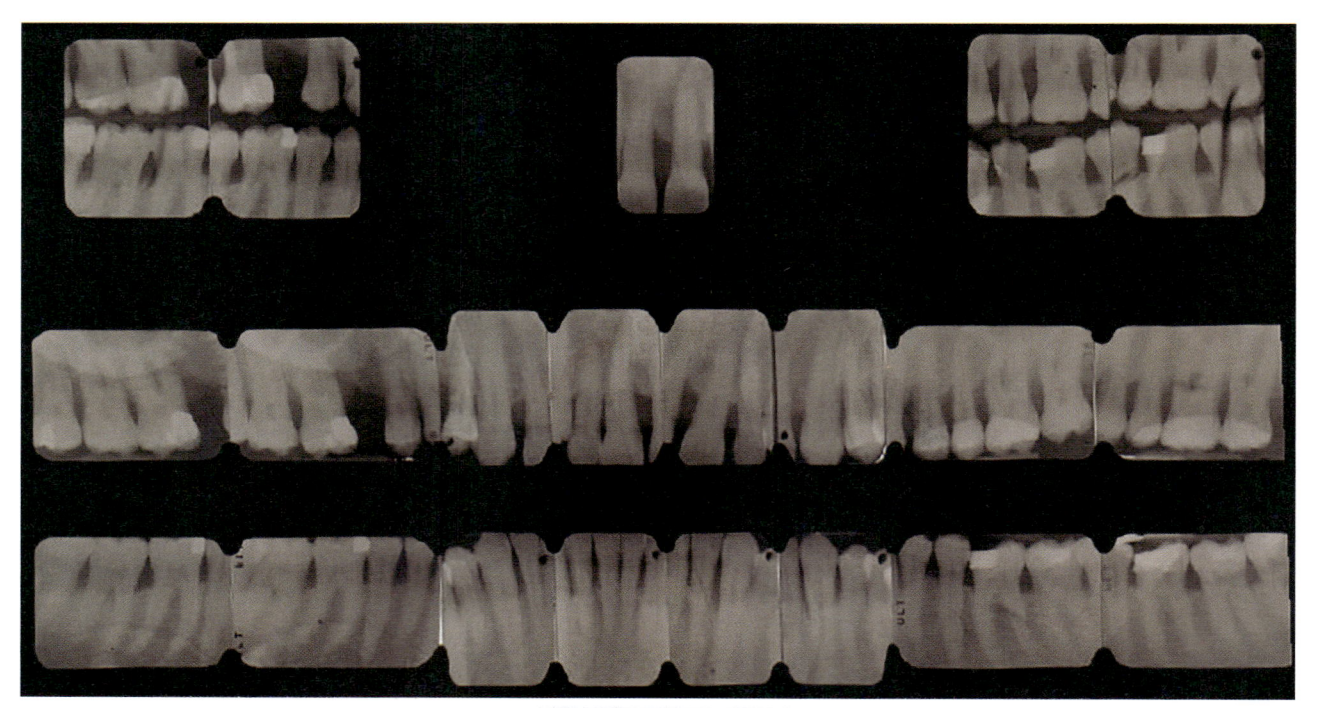

Fig. 16.16 Baseline status.

16 • Clear Aligner Orthodontic Treatment of Patients with Periodontitis

BASELINE PERIODONTAL CHART (FIG. 16.17)

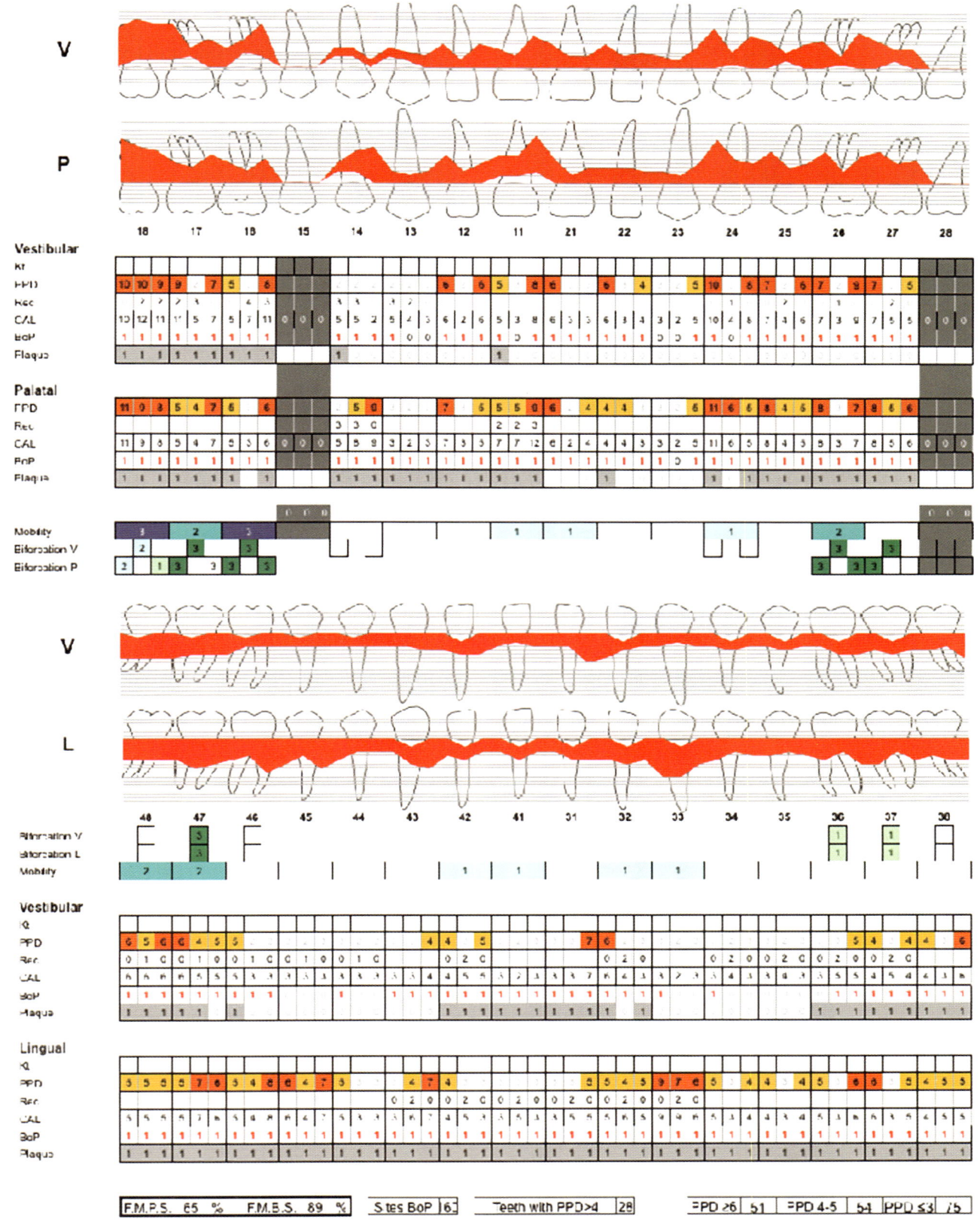

Fig. 16.17 Baseline periodontal chart.

PERIODONTAL EXAMINATION

- N. teeth: 30
- N. teeth with PPD ≥4 mm: 28

PD
- ≤ 3 mm: 75
- 4–5 mm: 54
- ≥ 6 mm: 51

PERIODONTAL REEVALUATION (FIGS. 16.18 and 16.19)

DIAGNOSIS

Generalized chronic severe periodontitis level 2 (presence of proximal attachment loss of ≥ 5 mm in two or more non-adjacent teeth)

Stage III grade B (Tables 16.4 and 16.5)

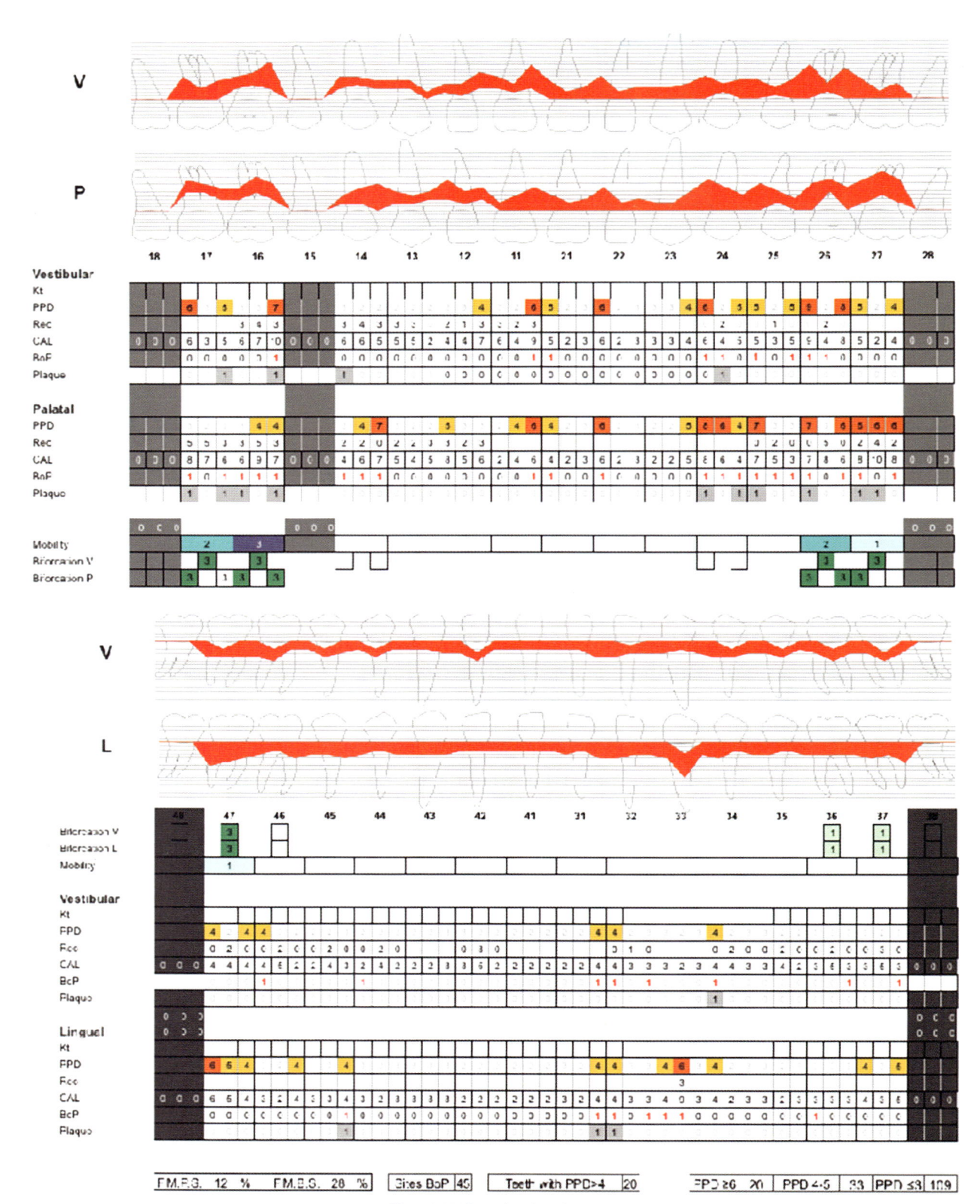

Fig. 16.18 Reevaluation chart.

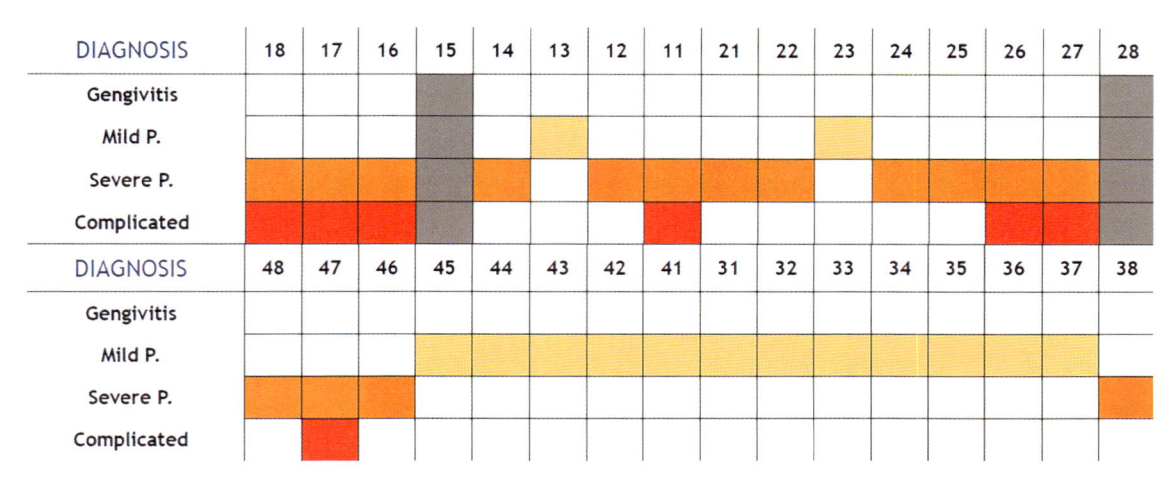

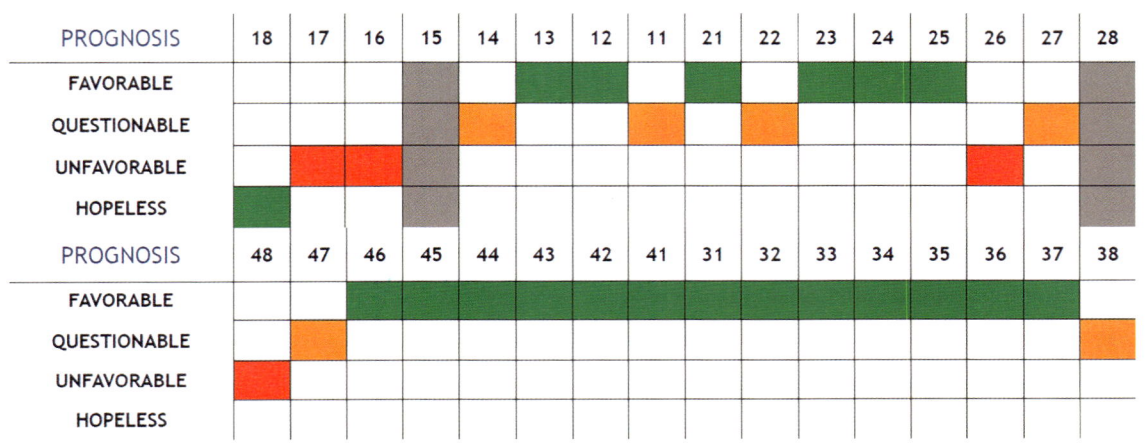

16 • Clear Aligner Orthodontic Treatment of Patients with Periodontitis   219

A

Fig. 16.19 (A) Tooth-by-tooth diagnosis. (B) Tooth-by-tooth prognosis. (From Kwok V, Caton JG. Commentary: prognosis revisited: a system for assigning periodontal prognosis. *J Periodontol*. 2007;87[11]:2063-2071.)

Table 16.4 Stages of Periodontitis

PERIODONTITIS STAGE		Stage I	Stage II	Stage III	Stage IV
Severity	Interdental CAL at site of greater loss	1–2 mm	3–4 mm	≥5 mm or extending to the middle third of the root	≥5 mm or extending to the apical third of the root
	Radiographic bone loss	Coronal (<15%)	Coronal third (15%–33%)	Extending to middle third	Extending to the apical third
	Tooth loss	No tooth loss due to periodontitis		Tooth loss due to periodontitis of ≤4 teeth	Tooth loss due to periodontitis of ≥5 teeth
Complexity	Local	• Maximum probing depth of 3–4 mm • Mostly horizontal bone loss	• Maximum probing depth 4–5 mm • Mostly horizontal bone loss	In addition to stage II complexity: • Probing depth ≥6 mm • Vertical bone loss ≥3 mm • Furcation involvement • Class II or III moderate ridge defect	In addition to stage III complexity: • Need for complex rehabilitation due to masticatory dysfunction • Secondary occlusal trauma (tooth mobility degree ≥2) • Bite collapse • Drifting • Flaring • <20 remaining teeth • Severe ridge defect
Extent and Distribution	Add to stage as descriptor	For each stage, describe extent as localized (<30% of teeth involved), generalized, or molar incisor pattern			

CAL, Clinical attachment level.

Table 16.5 Grades of Periodontitis

PERIODONTITIS GRADE			Grade A Slow Rate of Progression	Grade B Moderate Rate of Progression	Grade C Rapid Rate of Progression
Primary Criteria	Direct evidence of progression	Longitudinal data (PA radiographs or CAL loss)	Evidence of no loss over 5 years	<2 mm over 5 years	≥2 mm over 5 years
	Indirect evidence of progression	Bone loss/age	<0.25	0.25–1.00	>1.0
		Case phenotype	Heavy biofilm deposits with low level of destruction	Destruction commensurate with biofilm deposits	Destruction exceeds expectation given biofilm deposits, specific clinical patterns suggestive of periods of rapid progression and/or early onset disease, lack of expected response to standard bacterial control therapies
Grade Modifiers	Risk factors	Smoking	Nonsmoker	Smoker <10 cigarettes/day	Smoker ≥10 cigarettes/day
	Diabetes	Diabetes	Normoglycemic with or without prior diagnosis of diabetes	HbA1c <7.0 in diabetes patients	HbA1c ≥7.0 in diabetes patients

CAL, Clinical attachment loss; *PA*, periapical; *HbA1c*, refers to glycated haemoglobin

PERIO TREATMENT GOALS

1. Control of supragingival and subgingival infection
2. FMPS/FMBS <20%
3. Arrest of the progression of periodontitis
4. Extraction of hopeless teeth

TREATMENT PLAN

Etiologic therapy

1. Oral hygiene instructions and motivation
2. Nonsurgical therapy: Scaling and root planing (quadrant by quadrant) protocol
3. Extraction of 1.8, 3.8, 4.8
4. Change of filling: 3.6, 4.6

CLINICAL EXAMINATION REEVALUATION
(FIG. 16.20)

- N. teeth: 27
- N. teeth with PPD ≥4 mm: 20

PD
- ≤3 mm: 109
- 4–5 mm: 33
- ≥6 mm: 20

TREATMENT PLAN AFTER ETIOLOGIC THERAPY

- Regenerative therapy: 1.4, extraction: 1.6, 1.7
- Regenerative surgery: 1.1, 1.2, 2.2
- Extraction: 2.6, mesial root resection: 2.7
- Regenerative surgery: 2.4, 2.5
- Osseous resective surgery with tunnel preparation: 4.7
- Supportive periodontal treatment

Orthodontic

Alignment and space closure on upper arch

Implant Therapy

- 1.5, 1.7, 2.6

Periodontal Supportive Therapy

Every 3 months (Figs. 16.21 through 16.27)
The periodontal therapy was performed by Prof. Mario Aimetti, head of the Department of Periodontology of the Dental School of the University of Torino, Torino, Italy.

Orthodontic Diagnosis (Fig. 16.28)

Skeletal
- SKL CL 1, SKL NORMO

Dental
- Molar CL nonassessable, canine CL 1, deep bite, increased OVJ, spaces between teeth and black triangles, medial line deviated

Facial
- Convex profile

Specific Objectives of Treatment (Figs. 16.29 through 16.39)

- Maxilla: Align and intrude the teeth, close spaces, correct the midline
- Mandible: Close spaces, intrude lower incisors, correct the midline
- Facial esthetics: Improve esthetic smile line

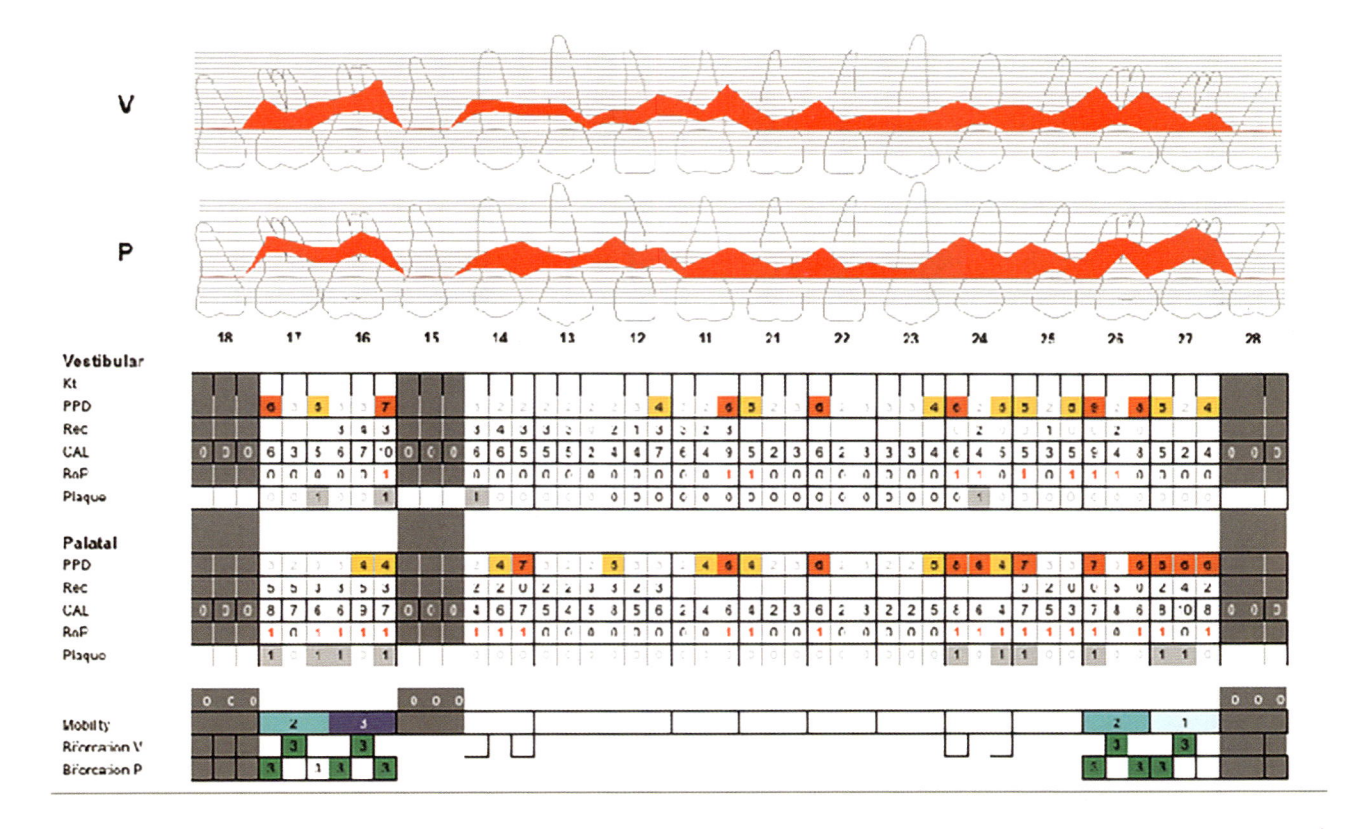

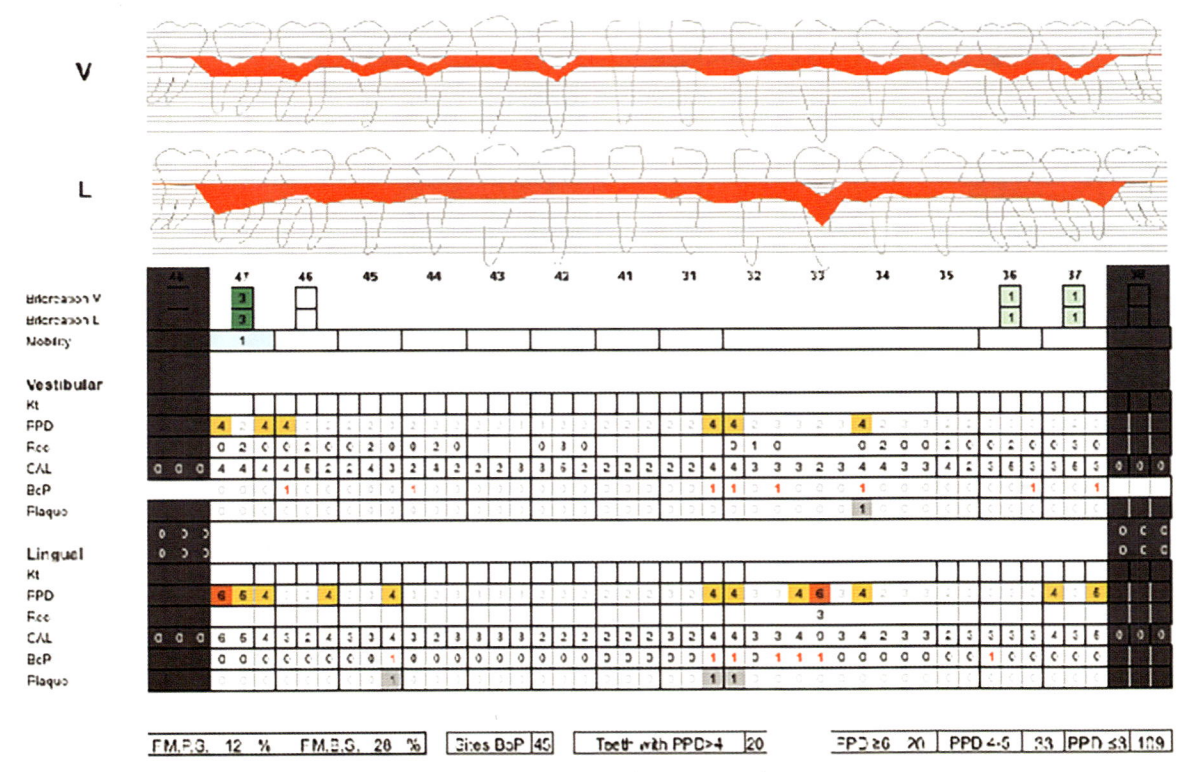

16 • Clear Aligner Orthodontic Treatment of Patients with Periodontitis

Fig. 16.20 Periodontal status and chart at reevaluation.

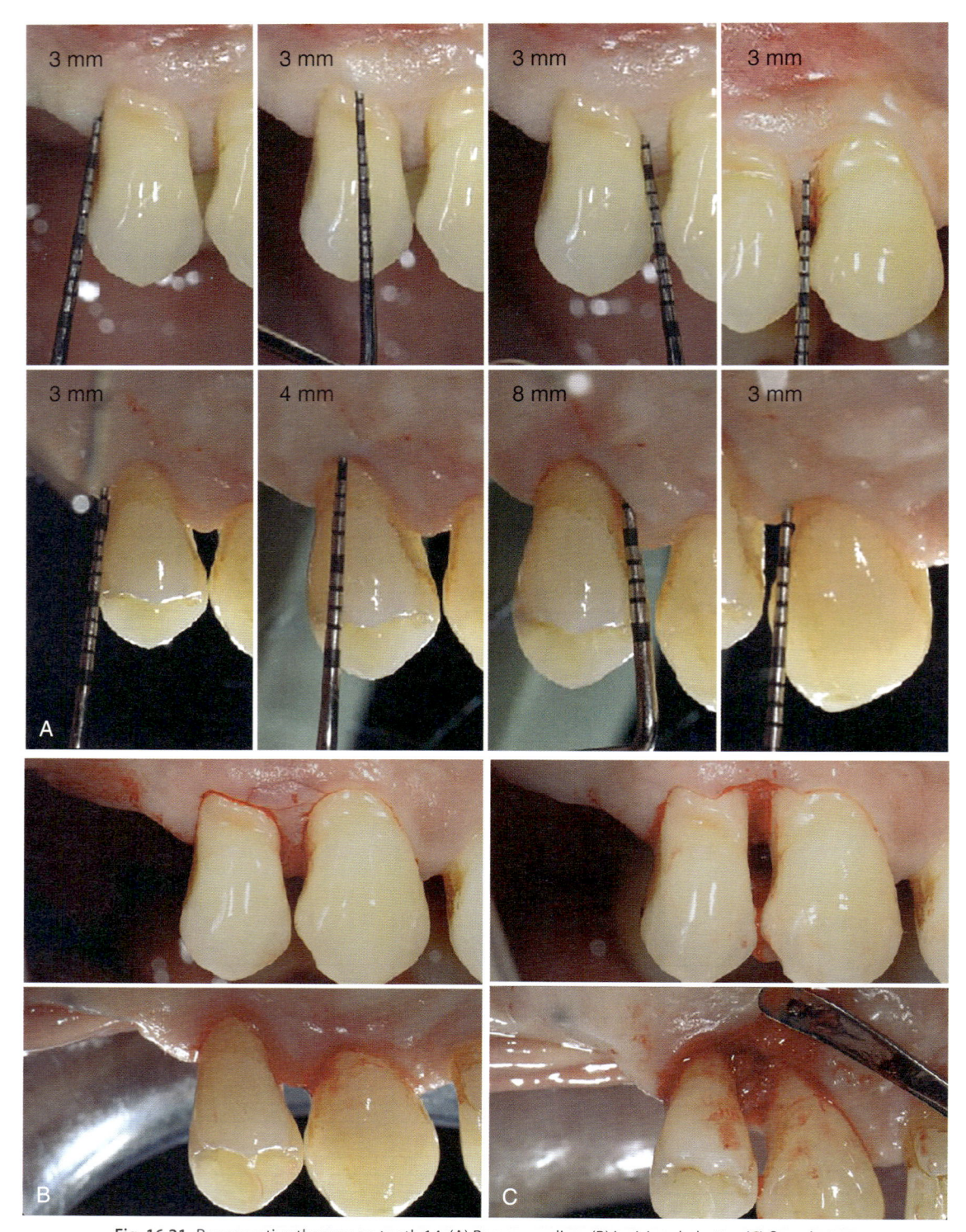

Fig. 16.21 Regenerative therapy on tooth 14. (A) Bone sounding, (B) incisional photos, (C) flap photos.

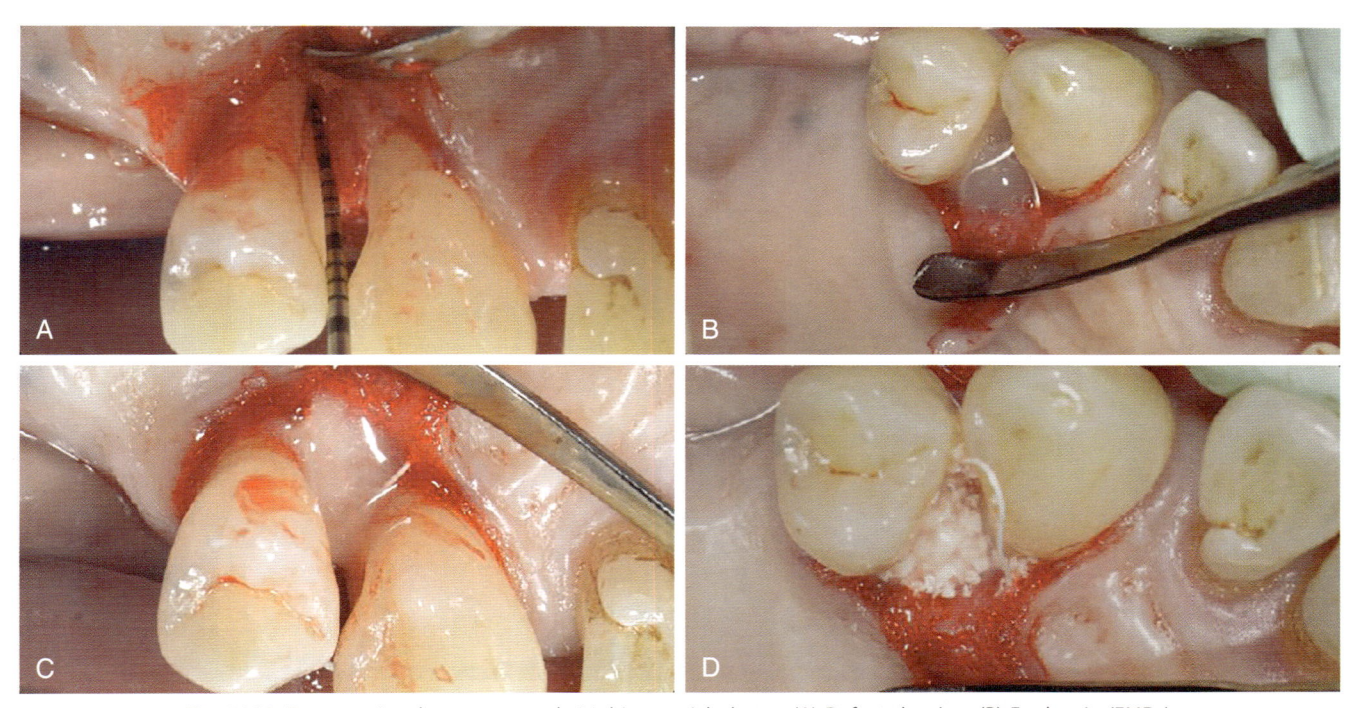

16 • Clear Aligner Orthodontic Treatment of Patients with Periodontitis   223

Fig. 16.22 Regenerative therapy on tooth 14: biomaterial photos. (A) Defect cleaning. (B) Emdogain (EMDs). (C) Pref Gel (EDTA). (D) BioOss.

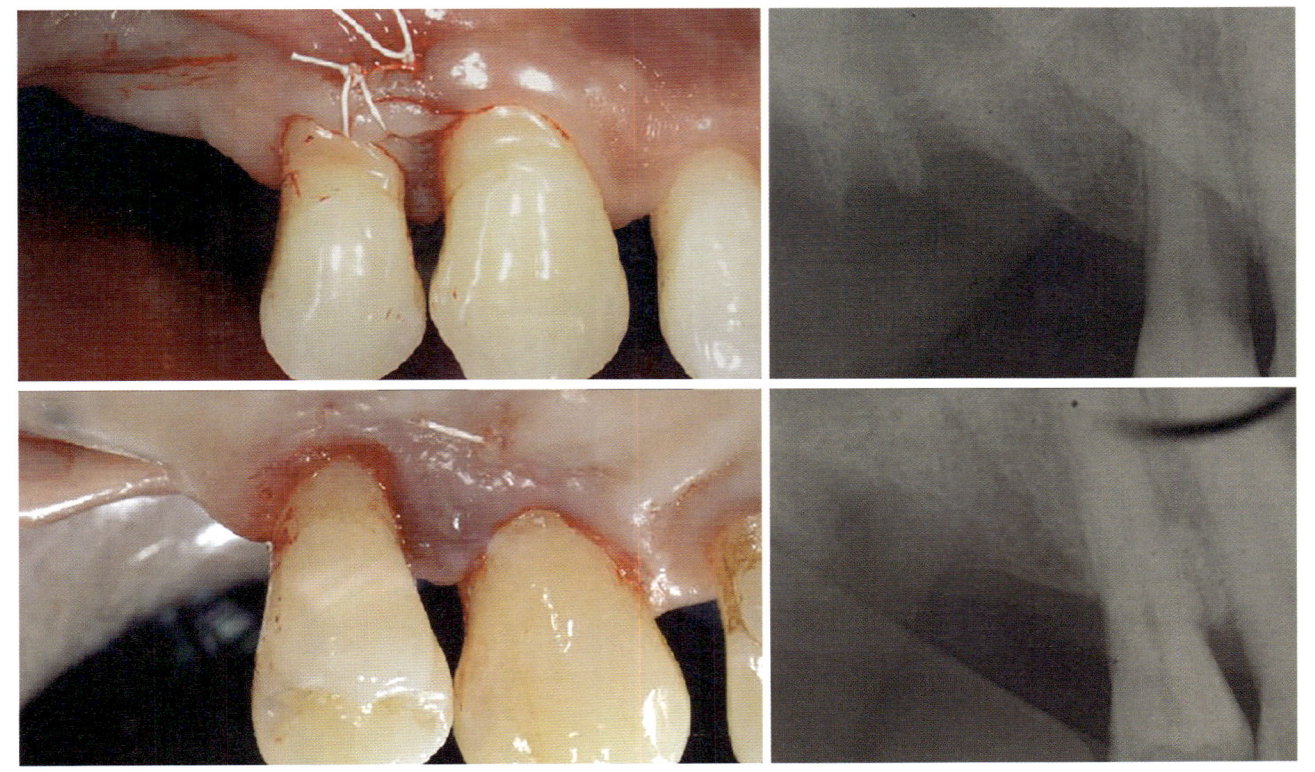

Fig. 16.23 Regenerative therapy on tooth: suture photos.

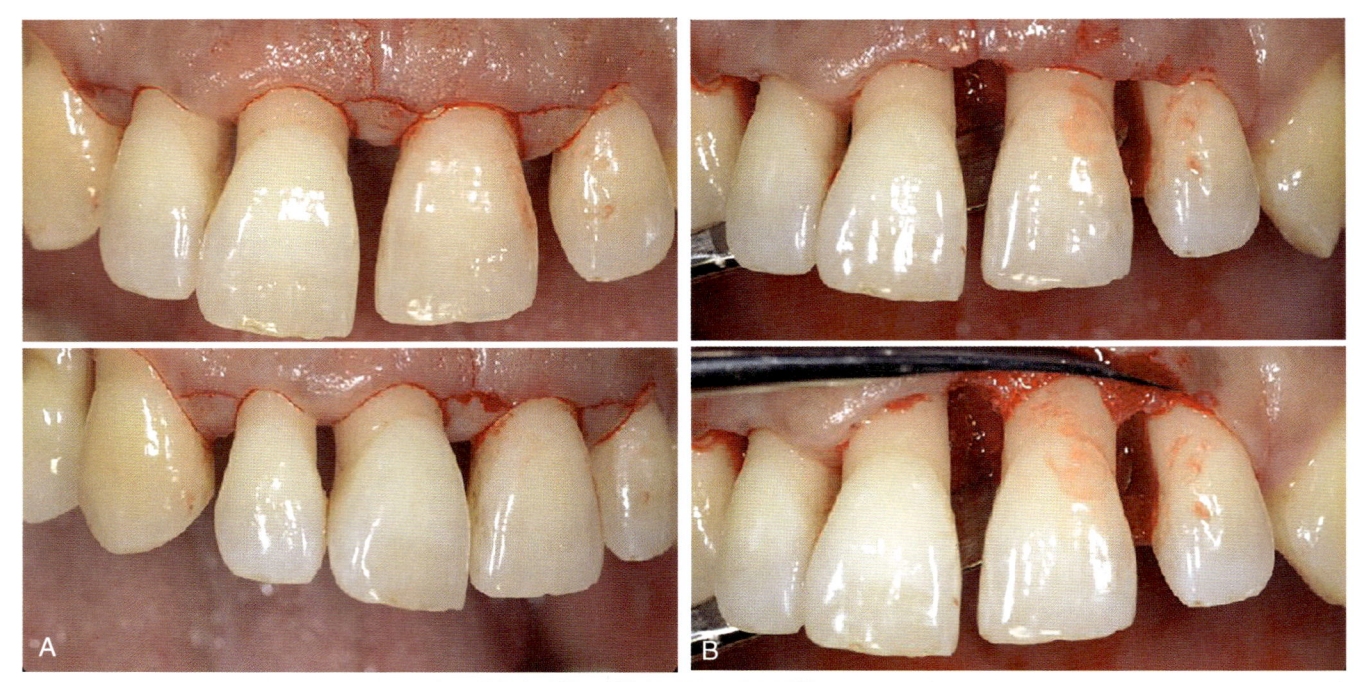

224 Principles and Biomechanics of Aligner Treatment

Fig. 16.24 Regenerative therapy on incisors. (A) Incision pfotos and, (B) flap photos.

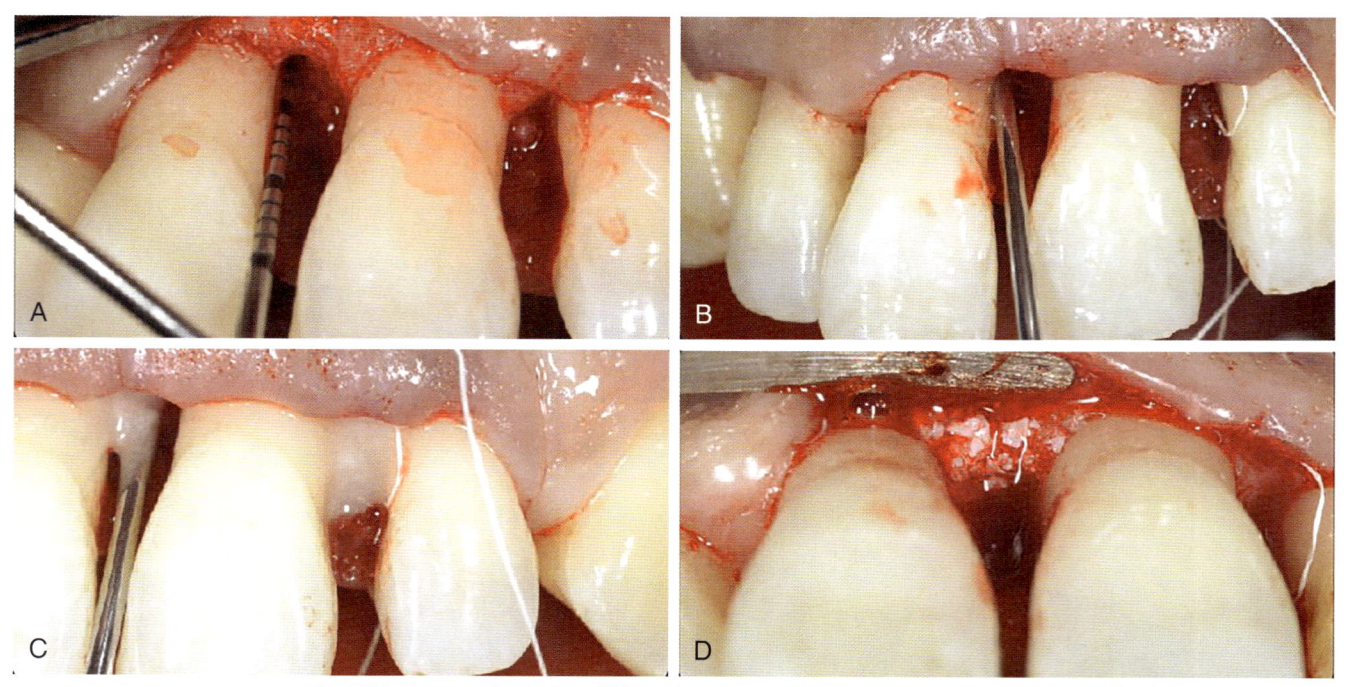

Fig. 16.25 Regenerative therapy on incisors: biomaterial photos. (A) Defect cleaning. (B) Emdogain (EMDs). (C) Pref Gel (EDTA). (D) BioOss.

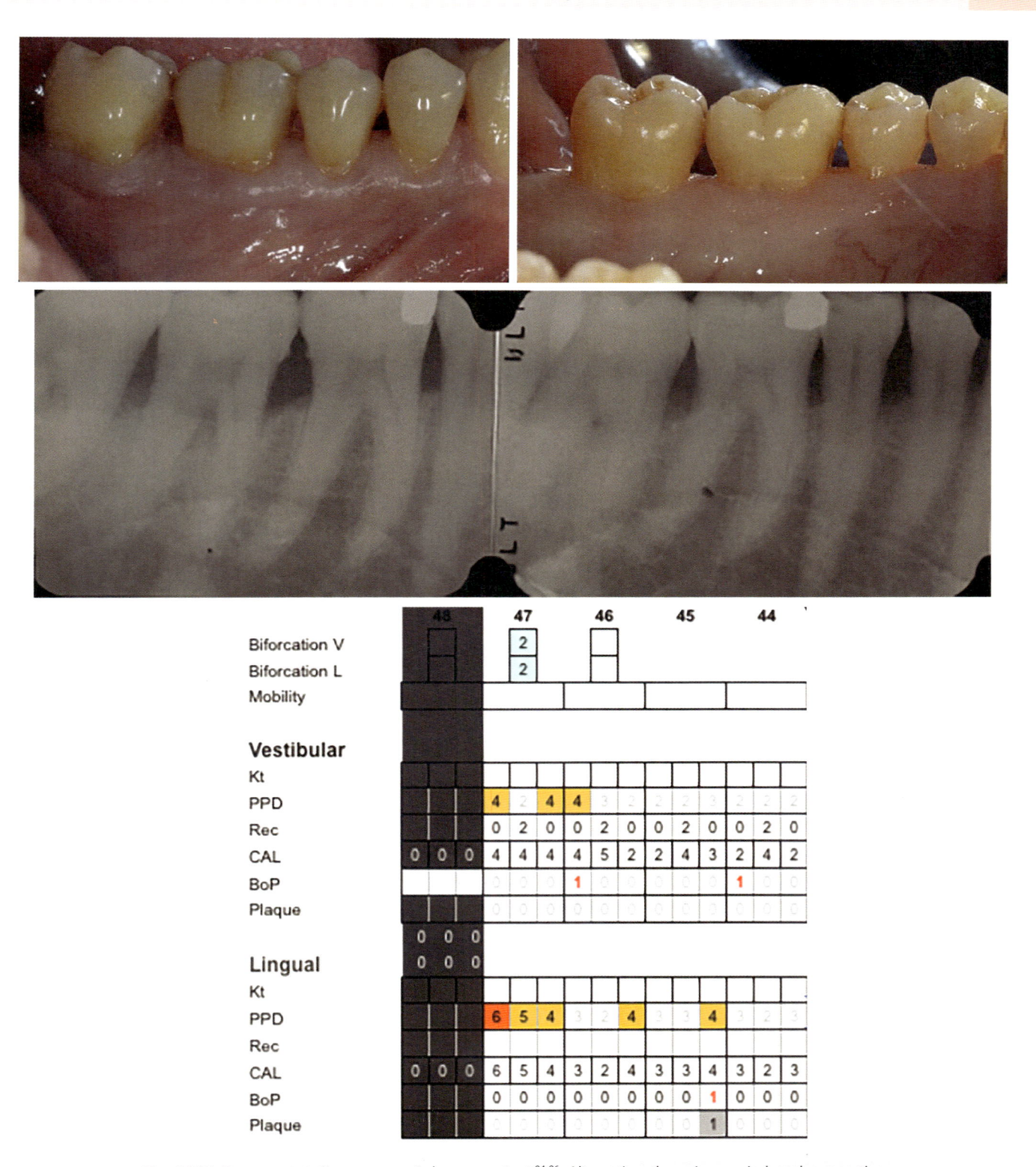

Fig. 16.26 Osseous resective surgery 6-degree sextant.[94-96] Alternative therapies: periodontal supportive therapy,[85,91,97] conservative surgery,[98-101] resective bone surgery.[94-96]

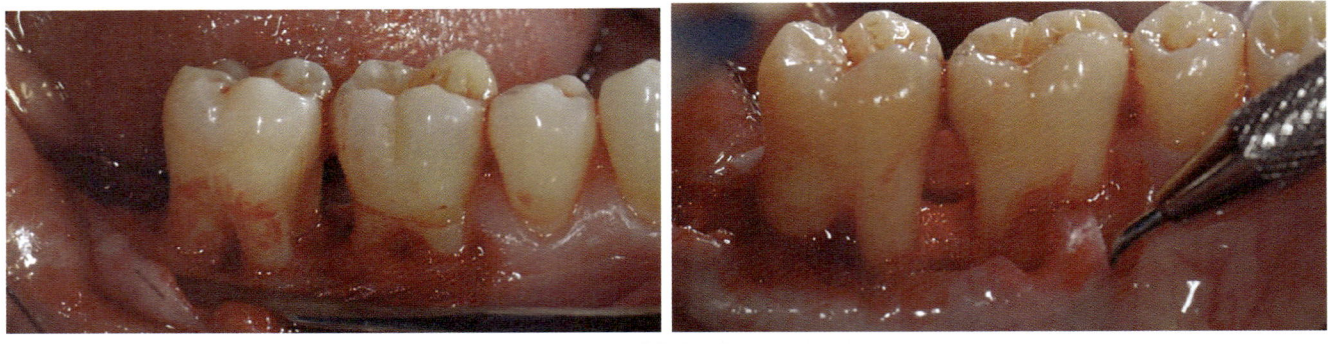

226 Principles and Biomechanics of Aligner Treatment

Fig. 16.27 Resective surgery: bone remodeling.

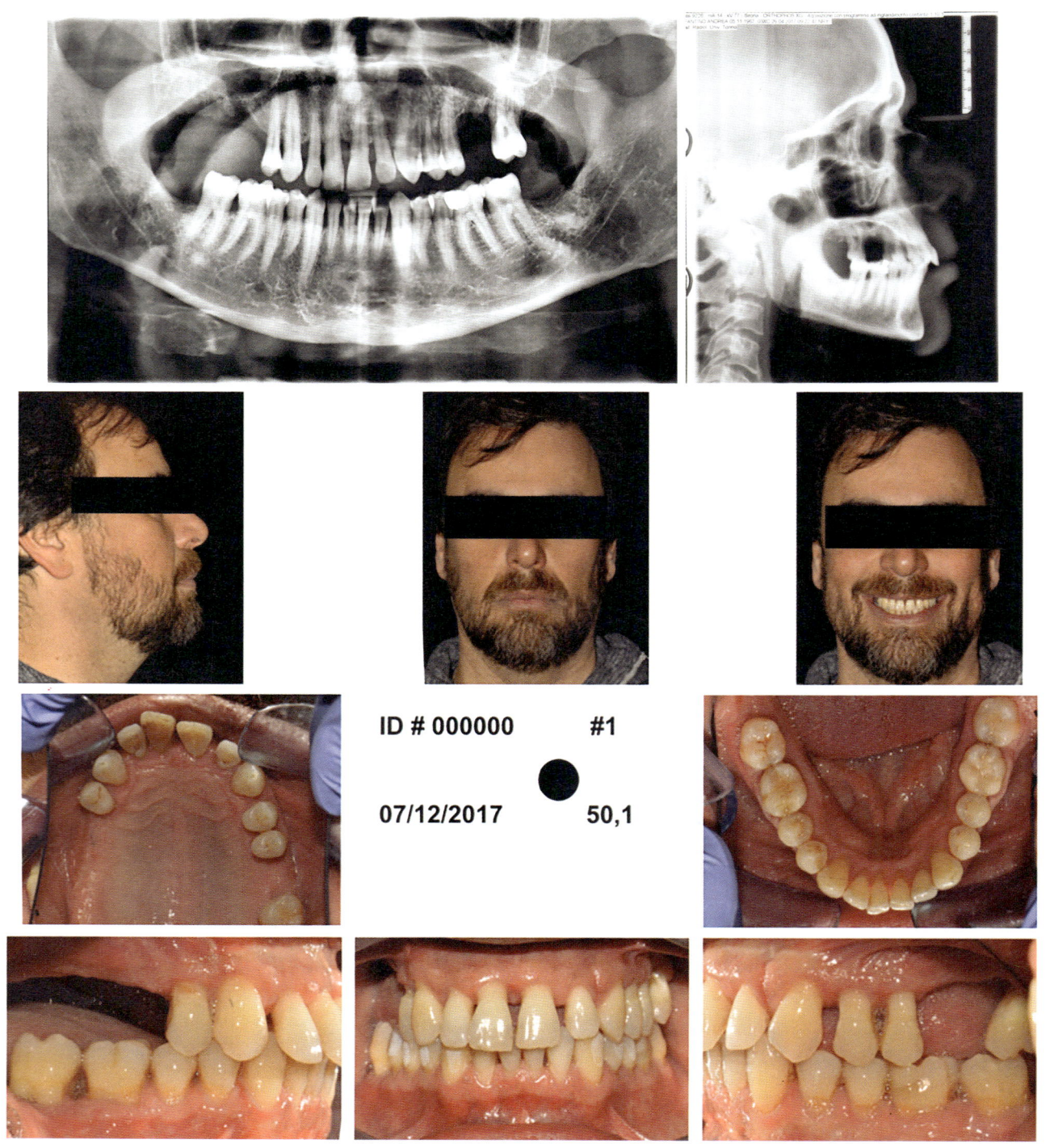

Fig. 16.28 Orthodontic records.

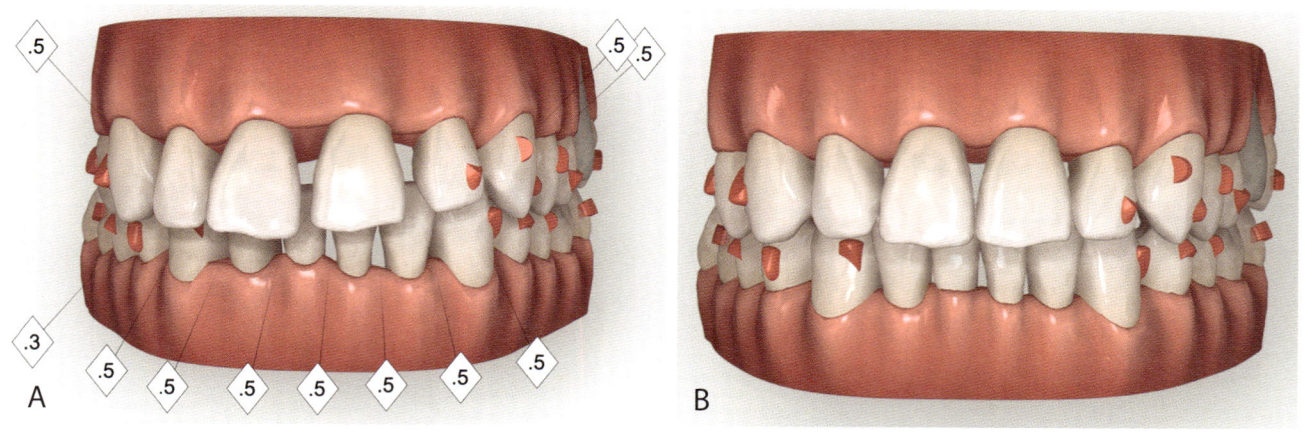

16 • Clear Aligner Orthodontic Treatment of Patients with Periodontitis   227

Fig. 16.29 ClinCheck beginning (A) and end (B): frontal view.

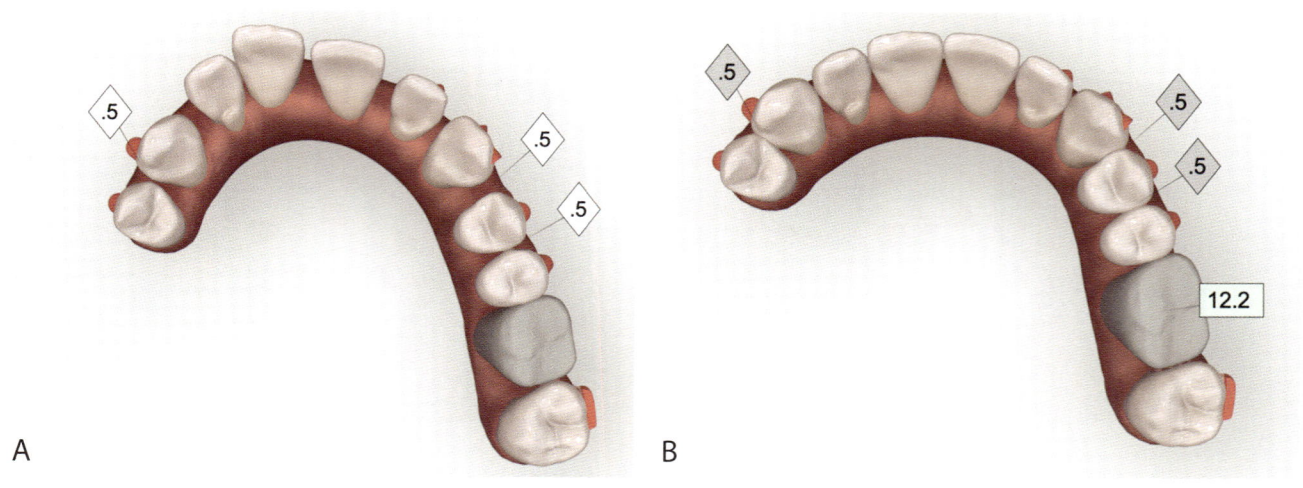

Fig. 16.30 ClinCheck beginning (A) and end (B): upper arch.

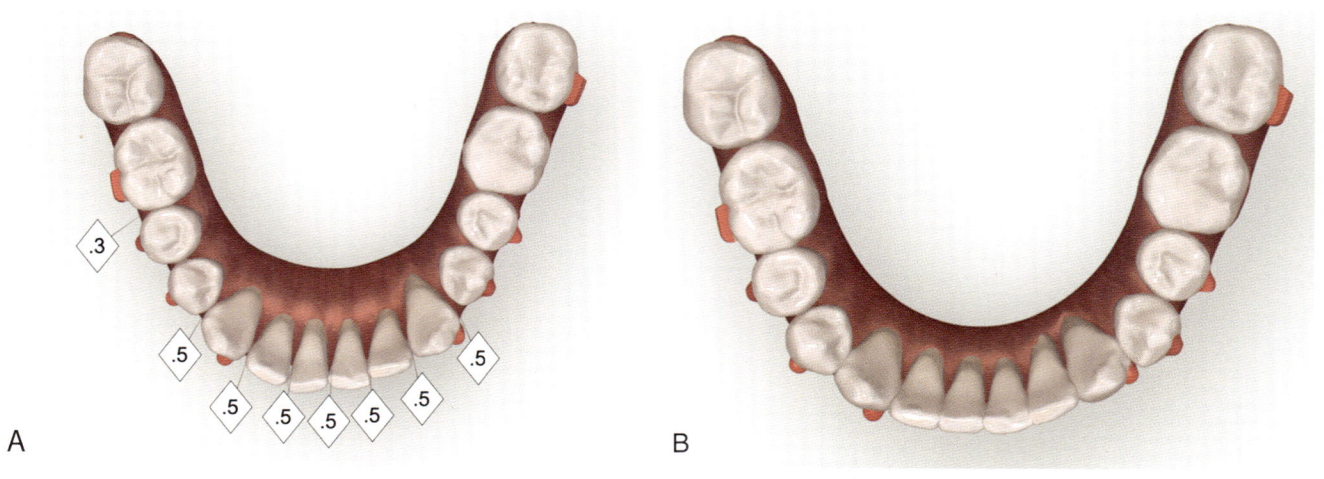

Fig. 16.31 ClinCheck beginning (A) and end (B): lower arch.

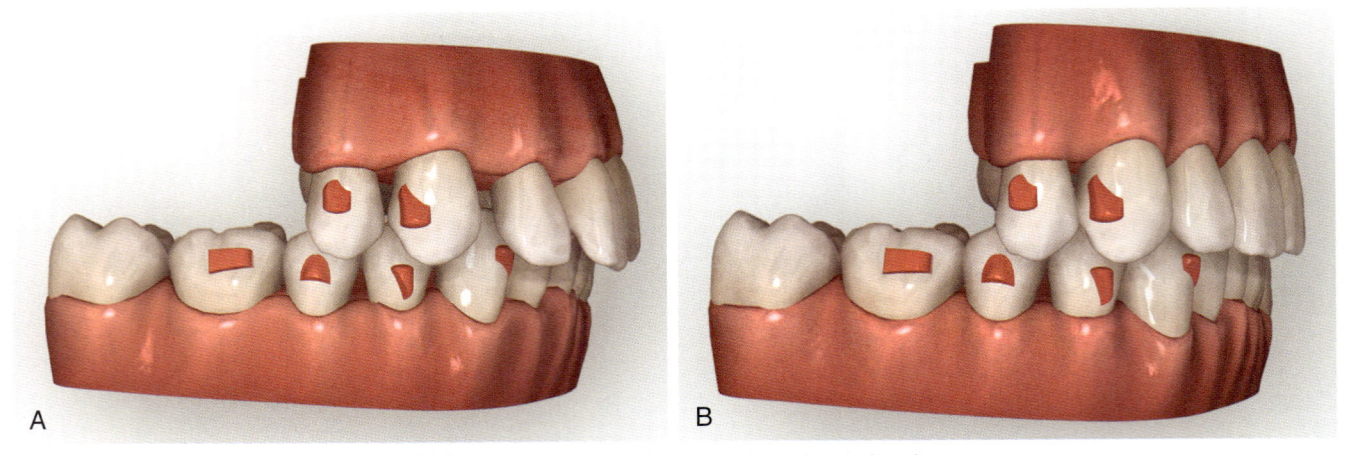

228 Principles and Biomechanics of Aligner Treatment

Fig. 16.32 ClinCheck beginning (A) and end (B): right side.

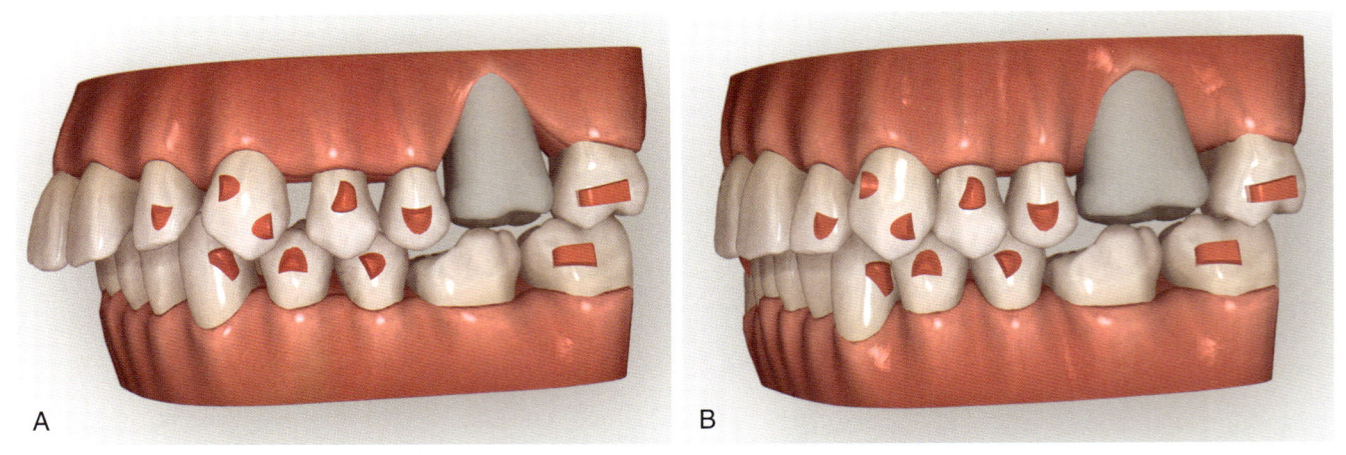

Fig. 16.33 ClinCheck beginning (A) and end (B): left side.

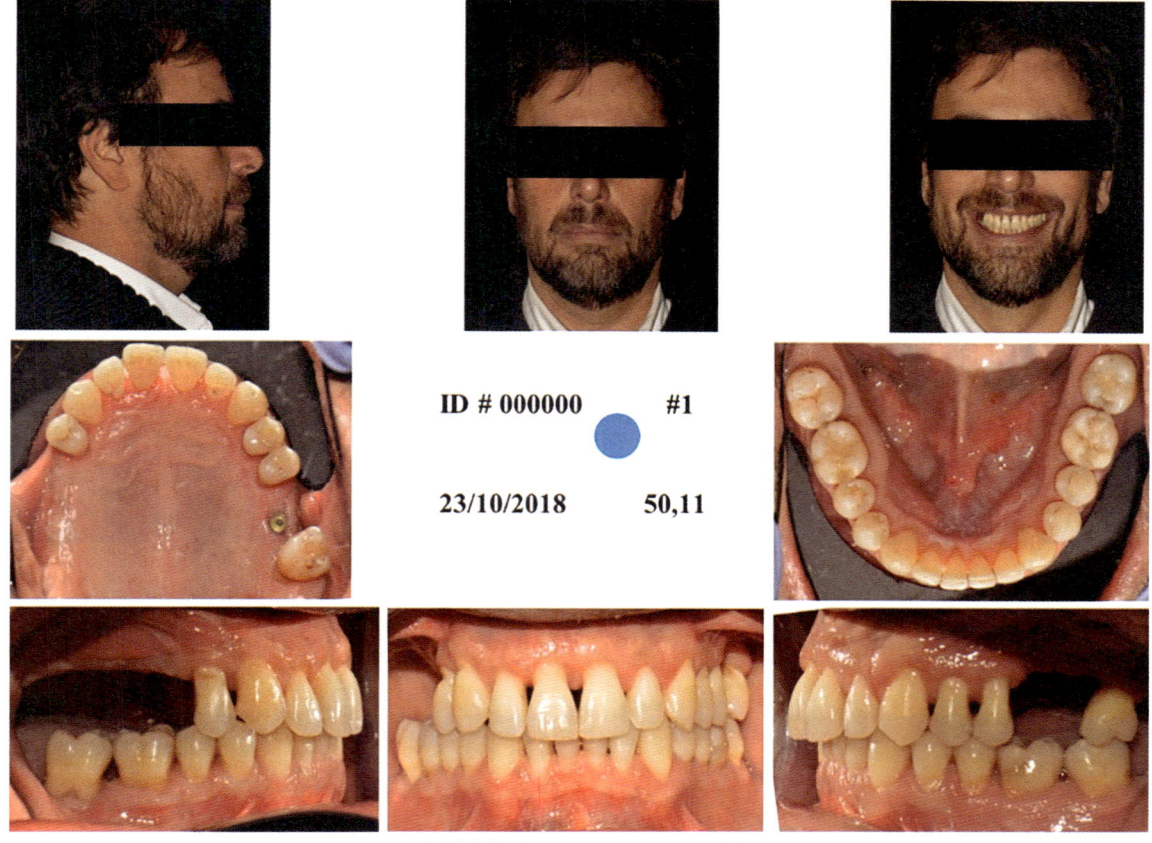

16 • Clear Aligner Orthodontic Treatment of Patients with Periodontitis   229

Fig. 16.34 End of preprosthetic orthodontics.

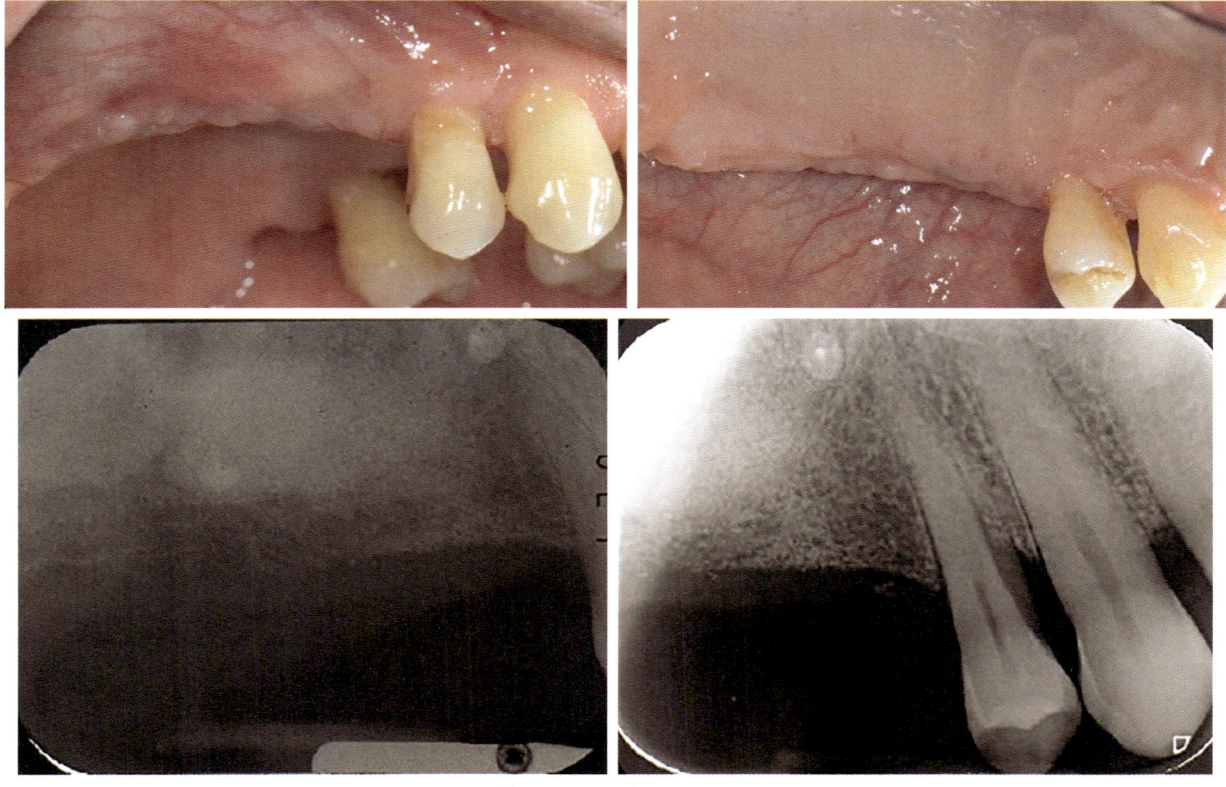

Fig. 16.35 Implant 1.5, 1.7.

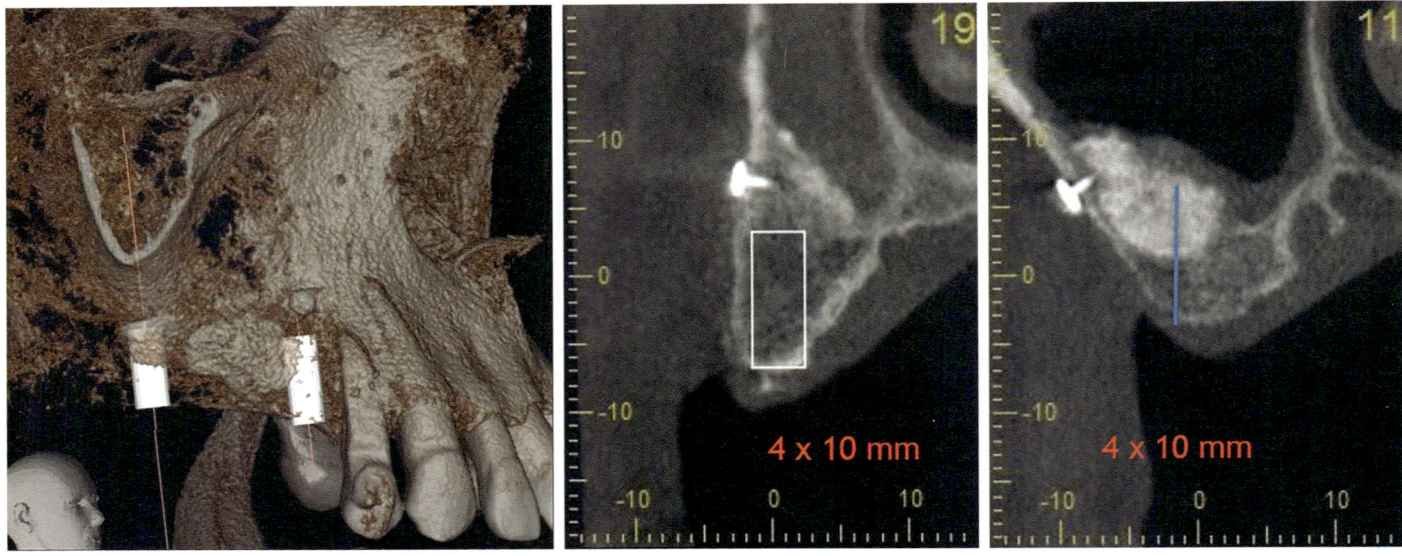

230 Principles and Biomechanics of Aligner Treatment

Fig. 16.36 Implant placement.

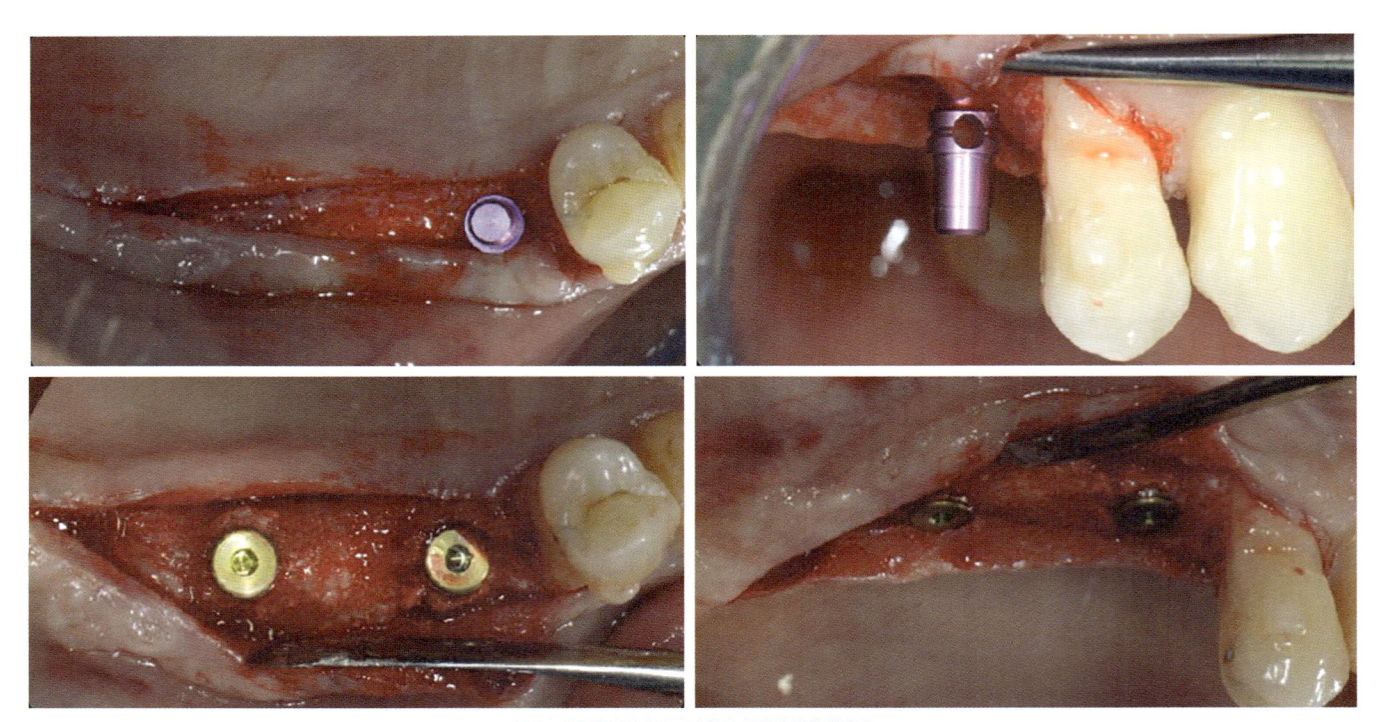

Fig. 16.37 Implant placement photos.

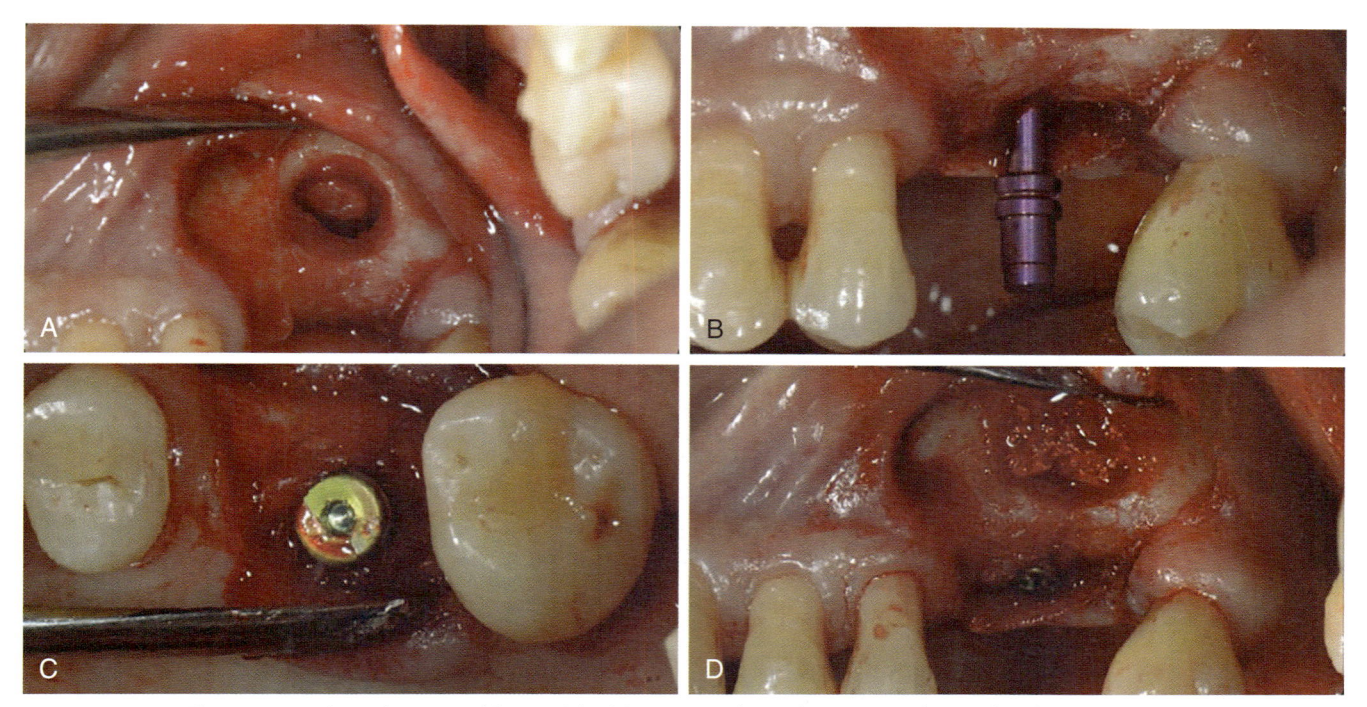

16 • Clear Aligner Orthodontic Treatment of Patients with Periodontitis   231

Fig. 16.38 Implant placement: biomaterials. (A) Bony window. (B) Sinus membrane elevation. (C) BioOss. (D) BioOss and membrane positioning.

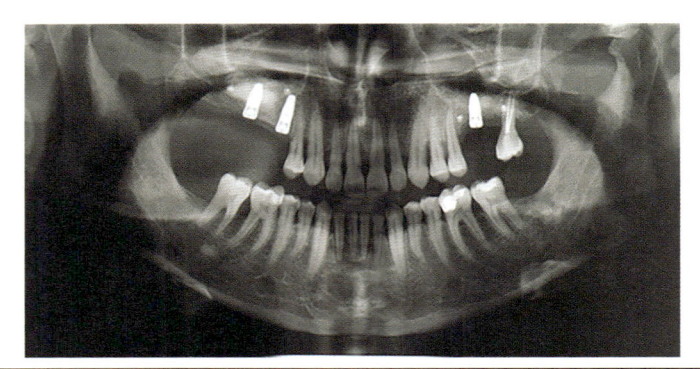

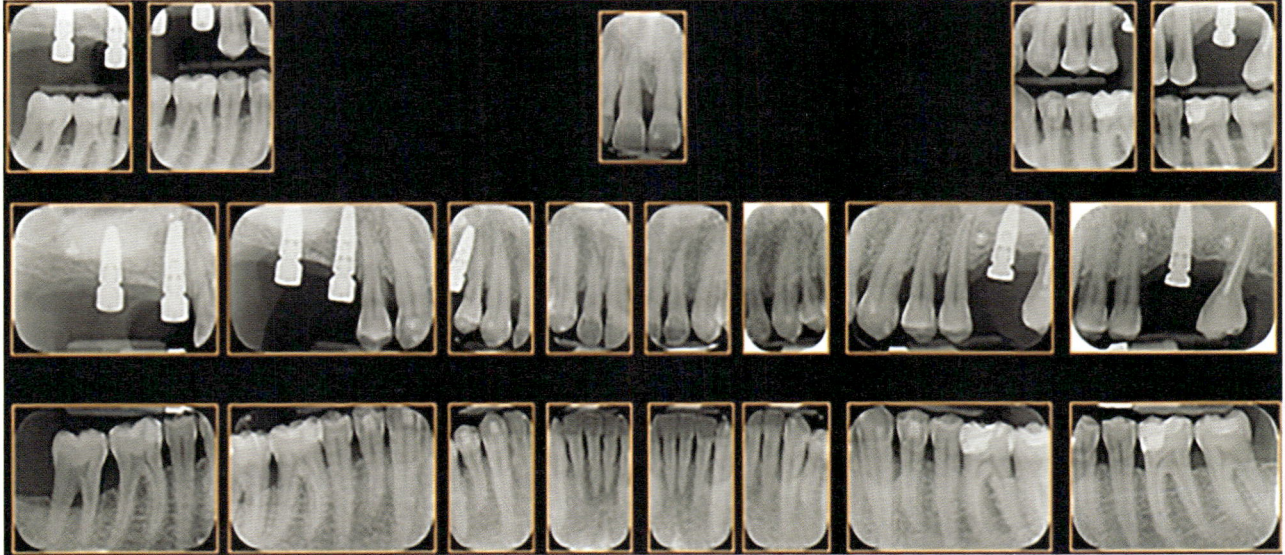

Fig. 16.39 Final orthodontic x-rays.

Continued

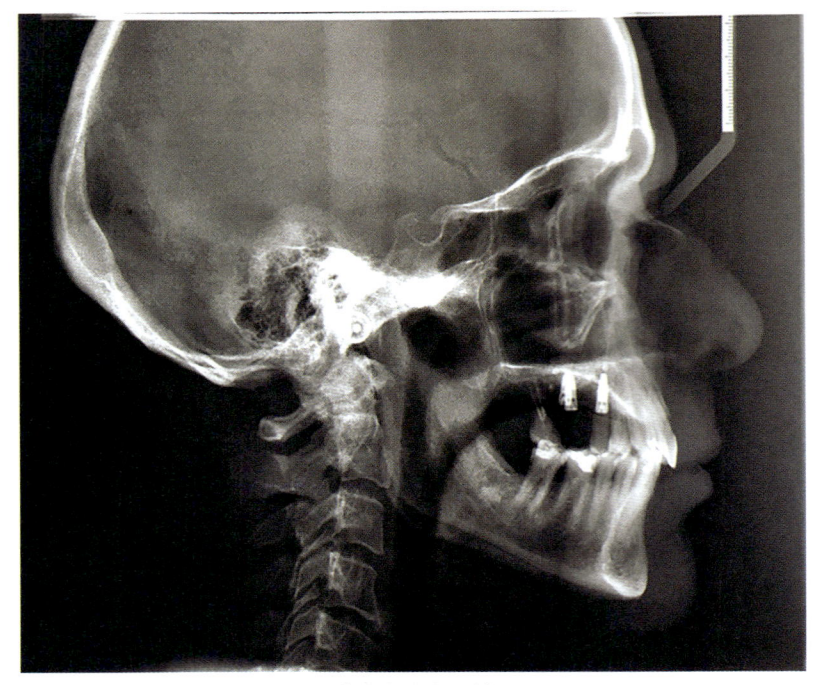

Fig. 16.39, cont'd

References

1. Geiger AM, Wasserman BH, Thompson Jr RH, et al. Relationship of occlusion and periodontal disease. V. Relation of classification of occlusion to periodontal status and gingival inflammation. *J Periodontol.* 1972;43:554-560.
2. Melsen B. *Adult Orthodontics.* 1st ed. Hoboken, NJ: Blackwell; 2013:205.
3. Buckley LA. The relationships between malocclusion, gingival inflammation, plaque and calculus. *J Periodontol.* 1981;52:35-40.
4. Chung CH, Vanarsdall RL, Cavalcanti EA, et al. Comparison of microbial composition in the subgingival plaque of adult crowded versus non-crowded dental regions. *Int J Adult Orthod Orthog Surg.* 2000;15:321-330.
5. Diedrich P. Periodontal relevance of anterior crowding. *J Orofac Orthop.* 2000;61:69-79.
6. Towfighi PP, Brunsvold MA, Storey AT, et al. Pathologic migration of anterior teeth in patients with moderate to severe periodontitis. *J Periodontol.* 1997;68:967-972.
7. Sanavi F, Weisgold AS, Rose LF. Biologic width and its relation to periodontal biotypes. *J Esthet Dent.* 1998;10:157-163.
8. Harrel SK, Nunn ME. The association of occlusal contacts with the presence of increased periodontal probing depth. *J Clin Periodontol.* 2009;36:1035-1042.
9. Geiger AM, Wasserman BH. Relationship of occlusion and periodontal disease: part IX-incisor inclination and periodontal status. *Angle Orthod.* 1976;46(2):99-110.
10. Gorbunkova A, Pagni G, Brizhak A, et al. Impact of orthodontic treatment on periodontal tissues: a narrative review of multidisciplinary literature. *Int J Dent.* 2016;2016:4723589.
11. Brunsvold MA. Pathologic tooth migration. *J Periodontol.* 2005;76(6):859-866.
12. Khorshidi H, Moaddeli MR, Golkari A, et al. The prevalence of pathologic tooth migration with respect to the severity of periodontitis. *J Int Soc Prev Community Dent.* 2016;6:S122-S125.
13. Gaumet PE, Brunsvold MI, McMahan CA. Spontaneous repositioning of pathologically migrated teeth. *J Periodontol.* 1999;70(10):1177-1184.
14. Diedrich P. The eleventh hour or where are our orthodontic limits? Case report. *J Orofac Orthop.* 1999;60:60-65.
15. Wennström JL, Stokland BL, Nyman S, et al. Periodontal tissue response to orthodontic movement of teeth with infrabony pockets. *Am J Orthod Dentofacial Orthop.* 1993;103:313-319.
16. Zhang J, Zhang AM, Zhang ZM, et al. Efficacy of combined orthodontic-periodontic treatment for patients with periodontitis and its effect on inflammatory cytokines: a comparative study. *Am J Orthod Dentofacial Orthop.* 2017;152(4):494-500.
17. Ricci G, Aimetti M. *Diagnosi e Terapia Parodontale.* 1st ed. Rho: Quintessence; 2012:565-567.
18. Nanda R. *Esthetics and Biomechanics in Orthodontics.* 2nd ed. St. Louis, MO: Elsevier; 2015:500.
19. Pabari S, Moles DR, Cunningham SJ. Assessment of motivation and psychological characteristics of adult orthodontic patients. *Am J Orthod Dentofacial Orthop.* 2011;140(6):263-272.
20. Cao T, Xu L, Shi J, et al. Combined orthodontic-periodontal treatment in periodontal patients with anteriorly displaced incisors. *Am J Orthod Dentofacial Orthop.* 2015;148:805-813.
21. Mathews DP, Kokich VG. Managing treatment for the orthodontic patient with periodontal problems. *Semin Orthod.* 1997;3(1):21-38.
22. Tonetti MS, Greenwell H, Kornman KS. Staging and grading of periodontitis: framework and proposal of a new classification and case definition. *J Periodontol.* 2018;89(1):S159-S172.
23. Kokich VG, Spear FM. Guidelines for managing the orthodontic restorative patient. *Semin Orthod.* 1997;3(1):3-20.
24. Evans M. 3D guided comprehensive approach to mucogingival problems in orthodontics. *Semin Orthod.* 2016;22:52-63.
25. Vanchit J, Langer L, Rasperini G. Periodontal soft tissue non-root coverage procedures: practical applications from the AAP regeneration workshop. *Clin Adv Periodontics.* 2015;5:11-20.
26. Kloukos D, Eliades T, Sculean A, et al. Indication and timing of soft tissue augmentation at maxillary and mandibular incisors in orthodontic patients. A systematic review. *Eur J Orthod.* 2014;36(4):442-449.
27. Kokich V. Enhancing restorative, esthetic and periodontal results with orthodontic therapy. In: Schluger S, Youdelis R, Page R, et al., eds. *Periodontal Therapy.* Philadelphia, PA: Lea and Febiger; 1990:433-460.
28. Becker W, Becker BE. Treatment of mandibular 3-wall intrabony defects by flap debridement and expanded polytetrafluoroethylene barrier membranes: long-term evaluation of 32 treated patients. *J Periodontol.* 1993;64:1138-1144.
29. Roccuzzo M, Marchese S, Dalmasso P, et al. Periodontal regeneration and orthodontic treatment of severely periodontally compromised teeth: 10-year results of a prospective study. *Int J Periodontics Restorative Dent.* 2018;38(6):801-809.

30. Matarasso M, Iorio-Siciliano V, Blasi A, et al. Enamel matrix derivative and bone grafts for periodontal regeneration of intrabony defects. A systematic review and meta-analysis. *Clin Oral Investig.* 2015;19:1581-1593.
31. Ogihara S, Wang HL. Periodontal regeneration with or without limited orthodontics for the treatment of 2- or 3-wall infrabony defects. *J Periodontol.* 2010;81(12):1734-1742.
32. Araújo MG, Carmagnola D, Berglundh T, et al. Orthodontic movement in bone defects augmented with Bio-Oss. An experimental study in dogs. *J Clin Periodontol.* 2001;28(1):73-80.
33. Sanz M, Martin C. Tooth movement in the periodontally compromised patient. In: Lang PN, Lindhe J, eds. *Clinical Periodontology and Implant Dentistry.* 6th ed. Hoboken, NJ: John Wiley & Sons; 2015 [vol 2].
34. Wennström JL. Mucogingival considerations in orthodontic treatment. *Semin Orthod.* 1996;2(1):46-54.
35. Vanarsdall RL, Secchi AG. Periodontal-orthodontic interrelationship. In: Graber LW, Vanarsdall RL, Vig WL, eds. *Orthodontics: Current Principles and Techniques.* Philadelphia, PA: Mosby; 2012:807-841.
36. Miner RM, Al Qabandi S, Rigali PH, et al. Cone-beam computed tomography transverse analysis. Part I: normative data. *Am J Orthod Dentofacial Orthop.* 2012;142(3):300-307.
37. Morais JF, Melsen B, de Freitas KMS, et al. Evaluation of maxillary buccal alveolar bone before and after orthodontic alignment without extractions: a cone beam computed tomographic study. *Angle Orthod.* 2018;88(6):748-756.
38. Artun J, Grobéty D. Periodontal status of mandibular incisors after pronounced orthodontic advancement during adolescence: a follow-up evaluation. *Am J Orthod Dentofacial Orthop.* 2001;119(1):2-10.
39. Steiner GG, Pearson JK, Ainamo J. Changes of the marginal periodontium as a result of labial tooth movement in monkeys. *J Periodontol.* 1981;52(6):314-320.
40. Diedrich P. Guided tissue regeneration associated with orthodontic therapy. *Semin Orthod.* 1996;2:39-45.
41. Kalina E, Zadurska M, Sobieska E, et al. Relationship between periodontal status of mandibular incisors and selected cephalometric parameters: preliminary results. *J Orofac Orthop.* 2019;80(3):107-115.
42. Melsen B, Allais D. Factors of importance for the development of dehiscences during labial movement of mandibular incisors: a retrospective study of adult orthodontic patients. *Am J Orthod Dentofacial Orthop.* 2005;127(5):552-561.
43. Melsen B. Biological reaction of alveolar bone to orthodontic tooth movement. *Angle Orthod.* 1999;69(2):151-158.
44. Artun J, Urbye KS. The effect of orthodontic treatment on periodontal bone support in patients with advanced loss of marginal periodontium. *Am J Orthod Dentofac Orthop.* 1988;93:143-148.
45. Re S, Corrente G, Abundo R, et al. Orthodontic treatment in periodontally compromised patients: a 12-years report. *Int J Periodontics Restorative Dent.* 2000;20:31-39.
46. Thornberg MJ, Riolo CS, Bayirli B, et al. Periodontal pathogen levels in adolescents before, during, and after fixed orthodontic appliance therapy. *Am J Orthod Dentofacial Orthop.* 2009;135(1):95-98.
47. Gomes SC, Varela CC, da Veiga SL, et al. Periodontal conditions in subjects following orthodontic therapy. A preliminary study. *Eur J Orthod.* 2007;29(5):477-481.
48. Rossini G, Parrini S, Castroflorio T, et al. Periodontal health during clear aligners treatment: a systematic review. *Eur J Orthod.* 2015;37(5):539-543.
49. Azaripour A, Weusmann J, Mahmoodi B, et al. Braces versus Invisalign: gingival parameters and patients' satisfaction during treatment: a cross-sectional study. *BMC Oral Health.* 2015;24:15:69.
50. Abbate GM, Caria MP, Montanari P, et al. Periodontal health in teenagers treated with removable aligners and fixed orthodontic appliances. *J Orofac Orthop.* 2015;76(3):240-250.
51. Chhibber A, Agarwal S, Yadav S, et al. Which orthodontic appliance is best for oral hygiene? A randomized clinical trial. *Am J Orthod Dentofacial Orthop.* 2018;153(2):175-183.
52. Simon M, Keilig L, Schwarze J, et al. Forces and moments generated by removable thermoplastic aligners: incisor torque, premolar derotation, and molar distalization. *Am J Orthod Dentofacial Orthop.* 2014;145(6):728-736.
53. Hahn W, Zapf A, Dathe H, et al. Torquing an upper central incisor with aligners—acting forces and biomechanical principles. *Eur J Orthod.* 2010;32(6):607-613.
54. Castroflorio T, Garino F, Lazzaro A, et al. Upper-incisor root control with Invisalign appliances. *J Clin Orthod.* 2013;47(6):346-351.
55. Bowman SJ, Celenza F, Sparaga J, et al. Creative adjuncts for clear aligners, part 3: extraction and interdisciplinary treatment. *J Clin Orthod.* 2015;49(4):249-262.
56. Simon M, Keilig L, Schwarze J, et al. Treatment outcome and efficacy of an aligner technique—regarding incisor torque, premolar derotation and molar distalization. *BMC Oral Health.* 2014;14:68.
57. Grünheid T, Loh C, Larson BE. How accurate is Invisalign in nonextraction cases? Are predicted tooth positions achieved? *Angle Orthod.* 2017;87(6):809-815.
58. Lombardo L, Arreghini A, Ramina F, et al. Predictability of orthodontic movement with orthodontic aligners: a retrospective study. *Prog Orthod.* 2017;13;18(1):35.
59. Sfondrini MF, Gandini P, Castroflorio T, et al. Buccolingual inclination control of upper central incisors of aligners: a comparison with conventional and self-ligating brackets. *Biomed Res Int.* 2018;2018:9341821.
60. Tepedino M, Paoloni V, Cozza P, et al. Movement of anterior teeth using clear aligners: a three-dimensional, retrospective evaluation. *Prog Orthod.* 2018;19(1):9.
61. Mantovani E, Castroflorio E, Rossini G, et al. Scanning electron microscopy evaluation of aligner fit on teeth. *Angle Orthod.* 2018;88(5):596-601.
62. Mantovani E, Castroflorio E, Rossini G, et al. Scanning electron microscopy analysis of aligner fitting on anchorage attachments. *J Orofac Orthop.* 2019;80(2):79-87.
63. Katsaros C, Livas C, Renkema AM. Unexpected complications of bonded mandibular lingual retainers. *Am J Orthod Dentofacial Orthop.* 2007;132(6):838-841.
64. Tarnow DP, Magner AW, Fletcher P. The effect of the distance from the contact point to the crest of bone on the presence or absence of the interproximal dental papilla. *J Periodontol.* 1992;63(12):995-996.
65. Verna CA, Bassarelli T. Orthodontic mechanics in patient with periodontal disease. In: Eliades T, Katsaros C, eds. *The Ortho-Perio Patient.* Batavia, IL: Quintessence; 2019:175.
66. Zachrisson BU, Lindhe J. Orthodontics and periodontics tooth movements in the periodontally compromised patient. In: Lindhe J, ed. *Clinical Periodontology and Implant Therapy.* 5th ed. Wiley Blackwell; 2008:1241-1279.
67. Spear FM, Mathews DM, Kokich VG. Interdisciplinary management of single tooth implants. *Semin Orthod.* 1997;3:45-72.
68. Uribe F, Chau V, Padala S, et al. Alveolar ridge width and height changes after orthodontic space opening in patients congenitally missing maxillary lateral incisors. *Eur J Orthod.* 2011;35(1). doi:10.1093/ejo/cjr072.
69. Lundgreen D, Kurol J, Thorstensson B, et al. Periodontal conditions around tipped and upright molars in adults. A intra-individual retrospective study. *Eur J Orthod.* 1992;14:449-455.
70. Lindskog-Stokland B, Wenstrom JL, Nyman S, et al. Orthodontic tooth movement into edentulous areas with reduced bone height. An experimental study in the dog. *Eur J Orthod.* 1993;15:89-96.
71. Joss-Vassalli I, Grebenstein C, Topouzelis N, et al. Orthodontic therapy and gingival recession: a systematic review. *Orthod Craniofac Res.* 2010;13:127-141.
72. Gil APS, Haas Jr OL, Méndez-Manjón I, et al. Alveolar corticotomies for accelerated orthodontics: a systematic review. *J Craniomaxillofac Surg.* 2018;46(3):438-445.
73. Diedrich P, Fritz U, Kinzinger G, et al. Movement of periodontally affected teeth after guided tissue regeneration (GTR)—an experimental pilot study in animals. *J Orofac Orthop.* 2003;64(3):214-227.
74. Melsen B, Agerbaek N, Eriksen J, et al. New attachment through periodontal treatment and orthodontic intrusion. *Am J Orthod Dentofacial Orthop.* 1998;94(2):104-116.
75. Melsen B, Agerbaek N, Markenstam G. Intrusion of incisors in adult patients with marginal bone loss. *Am J Orthod Dentofacial Orthop.* 1989;96:232-241.
76. Cardaropoli D, Re S, Corrente G, et al. Intrusion of migrated incisors with infrabony defects in adult periodontal patients. *Am J Orthod Dentofacial Orthop.* 2001;120:671-675.
77. Corrente G, Re S, Abundo R, et al. Orthodontic movement into infrabony defects in patients with advanced periodontal disease: a clinical and radiological study. *J Periodontol.* 2003;74:1104-1109.

78. Melsen B, Fiorelli G. Upper molar intrusion. *J Clin Orthod.* 1996; 30(2):91-96.
79. Re S, Cardaropoli D, Abundo R, et al. Reduction of gingival recession following orthodontic intrusion in periodontally compromised patients. *Orthod Craniofac Res.* 2004;7:35-39.
80. Cardaropoli D, Re S, Corrente G, et al. Intrusion of migrated incisors with infrabony defects in adult periodontal patients. *Am J Orthod Dentofacial Orthop.* 2001;120:671-675.
81. Corrente G, Abundo R, Re S, et al. Orthodontic movement into infrabony defects in patients with advanced periodontal disease: a clinical and radiological study. *J Periodontol.* 2003;74:1104-1109.
82. Ericsson I, Thilander B, Lindhe J. Periodontal condition after orthodontic tooth movements in the dog. *Angle Orthod.* 1978;48:201-218.
83. Oyama K, Motoyoshi M, Hirabayashi M, et al. Effects of root morphology on stress distribution at the root apex. *Eur J Orthod.* 2007;29(2): 113-117.
84. Potashnick SR, Rosenberg ES. Forced eruption: principles in periodontics and restorative dentistry. *J Prosthet Dent.* 1982;48(2):141-148.
85. Pontoriero R, Celenza F, Ricci G, et al. Rapid extrusion with fiber resection: a combined orthodontic-periodontic treatment modality. *Int J Periodontics Restorative Dent.* 1987;7:30-43.
86. Melsen B, Costa A. Immediate loading of implants used for orthodontic anchorage. *Clin Orthod Res.* 2000;3:23-28.
87. Rothe LE, Bollen AM, Little RM, et al. Trabecular and cortical bone as risk factors for orthodontic relapse. *Am J Orthod Dentofacial Orthop.* 2006;130(4):476-484.
88. Gkantidis N, Christou P, Topouzelis N. The orthodontic-periodontic interrelationship in integrated treatment challenges: a systematic review. *J Oral Rehabil.* 2010;37:377-390.
89. Rody Jr WJ, Elmaraghy S, McNeight AM, et al. Effects of different orthodontic retention protocols on the periodontal health of mandibular incisors. *Orthod Craniofac Res.* 2016;19(4):198-208.
90. Shaughnessy T, Proffit W, Samar S. Inadvertent tooth movement with fixed lingual retainers. *Am J Orthod Dentofacial Orthop.* 2016; 149:277-286.
91. Matuliene G, Pjetursson BE, Salvi GE. Influence of residual pockets on progression of periodontitis and tooth loss: results after 11 years of maintenance. *J Clin Periodontol.* 2008;35:685-695.
92. Salvi GE, Mischler DC, Schmidlin K. Risk factors associated with the longevity of multi-rooted teeth. Long-term outcomes after active and supportive periodontal therapy. *J Clin Periodontol.* 2014;41: 701-707.
93. Lee CT, Huang HY, Sun TC, et al. Impact of patient compliance on tooth loss during supportive periodontal therapy: a systematic review and metaanalysis. *J Dent Res.* 2015;94:777-786.
94. Ochsenbein C. Osseous resection in periodontal surgery. *J Periodontol.* 1958;29(1):15-26.
95. Carnevale G, Kaldahl WB. Osseous resective surgery. *Periodontol 2000.* 2000;22:59-87. doi:10.1034/j.1600-0757.2000. 2220106.x.
96. Carnevale G. Fibre retention osseous resective surgery: a novel conservative approach for pocket elimination. *J Clin Periodontol.* 2007;34(2):182-187. doi:10.1111/j.1600-051X.2006.01027.x.
97. Renvert S, Persson GR. A systematic review on the use of residual probing depth, bleeding on probing and furcation status following initial periodontal therapy to predict further attachment and tooth loss. *J Clin Periodontol.* 2002;29(3):S82-S91. doi:10.1034/ j.1600-051x.29.s-3.2.x.
98. Ramfjord SP, Nissle RR. The modified Widman flap. *J Periodontol.* 1974;45(8):601-607. doi:10.1902/jop.1974.45.8.2.601.
99. Lang NP. Focus on intrabony defects—conservative therapy. *Periodontol 2000.* 2000;22:51-58. doi:10.1034/j.1600-0757. 2000.2220105.x.
100. Heitz-Mayfield LJ, Trombelli L, Heitz F, et al. A systematic review of the effect of surgical debridement vs non-surgical debridement for the treatment of chronic periodontitis. *J Clin Periodontol.* 2002;29(3):S92-S162. doi:10.1034/j.1600-051x.29.s3.5.x.
101. Trombelli L, Farina R, Franceschetti G, et al. Single-flap approach with buccal access in periodontal reconstructive procedures. *J Periodontol.* 2009;80(2):353-360. doi:10.1902/jop.2009.080420.

17 Surgery First with Aligner Therapy

FLAVIO URIBE and RAVINDRA NANDA

HISTORIC BACKGROUND

The treatment of moderate to severe dentofacial deformity is usually addressed by means of orthognathic surgery. The objectives of orthognathic surgery are to accomplish adequate facial esthetics while achieving a functional occlusion. The occlusal relationship serves as a guide for the skeletal movements and therefore is an important element in orthognathic surgery. Fixed orthodontic appliances in the presurgical phase have historically been used to prepare the dentition for the skeletal movements and to fine-tune the occlusion after orthognathic surgery. Specifically, labial fixed appliances in the presurgical phase eliminate dental compensations and prepare the arches for surgery. Bonded orthodontic brackets on the labial surfaces of the teeth and wires are the orthodontic appliances of choice by clinicians in orthognathic surgery as treatment complexity is high in these patients.

Clear aligner therapy (CAT), with Invisalign (Align Technologies, San Jose, CA, USA) at the forefront, has become a treatment modality in orthodontics that has gained acceptance by practitioners after the significant improvements in the appliance over the last few years. More complex malocclusions have been able to be treated with this appliance with the addition of attachments that optimize tooth movements. An example of more complex approaches with the Invisalign appliance is evident in its use in tandem with orthognathic surgery instead of the conventional labial fixed appliances.

Orthognathic surgery in conjunction with the Invisalign appliance is well accepted by patients with dentofacial deformity for two main reasons. First, most of these patients are usually adults who understandably favor the inconspicuousness of clear aligners over fixed labial appliances. Second, often patients undergoing orthognathic surgery have received orthodontic treatment with fixed appliances during their early teenage years. This treatment has usually been long as the orthodontic therapy may have tried to camouflage the effects of abnormal growth. The net effect is a burnout of the patient who does not want to receive any more orthodontic therapy.

Orthognathic surgery has three specific stages, which include a presurgical orthodontic phase, the surgical procedure, and a postsurgical orthodontic finishing phase. The incorporation of Invisalign in orthognathic surgery can be accomplished in different ways, depending on which stage of treatment it will be used and the type surgical approach (surgery first or conventional approach). For example, one of the approaches is to limit the Invisalign appliance to the presurgical phase. Typically this phase is the longest in orthognathic surgery, lasting approximately from 12 to 25 months.[1,2] Therefore if patients receive CAT on the presurgical phase, fixed appliances will be only used for a short period of time during the postsurgical phase. This approach is often preferred since the labial fixed appliances used in the postsurgical phase typically have better finishing control of the occlusion. The labial orthodontic appliances are placed just before surgery, thereby facilitating the conventional approach during surgery that ties the interocclusal surgical splint to the orthodontic bonded appliances, required for fixation of the proximal and distal bone segments after the osteotomies. The second approach uses the Invisalign system for both pre- and postsurgical phases, with no fixed labial appliances, which has the challenge of limited areas available to securely tie the surgical splint for maxillary and mandibular fixation.

Although clinicians are using Invisalign in conjunction with orthognathic surgery, no studies have been conducted evaluating the outcomes with this approach. In fact, most of the published literature has been in the form of case reports. The first report of this approach was published in 2005 using Invisalign in combination to orthognathic surgery.[3] The treatment of two patients was described in which Invisalign was used for the presurgical phase of aligning and leveling the arches. Segmental fixed appliances were also used as adjuncts to the clear aligners to derotate some teeth, since at that point in time the Invisalign appliance had not developed the optimized attachments that facilitated these corrections. Fixed appliances were placed just before the surgical procedure and maintained through the postsurgical detailing phase. The total treatment time for one patient was 44 months (20 months for the presurgical phase with Invisalign) and 31 months for the other (27 months for the presurgical phase with Invisalign). The reason for one of the patients having undergone almost 4 years of treatment was attributed to insurance approval and scheduling the surgery date. Additionally, the patients were changing aligners every 2 weeks. Finally, the author suggested that in patients with single jaw surgery, fixed appliances would not be necessary, being managed fully with the Invisalign appliance.

In 2008, Womack and Day[4] reported on another patient treated with Invisalign and orthognathic surgery who had class II malocclusion and sleep apnea. In this report, bimaxillary advancement with a two-piece-maxilla for transverse correction was executed. Both the pre- and postsurgical phases were completed with the Invisalign appliance. The duration of the presurgical phase was 8 months for this patient. The fixation during surgery of the maxilla and the mandible after the osteotomies was achieved by means of archbars tied to the splint. Since the maxilla was split for transverse expansion, a soft tissue splint was placed during surgery and left for 6 weeks for stabilization of the two maxillary halves. After the surgical procedure, polyvinyl siloxane (PVS) impressions were taken for refinement of the occlusion, which took another 6 months of treatment. The total treatment time was 22 months, which included a period in which the patient was not seen due to unavailability related to a work schedule. During this finishing phase, buttons were bonded to the posterior teeth to settle the occlusion with elastics.

Mancuzzi et al.[5] in 2010 reported on the treatment of a patient who had multiple missing teeth and class III malocclusion who underwent orthognathic surgery with Invisalign. Both pre- and postsurgical phases were performed with the Invisalign appliance. The presurgical phase lasted 6 months. For the fixation of the maxilla and mandible into their new positions, buttons were bonded to the labial surfaces of the majority of the posterior teeth. The authors maintained the patient on the splint for 4 weeks after surgery and then delivered a dynamic functional positioner for 3 months. Some ceramic brackets were bonded to help with the seating of the occlusion. The total treatment time was 10 months.

Pagani et al.[6] in 2016 reported on another patient with a class III malocclusion treated with Invisalign in the pre- and postsurgical phases. A total of 10 months was the duration of the presurgical alignment phase. The day before surgery, fixed appliances were bonded, which were removed 1 month after surgery. The total duration of treatment was 12 months.

Splint-Aided Maxillary and Mandibular Fixation Without Labial Fixed Appliances

When labial fixed orthodontic appliances are not present, the stabilization of the surgical splint after the osteotomies can be troublesome. The maxilla and mandible need to be securely tied to the surgical splint to ensure proper referencing the jaws to each other to achieve the planned outcome after surgery. The surgical splint transfers the information of the virtual three-dimensional (3D) plan to guide the free osteotomized segment to a stable reference skeletal region. The splint must be tied to the dentition or denture bases to reference maxilla and mandible to each other. The connection of the splint to the teeth is usually facilitated when orthodontic appliances are bonded to the labial surfaces of the teeth. With Invisalign there are no labial appliances to enable this connection (Fig. 17.1). Different approaches have been described in the literature to overcome this problem.[7] Archbars used for maxillary and mandibular fracture fixation are one of the earliest adopted approaches. The problem with this approach is it is time consuming, thereby extending the duration of time the patient is under anesthesia, which increases the risks of the surgical procedure. Another approach is to bond multiple buttons on the labial surfaces of teeth, specifically to be used for the surgical procedure. This was reported by Hong et al.[8] when using lingual orthodontic appliances in orthognathic surgery.

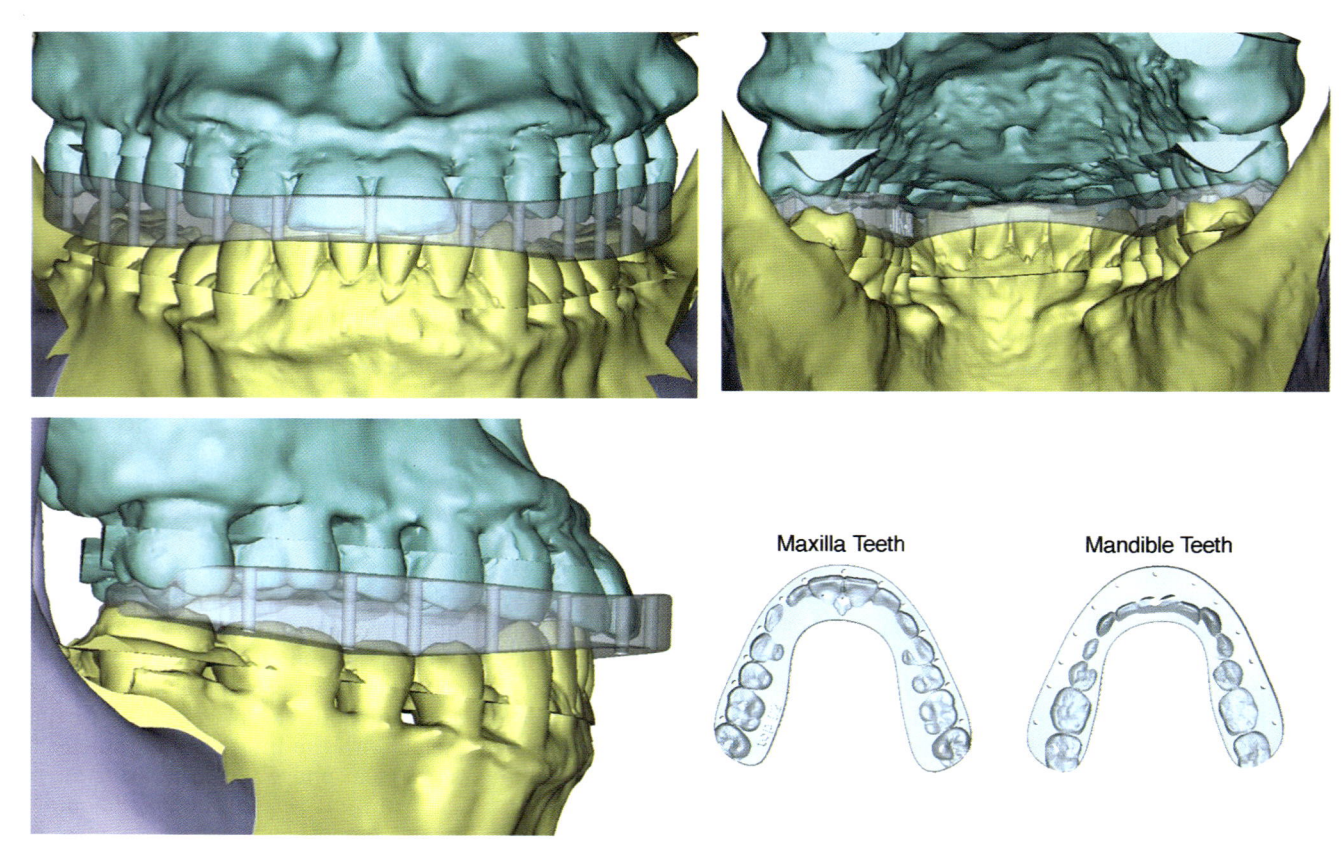

Fig. 17.1 Surgical splint with holes to be used in a patient undergoing orthognathic surgery using Invisalign as the only appliance for orthodontic treatment. Note that no labial orthodontic appliances are present.

However, since no archwires are present connecting the bonded buttons, bonding failure could occur during the operation while the jaws are being tractioned to seat them into the splint. Furthermore, the breakage of one of these attached buttons may end up entrapped in the mucoperiosteal flaps, causing a significant complication to the surgical procedure.

With the advent of miniscrews in orthodontics, the connection of the dentition to the surgical splint has been facilitated. This was reported by Paik et al.[9] who added two miniscrews in each of the quadrants, mesial to the first molars and premolars. These miniscrews are used to secure the splint tightly to the teeth and can be used after surgery to support the use of intermaxillary elastics to keep the teeth in the postsurgical planned occlusion. A more complex setup that connects the miniscrews through a bar framework is commercially available.[7] The Smartlock hybrid MMF from Stryker (Kalamazoo, MI, USA) and the MatrixWAVE MMF from Depuy Synthes Craniomaxillofacial (West Chester, PA, USA) are similar bone-supported archbars to be used during surgery. This framework is secured to the labial alveolar bone of the dentition through four to six miniscrews per arch. The main advantage of these two products over an approach that uses only the miniscrews is that more locations are available to connect the surgical splint to the maxilla and mandible through ligatures. This may facilitate more tight adaptation of the osteotomized segments into the surgical splint. Typically, the mesh (including the miniscrews) is removed after the osteotomized maxilla and mandible are secured with hardware, which has the drawback that intermaxillary elastic wear in the postsurgical stage will require to be delivered from the teeth, which could have an unfavorable extrusive effect on the specific teeth from which the elastics are being worn.

Transitioning Into and Out of Surgery With Clear Aligners

As mentioned, the major difference in the execution of surgery in patients with CAT is the absence of labial fixed orthodontic appliances typically necessary for securing the surgical splint. These patients are typically wearing a series of sequential aligners as part of the presurgical phase and will transition to the aligners in the postsurgical phase to complete orthodontic treatment. If the patient is wearing aligners in the presurgical phase, the surgical plan will consist of maxillomandibular movements that will achieve a result close to the final idealized occlusion. Prior to surgery, a scan or impression is taken to plan the tooth movements after surgery to detail the occlusion, which will be used for fabrication of the aligners. An alternative is to take this scan or PVS impression after surgery. However, the acquisition of a scan or impression after surgery is somewhat difficult due the limited mouth opening observed during the first 2 months after surgery. Therefore taking the scan prior to surgery may be advocated to be able to start wearing the aligners soon after surgery (approximately 2 weeks after). Although this approach may expedite treatment there still may be a slight unpredictability in the planned occlusion, and the actual postsurgical occlusion if different may require different movements than originally planned. However, since the teeth would be usually well aligned after the presurgical phase, any inaccuracies between the planned and the obtained occlusion can be managed with intermaxillary elastics.

On the other hand, the predictability of the planned final occlusal outcome for the fabrication of the postsurgical aligners could be more difficult in patients where the maxilla will require segmentation in two or more pieces. In these situations it is still possible that the presurgical dental models could be segmented to the planned outcome, and a scan of this model could be used for the fabrication of the surgical splint and the postsurgical aligners. However, it is better recommended to take the scan or impressions after the surgery to ensure a more precise fit of the aligners, especially if the segmentation is more that two pieces.

Another important consideration when segmenting the maxilla is that the patient typically will have to maintain the splint after surgery for 4 to 6 weeks prior to resuming orthodontic movements. A splint covering the incisal and occlusal surfaces of the teeth is bulky and cumbersome for a patient in recovery after surgery. A splint not covering the occlusal surfaces is typically recommended for the postsurgical phase prior to resuming the new aligners (Fig. 17.2).

An example of management of a patient with Invisalign appliances into and out of the surgical procedure is illustrated in Figs. 17.3, 17.4, and 17.5. This patient received a LeForte I osteotomy with a three-piece segmentation for transverse expansion and vertical impaction of the posterior segments (see Fig. 17.3). The occlusion 5 weeks after surgery at the splint removal visit shows a slight discrepancy between the surgical plan and the achieved outcome (see Fig. 17.4). The patient was scanned 3 weeks later when she was able to achieve enough range of motion. The aligners were delivered in conjunction with vertical elastics from the miniscrews used during surgery. The occlusion was nicely established to the projected outcome approximately 3 months after surgery (see Fig. 17.5).

A surgical intermaxillary splint has been designed by 3D Systems (Rockville, SC, USA), which consists of 3D-printed, thin, hard acrylic templates of the maxillary and mandibular arches attached together registering the final occlusion after the osteotomies.[10] There is no need for wires or miniscrews to tie the osteotomized dentition to the splint. The teeth fit into the splint by snapping physically into place. By using this splint, a transition to the postsurgical aligners may be more easily achieved. This clear aligner orthodontic splint was recently reported by Caminiti and Lou,[10] who also described a reduced cost version produced by splinting Essix-type trays through clear denture repair acrylic. One major disadvantage of this new type of intermaxillary splint is that the miniscrews are typically not placed, therefore intermaxillary elastics to maintain the occlusal result after surgery require either hooks on the clear aligners or cutouts for bonding buttons or brackets to the labial surfaces of some teeth.

Surgery First and CAT

A very novel approach to the application of the Invisalign system in orthognathic surgery is its integration to the

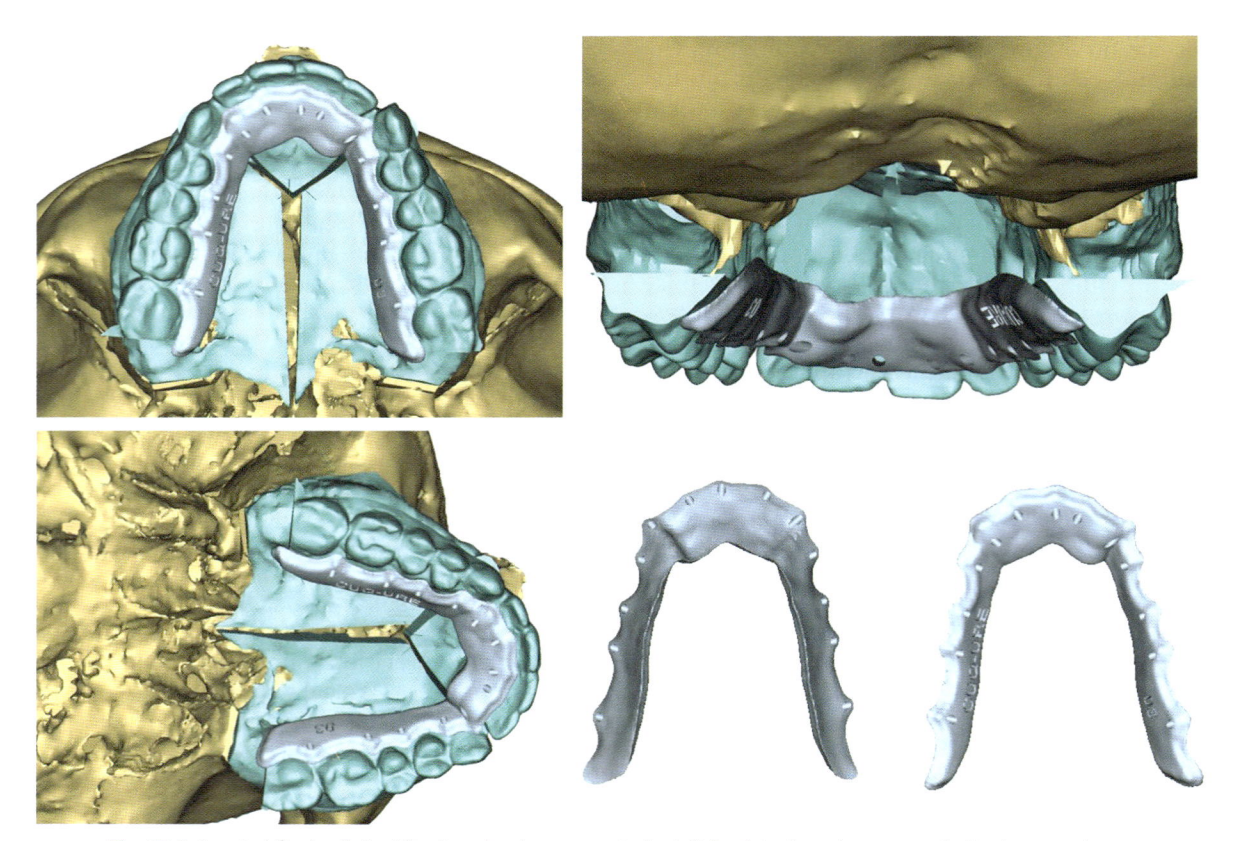

238 Principles and Biomechanics of Aligner Treatment

Fig. 17.2 Surgical final splint without occlusal coverage to be left for 4 to 5 weeks postsurgically due to a three-piece-maxilla osteotomy.

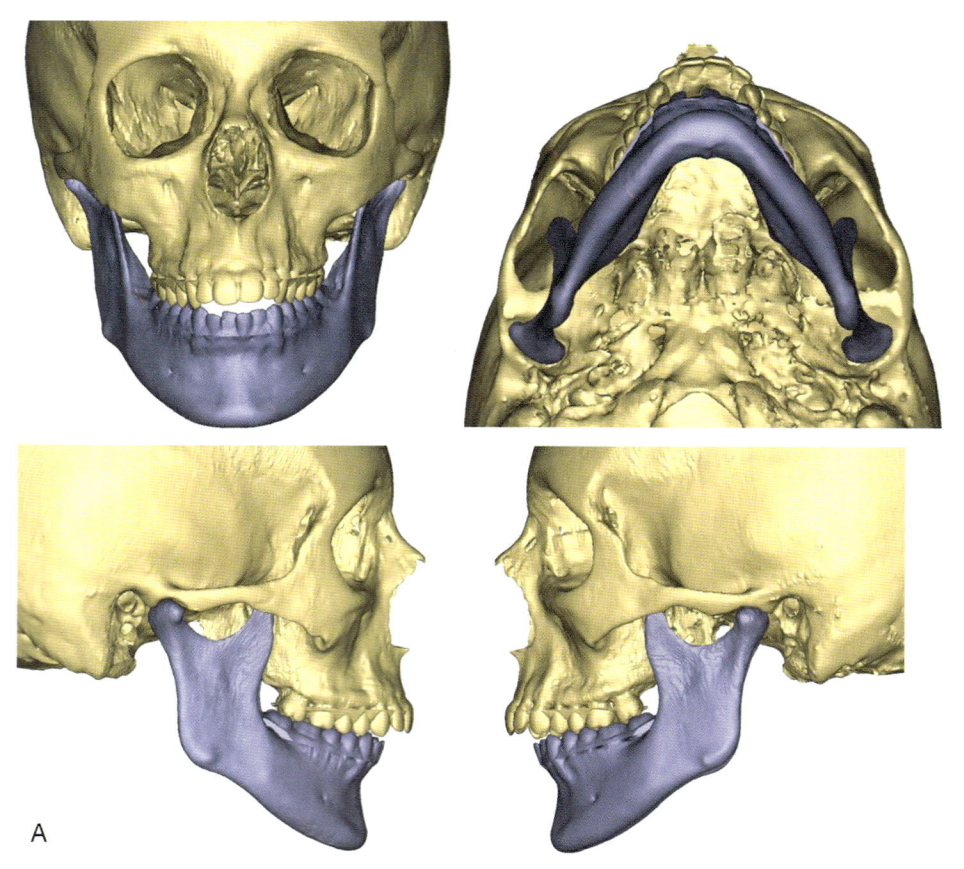

A

Fig. 17.3 Three-dimensional virtual surgical plan. (A) Presurgery.

17 • Surgery First with Aligner Therapy   239

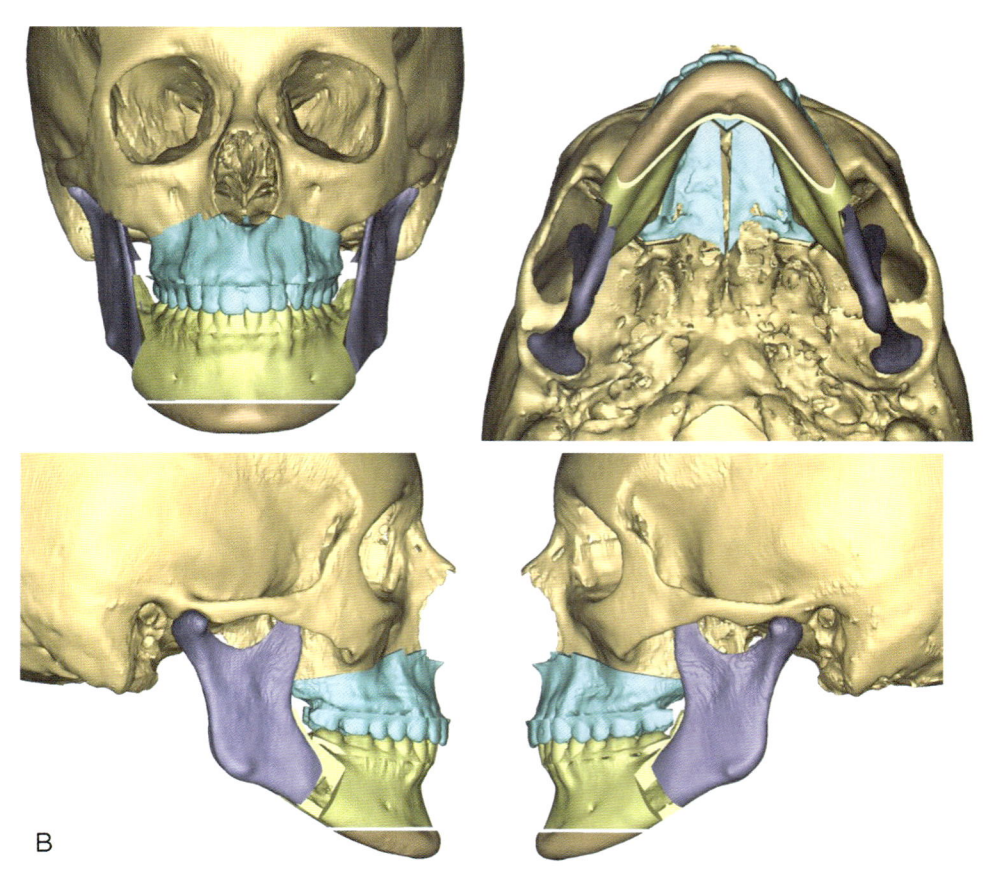

Fig. 17.3, cont'd (B) Planned osteotomies consisting of three-piece-maxilla with impaction of the posterior segments and mandibular advancement with genioplasty.

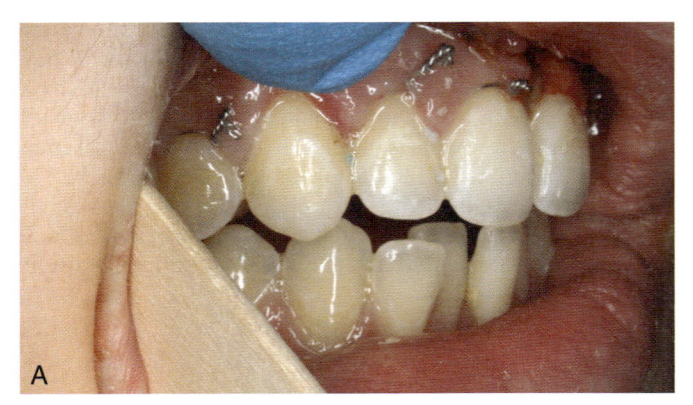

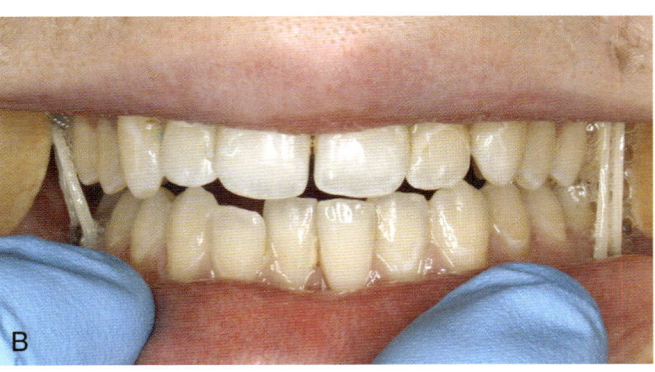

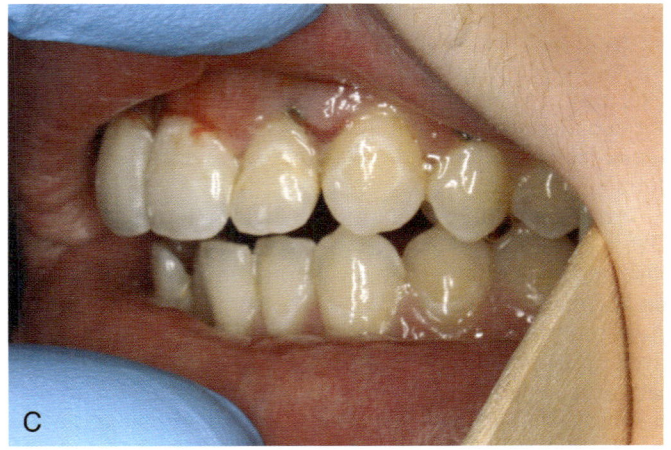

Fig. 17.4 Postsurgical occlusion deviating slightly from the planned occlusion. A) Right buccal, B) Left buccal, C) frontal occlusal views.

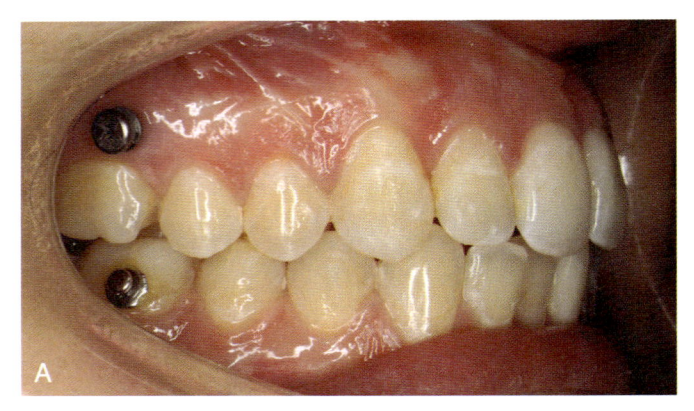

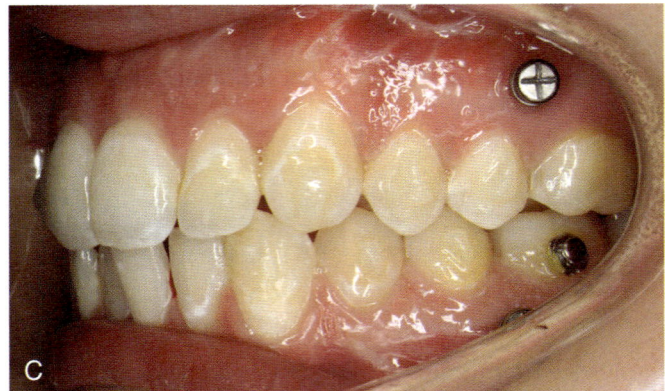

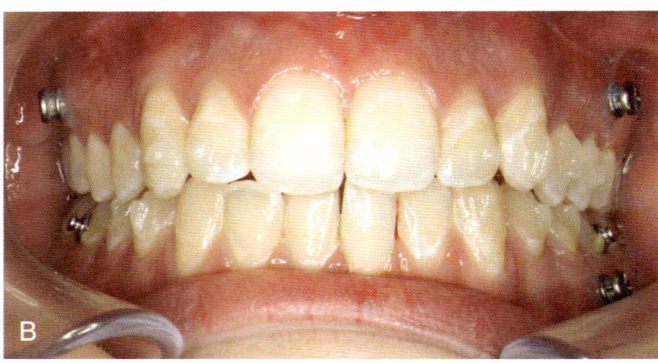

Fig. 17.5 Occlusion seated with intermaxillary elastics and clear aligners to the planned outcome after 3 months. A) Right buccal, B) Left buccal, C) frontal occlusal views.

surgery first approach (SFA). Perhaps this is one of the most attractive options for patients with dentofacial deformity where the facial and smile esthetics drive their chief complaint. Surgery first addresses the dentofacial deformity from the beginning of treatment without any presurgical orthodontics. By performing orthognathic surgery in this manner, it has been shown that patient satisfaction is higher than with the conventional approach.[11] This is understandable since obviating the presurgical phase, the typical decompensations that accentuate the dentofacial deformity are eliminated. Furthermore, the chief complaint of the patient is immediately addressed without being postponed for a year or more as is the case with the conventional approach.

Another condition where the combination of SFA and CAT is largely indicated is in the treatment of patients with obstructive sleep apnea who will undergo maxillomandibular advancement surgery. First, the surgery addresses immediately the medical functional condition without a delayed presurgical orthodontic phase; secondly, these patients can achieve a good occlusion after surgery with the use of clear appliances, which are more acceptable to this population particularly composed of adult patients.

In the SFA/CAT (Invisalign) approach, two common treatment modalities have been applied. The first consists of placing labial orthodontic appliances, including a wire, prior to surgery (1–2 weeks before). These fixed appliances are used for 2 to 4 months after surgery, during which time major intraarch movements are accomplished and intermaxillary vertical elastics are used to seat the occlusion. This approach also has the advantage for the surgeon of being able to tie the surgical splint to the orthodontic appliances during maxillary and mandibular osseous fixation.

The appliances are then removed after this short phase of orthodontic fixed therapy and Invisalign trays are given to the patient until treatment completion. The second treatment modality uses Invisalign as the only appliance for orthodontic movement after surgery without the use of any fixed labial appliances. This approach unfortunately poses the same challenge on maxillary and mandibular fixation for patients who do not have labial orthodontic appliances during surgery. Nonetheless, different alternatives have been designed to facilitate and increase the predictability of the fixation with Invisalign appliances as described earlier.

A patient who underwent SFA in conjunction with Invisalign is presented to illustrate this specific approach. This case report also illustrates how the 3D virtual plan for the surgical treatment can be integrated to the orthodontic 3D dental plan represented in the ClinCheck (Align Technologies, San Jose, CA, USA).

Case Study

A 19-year-old female patient presented to the oral maxillofacial surgeon with the goal of improving her facial esthetics (Fig. 17.6). She had received orthodontic treatment during her adolescence consisting of camouflage treatment for a class II skeletal relationship addressed through the extraction of maxillary first premolars. The patient had close to adequate arch alignment and a class II occlusion with a 5-mm overjet (Fig. 17.7); however, there was a significant facial convexity related to a large mandibular deficiency. The denture base was anteriorly positioned to the apical base in the mandible, and the lower incisors were significantly labially inclined. The patient also had steep

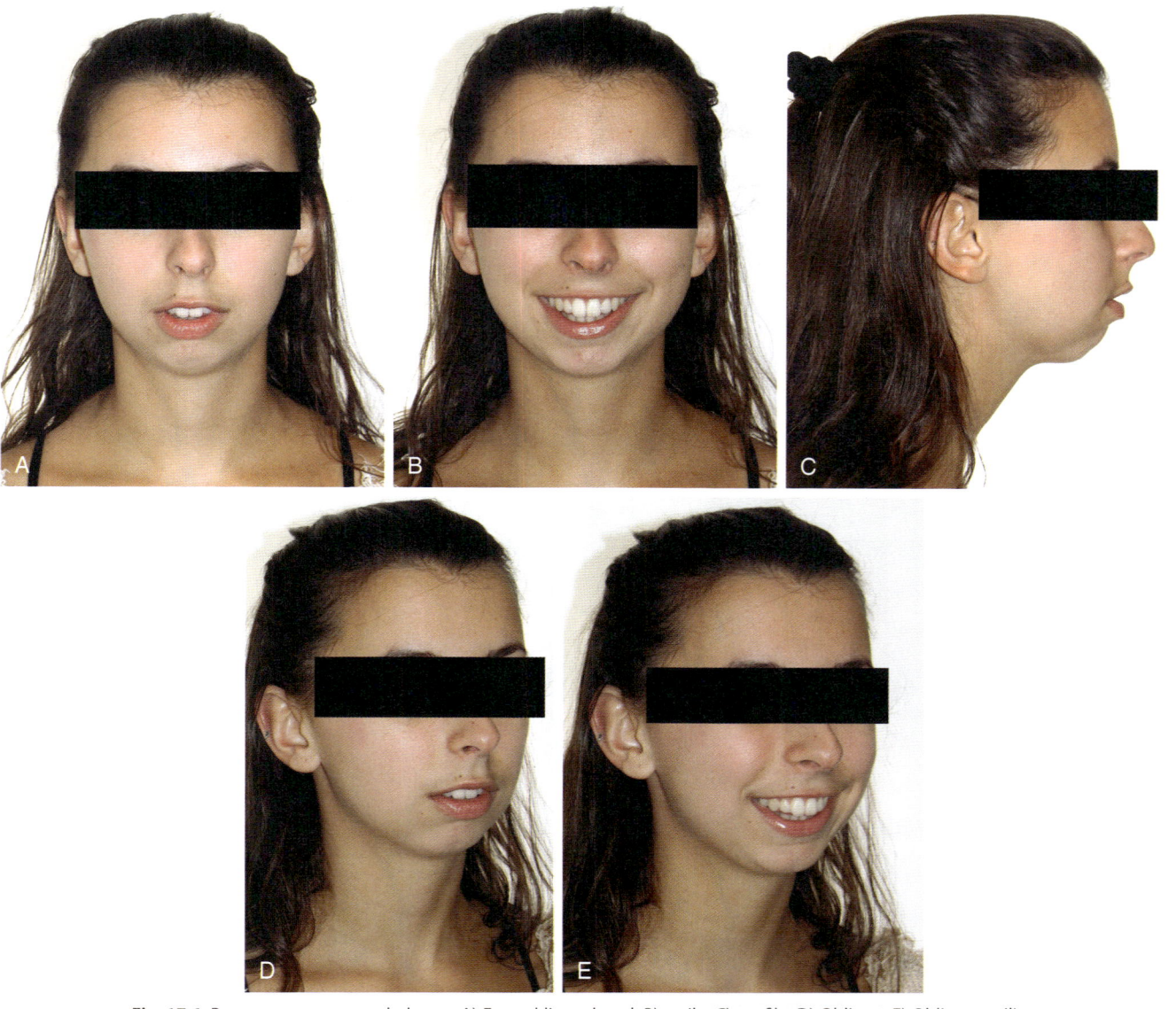

Fig. 17.6 Pretreatment extraoral photos. A) Frontal lips relaxed, B) smile, C) profile, D) Oblique, E) Oblique smiling views. (A-C from Chang J, Steinbacher D, Nanda R, et al. "Surgery-first" approach with Invisalign therapy to correct a class II malocclusion and severe mandibular retrognathism. *J Clin Orthod*. 2019;53[7]:397–404.)

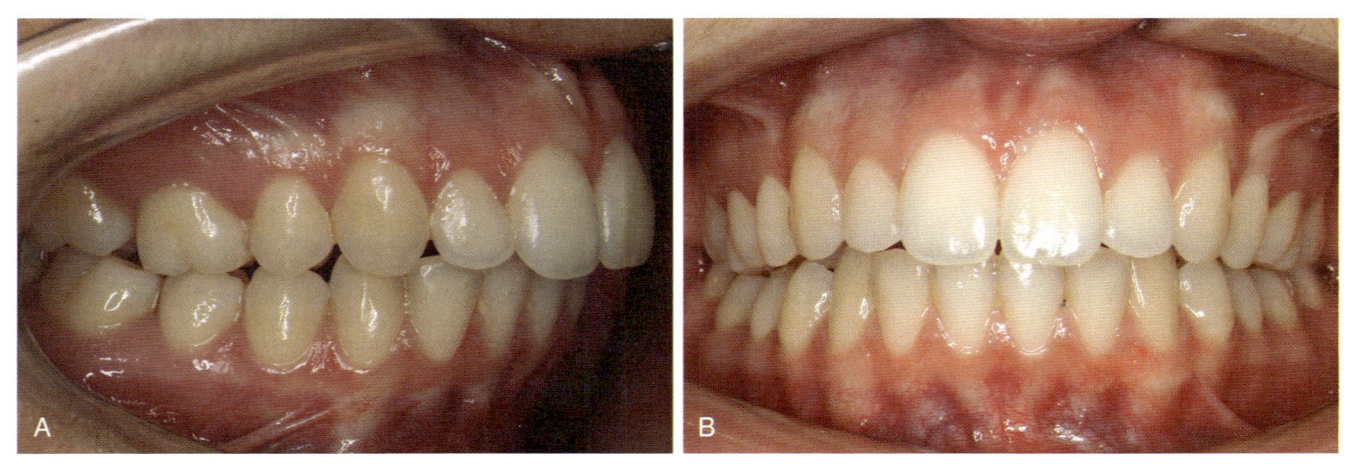

Fig. 17.7 Pretreatment intraoral photos. A) Right buccal, B) Frontal,

Continued

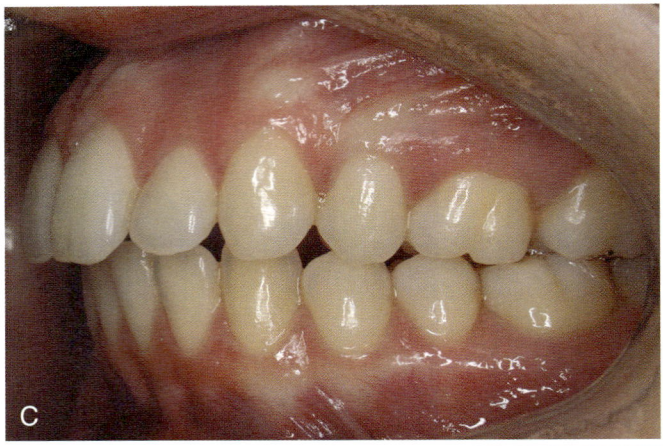

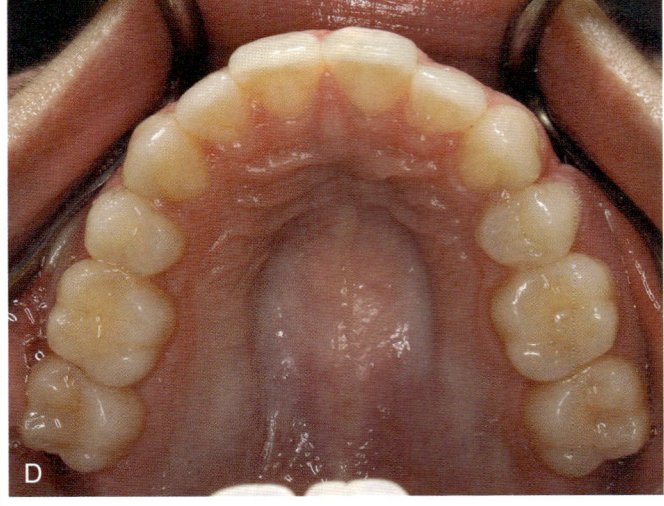

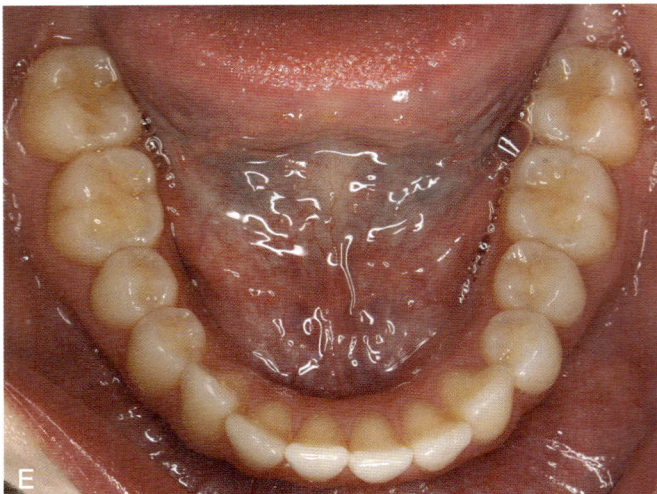

Fig. 17.7, cont'd C) Left buccal occlusion. D) Maxillary and E) Mandibular occlusal views. (From Chang J, Steinbacher D, Nanda R, et al. "Surgery-first" approach with Invisalign therapy to correct a class II malocclusion and severe mandibular retrognathism. *J Clin Orthod.* 2019;53[7]: 397–404.)

lower mandibular and occlusal planes. The maxillary position of the incisors was overall adequate in the vertical and anteroposterior dimensions and included a good inclination in reference to the cranial base (Fig. 17.8). All third molars had been extracted, and the roots had adequate root parallelism (Fig. 17.9).

To maximize the mandibular projection, two options were available. The first one required the extraction of two mandibular premolars to retract the mandibular incisors,

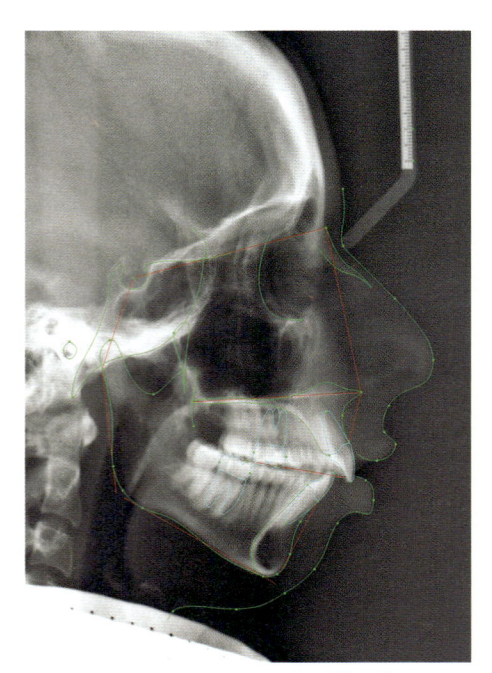

Fig. 17.8 Pretreatment digitized lateral cephalogram. (From Chang J, Steinbacher D, Nanda R, et al. "Surgery-first" approach with Invisalign therapy to correct a class II malocclusion and severe mandibular retrognathism. *J Clin Orthod.* 2019;53[7]:397-404.)

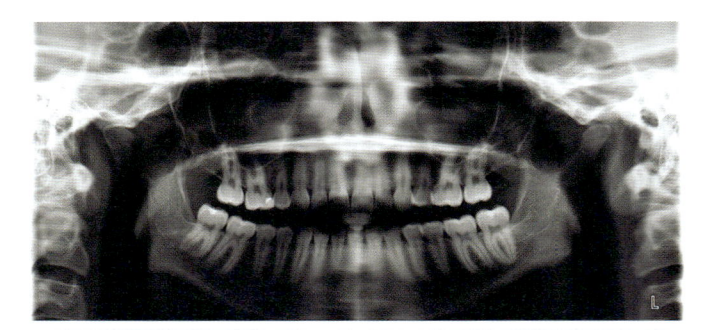

Fig. 17.9 Pretreatment panoramic radiograph. (From Chang J, Steinbacher D, Nanda R, et al. "Surgery-first" approach with Invisalign therapy to correct a class II malocclusion and severe mandibular retrognathism. *J Clin Orthod.* 2019;53[7]:397-404.)

achieving a large overjet to obtain a significant mandibular advancement with surgery. The second option was a nonextraction approach with a counterclockwise rotation of the maxillomandibular complex in conjunction with a genioplasty. The patient opted for the second option as she did not want any more tooth extractions and did not want a prolonged presurgical orthodontic phase of space closure. Additionally, with a nonextraction approach, surgery first was indicated as it addressed her chief complaint of optimizing her facial esthetics.

A virtual 3D plan was made for the surgical movements (Fig. 17.10). When her stone models were occluded in the planned occlusion after surgery, no transverse problems were observed; therefore no maxillary segmentation was planned (Fig. 17.11). Figures 17.10B and C shows the specific movements that were planned for this patient. The counterclockwise rotation of the maxillomandibular complex in conjunction with the genioplasty gave her approximately 19 mm of projection at menton.

Prior to surgery, PVS impressions were taken for fabrication of the aligners that would address the mild crowding and would also serve to detail the occlusion in the postsurgical phase.

The patient was advanced into an edge-to-edge incisor overcorrection relationship. Four miniscrews on each quadrant were placed interradicularly to be used during surgery for intermaxillary fixation. Two weeks after surgery, facial esthetics were greatly improved with the surgical procedure (Fig. 17.12). At the occlusal level, a slight lateral open bite was noticed on the right side, which was expected based on the planned postsurgical occlusion (Fig. 17.13). The patient was wearing intermaxillary elastics in a class II direction from the more anterior miniscrews in the maxilla to the most posterior miniscrews in the mandible. Two months after surgery, the facial swelling had reduced significantly (Fig. 17.14), and the patient had almost 90% of mandibular range of motion. All the attachments from the Invisalign appliance were bonded, and small tubes bonded to the mandibular first molars. The patient started the first phase of aligners changing them on a weekly basis. Intermaxillary elastics from the right maxillary miniscrew implants were used to erupt the mandibular teeth on this opposing quadrant into occlusion (Fig. 17.15). Five months after surgery, the lateral open bite on the right buccal segment was still evident (Fig. 17.16). A cantilever arm was extended from the lower right first molar to engage an elastic extending from the maxillary right posterior miniscrew (Fig. 17.17). The objective of this cantilever arm was to provide an uprighting moment to the right lower molar, which was mesially tipped. Intermaxillary elastics were also

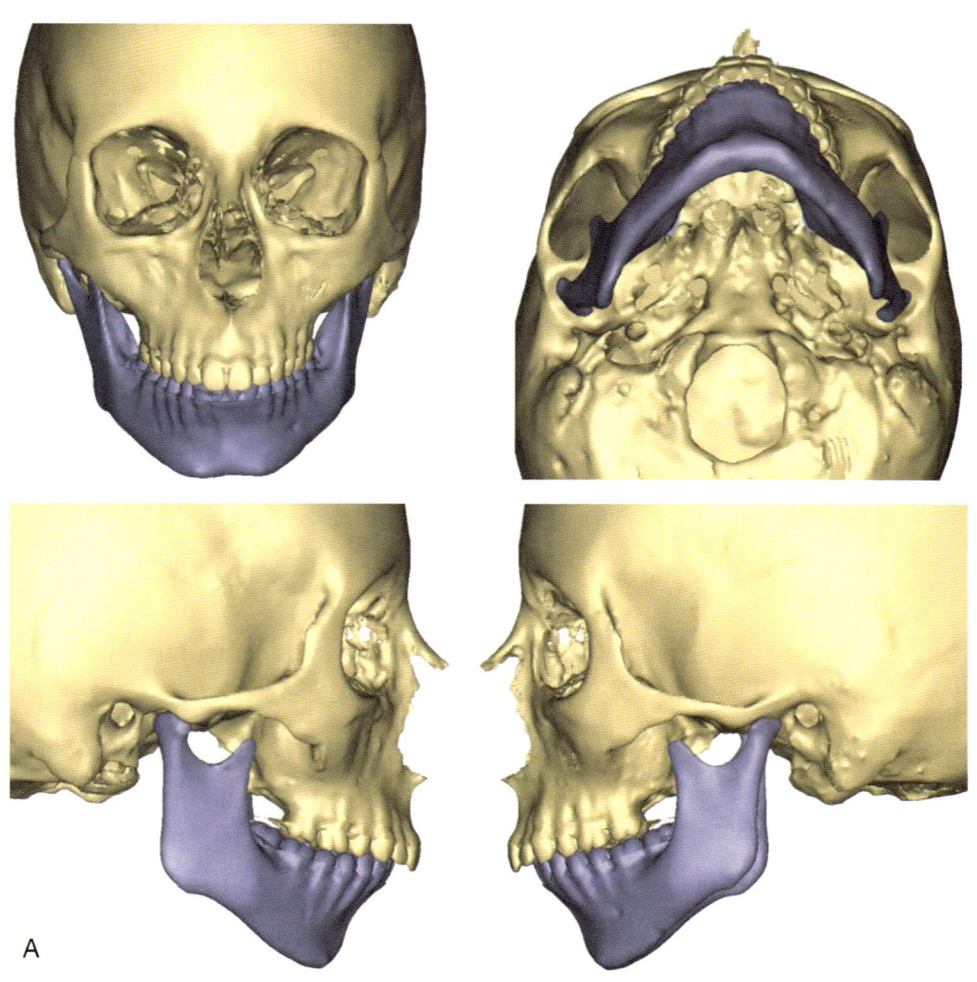

Fig. 17.10 (A) Three-dimensional (3D) virtual surgical plan presurgery.

Continued

Name	Left/Right (mm)	Ant/Post (mm)	Up/Down (mm)
A	1.3 L	1.0 Ant	0.7 Down
ANS	1.4 L	0.1 Post	0.0 Up
Maxilla 1st Molar L	0.8 L	2.9 Ant	4.3 Down
Maxilla 1st Molar R	0.8 L	4.1 Ant	4.2 Down
Maxilla Canine L	1.2 L	3.6 Ant	1.6 Down
Maxilla Canine R	1.2 L	4.3 Ant	1.5 Down
Maxilla Incisor Midline	1.3 L	4.2 Ant	0.3 Down
Maxilla Medial L	1.2 L	1.1 Post	1.4 Down
Maxilla Lateral L	0.8 L	0.0 Ant	4.3 Down
Maxilla Medial R	1.3 L	0.9 Post	1.2 Down
Maxilla Lateral R	0.8 L	1.1 Ant	4.5 Down
Mandible 1st Molar L	0.5 L	6.6 Ant	6.2 Down
Mandible 1st Molar R	0.6 L	8.5 Ant	6.9 Down
Mandible Canine L	1.4 L	7.3 Ant	2.8 Down
Mandible Canine R	1.4 L	8.4 Ant	3.4 Down
Mandible Incisor Midline	1.7 L	8.1 Ant	2.2 Down
Me	1.4 L	18.5 Ant	6.1 Down
Pog	1.6 L	18.2 Ant	5.8 Down

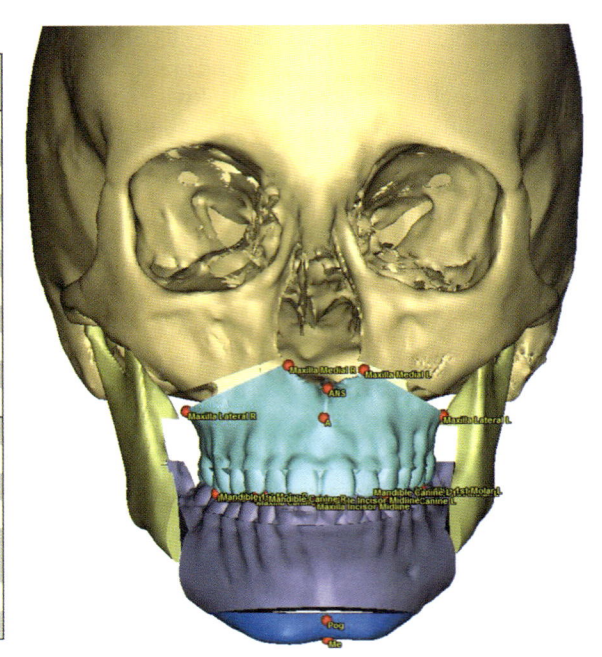

B

C

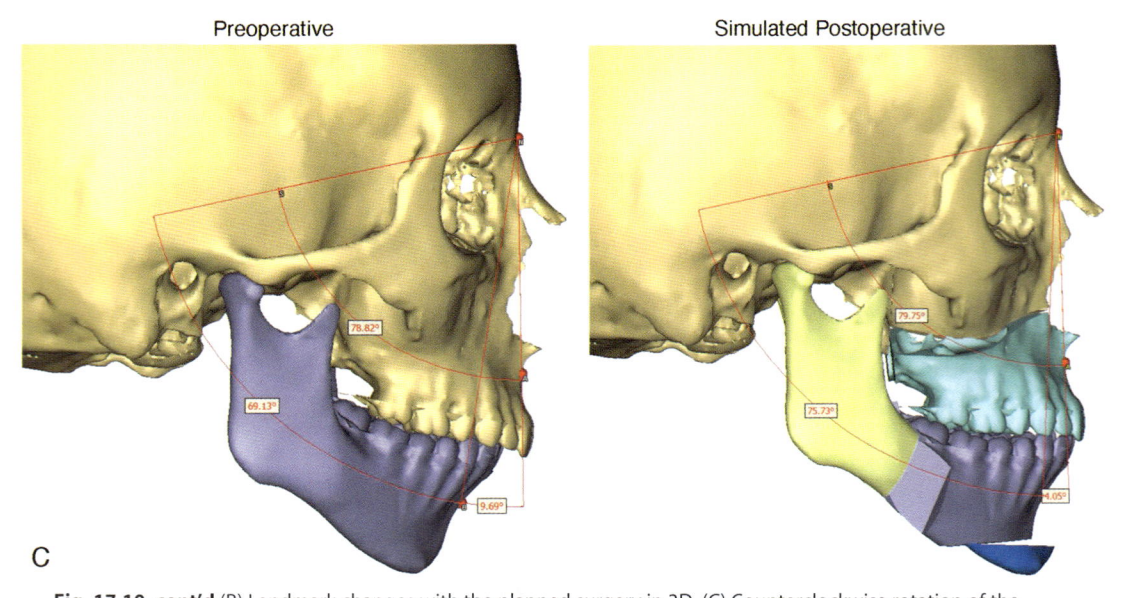

Fig. 17.10, cont'd (B) Landmark changes with the planned surgery in 3D. (C) Counterclockwise rotation of the maxillomandibular complex. (A from Chang J, Steinbacher D, Nanda R, et al. "Surgery-first" approach with Invisalign therapy to correct a class II malocclusion and severe mandibular retrognathism. *J Clin Orthod*. 2019;53[7]:397-404.)

worn from two mandibular buttons on the premolars to a hook in the maxillary aligner. Distal to the mandibular right canine, the aligner was cut to allow for extrusion on the mandibular buccal segment.

Twelve months after surgery, the swelling had completely resolved (Fig. 17.18). The occlusion was almost ideal at this point, with some minor refinement required (Fig. 17.19).

After another aligner refinement phase, the orthodontic treatment was finished to a good occlusal and facial result (Figs. 17.20 and 17.21). The lateral cephalogram depicts the sagittal soft and hard tissue changes (Fig. 17.22), while the panoramic radiograph shows adequate root parallelism (Fig. 17.23). The superimposition reveals the remarkable soft and hard tissue mandibular advancement (Fig. 17.24).

As part of her enhancing the patient's facial esthetics, a rhinoplasty was performed approximately 6 months after orthognathic surgery. A very nice esthetic and occlusal outcome was achieved in this patient with the SFA/CAT approach.

Interestingly, this patient was attending college in a location that was at a far distance from our institution. Most of her visits were carried during the summer when she was off school. During the academic year she was provided with the aligners, and her progress was monitored through photos she provided to our office every 2 months. The patient had approximately 10 orthodontic visits.

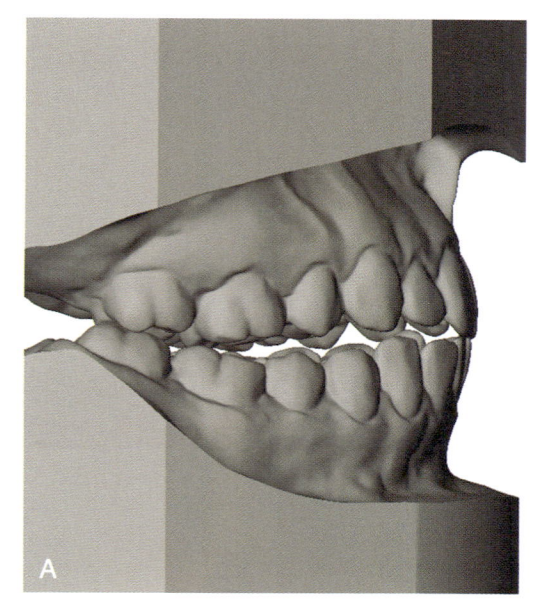

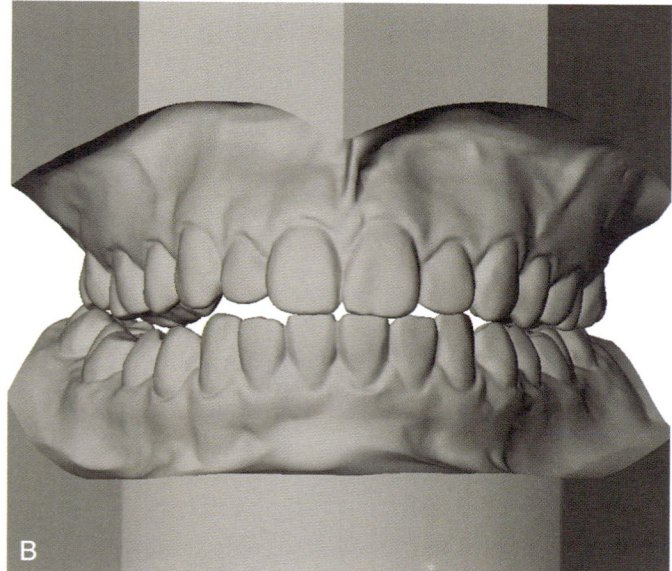

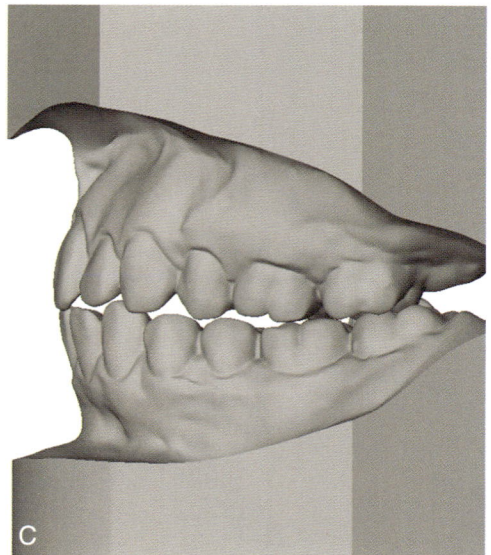

Fig. 17.11 Planned postsurgical occlusion with overcorrection. A) Right buccal, B) Frontal, C) Left Buccal views of the planned occlusion

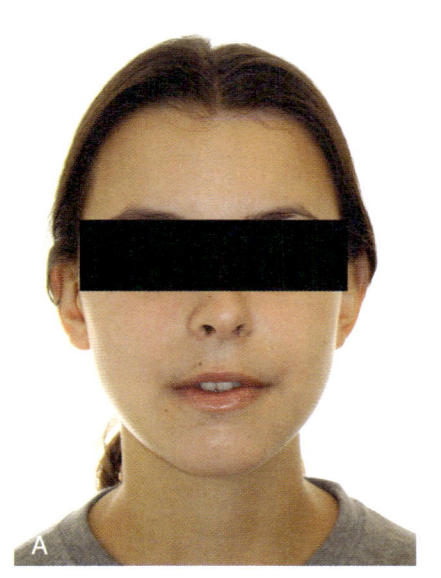

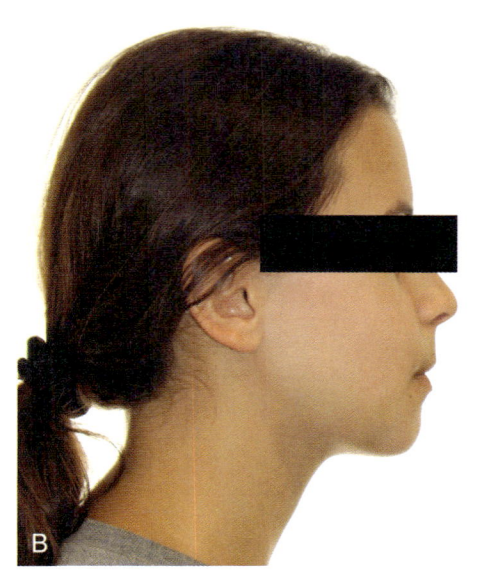

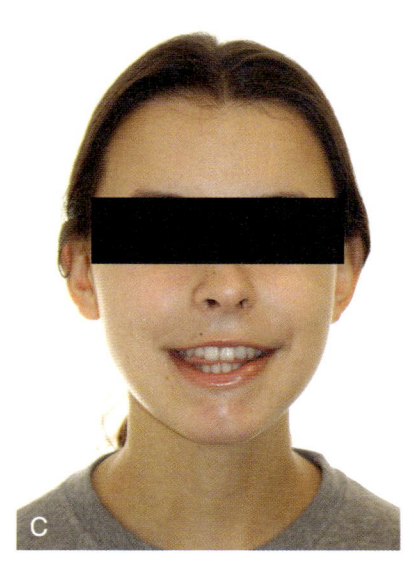

Fig. 17.12 Extraoral photos 2 weeks postsurgery. A) Frontal, B) Profile, and C) Smiling views.

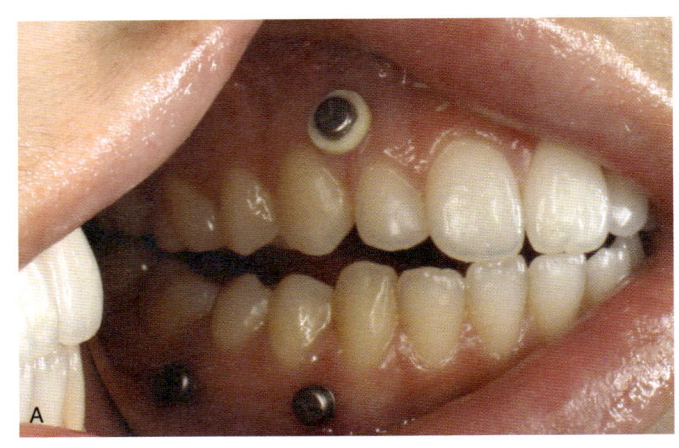

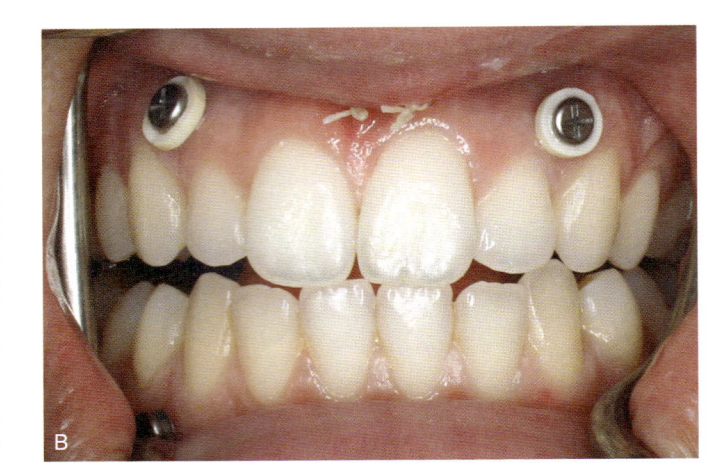

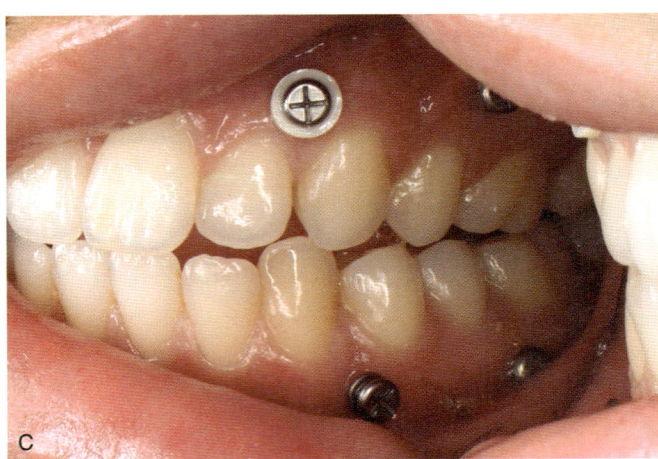

Fig. 17.13 Intraoral photos 2 weeks postsurgery. A) Right buccal, B) Frontal and C) Left buccal views of patient in occlusion.

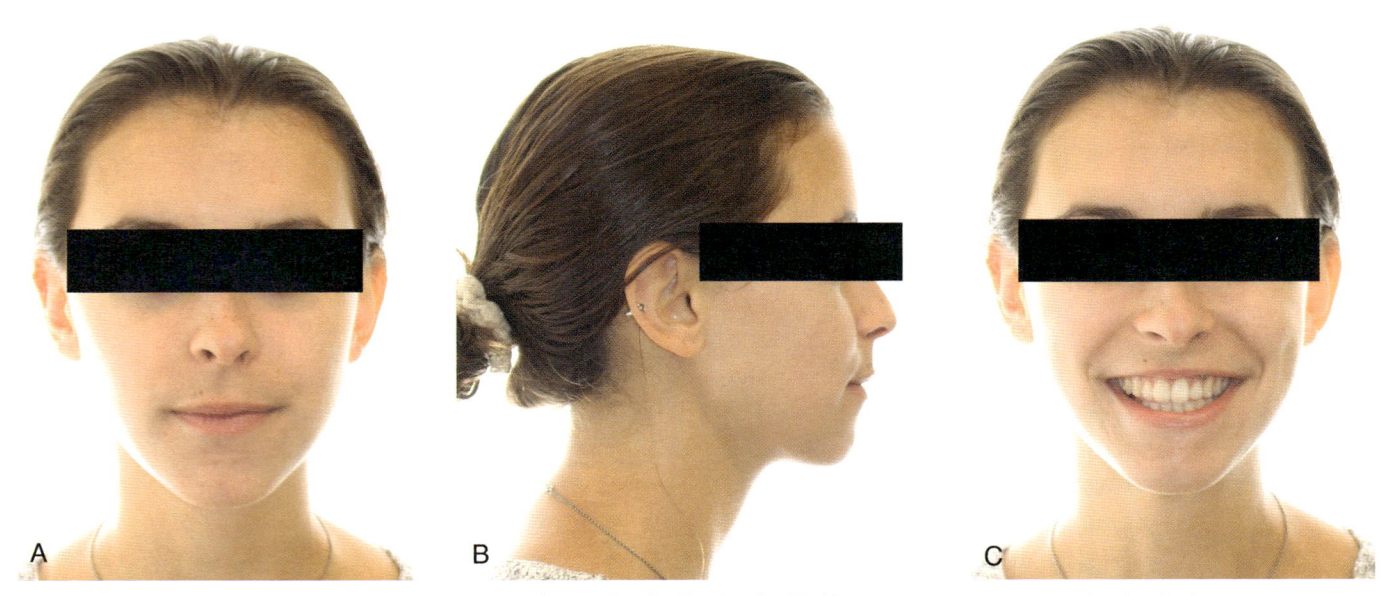

Fig. 17.14 Reduction of facial swelling 2 months postsurgery. A) Frontal, B) Profile, and C) Smiling views. (From Chang J, Steinbacher D, Nanda R, et al. "Surgery-first" approach with Invisalign therapy to correct a class II malocclusion and severe mandibular retrognathism. *J Clin Orthod*. 2019;53[7]:397-404.)

17 • Surgery First with Aligner Therapy 247

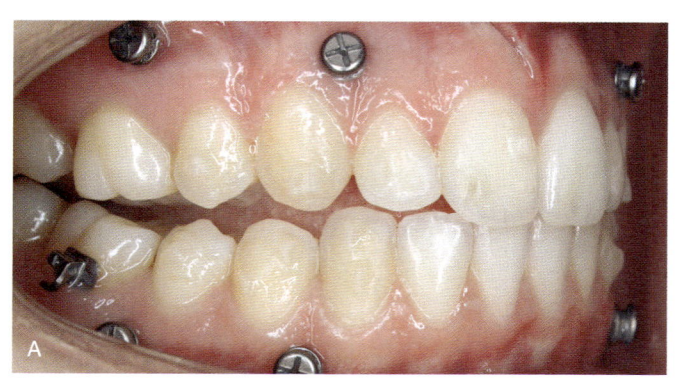

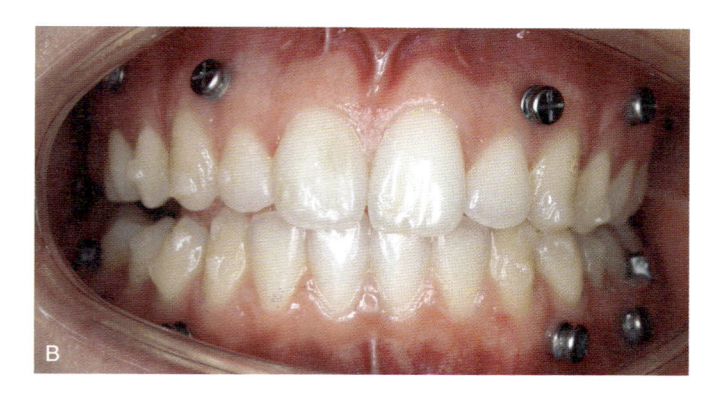

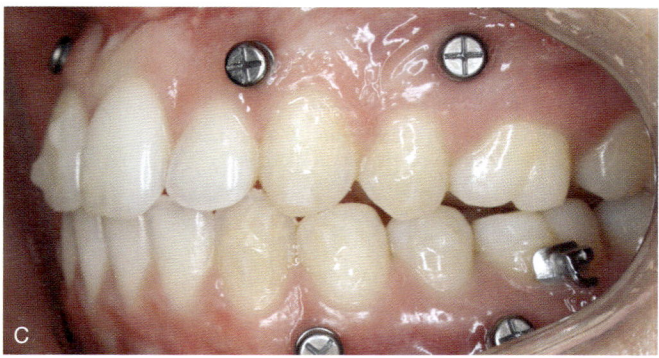

Fig. 17.15 Intraoral photos 2 months postsurgery. A) Right buccal, B) Frontal, and C) Left buccal views. (From Chang J, Steinbacher D, Nanda R, et al. "Surgery-first" approach with Invisalign therapy to correct a class II malocclusion and severe mandibular retrognathism. *J Clin Orthod.* 2019;53[7]:397-404.)

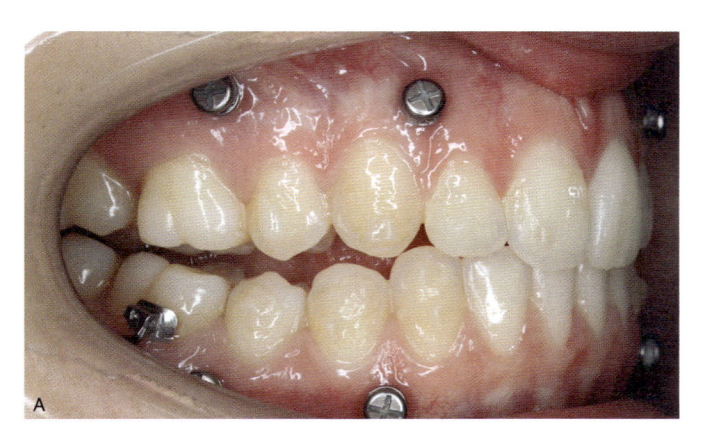

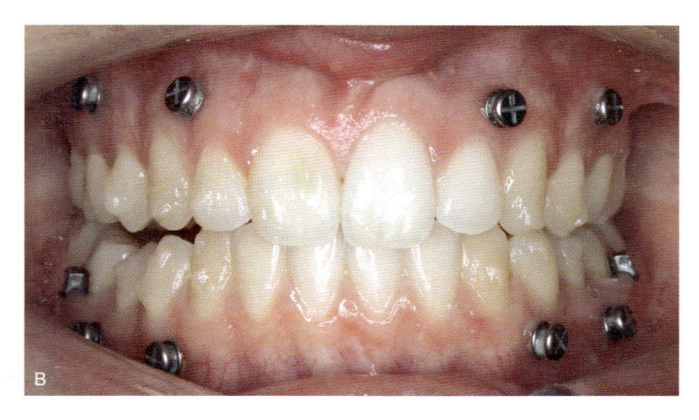

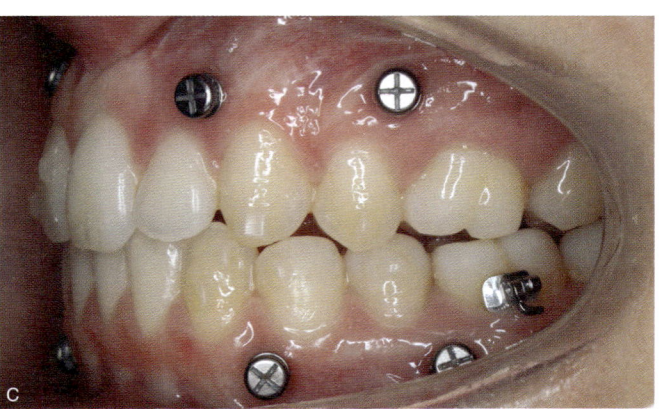

Fig. 17.16 Lateral open bite on the right is still present 5 months after surgery. A) Right buccal, B) Frontal, and C) Left buccal views of patient in occlusion.

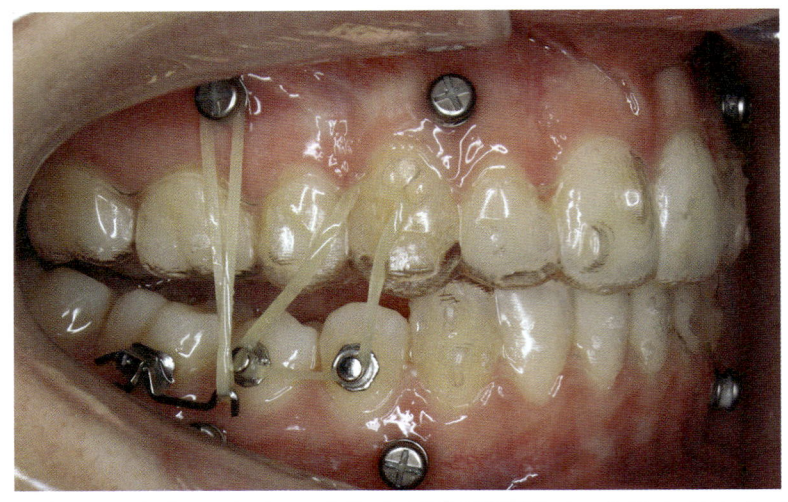

248   Principles and Biomechanics of Aligner Treatment

Fig. 17.17 Cantilever arm extended from bonded lower right molar tube to upright this tooth using an elastic from the maxillary miniscrews; aligner cut distal to the lower right canine to allow eruption of the buccal segment.

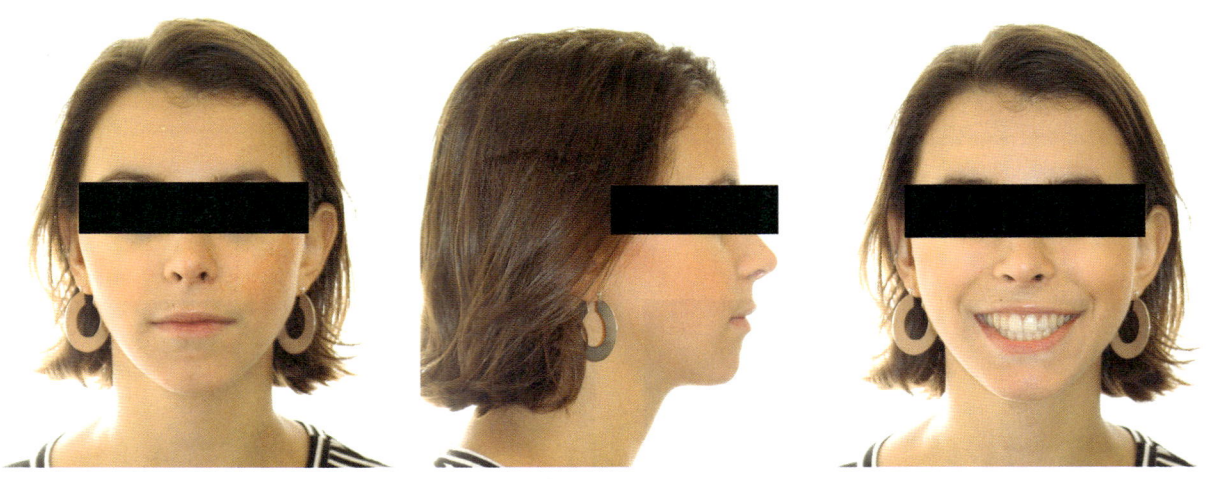

Fig. 17.18 Extraoral photos 12 months postsurgery.

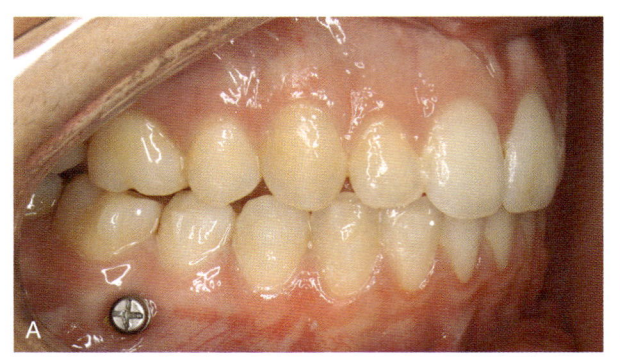

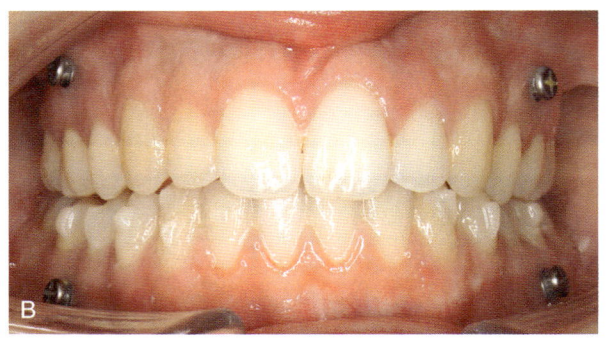

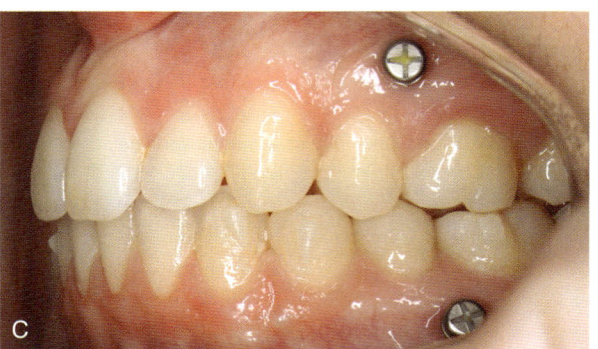

Fig. 17.19 Intraoral photos 12 months postsurgery. A) Right buccal, B) Frontal, and C) Left buccal views of patient in occlusion.

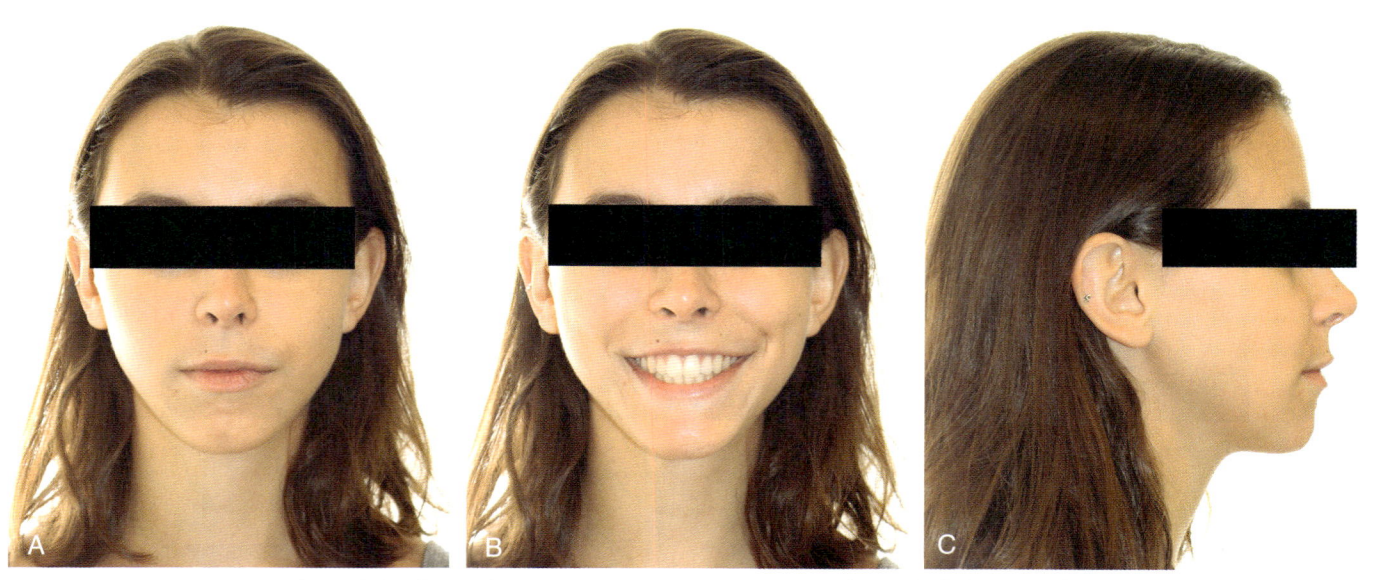

Fig. 17.20 Posttreatment extraoral photos. A) Frontal, B) Smiling and C) Profile views. (From Chang J, Steinbacher D, Nanda R, et al. "Surgery-first" approach with Invisalign therapy to correct a class II malocclusion and severe mandibular retrognathism. *J Clin Orthod*. 2019;53[7]:397-404.)

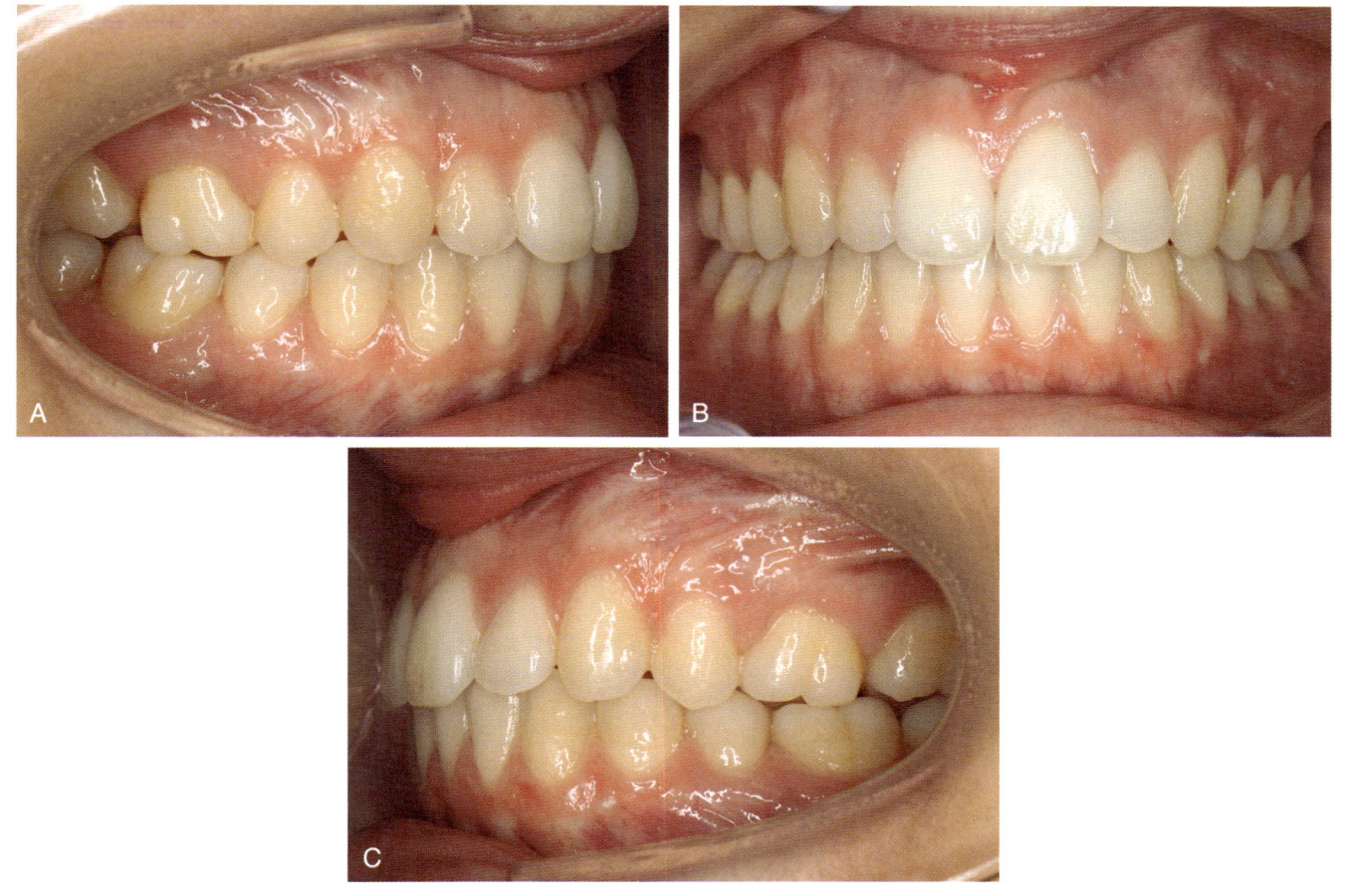

Fig. 17.21 Posttreatment intraoral photos. A) Right buccal, B) Frontal, and C) Left buccal views of patient in occlusion.

Continued

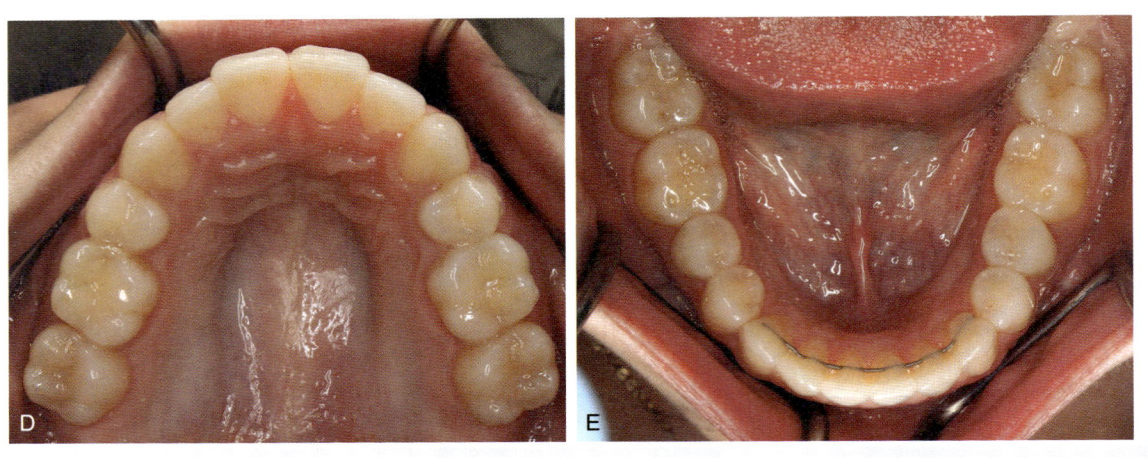

250 Principles and Biomechanics of Aligner Treatment

Fig. 17.21, cont'd D) Maxillary and E) Mandibular occlusal views. (From Chang J, Steinbacher D, Nanda R, et al. "Surgery-first" approach with Invisalign therapy to correct a class II malocclusion and severe mandibular retrognathism. *J Clin Orthod.* 2019;53[7]:397-404.)

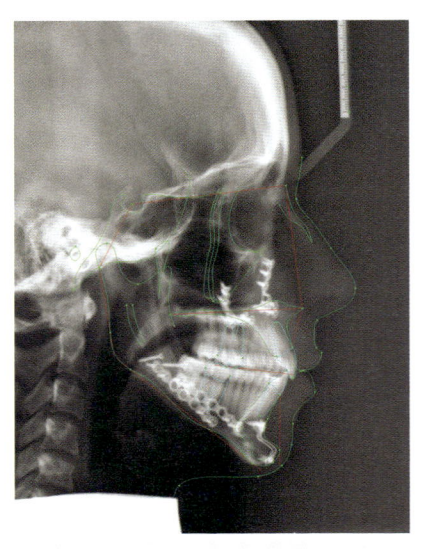

Fig. 17.22 Posttreatment lateral cephalogram. (From Chang J, Steinbacher D, Nanda R, et al. "Surgery-first" approach with Invisalign therapy to correct a class II malocclusion and severe mandibular retrognathism. *J Clin Orthod.* 2019;53[7]:397-404.)

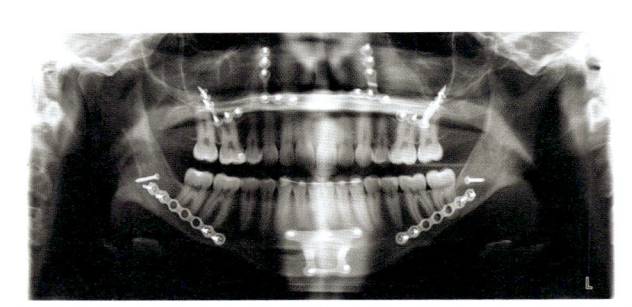

Fig. 17.23 Posttreatment panoramic radiograph. (From Chang J, Steinbacher D, Nanda R, et al. "Surgery-first" approach with Invisalign therapy to correct a class II malocclusion and severe mandibular retrognathism. *J Clin Orthod.* 2019;53[7]:397-404.)

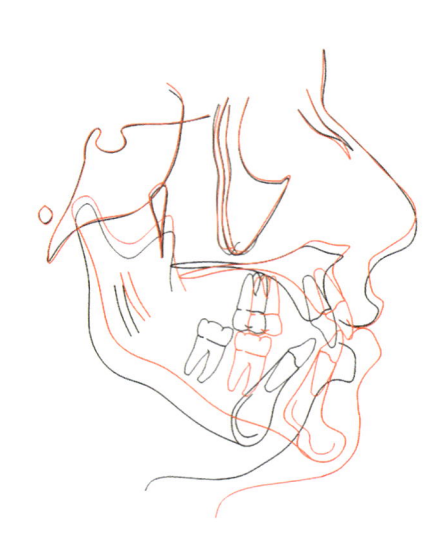

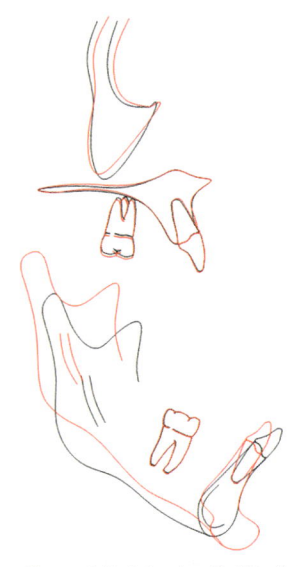

Fig. 17.24 Superimposition of the skeletal and soft tissue changes. (From Chang J, Steinbacher D, Nanda R, et al. "Surgery-first" approach with Invisalign therapy to correct a class II malocclusion and severe mandibular retrognathism. *J Clin Orthod.* 2019;53[7]:397-404.)

Conclusions

SFA/CAT is a very appealing approach for adult patients undergoing orthognathic surgery. A 3D plan for the skeletal movements in conjunction with a 3D plan for the dental movements can be interconnected to achieve excellent occlusal and esthetic results. Furthermore, the presurgical orthodontic phase can be obviated, with the immediate resolution of the dentofacial deformity. This approach may become mainstream in the future as refinements in the techniques and improvements in the Invisalign appliance are developed to increase predictability.

References

1. Dowling PA, Espeland L, Krogstad O, et al. Duration of orthodontic treatment involving orthognathic surgery. *Int J Adult Orthodon Orthognath Surg.* 1999;14:146-152.
2. Luther F, Morris DO, Hart C. Orthodontic preparation for orthognathic surgery: how long does it take and why? A retrospective study. *Br J Oral Maxillofac Surg.* 2003;41:401-406.
3. Boyd RL. Surgical-orthodontic treatment of two skeletal class III patients with Invisalign and fixed appliances. *J Clin Orthod.* 2005;39:245-258.
4. Womack WR, Day RH. Surgical-orthodontic treatment using the Invisalign system. *J Clin Orthod.* 2008;42:237-245.
5. Marcuzzi E, Galassini G, Procopio O, et al. Surgical-Invisalign treatment of a patient with class III malocclusion and multiple missing teeth. *J Clin Orthod.* 2010;44:377-384.
6. Pagani R, Signorino F, Poli PP, et al. The use of Invisalign system in the management of the orthodontic treatment before and after class III surgical approach. *Case Rep Dent.* 2016;2016:9231219.
7. Taub DI, Palermo V. Orthognathic surgery for the Invisalign patient. *Semin Orthod.* 2017;23:99-102.
8. Hong RK, Lee JG, Sunwoo J, et al. Lingual orthodontics combined with orthognathic surgery in a skeletal class III patient. *J Clin Orthod.* 2000;34:403-408.
9. Paik CH, Woo YJ, Kim J, et al. Use of miniscrews for intermaxillary fixation of lingual-orthodontic surgical patients. *J Clin Orthod.* 2002;36:132-136, quiz 145.
10. Caminiti M, Lou T. Clear aligner orthognathic splints. *J Oral Maxillofac Surg.* 2019;77:1071.
11. Pelo S, Gasparini G, Garagiola U, et al. Surgery-first orthognathic approach vs traditional orthognathic approach: oral health-related quality of life assessed with 2 questionnaires. *Am J Orthod Dentofacial Orthop.* 2017;152:250-254.

18 Pain During Orthodontic Treatment: Biologic Mechanisms and Clinical Management

TIANTONG LOU, JOHNNY TRAN, ALI TASSI, and IACOPO CIOFFI

The Importance of Orthodontic Pain

Pain, as defined by the International Association for the Study of Pain, is "an unpleasant and emotional experience associated with actual or potential tissue damage or described in terms of such damage."[1] The majority of patients will experience varying intensities and frequencies of pain during their course of orthodontic treatment.[2] Pain is a highly complex experience[3] and is frequently an area of concern among patients undergoing orthodontic treatment.[2,4-7] The experience of pain is modulated by several factors, such as the magnitude of noxious stimuli, emotions, cognition, past experience and memories of pain, and other concomitant sensory experiences.[8]

Orthodontic pain (i.e., dental pain associated with orthodontic tooth movement) can negatively impact patient compliance and oral hygiene,[8-10] lead to increased frequency of missed appointments,[11] and compromise the overall treatment result.[12,13] Fear of pain is a major reason for patients to forego orthodontic treatment.[6,14,15] In one particular survey, patients rated pain as the highest area of dislike in regard to orthodontic treatment and ranked pain fourth among major fears and apprehensions.[16] Not surprisingly, patients who experience reduced levels of orthodontic pain tend to have an improved level of cooperation in treatment.[12,17,18] Therefore, practitioners should aim to reduce the pain experience to improve patient compliance, decrease treatment times, and increase overall patient satisfaction.

Over the last few decades, there has been an increased demand from prospective orthodontic patients for more esthetic alternatives to traditional metal brackets and wires.[19,20] Orthodontic appliances that are less visible may lead to improved patient acceptance and improved quality of life.[21-23] More recent advancements in the specialty have led to the use of computer-aided design and computer-aided manufacturing (CAD/CAM) technology to fabricate orthodontic appliances. This has allowed clear aligner therapy (CAT) to become available to the mass market and emerge as a desirable treatment option for orthodontic patients.[24] Since its initial introduction in 1997, CAT has rapidly increased in popularity, and many orthodontists are utilizing clear aligners instead of conventional multibracket appliances to treat patients with a wide variety of malocclusions.[25]

This chapter aims to provide an overview regarding orthodontic pain, its relation to clear aligner therapy, as well as the pharmacologic and nonpharmacologic clinical management of pain experienced during orthodontic treatment.

Biologic Mechanisms of Orthodontic Pain and Clinical Correlates

The underlying mechanism of pain during orthodontic tooth movement is a result of the complex interplay between vast numbers of neurons and chemical mediators in both the central and peripheral nervous systems. It is well known that orthodontic pain is primarily due to an inflammatory reaction in the periodontium, which accompanies orthodontic tooth movement.[12] The application of orthodontic force results in a localized region induces ischemia, inflammation, and edema in the periodontal ligament space[26] and activates a cascade of proinflammatory mediators. One of these mediators is the enzyme cyclooxygenase-2 (COX-2), a critical component in the synthesis of prostaglandin,[27] which is targeted by nonsteroidal antiinflammatory drugs (NSAIDs). Nociceptive stimuli exerted by orthodontic appliances are primarily detected by sensory fibers[28] such as C fibers (unmyelinated) and thinly myelinated Aδ fibers in the pulp and periodontal ligament.[29] Other substances that either activate or sensitize nociceptors during inflammation include tumor necrosis factor-α (TNF-α), interleukin 6 (IL-6), IL-1β, bradykinin, enkephalin, serotonin, dopamine, glutamate γ-amino butyric acid, and histamine.[30-34] Studies have demonstrated that elevated levels of these compounds are associated with hyperalgesia.[35,36] In addition, the activated proinflammatory mediators can stimulate the release of neuropeptides from the afferent nerve endings into the surrounding tissues.[37] Substance P and calcitonin gene-related peptide (CGRP) are two potent neuropeptides that cause neurogenic inflammation.[37-42] These sensory neuropeptides enhance inflammation through interactions with epithelial cells to induce vasodilation and increase blood vessel permeability.[43,44] They also lead to mast cell degranulation and further release of proinflammation mediators such as histamine and serotonin.[45] These inflammatory mediators trigger the release of more neuropeptides, contributing to a continuation and intensification of the inflammatory process.[28] Substance P also increases the levels of various cytokines, such as TNF-α, IL-1β, and IL-6.[33,42] CGRP stimulates the release of IL-6, IL-8, and TNF-α.[42] These cytokines serve as signaling messengers between immune cells and are important in bone resorption, deposition, and remodeling.[46] IL-1β is released by fibroblasts of the gingiva surrounding the teeth during orthodontic tooth movement and is involved in bone remodeling.[47,48] IL-6 is a regulator of the immune response during inflammation and the formation and activity of osteoclasts.[49-51] TNF-α is synthesized and released by monocytes and macrophages and may be related to bone remodeling.[52]

The afferent fibers have their cell bodies residing in the trigeminal ganglion of Meckel cave and transmit electrical signals to the central nervous system. They ascend the trigeminal spinal tract and enter the trigeminal sensory nuclear complex. From the trigeminal brainstem complex, the nociceptive signal is transmitted to the thalamus and eventually to the cerebral primary somatosensory cortex, where the location of the signal is discriminated. Top-down neural pathways modulate the nociceptive stimuli coming from the periphery.[53] Although several brain areas are involved in pain processing, still little is known about how pain is encoded in the brain. However, it is clear that the pain and salience brain networks overlap.[54]

The initial pattern of pain experienced by patients undergoing traditional multibracket orthodontic appliance therapy has been long studied and well documented.[2,9,55-58] Pain appears approximately 2 to 3 hours after orthodontic forces are applied to the teeth, with peak levels frequently occurring within the first 24 hours after archwire placement, followed by a steady decrease toward baseline levels within 7 days (Fig. 18.1).[2,59-63] These findings have been confirmed in several racial and ethnic groups[56,64-67] and through the use of ecologic momentary assessment.[68] There also appears to be a diurnal variation in pain experienced by patients, with higher levels occurring in the evenings and nights.[69]

Overall, patients are generally able to tolerate and adapt to new appliances within 1 week after placement.[70] However, female patients in middle adolescence have been reported to experience more pain than age-matched males and younger patients when exposed to orthodontic procedures.[71] In addition, orthodontic pain is significantly affected by menstrual phase, with the pain levels being higher in the luteal phase.[72] While there is conflicting reports on the effect of age on orthodontic pain perception,[3] there is substantial evidence that the type of malocclusion and the amount of crowding have little effect on pain experienced during orthodontic treatment.[73,74] These findings suggest that pain is likely most affected by other factors, including hormonal and psychological variables.[12] One such example is anxiety,[75] which among other things can be dependent on the relationship with the orthodontic care provider.[76]

Orthodontic Tooth Pain in Clear Aligner Therapy

Orthodontic pain associated with CAT has been investigated in a limited number of studies. CAT appears to follow a similar pattern of pain progression in terms of peaking at 24 hours and trending toward baseline levels after 7 days.[21,60-62,77] However, to date, CAT has mainly been associated with more intermittent forces as compared to conventional treatment with multibracket appliances, although several companies are focusing on developing materials that may provide more gentle and continuous forces. Only a limited number of studies exist that examine orthodontic pain in patients undergoing CAT with Invisalign's latest generation multilayered polyurethane-based polymer, SmartTrack. These studies show a maximum patient-reported pain score of 20 mm on a 100-mm visual analogue scale (VAS), which may be considered mild and of limited clinical significance.[62,77] In previous literature, Exceed-30 thermoplastic material was used in the older generation, and coincidently these studies showed significantly higher reported pain scores in the first week of treatment (up to 40 mm on VAS).[21,60,61] Limited evidence suggests SmartTrack may be more comfortable than older generation materials,[78] but further studies are needed to validate this.

Interestingly, with continued active tooth movements of the subsequent aligner stages, there is less pain reported by patients compared to the first stage aligners even if the first stage aligners are programmed to be passive (without active tooth movements).[77] This perhaps could be a result of the accuracy, fit, and deformation of the first trays,[61] the introduction of iatrogenic posterior occlusal interferences,[79,80] or the apprehension and stress involved with starting orthodontic treatment with a new appliance.[16,75] Indeed, pain perception with CAT, especially during the first stage, is significantly related to an individual's psychological stress and anxiety.[77]

In general, when compared to traditional multibracket appliances, CAT results in less reported pain and improved patient experience. Miller et al.[60] conducted the first study evaluating the differences in pain and impact on quality of life experienced by patients undergoing CAT versus multibracket appliance therapy. This was a prospective longitudinal cohort study with 33 CAT patients and 27 multibracket appliance patients. The participants were asked to use a daily diary for 7 days, measuring functional, psychosocial, and pain-related impacts.[81] The diary consisted of questions adapted from the Geriatric Oral Health Assessment Index,[82] a 5-point Likert scale for demographic data, and a visual analog scale for pain. The results showed that the

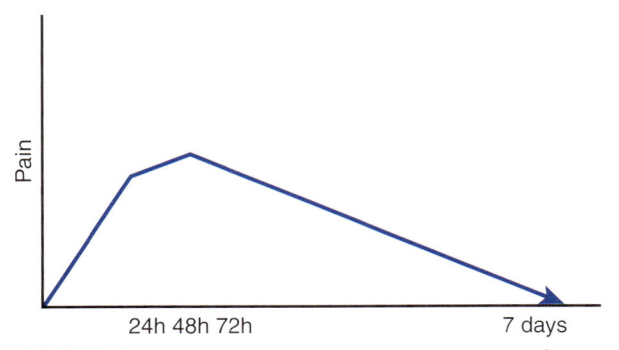

Fig. 18.1 Trajectory of dental pain after orthodontic procedures.

progression of pain in aligner treatment followed a similar pattern to multibracket appliances, in which pain peaked after 24 hours and gradually returned to normal. Additionally, although the initial levels of pain were higher for the multibracket appliance group, along with higher levels of analgesic consumption, both groups recovered to baseline within 7 days.

In a subsequent study by Shalish et al.,[21] 68 patients being treated by either buccal multibracket appliances, lingual multibracket appliances, or CAT were recruited to complete a health-related quality of life questionnaire[22,23,83-85] and a 5-point scale for dysfunction during the first week and on day 14. Their results showed the average initial pain levels were consistently higher in the lingual multibracket appliance and clear aligner groups, with analgesic consumption paralleling the dynamics of the pain levels (although the difference did not reach statistical significance). In all groups, the pain levels subsided within 1 week. These results contradict the findings by Miller et al.,[60] which the authors attributed to a greater mechanical force being applied in the aligner group compared to the buccal multibracket appliance group.

To further elucidate and compare pain levels between these orthodontic treatment modalities, Fujiyama et al.[61] conducted a prospective clinical trial with 145 patients receiving either CAT, multibracket appliance therapy, or a hybrid treatment combining both modalities. Using VAS, the participants were asked to record their pain levels at time points of 60 seconds, 6 hours, 12 hours, and 1 to 7 days post appliance insertion. This was repeated at weeks 3 and 5 after appliance delivery. Their results illustrated a similar pattern of pain progression during the first week of appliance delivery for all groups studied. However, the overall pain levels were significantly more intense and longer lasting for the multibracket appliance group than either the aligner or the hybrid group.[61]

In a recent study by White et al.,[62] patients were randomly allocated to either clear aligner or multibracket appliance treatment groups to investigate differences in their pain levels. The participants were asked to complete a daily diary with pain measured on VAS. The diary was completed at initial appliance delivery, daily for the first week, as well as the first 4 days after their next two follow-up appointments. The pattern of pain progression during the first week following initial appliance activation was in general agreement with previous studies.[2,21,55,56,60,86] The clear aligner group experienced consistently lower discomfort than the multibracket appliance group during most of the first week, with statistically significant differences observed after 2 to 3 days. Moreover, analgesic consumption was more frequent in the multibracket appliance group, and their rate of consumption closely mirrored the pattern of pain progression during the first week. Similarly, over a relatively longer term of 2 months, the level of pain was less in the aligner group than the multibracket appliance group. The patients in the multibracket appliance group may have experienced an increased initial inflammatory response, which led to increased sensitization of the nociceptors and higher pain sensation in subsequent follow-up appointments.[62]

The results of White et al.,[62] Fujiyama et al.,[61] and Miller et al.[60] comparing pain and discomfort between CAT and multibracket appliances are in general agreement with one another, as well as with past studies that demonstrated multibracket appliances may cause more pain than removable appliances.[12,70,87,88] As mentioned earlier, these results were in contrast to the findings from Shalish et al.,[21] who reported the pain was greater in patients treated with aligners than multibracket appliances. One possible explanation for this discrepancy could be the variations in the initial archwires used between the studies. For example, the classic nickel titanium (NiTi) or nitinol wires used in the Shalish et al. study have been shown to display higher peak discomfort than the superelastic copper NiTi wires used in White et al.[89,90] Furthermore, the White et al. study was the only one to utilize SmartTrack, a new aligner material brought to market by Align Technology in 2013,[91,92] whereas the previous studies used the older Exceed-30 aligner material. Limited evidence suggests SmartTrack may be more comfortable than previous materials,[93] although further studies are needed to verify this.[62] Lastly, Shalish et al. speculated that the differences in pain levels observed may possibly have been due to a higher level of mechanical force being applied early in treatment for the aligner group.

In summary, although orthodontic pain exists with CAT, the current evidence seems to suggest it is of a lesser degree than multibracket appliances, especially during the first week. However, additional studies providing more substantial data are needed. As would be expected, activation in the aligner tray has been reported as the most frequent cause of pain and discomfort.[61] However, other issues leading to pain in association with clear aligners might include nonsmooth edges, tray, and attachment deformation.[61]

Modulators of Pain: Psychological Factors

Clinical and pain assessment literature continues to be focussed on identifying and managing specific cognitive and psychological factors that are related to the individual's experience of pain. In orthodontics, pain is a common sequela and expected with treatment. However, it is apparent clinically that the perception of pain varies considerably across individuals when the same stimulus, such as an initial light archwire, is activated. The expected pain from an orthodontic adjustment is generally believed to be relatively minor and self-limiting; however, some patients will report a much different experience.[75] It is generally accepted that particular affective and cognitive behavioral factors contribute to these differences in individual pain perception.[94] Specifically relevant to medical and dental settings, pain perception is influenced by factors such as somatosensory amplification, anxiety, depression, and catastrophizing.[95-104]

It has been shown that patients with prolonged pain during orthodontic treatment exhibit higher levels of anxiety than individuals with pain of short duration.[105] Furthermore, experimentally induced orthodontic pain via elastomeric separators is greater in individuals who exhibit higher levels of trait anxiety and somatosensory amplification—a tendency to perceive normal somatic and visceral sensations as being relatively intense, noxious, and disturbing[106]—as compared to individuals with low levels of both.[75] Of importance, anxiety and other mood disorders have been found to be related to increased frequencies of waking-state oral parafunctional behaviors, such as waketime tooth clenching,[107-109] which are also associated with temporomandibular disorders.[79,110,111] Therefore, it might be questioned whether anxiety, orthodontic pain, and jaw motor behavior are intertwined.

Recently, we performed a large web survey[112] and recruited 45 individuals subdivided into groups with high, intermediate, and low levels of trait anxiety.[113,114] Elastomeric separators were applied to the molars and pain and frequency of tooth clenching episodes were recorded for 5 days. A significant correlation orthodontic pain and frequency of tooth clenching was observed. In participants with high anxiety, the decrease in orthodontic pain was paralleled by a decrease in the frequency of waketime tooth clenching episodes. These results suggest that individuals with high trait anxiety may respond with an avoidance behavior (decrease of jaw motor activity) to orthodontic stimuli as a method to reducing their pain experience. The relationship between jaw motor activity and orthodontic pain is supported by a recent study that demonstrated a reduced masticatory performance in orthodontic patients during the period in which they reported the maximum levels of pain and crevicular IL-1β.[115] However, there is some evidence of increased jaw muscle activity with CAT,[116,117] leading to jaw muscle tenderness of limited clinical significance.[77]

Beck et al. estimated the contribution of psychological factors to orthodontic pain.[96] Of interest, for every pain catastrophizing scale (PCS) magnification score of 1 unit higher, the relative risk of being a high-pain responder was 1.6.[96] Magnification refers to an individual's tendency to exaggerate the threat value of nociceptive inputs.[95] In this study, the authors showed that cold sensitivity significantly predicts the pain experienced, with those reporting greater scores for cold sensitivity having greater orthodontic pain. This result supports the hypothesis that somatosensory amplification plays a major role in orthodontic pain experience.[75] Evaluation of the abovementioned psychological constructs in a clinical setting utilizing validated questionnaires is advisable to identify individuals who may be more sensitive to pain and discomfort during orthodontic therapy. Anxiety and symptom perception management might be recommended for those susceptible individuals.

Clinical Considerations for the Management of Orthodontic Pain

In the last decade, several reviews and clinical studies have been published on the management of orthodontic pain. It is well known that pharmacologic approaches with over-the-counter analgesics are effective in managing orthodontic pain. In particular, acetaminophen (paracetamol) is usually prescribed in place of NSAIDs to avoid possible effects on the rate of tooth movement.[118,119] Indeed, NSAIDs have been reported to interfere with the synthesis of prostaglandin E2 (PGE2), which is known to be an important chemical mediator during the bone remodeling process.[120,121] A recent Cochrane review,[122] including 32 randomized controlled trials (RCTs) and 3,110 participants aged 9 to 34 years, did not find any evidence of a difference in efficacy between NSAIDs and paracetamol at 2, 6, or 24 hours postintervention. They concluded that analgesics are more effective at reducing orthodontic pain than placebo or no treatment.

Sandhu and Leckie[123] examined the diurnal variation of pain in 85 orthodontic patients. Consistent with the abovementioned studies, pain was reported to peak after 24 hours. Interestingly, during the peak period, orthodontic pain was lower during the afternoon as compared to the night and morning. Therefore, the authors suggested that patients should be advised to take analgesics accordingly and need not be prescribed routine analgesics to be taken every 6 to 8 hours. In addition, they suggested that preemptive administration of analgesics may be more effective than posttreatment administration, as the traditional administration at regular intervals does not consider temporal variations in orthodontic pain. However, the previously mentioned review[122] indicated there is very low evidence suggesting preemptive ibuprofen gives better pain relief at 2 hours than ibuprofen taken posttreatment. Finally, it must be noted that the combination of acetaminophen plus ibuprofen provides greater analgesic efficacy than acetaminophen or ibuprofen alone.[124]

Special considerations should be made for patients with a history of regularly taking pain medications. Indeed, a recent literature review (which included animal studies) suggested that long-term consumption of pain relievers can significantly affect the rate of orthodontic tooth movement.[125] Surprisingly, they found that animals in treatment with ibuprofen did not show a significant decrease in orthodontic tooth movement, as some previous human studies had shown. On the other hand, long-term administration of indomethacin, ketorolac, and high doses of etoricoxib decreased the amount of tooth movement. However, caution should be taken when interpreting these results due to the questionable quality of evidence that is available.

Several nonpharmacologic approaches have been considered to manage orthodontic pain. In another recent Cochrane review,[126] Fleming et al. included 14 RCTs with 931 participants and analyzed the effects of low-level laser therapy (LLLT), vibratory adjuncts, experimental chewing adjuncts (e.g., bite wafers and chewing gum), and psychosocial and physical interventions on orthodontic pain. They concluded that laser irradiation may help reduce orthodontic pain in the short term. On the other hand, evidence to support other methods is of low quality.

It is the opinion of the authors that nonpharmacologic interventions should be used whenever possible to reduce orthodontic pain (Table 18.1), provided they do not expose patients to harm or additional costs during treatment; they should be used especially when a medical condition prevents the use of recommended analgesics. Of foremost importance, clinicians should establish a relationship of trust with patients and improve their communication skills to reduce nocebo and favor placebo effects. Overall, a proper pain management approach would require a careful baseline assessment of pain predictors, psychological factors, and patient expectations. Moreover, placebo and nocebo effects should be considered when communicating with

Table 18.1 Strategies to Reduce Pain During Orthodontic Treatment

Pharmacologic	Acetaminophen or ibuprofen PRN	High level of evidence to support pain reduction with this treatment
Nonpharmacologic	• Chewing adjuncts • Low-level laser therapy • Vibratory stimulation	Low level of evidence to support orthodontic pain reduction with this treatment
Doctor-patient communication	Improve pre- and posttreatment communication	High level of evidence to support pain reduction with this approach

PRN, Pro re nata (As necessary).

patients. Blasini et al. highlighted that negative patient-practitioner interaction should be avoided and that communication with patients should be well-balanced by not providing excessive negative information with regard to side effects and limiting information regarding benefits.[127]

References

1. Merskey H, Albe Fessard D, Bonica J, et al. Pain terms: a list with definitions and notes on usage. Recommended by the IASP Subcommittee on Taxonomy. *Pain.* 1979;6:249.
2. Scheurer PA, Firestone AR, Bürgin WB. Perception of pain as a result of orthodontic treatment with fixed appliances. *Eur J Orthod.* 1996;18: 349-357.
3. Moayedi M, Davis KD. Theories of pain: from specificity to gate control. *J Neurophysiol.* 2013; 109(1):5-12.
4. Kvam E, Gjerdet NR, Bondevik O. Traumatic ulcers and pain during orthodontic treatment. *Community Dent Oral Epidemiol.* 1987;15:104-107.
5. Lew KK. Attitudes and perceptions of adults towards orthodontic treatment in an Asian community. *Community Dent Oral Epidemiol.* 1993;21:31-35.
6. Oliver RG, Knapman YM. Attitudes to orthodontic treatment. *Br J Orthod.* 1985;12:179-188.
7. Kluemper GT, Hiser DG, Rayens MK, et al. Efficacy of a wax containing benzocaine in the relief of oral mucosal pain caused by orthodontic appliances. *Am J Orthod Dentofacial Orthop.* 2002;122:359-365.
8. Chow J, Cioffi I. Pain and orthodontic patient compliance: a clinical perspective. *Semin Orthod.* 2018;24:242-247.
9. Sergl HG, Klages U, Zentner A. Pain and discomfort during orthodontic treatment: causative factors and effects on compliance. *Am J Orthod Dentofacial Orthop.* 1998;114:684-691.
10. Ukra A, Bennani F, Farella M. Psychological aspects of orthodontics in clinical practice. Part one: treatment-specific variables. *Prog Orthod.* 2011;12:143-148.
11. Krukemeyer AM, Arruda AO, Inglehart MR. Pain and orthodontic treatment. *Angle Orthod.* 2009;79:1175-1181.
12. Krishnan V. Orthodontic pain: from causes to management—a review. *Eur J Orthod.* 2007;29:170-179.
13. Cozzani M, Ragazzini G, Delucchi A, et al. Self-reported pain after orthodontic treatments: a randomized controlled study on the effects of two follow-up procedures. *Eur J Orthod.* 2016;38:266-271.
14. Asham AA. Readers' forum: orthodontic pain. *Am J Orthod Dentofacial Orthop.* 2004;125:18A.
15. Keim RG. Managing orthodontic pain. *J Clin Orthod.* 2004;38:641-642.
16. O'Connor PJ. Patients' perceptions before, during, and after orthodontic treatment. *J Clin Orthod.* 2000;34:591-592.
17. Albino JE, Lawrence SD, Lopes CE, et al. Cooperation of adolescents in orthodontic treatment. *J Behav Med.* 1991;14:53-70.
18. Giannopoulou C, Dudic A, Kiliaridis S. Pain discomfort and crevicular fluid changes induced by orthodontic elastic separators in children. *J Pain.* 2006;7:367-376.
19. Ziuchkovski JP, Fields HW, Johnston WM, et al. Assessment of perceived orthodontic appliance attractiveness. *Am J Orthod Dentofacial Orthop.* 2008;133:S68-S78.
20. Rosvall MD, Fields HW, Ziuchkovski JP, et al. Attractiveness, acceptability, and value of orthodontic appliances. *Am J Orthod Dentofacial Orthop.* 2009;135:276, e271-e212, discussion 276-277.
21. Shalish M, Cooper-Kazaz R, Ivgi I, et al. Adult patients' adjustability to orthodontic appliances. Part I: a comparison between labial, lingual, and Invisalign. *Eur J Orthod.* 2012;34:724-730.
22. O'Brien K, Kay L, Fox D, et al. Assessing oral health outcomes for orthodontics—measuring health status and quality of life. *Community Dent Health.* 1998;15:22-26.
23. Cunningham SJ, Hunt NP. Quality of life and its importance in orthodontics. *J Orthod.* 2001;28:152-158.
24. Wong BH. Invisalign A to Z. *Am J Orthod Dentofacial Orthop.* 2002;121: 540-541.
25. Morton J, Derakhshan M, Kaza S, et al. Design of the Invisalign system performance. *Semin Orthod.* 2017;23:3-11.
26. Park HJ, Baek KH, Lee HL, et al. Hypoxia inducible factor-1 alpha directly induces the expression of receptor activator of nuclear factor-kappa B ligand in periodontal ligament fibroblasts. *Mol Cells.* 2011;31:573-578.
27. Lee JJ, Natsuizaka M, Ohashi S, et al. Hypoxia activates the cyclooxygenase-2-prostaglandin E synthase axis. *Carcinogenesis.* 2010;31:427-434.
28. Kyrkanides S, Huang HC, Faber RD. Neurologic regulation and orthodontic tooth movement. In: Kantarci A, Will L, Yen S, eds. *Tooth Movement.* Basel: Karger; 2016:64-74.
29. Norevall LI, Matsson L, Forsgren S. Main sensory neuropeptides, but not VIP and NPY, are involved in bone remodeling during orthodontic tooth movement in the rat. *Ann N Y Acad Sci.* 1998; 865:353-359.
30. Yamasaki K, Shibata Y, Imai S, et al. Clinical-application of prostaglandin-E1 (PGE1) upon orthodontic tooth movement. *Am J Orthod.* 1984;85:508-518.
31. Walker JA, Tanzer FS, Harris EF, et al. The enkephalin response in human tooth-pulp to orthodontic force. *Am J Orthod Dentofacial Orthop.* 1987;92:9-16.
32. Davidovitch Z, Nicolay OF, Ngan PW, et al. Neurotransmitters, cytokines, and the control of alveolar bone remodeling in orthodontics. *Dent Clin North Am.* 1988;32:411-435.
33. Nicolay OF, Davidovitch Z, Shanfeld JL, et al. Substance-P immunoreactivity in periodontal tissues during orthodontic tooth movement. *Bone Miner.* 1990;11:19-29.
34. Alhashimi N, Frithiof L, Brudvik P, et al. Orthodontic tooth movement and de novo synthesis of proinflammatory cytokines. *Am J Orthod Dentofacial Orthop.* 2001;119:307-312.
35. Grieve III WG, Johnson GK, Moore RN, et al. Prostaglandin E (PGE) and interleukin-1 beta (IL-1 beta) levels in gingival crevicular fluid during human orthodontic tooth movement. *Am J Orthod Dentofacial Orthop.* 1994;105:369-374.
36. Vandevska-Radunovic V. Neural modulation of inflammatory reactions in dental tissues incident to orthodontic tooth movement. A review of the literature. *Eur J Orthod.* 1999;21:231-247.
37. Kato J, Ichikawa H, Wakisaka S, et al. The distribution of vasoactive intestinal polypeptides and calcitonin gene-related peptide in the periodontal-ligament of mouse molar teeth. *Arch Oral Biol.* 1990;35:63-66.
38. Kvinnsland I, Heyeraas KJ, Byers MR. Effects of dental trauma on pulpal and periodontal nerve morphology. *Proc Finn Dent Soc Suomen Hammaslaakariseuran Toimituksia.* 1992;88(1): S125-S132.
39. Kvinnsland I, Kvinnsland S. Changes in CGRP-immunoreactive nerve-fibers during experimental tooth movement in rats. *Eur J Orthod.* 1990;12:320-329.
40. Kvinnsland S, Heyeraas K, Ofjord ES. Effect of experimental tooth movement on periodontal and pulpal blood-flow. *Eur J Orthod.* 1989;11:200-205.
41. Saito I, Ishii K, Hanada K, et al. Responses of calcitonin gene-related peptide-immunopositive nerve-fibers in the periodontal-ligament of rat molars to experimental tooth movement. *Arch Oral Biol.* 1991;36:689-692.

42. Norevall LI, Forsgren S, Matsson L. Expression of neuropeptides (CGRP, substance P) during and after orthodontic tooth movement in the rat. *Eur J Orthod.* 1995;17:311-325.
43. Maggi CA, Giuliani S, Santicioli P, et al. Peripheral effects of neurokinins—functional evidence for the existence of multiple receptors. *J Auton Pharmacol.* 1987;7:11-32.
44. Gray DW, Marshall I. Human alpha-calcitonin gene-related peptide stimulates adenylate-cyclase and guanylate-cyclase and relaxes rat thoracic aorta by releasing nitric-oxide. *Br J Pharmacol.* 1992;107:691-696.
45. Assem ESK, Ghanem NS, Abdullah NA, et al. Substance-P and Arg-Pro-Lys-Pro-NH-C12-H25-induced mediator release from different mast-cell subtypes of rat and guinea-pig. *Immunopharmacology.* 1989;17:119-128.
46. Yamaguchi M, Kasai K. Inflammation in periodontal tissues in response to mechanical forces. *Arch Immunol Ther Exp (Warsz).* 2005;53:388-398.
47. Gowen M, Wood DD, Ihrie EJ, et al. An interleukin-1 like factor stimulates bone-resorption invitro. *Nature.* 1983;306:378-380.
48. Stashenko P, Obernesser MS, Dewhirst FE. Effect of immune cytokines on bone. *Immunol Invest.* 1989;18:239-249.
49. Ishimi Y, Miyaura C, Jin CH, et al. IL-6 is produced by osteoblasts and induces bone-resorption. *J Immunol.* 1990;145:3297-3303.
50. Kurihara N, Bertolini D, Suda T, et al. IL-6 stimulates osteoclast-like multinucleated cell-formation in long-term human marrow cultures by inducing IL-1 release. *J Immunol.* 1990;144:4226-4230.
51. Lowik C, van der Pluijm G, Bloys H, et al. Parathyroid-hormone (PTH) and PTH-like protein (PLP) stimulate interleukin-6 production by osteogenic cells—a possible role of interleukin-6 in osteoclastogenesis. *Biochem Biophys Res Commun.* 1989;162:1546-1552.
52. Takeichi O, Saito I, Tsurumachi T, et al. Expression of inflammatory cytokine genes in vivo by human alveolar bone-derived polymorphonuclear leukocytes isolated from chronically inflamed sites of bone resorption. *Calcif Tissue Int.* 1996;58:244-248.
53. Sessle BJ. The neurobiology of facial and dental pain: present knowledge, future directions. *J Dent Res.* 1987;66:962-981.
54. Davis KD, Moayedi M. Central mechanisms of pain revealed through functional and structural MRI. *J Neuroimmune Pharmacol.* 2013;8:518-534.
55. Jones M, Chan C. The pain and discomfort experienced during orthodontic treatment: a randomized controlled clinical trial of two initial aligning arch wires. *Am J Orthod Dentofacial Orthop.* 1992;102:373-381.
56. Ngan P, Kess B, Wilson S. Perception of discomfort by patients undergoing orthodontic treatment. *Am J Orthod Dentofacial Orthop.* 1989;96:47-53.
57. Wilson S, Ngan P, Kess B. Time course of the discomfort in young patients undergoing orthodontic treatment. *Pediatr Dent.* 1989;11:107-110.
58. Stewart FN, Kerr WJ, Taylor PJ. Appliance wear: the patient's point of view. *Eur J Orthod.* 1997;19:377-382.
59. Shalish M, Cooper-Kazaz R, Ivgi I, et al. Adult patients' adjustability to orthodontic appliances. Part I: a comparison between labial, lingual, and Invisalign. *Eur J Orthod.* 2012;34:724-730.
60. Miller KB, McGorray SP, Womack R, et al. A comparison of treatment impacts between Invisalign aligner and fixed appliance therapy during the first week of treatment. *Am J Orthod Dentofacial Orthop.* 2007;131:302, 301-e309.
61. Fujiyama K, Honjo T, Suzuki M, et al. Analysis of pain level in cases treated with Invisalign aligner: comparison with multibracket edgewise appliance therapy. *Prog Orthod.* 2014;15:64.
62. White DW, Julien KC, Jacob H, et al. Discomfort associated with Invisalign and traditional brackets: a randomized, prospective trial. *Angle Orthod.* 2017;87:801-808.
63. Bergius M, Kiliaridis S, Berggren U. Pain in orthodontics. A review and discussion of the literature. *J Orofac Orthop.* 2000;61:125-137.
64. Ngan P, Wilson S, Shanfeld J, et al. The effect of ibuprofen on the level of discomfort in patients undergoing orthodontic treatment. *Am J Orthod Dentofacial Orthop.* 1994;106:88-95.
65. Firestone AR, Scheurer PA, Bürgin WB. Patients' anticipation of pain and pain-related side effects, and their perception of pain as a result of orthodontic treatment with multibracket appliances. *Eur J Orthod.* 1999;21:387-396.
66. Erdinç AME, Dinçer B. Perception of pain during orthodontic treatment with fixed appliances. *Eur J Orthod.* 2004;26:79-85.
67. Polat O, Karaman AL. Pain control during fixed orthodontic appliance therapy. *Angle Orthod.* 2005;75:214-219.
68. Sew Hoy W, Anoun JS, Lin W, et al. Ecological momentary assessment of pain in adolescents undergoing orthodontic treatment using a smartphone app. *Semin Orthod.* 2018;24:209-216.
69. Jones ML, Chan C. Pain in the early stages of orthodontic treatment. *J Clin Orthod.* 1992;26:311-313.
70. Sergl HG, Zentner A. A comparative assessment of acceptance of different types of functional appliances. *Eur J Orthod.* 1998;20:517-524.
71. Sandhu SS, Sandhu J. Orthodontic pain: an interaction between age and sex in early and middle adolescence. *Angle Orthod.* 2013;83:966-972.
72. Long H, Gao M, Zhu Y, et al. The effects of menstrual phase on orthodontic pain following initial archwire engagement. *Oral Dis.* 2017;23:331-336.
73. Abdelrahman RSh, Al-Nimri KS, Al Maaitah EF. Pain experience during initial alignment with three types of nickel-titanium archwires: a prospective clinical trial. *Angle Orthod.* 2015;85:1021-1026.
74. Cioffi I, Piccolo A, Tagliaferri R, et al. Pain perception following first orthodontic archwire placement—thermoelastic vs superelastic alloys: a randomized controlled trial. *Quintessence Int.* 2012;43:61-69.
75. Cioffi I, Michelotti A, Perrotta S, et al. Effect of somatosensory amplification and trait anxiety on experimentally induced orthodontic pain. *Eur J Oral Sci.* 2016;124:127-134.
76. Roy J, Dempster L. Dental anxiety associated with orthodontic care: prevalence and contributing factors. *Semin Orthod.* 2018;24:233-241.
77. Tran J, Lou T, Nebiolo B, Castroflorio T, Tassi A, Cioffi I. Impact of clear aligner therapy on tooth pain and masticatory muscle soreness. *J Oral Rehabil.* 2020; 47(12):1521-1529.
78. Brascher AK, Zuran D, Feldmann RE, et al. Patient survey on Invisalign treatment compare the SmartTrack material to the previous aligner material. *J Orofac Orthop.* 2016;77:432-438.
79. Michelotti A, Cioffi L, Landino D, et al. Effects of experimental occlusal interferences in individuals reporting different levels of wake-time parafunctions. *J Orofac Pain.* 2012;26:168-175.
80. Clark GT, Tsukiyama Y, Baba K, et al. Sixty-eight years of experimental occlusal interference studies: what have we learned? *J Prosthet Dent.* 1999;82:704-713.
81. Carp FM, Carp A. The validity, reliability and generalizability of diary data. *Exp Aging Res.* 1981;7:281-296.
82. Atchison KA, Dolan TA. Development of the geriatric oral health assessment index. *J Dent Educ.* 1990;54:680-687.
83. Jokovic A, Locker D, Stephens M, et al. Validity and reliability of a questionnaire for measuring child oral-health-related quality of life. *J Dent Res.* 2002;81:459-463.
84. Locker D. Applications of self-reported assessments of oral health outcomes. *J Dent Educ.* 1996;60:494-500.
85. Locker D, Jokovic A. Using subjective oral health status indicators to screen for dental care needs in older adults. *Community Dent Oral Epidemiol.* 1996;24:398-402.
86. Young AN, Taylor RW, Taylor SE, et al. Evaluation of preemptive valdecoxib therapy on initial archwire placement discomfort in adults. *Angle Orthod.* 2006;76:251-259.
87. Caniklioglu C, Oztürk Y. Patient discomfort: a comparison between lingual and labial multibracket appliances. *Angle Orthod.* 2005;75:86-91.
88. Wu AK, McGrath C, Wong RW, et al. A comparison of pain experienced by patients treated with labial and lingual orthodontic appliances. *Eur J Orthod.* 2010;32:403-407.
89. Fernandes LM, Ogaard B, Skoglund L. Pain and discomfort experienced after placement of a conventional or a superelastic NiTi aligning archwire. A randomized clinical trial. *J Orofac Orthop.* 1998;59:331-339.
90. Nakano H, Satoh K, Norris R, et al. Mechanical properties of several nickel-titanium alloy wires in three-point bending tests. *Am J Orthod Dentofacial Orthop.* 1999;115:390-395.
91. Align Technology. Align Technology receives U.S. patents for SmartTrack Invisalign aligner material. https://www.invisalign.ca/the-invisalign-difference/smarttrack-material. Accessed May 24, 2017.
92. Align Technology. Align Technology announces January 21st availability of SmartTrack Invisalign aligner material. https://investor.aligntech.com/news-releases/news-release-details/align-technology-receives-us-patents-smarttrackr-invisalignr/. Accessed January 18, 2013.
93. Brascher AK, Zuran D, Feldmann Jr RE, et al. Patient survey on Invisalign treatment compare the SmartTrack material to the previous aligner material. *J Orofac Orthop.* 2016;77:432-438.

94. Sturgeon JA, Zautra AJ. Psychological resilience, pain catastrophizing, and positive emotions: perspectives on comprehensive modeling of individual pain adaptation. *Curr Pain Headache Rep.* 2013;17:317.
95. Sullivan M, Bishop S, Pivik J. The pain catastrophizing scale: development and validation. *Psychol Assess.* 1995;7:524-532.
96. Beck VJ, Farella M, Chandler NP, et al. Factors associated with pain induced by orthodontic separators. *J Oral Rehabil.* 2014;41:282-288.
97. Baeza-Velasco C, Gely-Nargeot MC, Vilarrasa AB, et al. Joint hypermobility syndrome: problems that require psychological intervention. *Rheumatol Int.* 2011;31:1131-1136.
98. Sullivan MJL, Thorn B, Haythornthwaite JA, et al. Theoretical perspectives on the relation between catastrophizing and pain. *Clin J Pain.* 2001;17:52-64.
99. Jacobsen PB, Butler RW. Relation of cognitive coping and catastrophizing to acute pain and analgesic use following breast cancer surgery. *J Behav Med.* 1996;19:17-29.
100. Turk DC, Rudy TE. Assessment of cognitive-factors in chronic pain—a worthwhile enterprise. *J Consult Clin Psychol.* 1986;54:760-768.
101. Heyneman NE, Fremouw WJ, Gano D, et al. Individual-differences and the effectiveness of different coping strategies for pain. *Cognit Ther Res.* 1990;14:63-77.
102. Katon WJ. Clinical and health services relationships between major depression, depressive symptoms, and general medical illness. *Biol Psychiatry.* 2003;54:216-226.
103. Beck AT. A systematic investigation of depression. *Compr Psychiatry.* 1961;2:163-170.
104. Wang J, Jian F, Chen J, et al. Cognitive behavioral therapy for orthodontic pain control: a randomized trial. *J Dent Res.* 2012;91:580-585.
105. Bergius M, Broberg AG, Hakeberg M, et al. Prediction of prolonged pain experiences during orthodontic treatment. *Am J Orthod Dentofacial Orthop.* 2008;133:339, e1-e8.
106. Barsky AJ, Goodson JD, Lane RS, et al. The amplification of somatic symptoms. *Psychosom Med.* 1988;50:510-519.
107. Markiewicz MR, Ohrbach R, McCall WD. Oral behaviors checklist: reliability of performance in targeted waking-state behaviors. *J Orofac Pain.* 2006;20:306-316.
108. Endo H, Kanemura K, Tanabe N, et al. Clenching occurring during the day is influenced by psychological factors. *J Prosthodont Res.* 2011;55:159-164.
109. Winocur E, Uziel N, Lisha T, et al. Self-reported bruxism—associations with perceived stress, motivation for control, dental anxiety and gagging. *J Oral Rehabil.* 2011;38:3-11.
110. Michelotti A, Cioffi I, Festa P, et al. Oral parafunctions as risk factors for diagnostic TMD subgroups. *J Oral Rehabil.* 2010;37:157-162.
111. Slade GD, Ohrbach R, Greenspan JD, et al. Painful temporomandibular disorder: decade of discovery from OPPERA studies. *J Dent Res.* 2016;95:1084-1092.
112. Chow JC, Cioffi I. Effects of trait anxiety, somatosensory amplification, and facial pain on self-reported oral behaviors. *Clin Oral Investig.* 2019;23:1653-1661.
113. Spielberg CD, Gorsuch RL, Re L. *Manual of the State-Trait Anxiety Inventory.* Palo Alto: Consulting Psychologists Press; 1970.
114. Chow J. *Effects of Anxiety and Daytime Clenching on Orthodontic Pain Perception.* University of Toronto; 2018.
115. Gameiro GH, Schultz C, Trein MP, et al. Association among pain, masticatory performance, and proinflammatory cytokines in crevicular fluid during orthodontic treatment. *Am J Orthod Dentofacial Orthop.* 2015;148:967-973.
116. Castroflorio T, Bargellini A, Lucchese A, et al. Effects of clear aligners on sleep bruxism: randomized controlled trial. *J Biol Regul Homeost Agents.* 2018;32:21-29.
117. Lou T, Tran J, Castroflorio T, Tassi A, Cioffi I. Evaluation of masticatory muscle response to clear aligner therapy using ambulatory electromyographic recording. *Am J Orthod Dentofacial Orthop.* 2021;159(1):e25-e33.
118. Arias OR, Marquez-Orozco MC. Aspirin, acetaminophen, and ibuprofen: their effects on orthodontic tooth movement. *Am J Orthod Dentofacial Orthop.* 2006;130:364-370.
119. Roche JJ, Cisneros GJ, Acs G. The effect of acetaminophen on tooth movement in rabbits. *Angle Orthod.* 1997;67:231-236.
120. Leiker BJ, Nanda RS, Currier GF, et al. The effects of exogenous prostaglandins on orthodontic tooth movement in rats. *Am J Orthod Dentofacial Orthop.* 1995;108:380-388.
121. Tyrovola JB, Spyropoulos MN. Effects of drugs and systemic factors on orthodontic treatment. *Quintessence Int.* 2001;32:365-371.
122. Monk AB, Harrison JE, Worthington HV, et al. Pharmacological interventions for pain relief during orthodontic treatment. *Cochrane Database Syst Rev.* 2017;11:CD003976.
123. Sandhu S, Leckie G. Diurnal variation in orthodontic pain: clinical implications and pharmacological management. *Semin Orthod.* 2018;24:217-224.
124. Ong CK, Seymour RA, Lirk P, et al. Combining paracetamol (acetaminophen) with nonsteroidal antiinflammatory drugs: a qualitative systematic review of analgesic efficacy for acute postoperative pain. *Anesth Analg.* 2010;110:1170-1179.
125. Makrygiannakis MA, Kaklamanos EG, Athanasiou AE. Does long-term use of pain relievers have an impact on the rate of orthodontic tooth movement? A systematic review of animal studies. *Eur J Orthod.* 2019;41(5):468-477.
126. Fleming PS, Strydom H, Katsaros C, et al. Non-pharmacological interventions for alleviating pain during orthodontic treatment. *Cochrane Database Syst Rev.* 2016;12:CD010263.
127. Blasini M, Movsas S, Colloca L. Placebo hypoalgesic effects in pain: potential applications in dental and orofacial pain management. *Semin Orthod.* 2018;28:259-268.

19 Retention and Stability Following Aligner Therapy

JOSEF KUČERA and IVO MAREK

Retention and Stability in Orthodontic Treatment

INTRODUCTION

Orthodontic treatment is an area of medicine and dentistry that has to address not just health and function but also aesthetics. It is usually the aesthetic considerations that make patients seek out orthodontic treatment in the first place. Achieving an excellent aesthetic and functional result can be lengthy and expensive, therefore it is in the interests of both the patient and the clinician that the result of orthodontic treatment remains stable in the long term. Unfortunately the importance of the retention phase is often underestimated, when in reality it is as important to the patients as the active orthodontic treatment itself.

The period after the completion of active treatment can be divided into a retention period and a postretention period. The purpose of the retention phase following active orthodontic treatment is to prevent relapse defined as the natural tendency of the teeth to migrate into their original position in the dental arch and to eliminate the influence of other factors that might destabilize the result. It is very difficult to say how long the retention phase should last. The literature offers many recommendations, although they vary considerably and are often vague. Some authors suggest that, following orthodontic treatment, teeth should be held in the position achieved by treatment for as long as it is necessary to sustain the result,[1] or that the retention phase should be as long as needed and as short as possible.[2] Others suggest that retainers should be used until the patient's growth is complete or the third molars erupt,[3] or for a period of 10 years[4] or even 20 years,[5] or simply as long as the patient wishes to keep the teeth aligned.[6]

It is generally recommended that nongrowing patients wear retainers for at least 1 year and is biologically defined as the completion of the reorganization of bone and periodontal ligaments around the teeth.[7] Collagen fibers are reorganized within the first 3 to 4 months.[6] This period is critical, and the wearing of retention appliances is essential because relapse is very likely at this stage; after this critical period the risk decreases substantially.[8] However, the reorganization of elastic supracrestal fibers may take more than 1 year, which makes the retention of severely rotated teeth particularly difficult; some authors recommend adjunctive surgical procedures such as fiberotomy to decrease the amount of relapse.[9,10] In growing patients retainers should be worn until the growth is complete.[6] At the time patients stop wearing the retention appliances, the postretention period begins, and it is only then that we get a true picture of the stability of the original result that had been achieved by the orthodontic treatment. During the postretention period numerous factors and the complexity of their interactions may ultimately destabilize treatment results.

FACTORS INFLUENCING LONG-TERM STABILITY

With regard to stability there are some general guidelines and recommendations for orthodontic treatment, and so long as these are respected when making and carrying out the treatment plan they tend to produce stable results with relatively little risk of relapse. In such cases, long-term changes in dental arches of treated patients are then similar to those occurring in untreated subjects.

Before starting treatment, orthodontists need to keep in mind that the position of the teeth and the shape of the dental arches are the balanced result of many factors, especially the influence of the forces exerted by the surrounding soft tissues (i.e., pressure from the cheeks, lips, and tongue) that create a "neutral zone" or "zone of stability." Orthodontic movement of the teeth outside of this neutral zone pushes them into an unbalanced zone, with consequent relapse.[6,11] The shape of the dental arch, particularly the mandibular arch, should therefore be respected in the planning and implementation of treatment because changes in arch shape tend to relapse into the original shape in the long term.[12,13] The upper dental arch may be expanded more than the lower arch in indicated cases (rapid maxillary expansion); however, even in these cases, the long-term stability appears to be quite problematic.[14] Any changes in the lower intercanine distance are also very prone to relapse,[15,16] partly because decrease in the lower intercanine distance is due to the natural changes that occur in the dental arch as a result of aging.[17,18] The quality of articulation and intercuspation can also be very important for the long-term stability.[16,19,20] The correct intercuspation of the teeth in lateral segments with high cusps itself provides the best retention, both in sagittal and transverse dimensions.[2] It is also important to achieve the correction in the vertical direction, and especially for sufficient correction of the deep bite, as its deepening reduces the space for the lower incisors.[20] Incisor shape can also be a source of posttreatment instability. In triangular-shaped incisors, recontouring of the approximal surfaces (i.e., interproximal enamel reduction, stripping) provides more stable contact between the incisors. According to some studies, this stabilizing effect of lower incisor stripping is comparable to the efficiency of bonded retainers.[21,22] Similarly, the adjustment of large proximal enamel ridges on the palatal surfaces of the upper incisors is also important for the stability of the incisor region.[23]

Continuing growth is a separate issue and needs to be addressed with particular attention in more pronounced skeletal malocclusions, especially in the sagittal and vertical dimensions, which continue to grow over a longer period than in the transverse dimension. Unfavorable growth of the jaws has a negative impact on the occlusal relationship and on the position of incisors due to the dentoalveolar compensation process.[24] This is one of the reasons why it is recommended to plan comprehensive treatment of severe skeletal malocclusions after the patient's growth is complete. However, even after growth completion, the dental arches are also subject to changes related to the patient's aging, and these processes are in fact lifelong and may result in the development of irregularities in the incisor segment[17,18,25,26] that often bring patients back for retreatment.

Retention Protocols and the Choice of Retention Appliance

RETENTION PROTOCOLS

To date, there is no universal retention protocol, and there is insufficient high-quality scientific literature to reliably establish such a protocol in terms of the length of the retention phase, the wearing regime, and the choice of type of retention device.[27,28] This is because we cannot generalize a single procedure for patients who differ in diagnosis, severity of the malocclusion, age, type of growth, treatment type, and quality of treatment result. Thus the choice of retention device should always be individualized, with consideration of all the potential factors of instability mentioned earlier. This approach is called "differential retention," meaning that for every patient, orthodontists must focus and aim the retention on those points that pose the greatest threat and risk of relapse in the individual patient (Fig. 19.1).[4]

According to surveys on retention protocols, the most common retention devices are the Hawley retainers and clear thermoplastic retainers. For the mandible, a fixed retainer is often indicated, either on its own or in combination with a removable appliance.[29,30] An increasing trend has been observed in the use of thermoplastic retainers, which patients prefer because of their good aesthetics and inconspicuousness.[31] A similar trend can also be observed with fixed retainers in both jaws. In terms of the frequency of use of the various retention devices, an indefinite use of fixed retainers is recommended by many clinicians.[29,32,33]

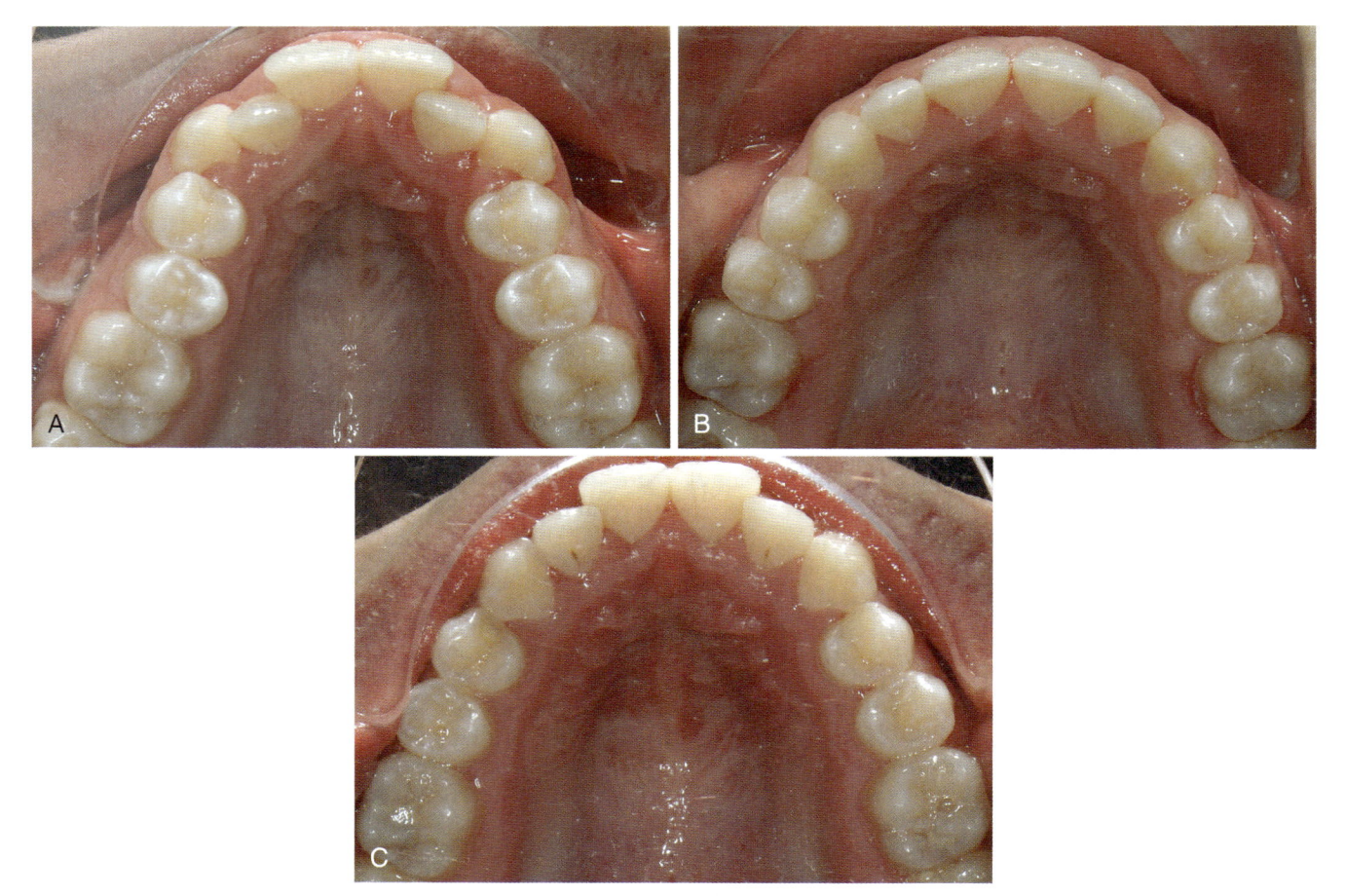

Fig. 19.1 Examples of relapse after orthodontic treatment, where either the patient failed to wear the retention appliances after rapid maxillary expansion (A-C) or the retention regime selected was insufficient for a noncompliant patient; the rotational relapse of lateral incisors

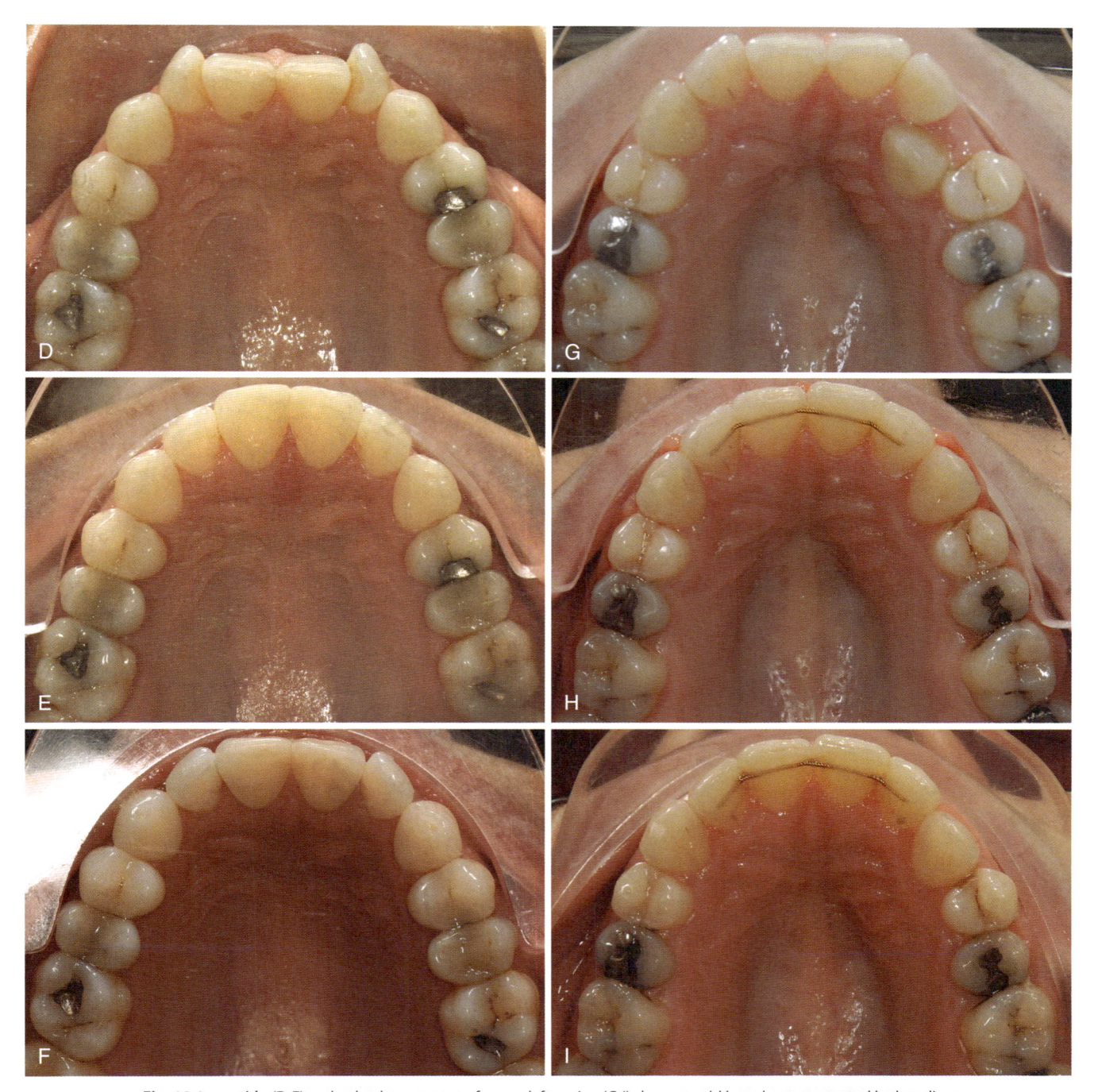

Fig. 19.1, cont'd (D-F) and palatal movement of upper left canine (G-I) shown could have been prevented by bonding a fixed retainer and including problematic teeth.

If the decision is made to use a retention appliance long term, a fixed retainer seems to be the best option mainly because it prevents relapse of the aesthetically important anterior teeth very efficiently and without any need for patient cooperation.[34,35] Bonded retainers have also been described in the literature as safe, predictable, and posing no health risks to the patient.[4,5,36] Some studies, however, have indicated that there is a tendency toward increased buildup of plaque and calculus around bonded retainers (Fig. 19.2), having negative consequences on the periodontium[37]; however, this can be minimized with regular care, exercised by the patient and a dental hygienist.

The biggest disadvantage of bonded retainers that impacts their long-term or lifelong use is failure rate. According to the literature, the failure rate varies widely, from 0.1% to 53%.[38,39] However, we believe that the occurrence of common failures, such as abrasion of the layer of adhesive resin caused by food attrition or occlusal contacts, is only a matter of time (Fig. 19.3). Other considerable risks associated with prolonged use of bonded retainers are the so-called unexpected complications, where unexpected tooth movement occurs, even when the integrity of the bonded retainer has not been compromised in any way. The incidence of these complications is quite small, occurring

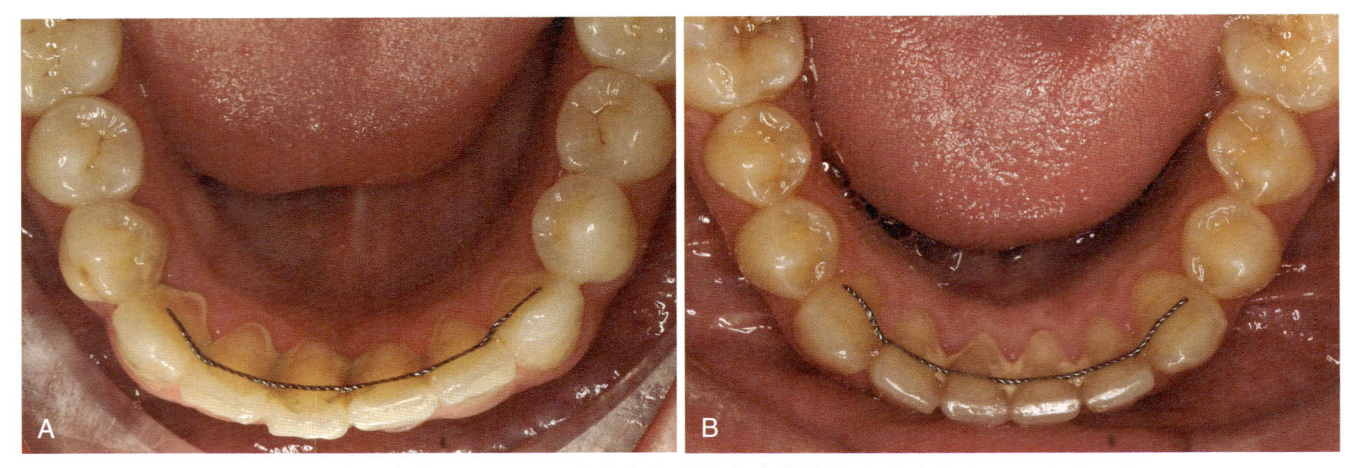

Fig. 19.2 Calculus accumulation and gingival inflammation around the lower bonded retainer (A and B).

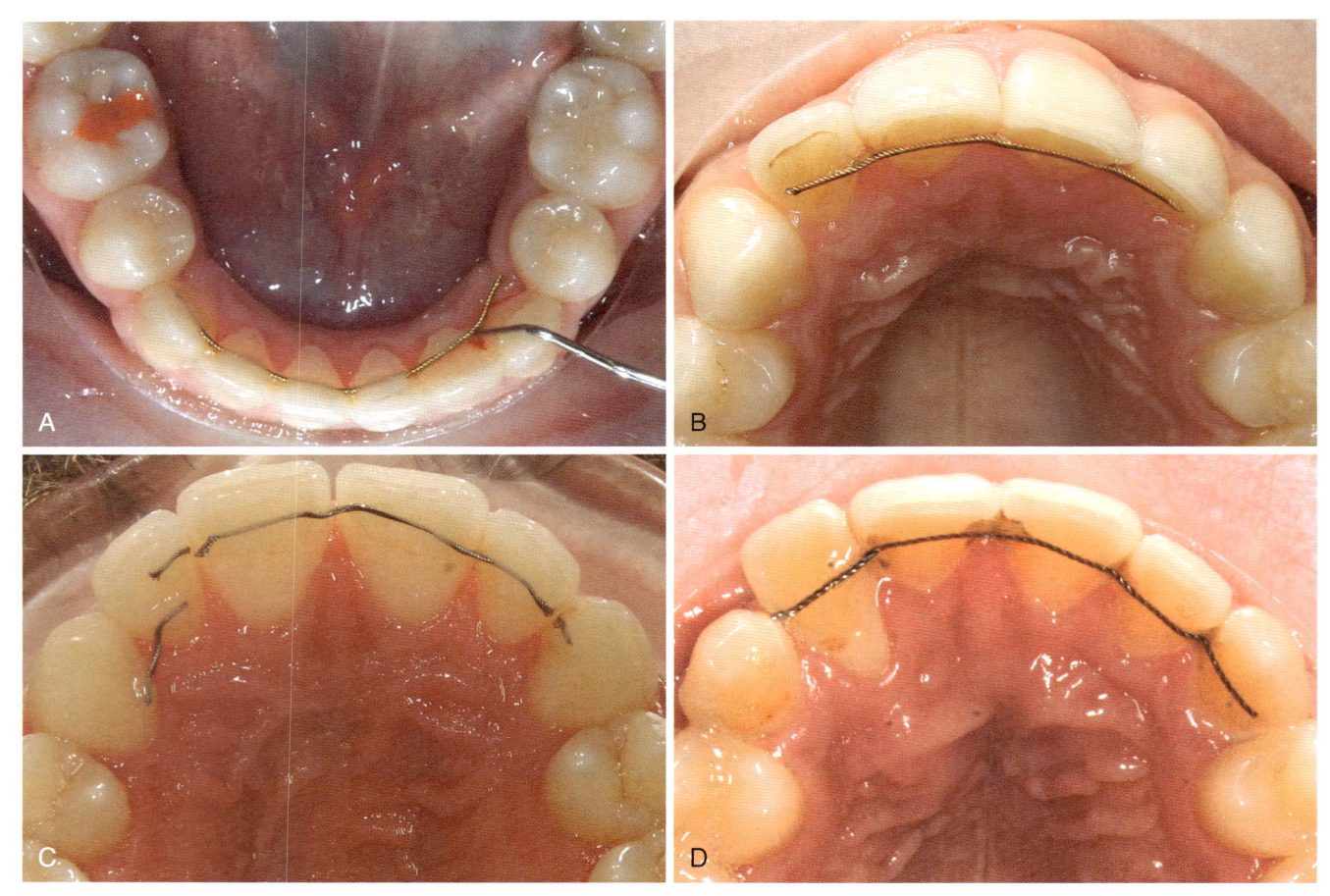

Fig. 19.3 Examples of failures of bonded retainers. (A) The detachment of a composite resin layer is usually a consequence of bonding errors. (B) The loss of the adhesive layer due to mastication or premature contact on the bonded retainer. (C) Premature contact on the retainer wire, wire fatigue, or selection of a wire with insufficient mechanical properties (small diameter dead-soft wire) resulting in fracture of the wire. (D) Extending the upper retainer to the canines increases the risk of fracture, with consequent wire activation and unwanted tooth movement. (Kučera J, Littlewood SJ, Marek I. *Fixed retention: pitfalls and complications*. British Dental Journal 2021; 230 (11): 703-708.)

in approximately 1% to 5% of cases,[40,41] but their clinical consequences can be very severe. In addition, it is estimated that up to 50% of such cases require retreatment.[41] There are two distinct types (Fig. 19.4), characterized by a torque difference between two adjacent incisors (X effect) or opposite inclination of contralateral canines (Twist effect).[40,42]

These complications are surprising because they may appear after a relatively long period of problem-free retention, often occurring after several years.[40,41,43] The unwanted tooth movement can be so pronounced that the root is moved outside of the alveolar bone (Fig. 19.5), which is in many cases accompanied by the occurrence of gingival

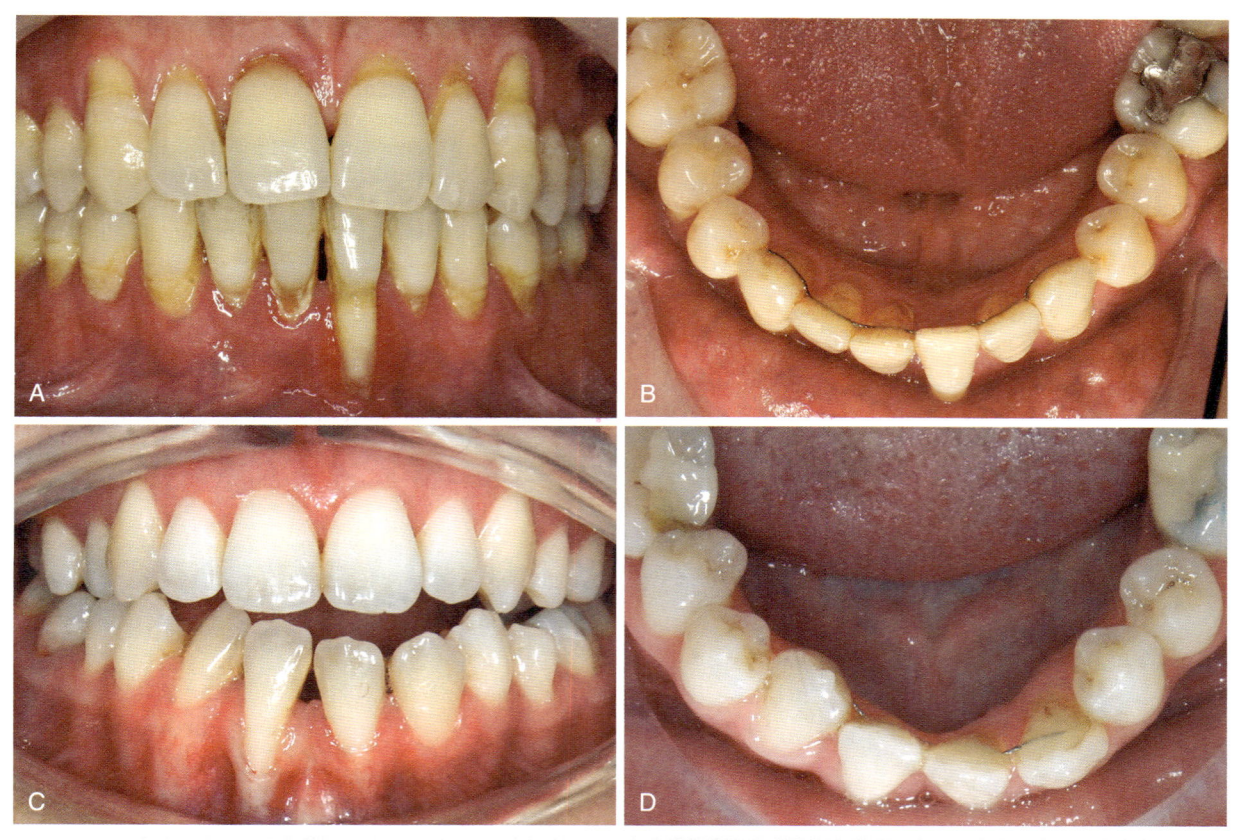

19 • Retention and Stability Following Aligner Therapy   263

Fig. 19.4 Two distinct types of unexpected complication of lower bonded retainers: opposite torque on two adjacent incisors (X effect; A, B) and opposite inclination of contralateral canines (Twist effect; C, D). Both X effect and Twist effect may be accompanied by severe gingival recession (A, C). (C, D from Kucera J, Streblov J, Marek I, et al. Treatment of complications associated with lower fixed retainers. *J Clin Orthod*. 2016;50[1]:54-59.)

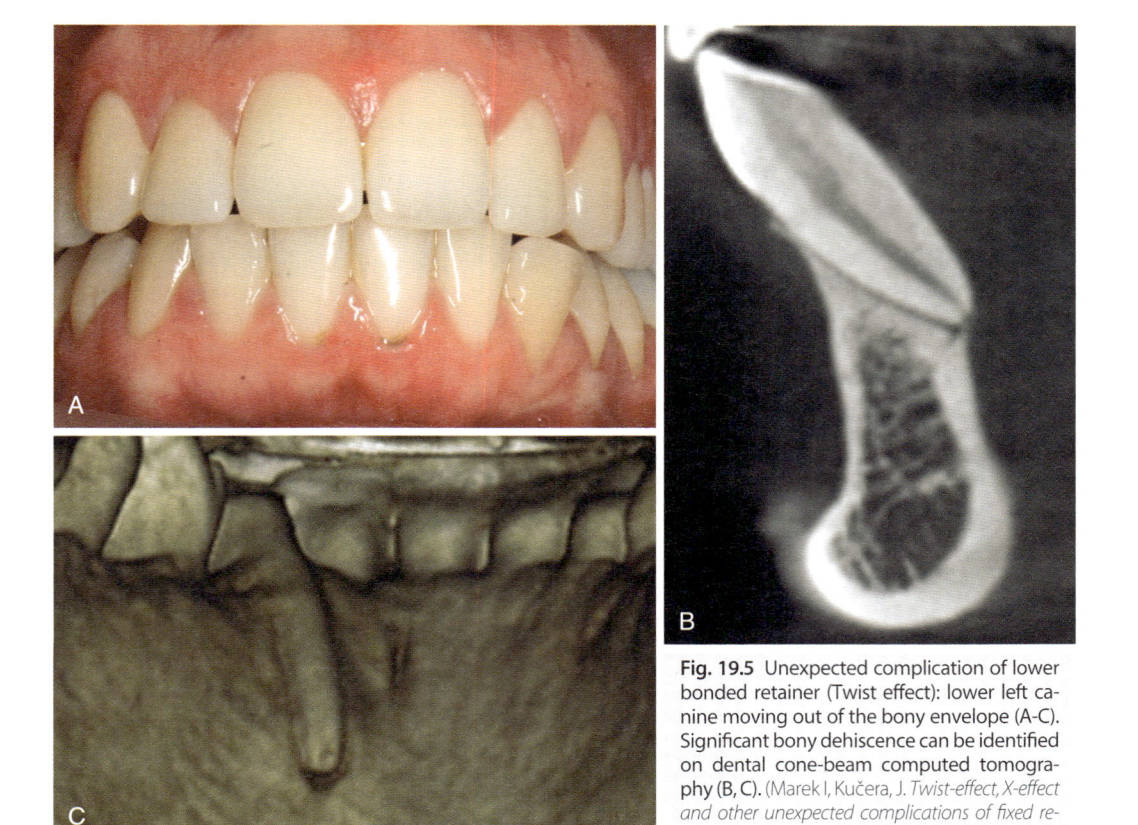

Fig. 19.5 Unexpected complication of lower bonded retainer (Twist effect): lower left canine moving out of the bony envelope (A-C). Significant bony dehiscence can be identified on dental cone-beam computed tomography (B, C). (Marek I, Kučera, J. *Twist-effect, X-effect and other unexpected complications of fixed retainers – original article*. LKS 2015, 25(5):98-106.)

recession. In such severe cases, orthodontic retreatment is necessary, and often a surgical periodontal intervention may also be needed (Fig. 19.6).[43,44]

Long-term or lifelong retention is not without risk. It should be indicated with caution, and it is essential that fixed retainers are regularly checked by an orthodontist or during regular dental or hygiene checkups. It is also very important that dentists and dental hygienists who see the patients most frequently are informed about the retention devices used and their associated risks, no matter how small. This is especially important for the dental health care providers to help their patients manage because many of the patients consider the orthodontic treatment completed when the fixed appliance is removed, and their regular attendance for checkups at the orthodontic office in the retention phase can be a problem (Fig. 19.7).[40] It is needless to say that early detection of these complications can minimize the damage to adjacent tissues and facilitate the subsequent care.

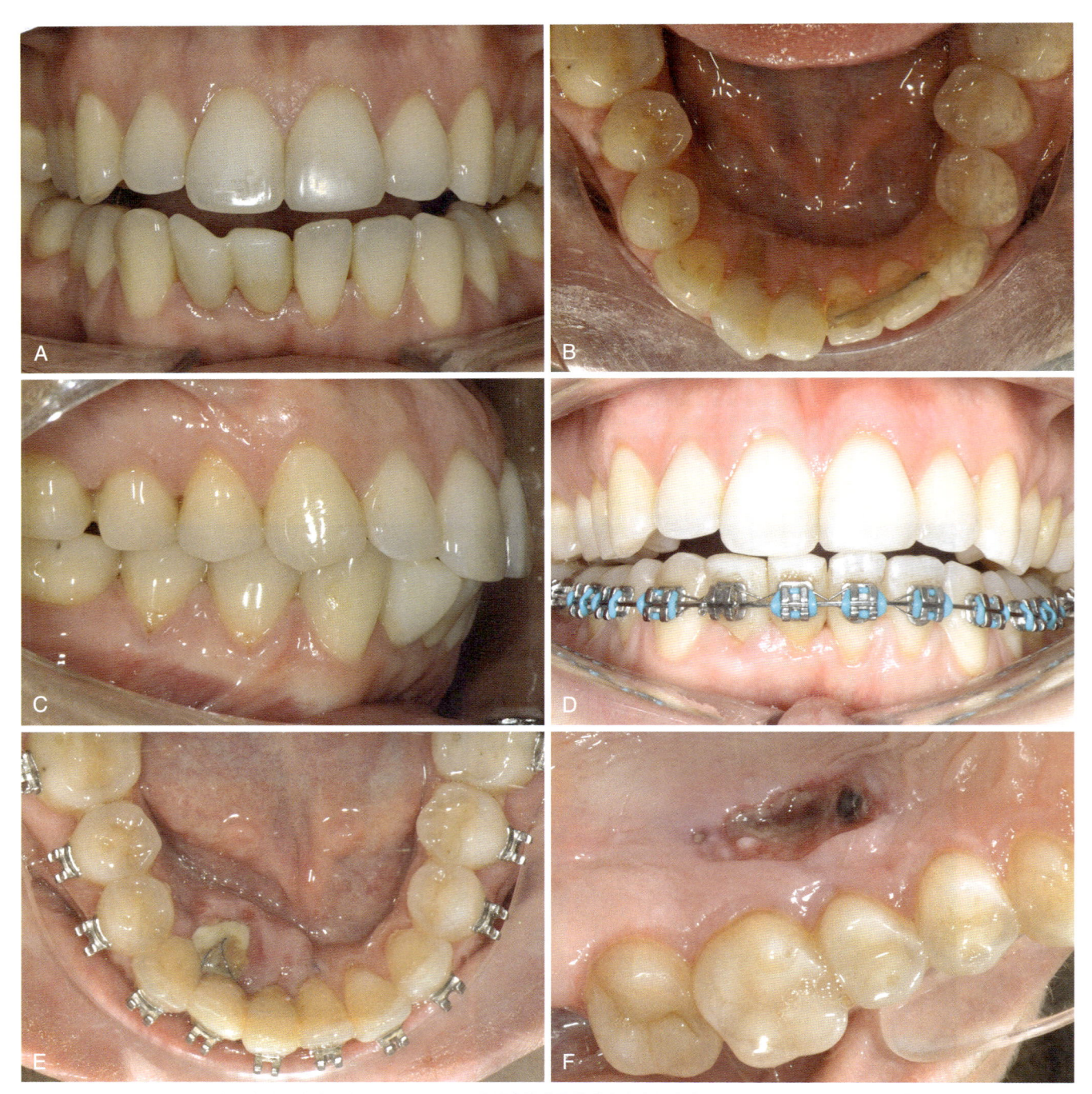

Fig. 19.6 Treatment of a complication associated with a lower bonded retainer. (A-C) Lower left central and lateral incisors severely proclined by a fractured bonded retainer and lingual gingival recessions occurring on both incisors. (D-F) Retreatment with a full lower fixed appliance corrected the torque of the incisors and was followed by a periodontal reconstructive surgery.

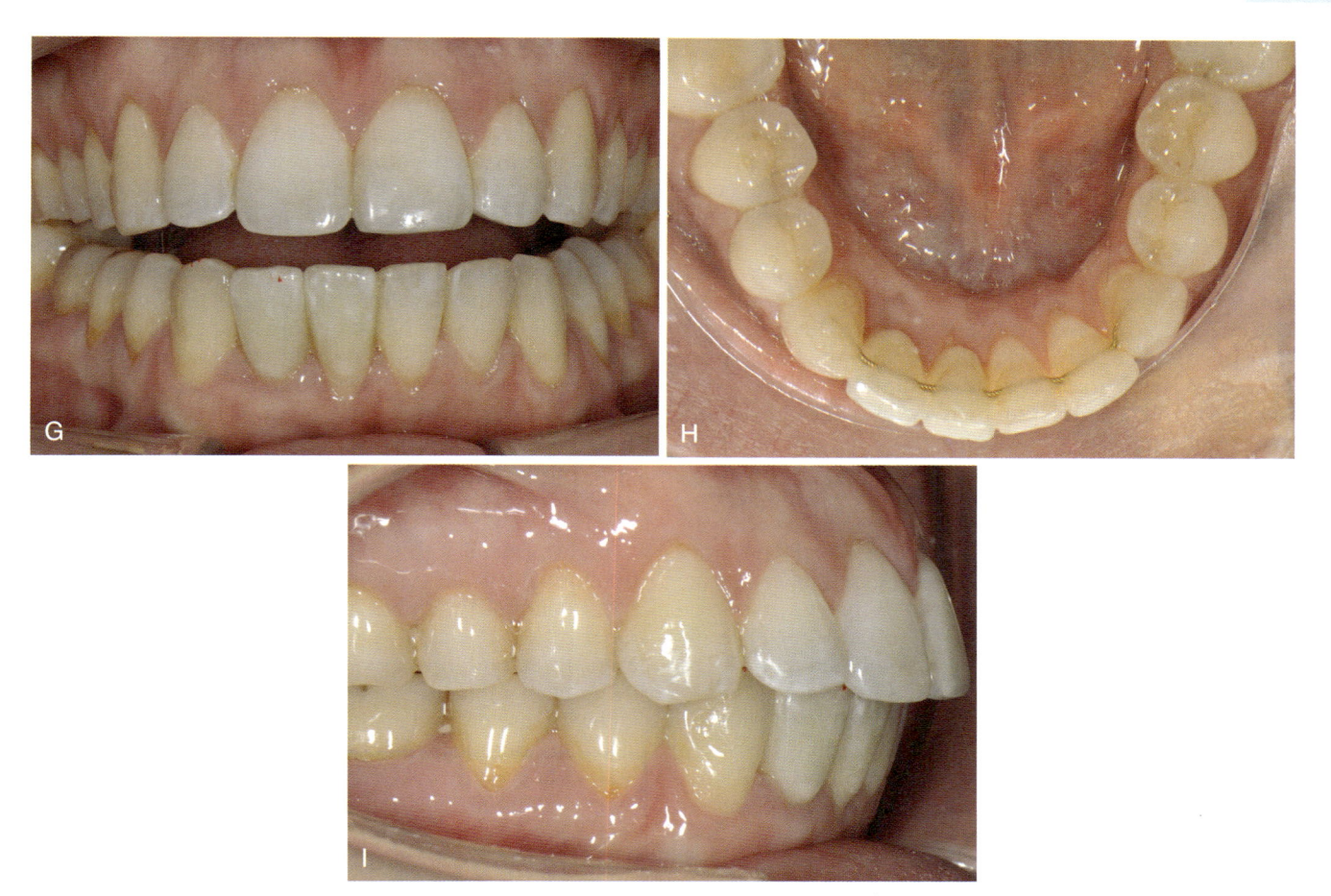

Fig. 19.6, cont'd (G-I) Final reconstruction with full porcelain crowns and bonding of a new lower fixed retainer.

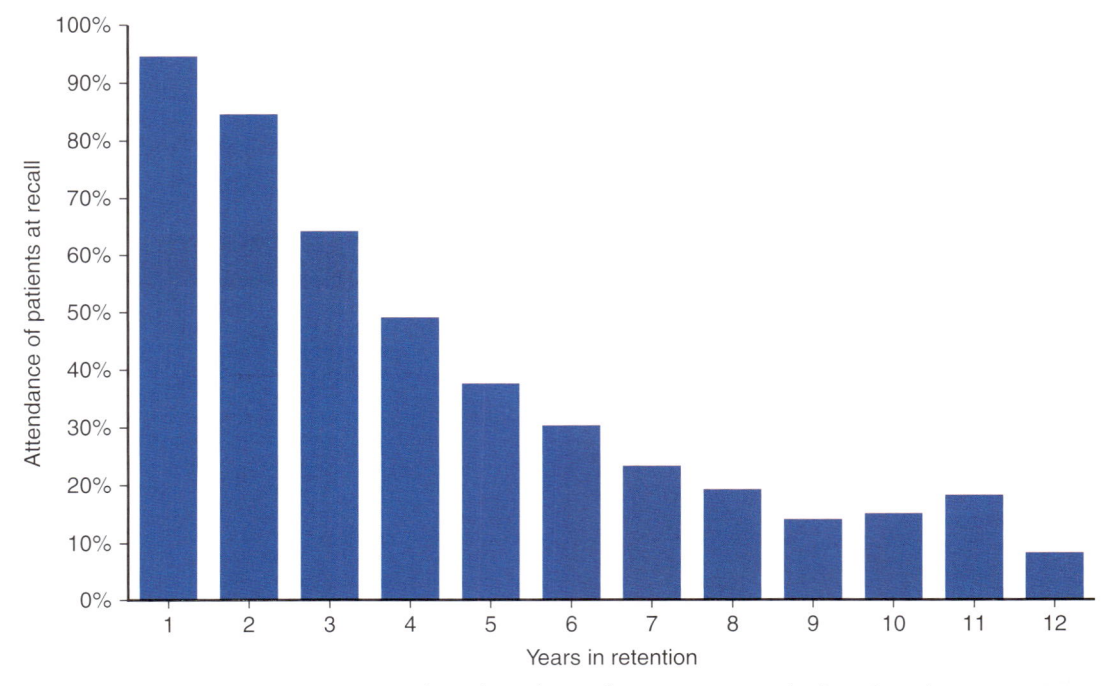

Fig. 19.7 When long-term retention is indicated, regular recalls are necessary to check retainers; however, attendance of patients decreases in the retention period, as seen on this graph. (From Kucera J, Marek I. Unexpected complications associated with mandibular fixed retainers: a retrospective study. *Am J Orthod Dentofacial Orthop*. 2016;149[2]:202-211.)

APPLIANCES FOR RETENTION AND INDICATIONS OF VARIOUS RETENTION DEVICES

Based on the biologic principles and knowledge of factors that influence the position of teeth in the retention phase, several combinations of retention appliances have been recommended. Most often a removable Hawley retainer with van der Linden labial bow and Adams clasps on the first molars is used for both the upper and lower jaws (Fig. 19.8). Hawley retainers are worn largely during the nighttime only. The second option is clear thermoplastic retainers, suitable for both night- and daytime wear (Fig. 19.9). Hawley retainers are indicated especially for patients who have need for an increased stabilization of the canine positions. Other typical indications are patients after transverse expansion or after treatment of a deep bite when the appliance is also serving as a bite plate. In class II cases where intermaxillary elastics or a bite-jumping device was used, an activator with van der Linden labial bow and Adams clasps on maxillary molars (Fig. 19.10) or two clear thermoplastic appliances with class II precision wings should be considered. In the majority of patients, each of these removable retainers is used in combination with an upper or lower bonded retainer. Bonded retainers are most often made of thin multistrand flexible steel archwires of various strengths and with various cross sections (most often the cross section varies between 0.0155 and 0.021in). The wire is shaped and passively attached by a flow composite resin to all anterior teeth in the lower jaw (canines and incisors) on the lingual surface, preferably in the apical third of teeth. Alternatively, thick monofilament stainless steel, cobalt-chromium or titanium-molybdenum wires bonded only to the canines can be used (cross section ranges between 0.025 and 0.036 in). In the upper arch, fixed retainers most often are limited only to the incisor segment, while in some patients with increased need for canine stabilization (e.g., palatally or buccally impacted canines) the canines are also included in the bonded retainer (Fig. 19.11). The use of fixed retainers is particularly necessary in patients with compromised periodontal health, where they also serve as periodontal splints, as well as in patients with spacing or midline diastemas, after complicated space closure following extractions, severe tooth rotations, open bite, or with impacted canines, or even as a space maintainer before dental implants are placed (Fig. 19.12).

SPECIFICS OF RETENTION FOLLOWING CLEAR ALIGNER THERAPY

General principles that apply in treatment planning and that fundamentally influence the occurrence of relapse and the stability of treatment are equally relevant in the treatment by fixed or clear aligner appliance treatment. However, the retention phase following orthodontic treatment using clear aligners is different to some extent from that following use of fixed appliances.

When planning retention after clear aligner therapy (CAT), the greatest disadvantage is the complicated achievement of final articulation and intercuspation in the posterior segments, as opposed to fixed appliance treatment, where an ideal occlusal contact can be achieved in the final

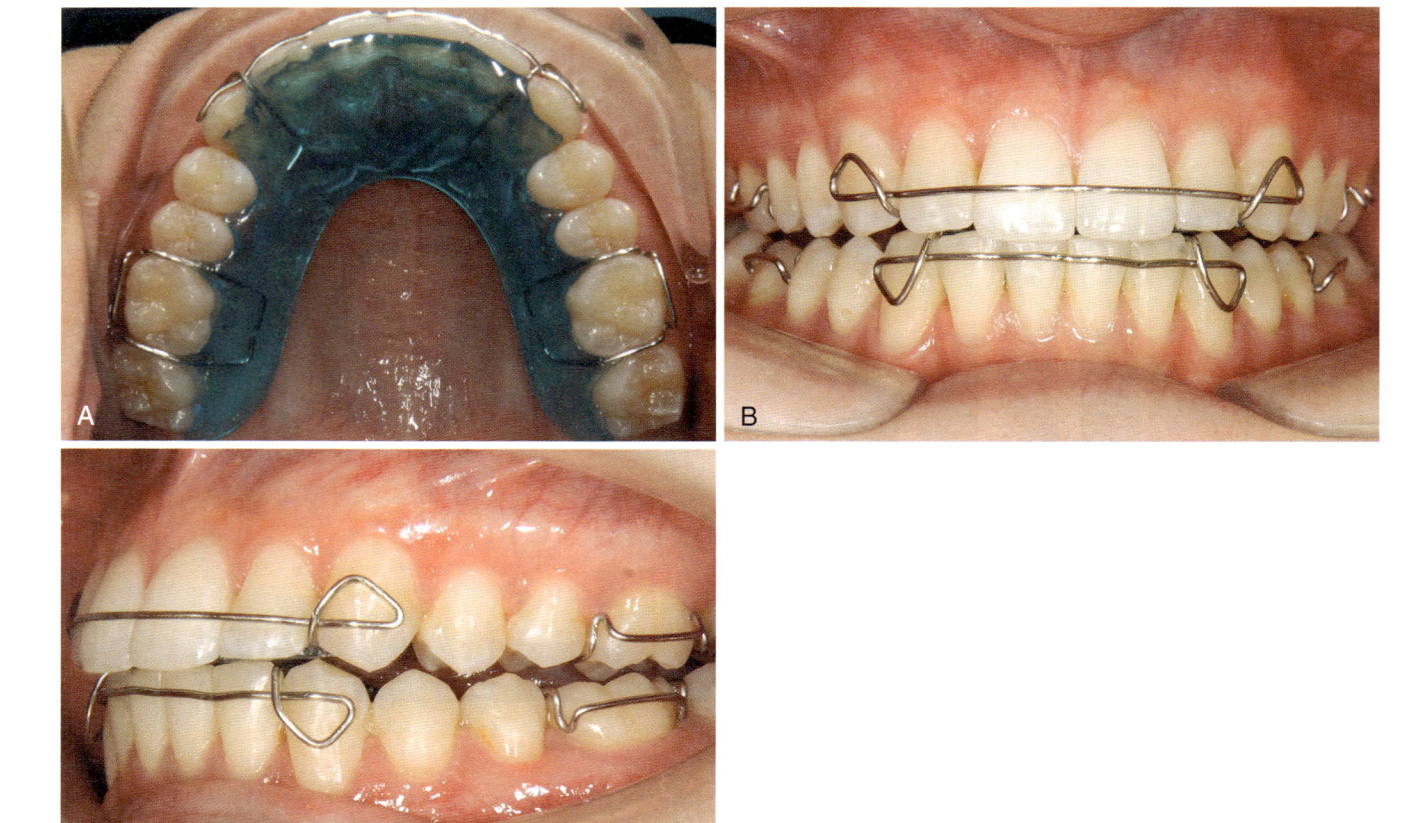

Fig. 19.8 Hawley retainer with frontal bite plane in occlusal (A), front (B), and lateral (C) views.

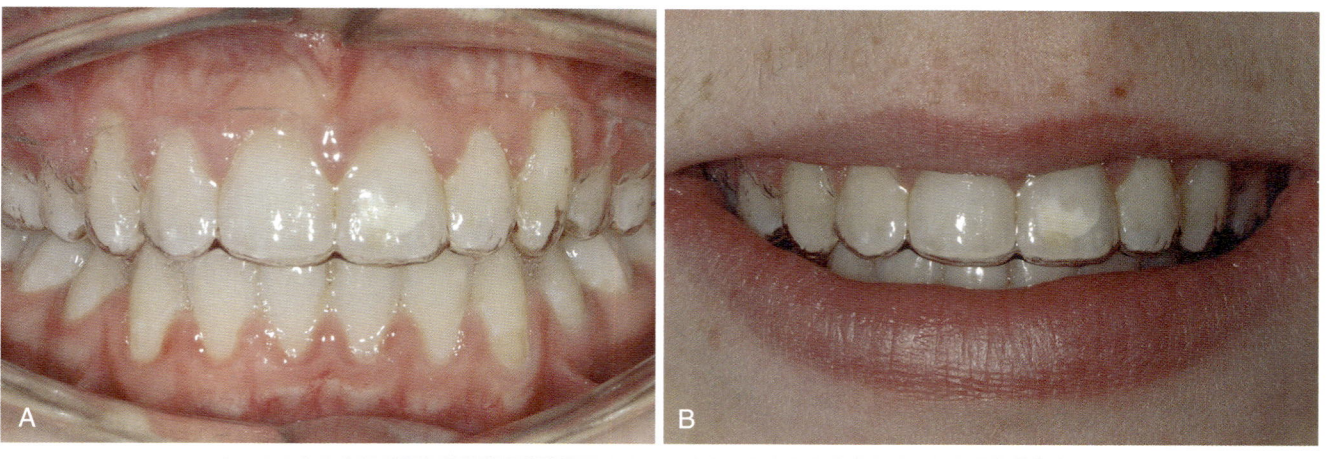

Fig. 19.9 Vacuum-formed thermoplastic retainer in the upper jaw in frontal view (A) and smile (B).

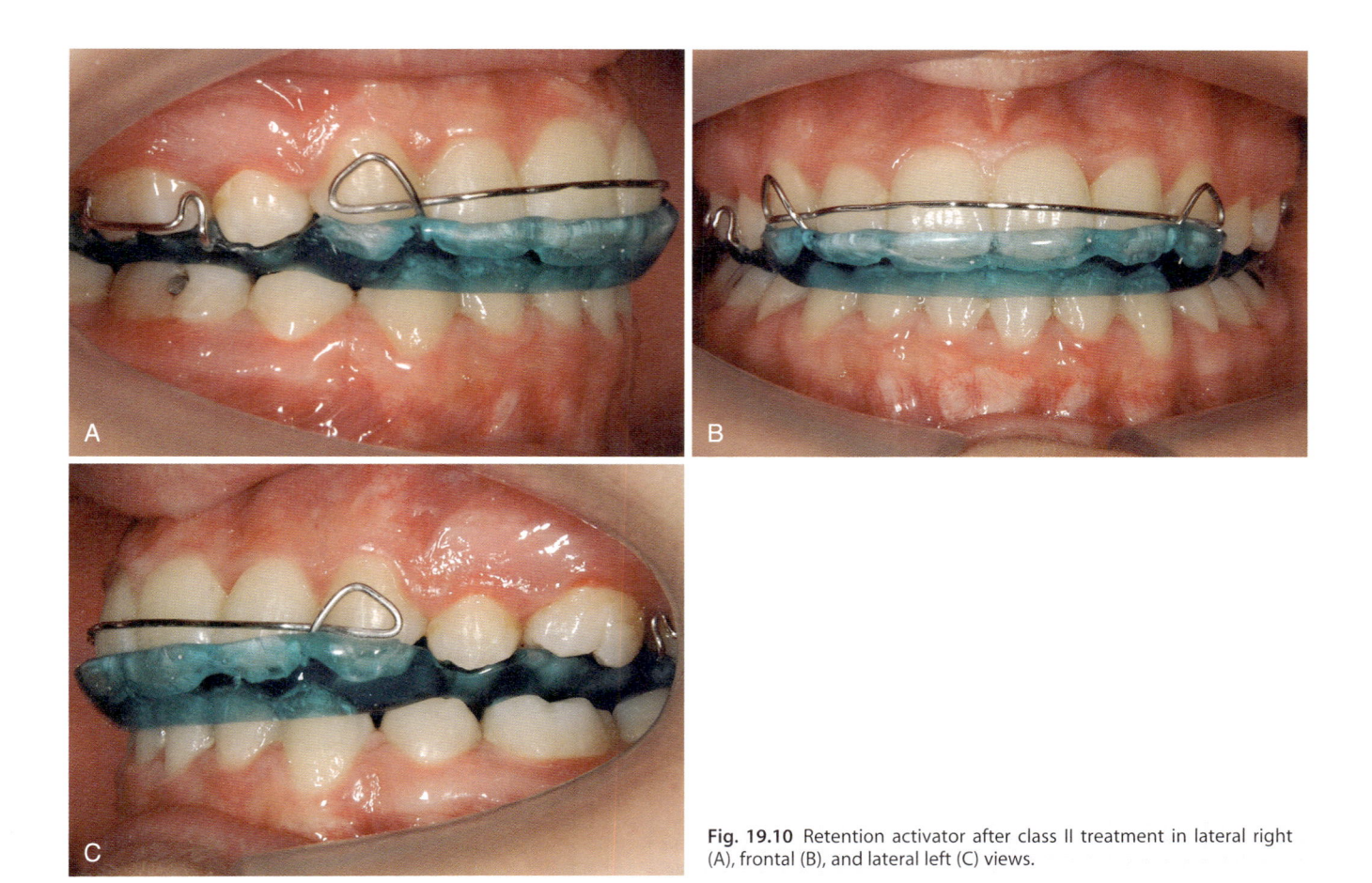

Fig. 19.10 Retention activator after class II treatment in lateral right (A), frontal (B), and lateral left (C) views.

stage of treatment by use of settling elastics. In CAT, a posterior open bite often occurs. This may be a consequence of various factors, including premature anterior contact of incisors (Fig. 19.13) due to insufficient intrusion of lower incisors or incorrect torque of upper or even lower incisors. In addition, the intrusive influence of masticatory forces on aligners in the posterior segments plays an important role. This situation can be solved by additional aligners; nevertheless, even then a slight open bite often persists. In these cases, posterior teeth need to be allowed to achieve their best possible contact (natural settling) with their antagonists. In this regard, the use of clear aligners for retention may not be appropriate, as it might hinder this natural process entirely, thereby making the settling less effective than when Hawley appliances are used (Fig. 19.14).[45]

On the other hand, the abovementioned intrusion effect of clear aligners on the posterior segments is advantageous when treating open-bite cases. Compared to the

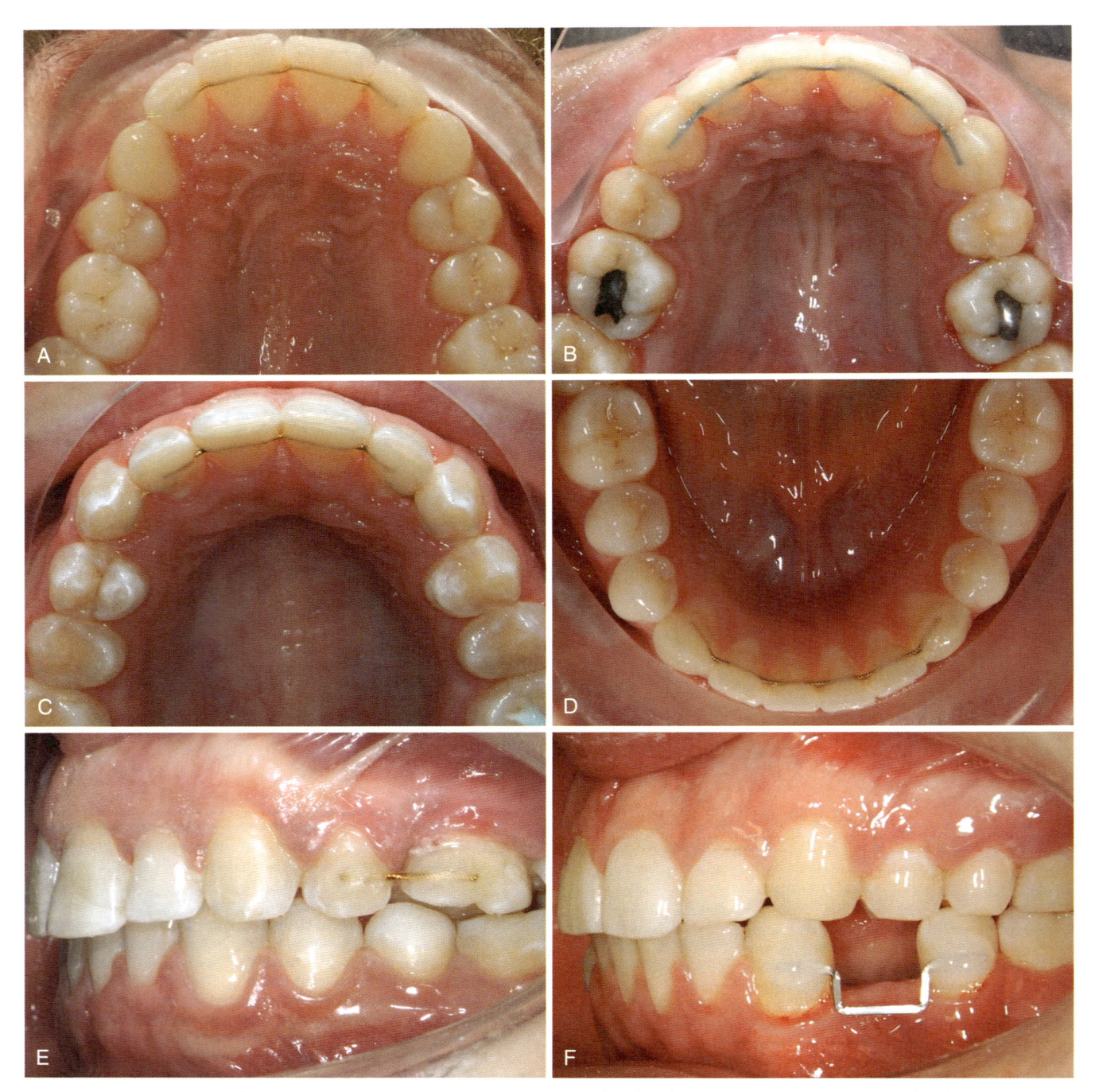

Fig. 19.11 Different types of commonly used fixed retainers. Upper retainers can include incisors only (A), or even both canines, either continuous (B) or segmented (C); the segmented version is more suitable because premature contact on the retainer can be avoided, thereby decreasing both the incidence of fracture and the adhesive layer. (D) Lower fixed retainer usually includes canines and incisors. Vestibular retainers can be used after difficult extraction space closure (E) or as a space maintainer prior to implant placement (F).

fixed appliance treatment, clinically significant intrusion of molars and premolars can be achieved even without using temporary anchorage devices. These intrusion movements also seem to be very stable, though valid data to verify this premise are lacking currently (Fig. 19.15) In open-bite cases where incisor extrusion is a part of the treatment, it is important that both upper and lower fixed retainers extending from canine to canine are used as part of the retention protocol. Additionally, it is essential that all teeth in the upper and lower arches are included in thermoplastic retainers to prevent unwanted eruption of the last molars and consequent reopening of the bite (Fig. 19.16).

The apparent advantage of CAT is the final position of the lower incisors can be predicted very precisely during treatment planning, allowing the clinician to predict and reduce unwanted proclination of incisors and thus expected relapse as well (Fig. 19.17).[46] Therefore functions

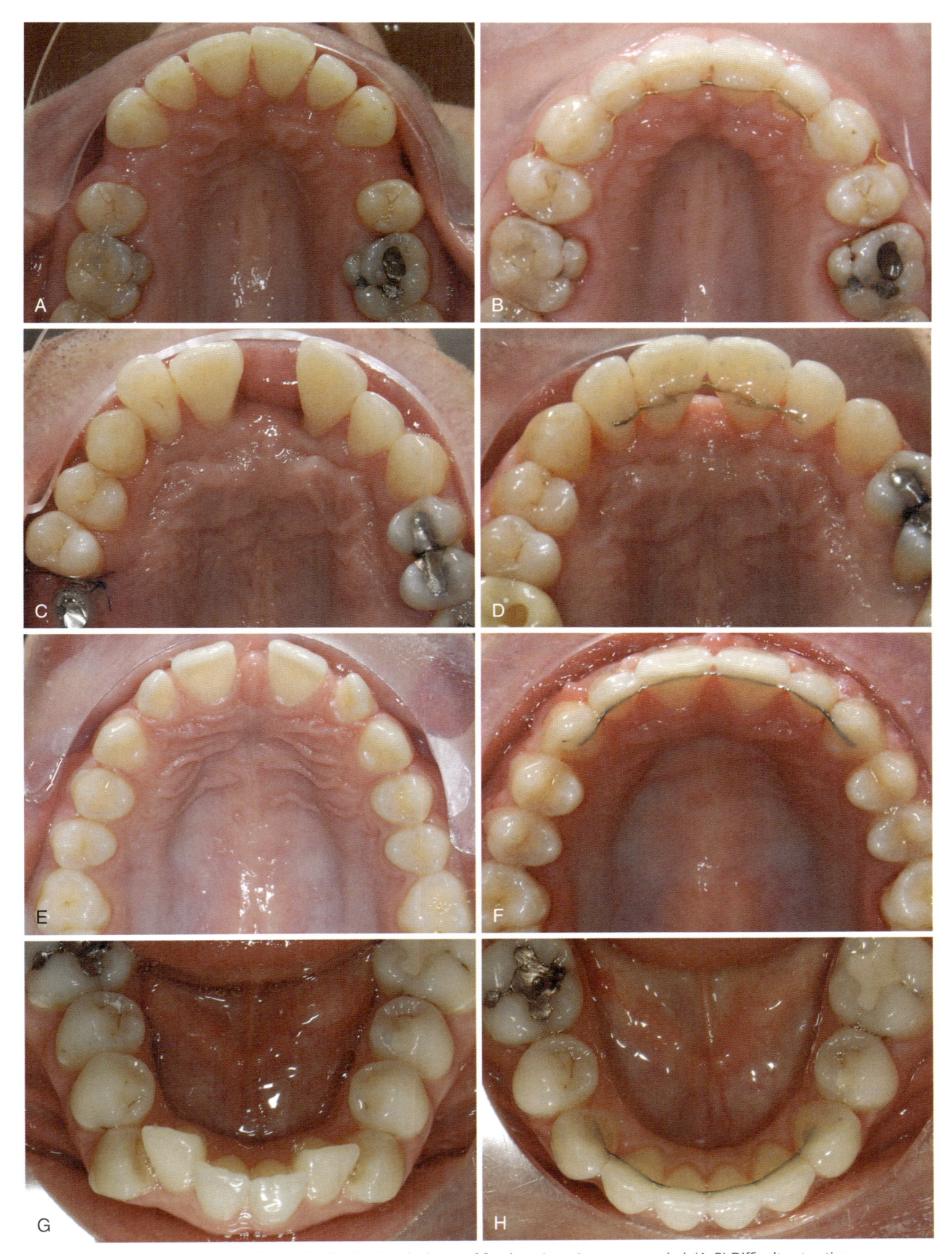

Fig. 19.12 Examples of typical indication in which use of fixed retainers is recommended. (A, B) Difficult extraction space closure. (C, D) Large midline diastema closure in a periodontally compromised patient. (E, F) Space closure in a patient with generalized spacing. (G, H) Severe crowding and tooth rotations.

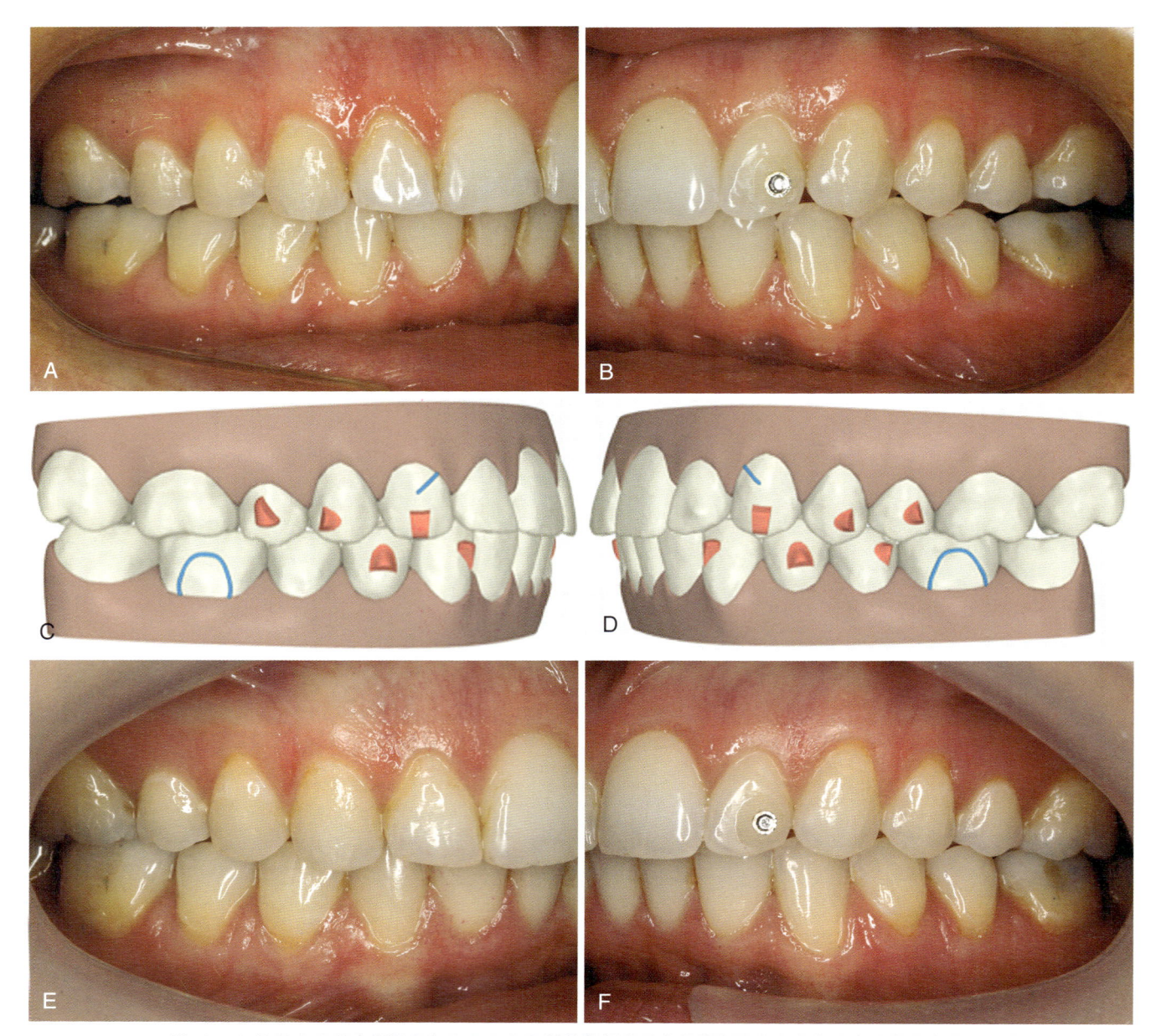

Fig. 19.13 (A, B) Lateral open bite often occurs after aligner treatment. (C, D) The clinical picture at the end of treatment may thus differ when compared to the final situation depicted in the treatment planning software. (E, F) However, the clinical situation after 2 years in recall shows that the teeth will eventually settle into the desired position.

like *grip* and *superimposition* in treatment planning software should be included in the standard protocol when planning nonextraction therapy in cases of crowding or in class II cases where use of elastics is planned. Despite providing exact control of the lower incisor position, fixed retainers may still be recommended as the most reliable retention method for stabilizing the position of the lower incisors in the long term. After class II treatment, the use of a retention activator in construction bite or thermoplastic retainers with precision wings should be considered to maintain the interarch occlusal change. In crossbite cases where transverse expansion was performed, it is more suitable to use a removable retention plate because it is more rigid and maintains the final transverse dimension better and can be easily adjusted by selective grinding where settling is needed to finalize the articulation.

RETENTION PROTOCOL AND SCHEDULE OF CHECKUPS IN THE RETENTION PERIOD

In standard cases the following retention protocol is used in our institution: In the rare cases when patients do not have a bonded maxillary fixed retainer, full-time wear of the retention appliance for the first 3 months is recommended (this most often involves a thermoplastic retainer during the day and a Hawley appliance overnight, achieving 24 hours of retainer wear, with the exception of time that the patient spends eating, drinking, teeth brushing, and possibly participating in sport activities); after the 3-month period, the patients are then asked to wear retention appliances overnight for the rest of the first year of retention, followed by every other night in the second year, twice a week in the third year, and once a week afterwards; when a fixed retainer is

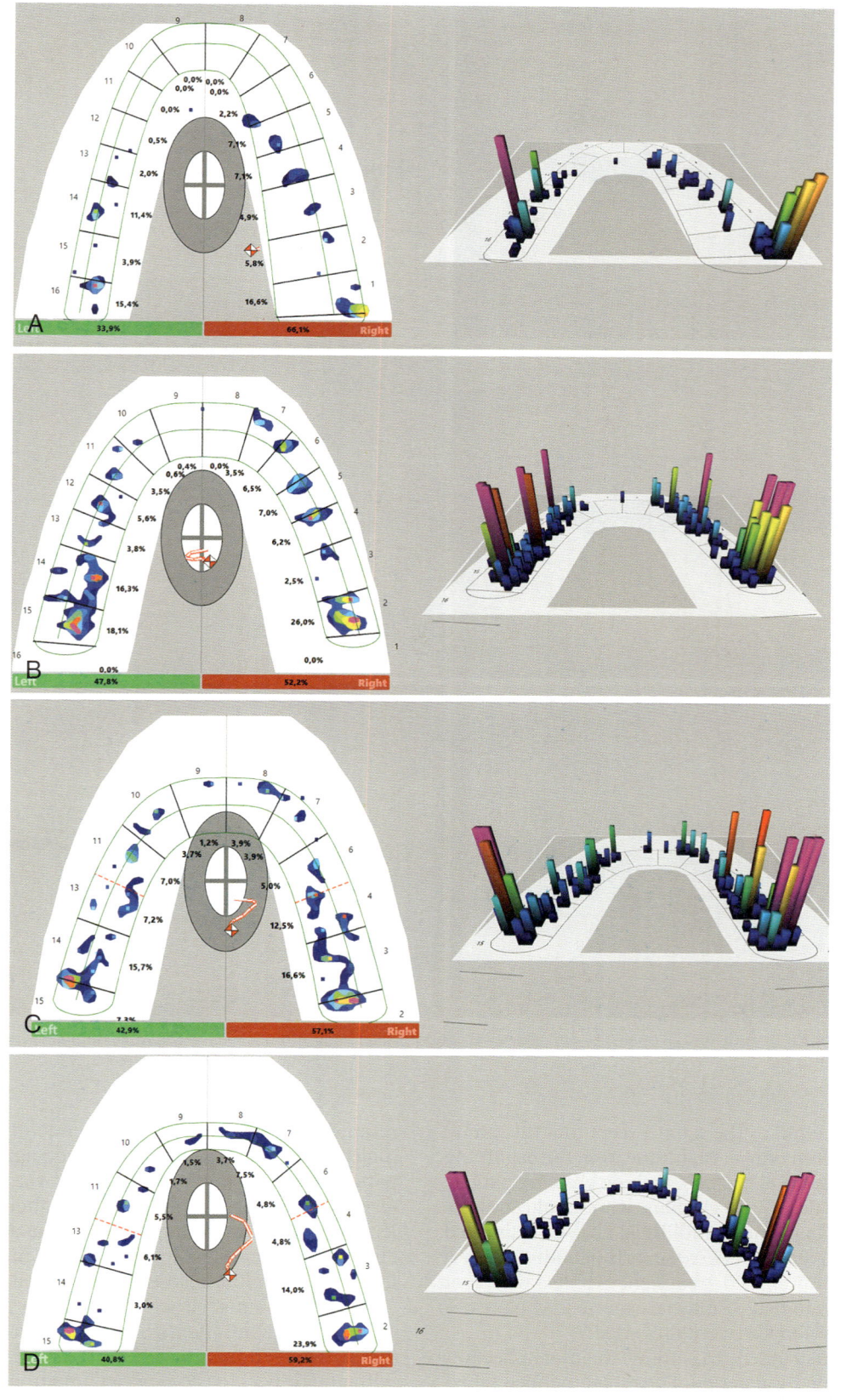

Fig. 19.14 Natural settling of teeth after orthodontic treatment in recall after 6 months, as visualized on T scans of a patient wearing a Hawley retainer at nighttime (A, B) and a thermoplastic retainer (C, D).

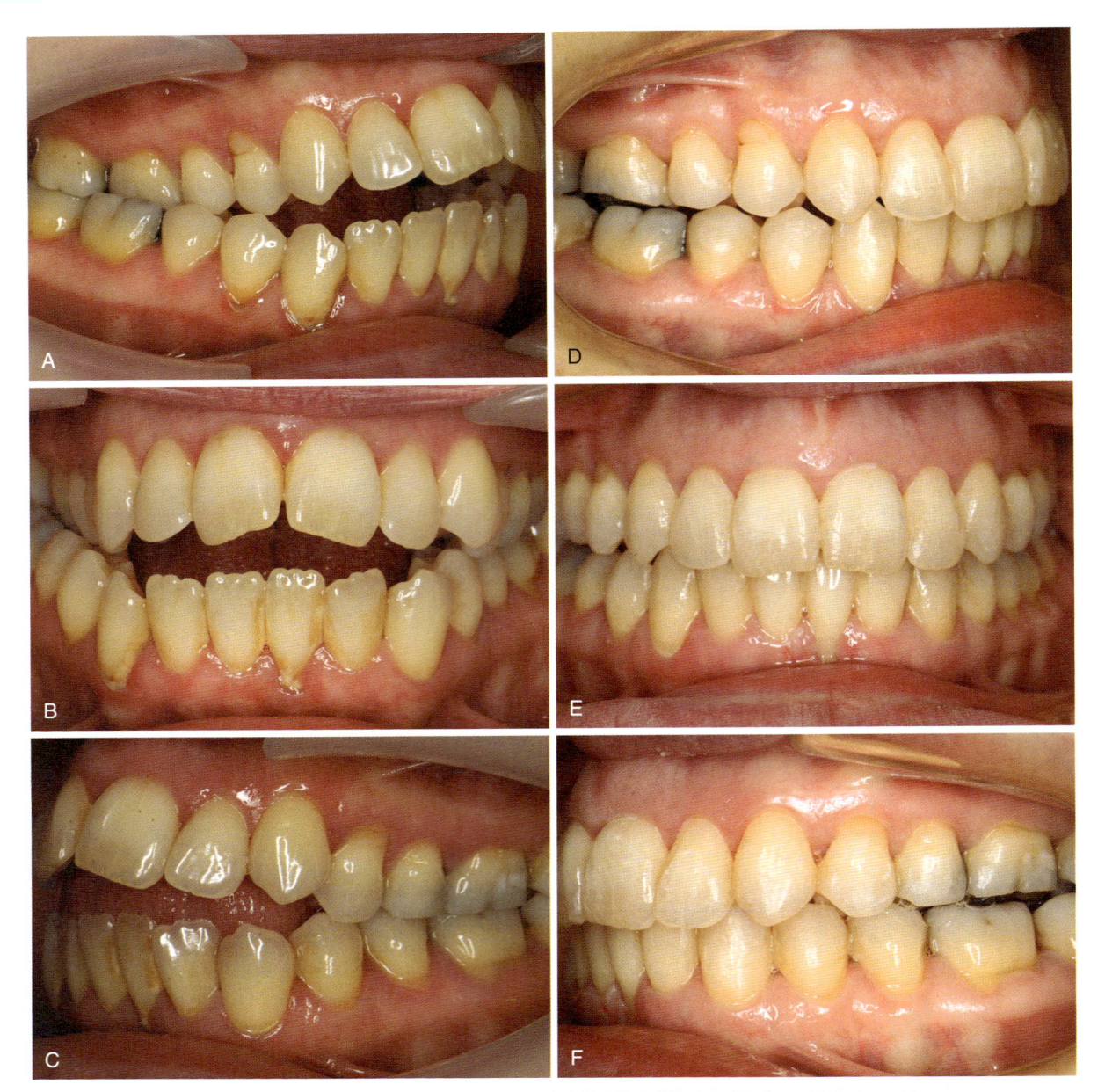

Fig. 19.15 Treatment of an open bite with aligners that was facilitated by intrusive force in the lateral segments.

used, the protocol remains the same, except that the removable appliance is worn only at nighttime from the beginning. Exceptions to the general protocol include growing patients with sagittal or vertical malocclusions, who should continue to wear retention appliances until their growth is finished, and patients who have undergone orthognathic surgery or those with compromised treatment results, where an increased tendency to relapse may be expected, who are also recommended a prolonged retention period.

Patients are instructed to attend regular checkups throughout the retention period. The recommended schedule is once every 3 or 4 months during the first year, twice a year in the second year, and at least once a year thereafter. Currently there is a tendency to maintain the bonded retainers indefinitely and independently of the original malocclusion but only after a prior agreement with the patient. Patients are instructed that the retention may be discontinued at some point but that their dentition is subject to continuous change throughout their lives, and this change may manifest itself in the occurrence of various irregularities in the aesthetically exposed anterior segment. Thus patients must either accept the risk of these changes or they must continue with a bonded or removable retainer if they want to maintain their teeth alignment. However, with due respect to the expected and unexpected complications associated with the prolonged use of a bonded retainer, they need to be checked regularly, at least once a year.

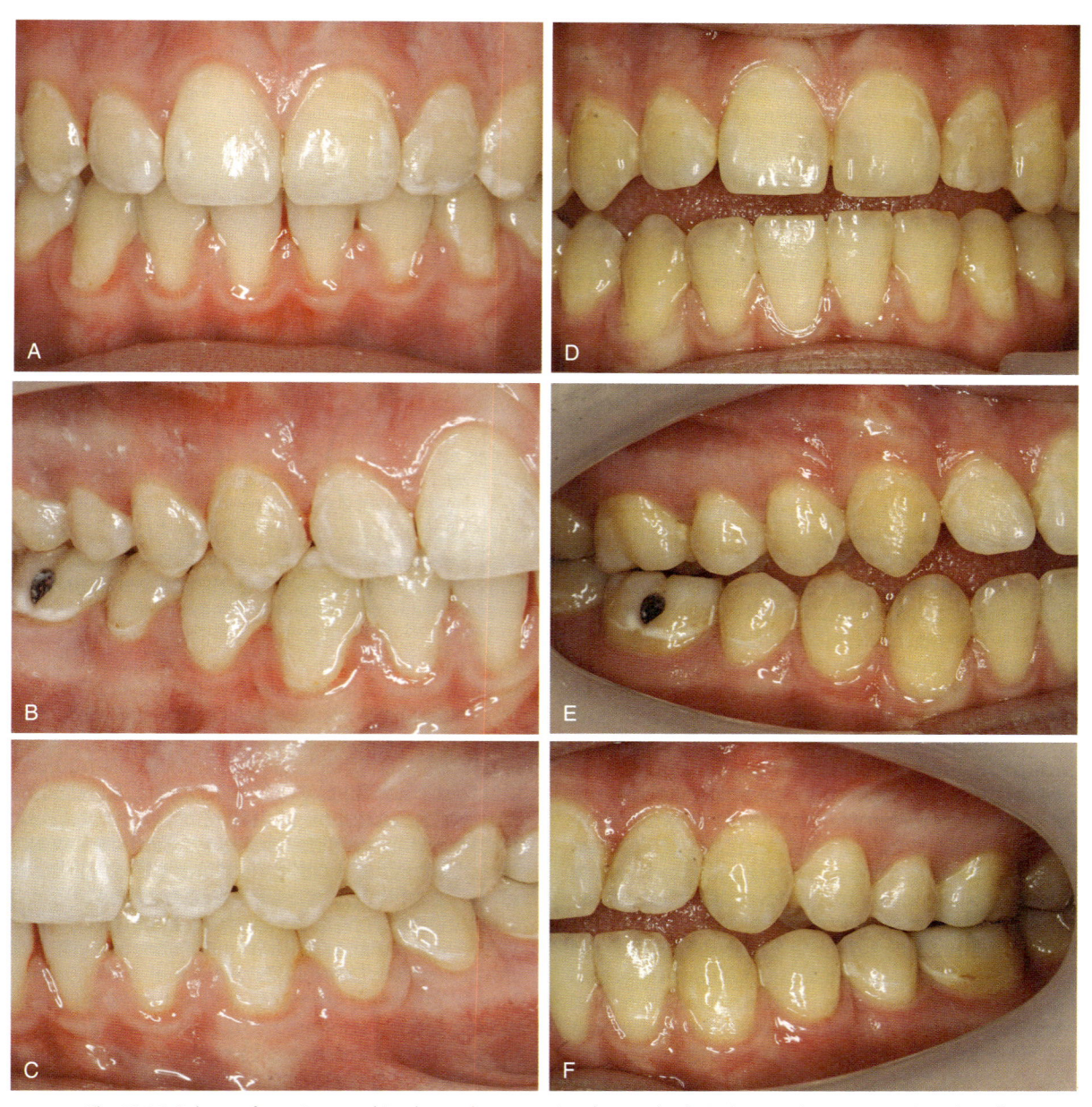

19 • Retention and Stability Following Aligner Therapy

Fig. 19.16 Relapse of anterior open bite due to short retention thermoplastic retainers and consequent extrusion of second molars. Situation after treatment (A-C) and 1.5 years in recall (D-F).

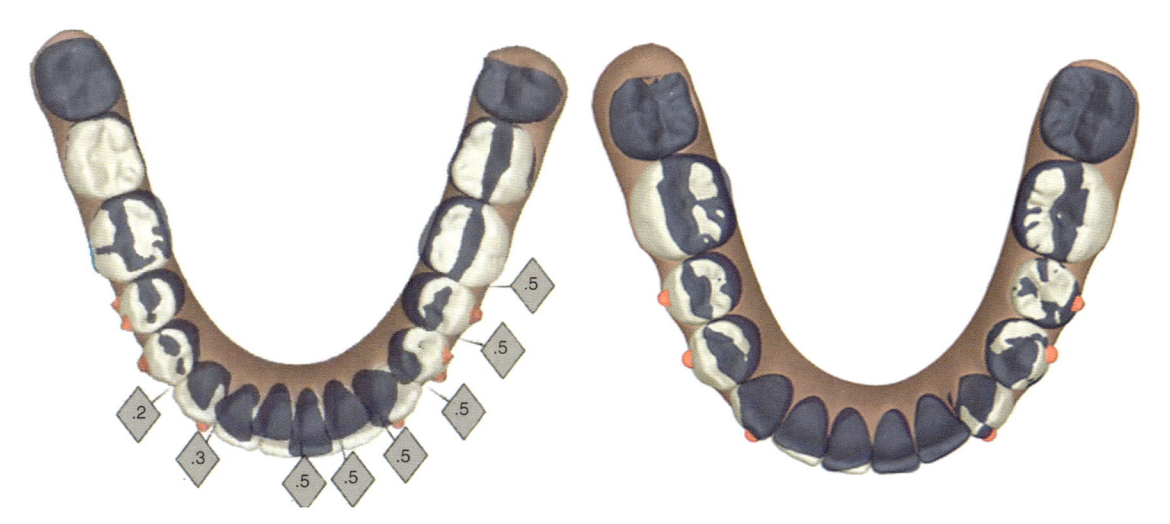

Fig. 19.17 Treatment planning software can be used to plan the position of lower incisors exactly, avoiding unwanted proclination of the lower incisors and thus preventing the risk of relapse.

References

1. Moyers RE. *Handbook of Orthodontics for the Student and General Practitioner*. 3rd ed. Chicago: Yearbook Medical Publishers; 1973.
2. Kamínek M. *Ortodoncie*. 1st ed. Praha: Galén; 2014.
3. Zachrisson BU, Büyükyilmaz T. Bonding in orthodontics. In: Graber LW, Vanarsdall RL, Vig KLW, eds. *Orthodontics Current Principles and Techniques*. 5th ed. Philadelphia, PA: Mosby Elsevier; 2012:727-784 [chap 21].
4. Zachrisson BU. Long-term experience with direct bonded retainers: update and clinical advice. *J Clin Orthod*. 2007;41(12):728-737.
5. Booth FA, Edelman JM, Proffit WR. Twenty-year follow-up of patients with permanently bonded mandibular canine-to-canine retainers. *Am J Orthod Dentofacial Orthop*. 2008;133(1):70-76.
6. Proffit WR, Fields HW, Sarver DM. *Contemporary Orthodontics*. 4th ed. St. Louis, MO: Mosby Elsevier; 2007.
7. Reitan K. Clinical and histologic observations on tooth movement during and after orthodontic treatment. *Am J Orthod*. 1967;53(10):721-745.
8. van Leeuwen EJ, Maltha JC, Kuijpers-Jagtman AM, et al. The effect of retention on orthodontic relapse after the use of small continuous or discontinuous forces. An experimental study in beagle dogs. *Eur J Oral Sci*. 2003;111(2):111-116.
9. Boese LR. Increased stability of orthodontically rotated teeth following gingivectomy in Macaca nemestrina. *Am J Orthod*. 1969;56(3):273-290.
10. Edwards JG. A long-term prospective evaluation of the circumferential supracrestal fiberotomy in alleviating orthodontic relapse. *Am J Orthod Dentofacial Orthop*. 1988;93(5):380-387.
11. Weinstein S, Haack DC, Morris LY, et al. On an equilibrium theory of tooth position. *Angle Orthod*. 1963;33(1):1-26.
12. de la Cruz A, Sampson P, Little RM, et al. Long-term changes in arch form after orthodontic treatment and retention. *Am J Orthod Dentofacial Orthop*. 1995;107(5):518-530.
13. Alexander RG. *The Alexander Discipline*: Long-Term Stability. Hanover Park: Quintessence; 2011.
14. Lagravére MO, Major PW, Flores-Mir C. Long-term dental arch changes after rapid maxillary expansion treatment: a systematic review. *Angle Orthod*. 2005;75(2):155-161.
15. Little RM, Riedel RA, Årtun J. An evaluation of changes in mandibular anterior alignment from 10-20 years post-retention. *Am J Orthod*. 1988;93(5):423-428.
16. Kahl-Nieke B, Fischbach H, Schwarze CW. Post-retention crowding and incisor irregularity: a long-term follow-up evaluation of stability and relaps. *Br J Orthod*. 1995;22(3):249-257.
17. Sinclair PM, Little RM. Maturation of untreated normal occlusions. *Am J Orthod*. 1983;83(2):114-123.
18. Bishara SE, Treder JE, Damon P, et al. Changes in the dental arches and dentition between 25 and 45 years of age. *Angle Orthod*. 1996;66(6):417-422.
19. de Freitas KM, Janson G, de Freitas MR, et al. Influence of the quality of the finished occlusion on postretention occlusal relapse. *Am J Orthod Dentofacial Orthop*. 2007;132(4):428.e9-428.e14.
20. Zachrisson BU. Important aspects of long-term stability. *J Clin Orthod*. 1997;31(9):562-83.
21. Aasen TO, Espeland L. An approach to maintain orthodontic alignment of lower incisors without the use of retainers. *Eur J Orthod*. 2005;27(3):209-214.
22. Edman Tynelius G, Petrén S, Bondemark L, et al. Five-year postretention outcomes of three retention methods—a randomized controlled trial. *Eur J Orthod*. 2015;37(4):345-353.
23. Zachrisson BU. Important aspects of long-term stability. *J Clin Orthod*. 1997;31(9):562-83.
24. Enlow DH, Kuroda T, Lewis AB. Intrinsic craniofacial compensations. *Am J Othod*. 1971;41(4):271-285.
25. Eslambolchi S, Woodside DG, Rossouw PE. A descriptive study of mandibular incisor alignment in untreated subjects. *Am J Orthod Dentofacial Orthod*. 2008;133(3):343-353.
26. Behrents RG. Growth in the aging craniofacial skeleton. Monograph 17, Craniofacial Growth series. Ann Harbour: Center for Human Growth and Development: University of Michigan; 1985. In: Nanda RS, Nanda SK. Considerations of craniofacial growth in long-term retention and stability: is active retention needed? *Am J Orthod Dentofacial Orthop*. 1992;101(4):297-302.
27. Littlewood SJ. Evidence-based retention: where are we now? *Semin Orthod*. 2017;23(2):229-236.
28. Littlewood SJ, Millett DT, Doubleday B, et al. Retention procedures for stabilising tooth position after treatment with orthodontic braces. *Cochrane Database Syst Rev*. 2016;29(1):1-139.
29. Pratt MC, Kluemper GT, Hartsfield Jr JK, et al. Evaluation of retention protocols among members of the American Association of Orthodontists in the United States. *Am J Orthod Dentofacial Orthop*. 2011;140(4):520-526.
30. Renkema AM, Sips ET, Bronkhorst E, et al. A survey on orthodontic retention procedures in the Netherlands. *Eur J Orthod*. 2009;31(4):432-437.
31. Rowland H, Hichens L, Williams A, et al. The effectiveness of Hawley and vacuum-formed retainers: a single-center randomized controlled trial. *Am J Orthod Dentofacial Orthop*. 2007;132(6):730-737.
32. Lai CS, Grossen JM, Renkema A-M, et al. Orthodontic retention procedures in Switzerland. *Swiss Dent J*. 2014;124(6):655-661.
33. Padmos JAD, Fudalej PS, Renkema AM. Epidemiologic study of orthodontic retention procedures. *Am J Orthod Dentofacial Orthop*. 2018;153(4):496-504.
34. Årtun J, Spadafora AT, Shapiro PA. A 3-year follow-up study of various types of orthodontic canine-to-canine retainers. *Eur J Orthod*. 1997;19(5):501-509.
35. Renkema AM, Renkema A, Bronkhorst E, et al. Long-term effectiveness of canine-to-canine bonded flexible spiral wire lingual retainers. *Am J Orthod Dentofacial Orthop*. 2011;139(5):614-621.
36. Årtun J. Caries and periodontal reactions associated with long-term use of different types of bonded lingual retainers. *Am J Orthod*. 1984;86(2):112-118.
37. Pandis N, Vlahopoulos K, Madianos P, et al. Long-term periodontal status of patients with mandibular lingual fixed retention. *Eur J Orthod*. 2007;29(5):471-476.
38. Rogers MB, Andrews LJ. Dependable technique for bonding a 3 x 3 retainer. *Am J Orthod Dentofacial Orthop*. 2004;126(2):231-233.
39. Störmann I, Ehmer U. A prospective randomized study of different retainer types. *J Orofac Orthop*. 2002;63(1):42-50.
40. Kučera J, Marek I. Unexpected complications associated with mandibular fixed retainers: a retrospective study. *Am J Orthod Dentofacial Orthop*. 2016;149(2):202-211.
41. Katsaros C, Livas C, Renkema AM. Unexpected complications of bonded mandibular lingual retainers. *Am J Orthod Dentofacial Orthop*. 2017;132(6):838-841.
42. Marek I, Kučera J. Twist-effect, X-effect and other unexpected complications of fixed retainers. *LKS*. 2015;25(5):98-106.
43. Pazera P, Fudalej P, Katsaros C. Severe complication of a bonded mandibular lingual retainer. *Am J Orthod Dentofacial Orthop*. 2012;142(3):406-409.
44. Kučera J, Streblov J, Marek I, et al. Treatment of complications associated with lower fixed retainers. *J Clin Orthod*. 2016;50(1):54-59.
45. Vrátná D, Marek I, Tycová H. Settling after orthodontic therapy according to type of retention. *Ortodoncie*. 2015;24(2):93-106.
46. Hannessy T, Garvey T, Al-Awadhi EA. A randomized clinical trial comparing mandibular incisor proclination produced by fixed labial appliances and clear aligners. *Angle Orthod*. 2016;86(5):706-712.

20 Overcoming the Limitations of Aligner Orthodontics: A Hybrid Approach

LUCA LOMBARDO and GIUSEPPE SICILIANI

Introduction

Aligners were first introduced by Kesling[1] in 1945 to correct crowding. Later, Ponitz[2] reported the use of a removable plastic retainer (Essix, Dentsply, York, PA, USA). However, it was not until the 1990s, when Sheridan et al.[3] combined these retainers with interproximal reduction (IPR), that they began to gain popularity. Then, in 1999, Zia Chishti and Kelsey Wirth, together with a computer specialist, founded Align Technology in Palo Alto, CA, USA.[4] Since they launched their Invisalign brand into the market, the demand for orthodontic aligners has been growing among patients; especially adults, thanks to their esthetic properties and clinical efficacy.[5]

At first, aligners were marketed as an alternative to traditional fixed appliances in simple malocclusion cases involving slight crowding or minor space closure.[6] Over time, however, the range of malocclusion cases that can be treated by means of invisible aligners has broadened. Clinical research has developed aligner-based solutions for even complex cases involving major rotation of the premolars, upper incisor torque, distalization, and/or extraction space closure.[7] Despite the claimed efficiency of aligner treatment, however, its clinical potential still remains controversial among clinicians. Its advocates are convinced by the clinical evidence arising from successfully treated cases, while skeptics point to the significant limitations of the technique, especially in the treatment of complex malocclusions.[8-11] Orthodontics companies claim that aligners can resolve, without the use of additional techniques, rotations of 40 degrees at the upper and lower central incisors, 45 degrees in canines and premolars, 30 degrees in lateral incisors, and 20 degrees in molars. Extrusions and intrusions of 2.5 mm have been achieved in anterior teeth, and root movements of 4 mm and 2 mm have been reported in posterior teeth.[12]

Nevertheless, few studies have been published to support these claims, which are not always supported by the experience of other clinical practitioners. In fact, some orthodontists indicate that the number of patients who require some unplanned correction or even recourse to fixed orthodontics is closer to 70% to 80%.[5,13] Kravitz reported that Invisalign aligners had a mean accuracy of 41% in terms of achieving planned outcomes, with the most predictable movement being lingual contraction (47.1%) and the least predictable extrusion (29.6%).[14]

In the attempt to clarify the situation, Lagravère and Flores-Mir[15] published the first systematic review on the subject in 2005. Since then, several authors have provided updated evidence on aligner efficacy.[12,16-18] The most recent systematic reviews into the accuracy of orthodontic movements achievable with aligners have concluded that they are able to produce distal movement of the upper molars and resolve anterior crowding issues through incisor protrusion and by increasing the intercanine, interpremolar, and intermolar distances. On the other hand, removable aligners are far less effective at achieving transverse expansion via bodily movement of the posterior teeth. Furthermore, they are unable to perform canine and premolar rotations satisfactorily, and seem to fall short in terms of extrusion movements and control of overbite and occlusal contacts.

Bearing in mind this evidence, our clinical experience, and the ever-growing popularity of aligner treatment, we have developed a new hybrid approach using a combination of different devices to overcome some of the most common limitations of removable appliances.

Transverse Expansion of the Posterior Teeth

Research has shown that aligners are unable to perform predictable bodily premolar and molar expansion. Digital setups tend to overestimate bodily expansion movements, and more tipping than planned occurs.[19-21] However, in clinical cases (Fig. 20.1) in which the posterior sectors are greatly negatively inclined, it is possible to plan uncontrolled tipping of the upper and lower canines, premolars, and molars. Furthermore, the space needed to resolve crowding can be created by using aligners alone (Fig. 20.2) to exert pressure on the lingual surfaces of the teeth; this improves the archform by significantly increasing the intercanine, interpremolar, and intermolar distances (Fig. 20.3). In fact, Lombardo et al.[22] have demonstrated that this vestibulolingual tipping can be achieved with a predictability of 72.9%.

That being said, in young patients with transverse deficits due to hypoplasia of the upper jaw (Fig. 20.4), it is not realistic to expect aligners to achieve skeletal alteration. Only an orthopedic approach, first on the deciduous teeth (Fig. 20.5) and then via skeletal anchorage[23] (Fig. 20.6), is able to normalize the maxillary dimensions and therefore

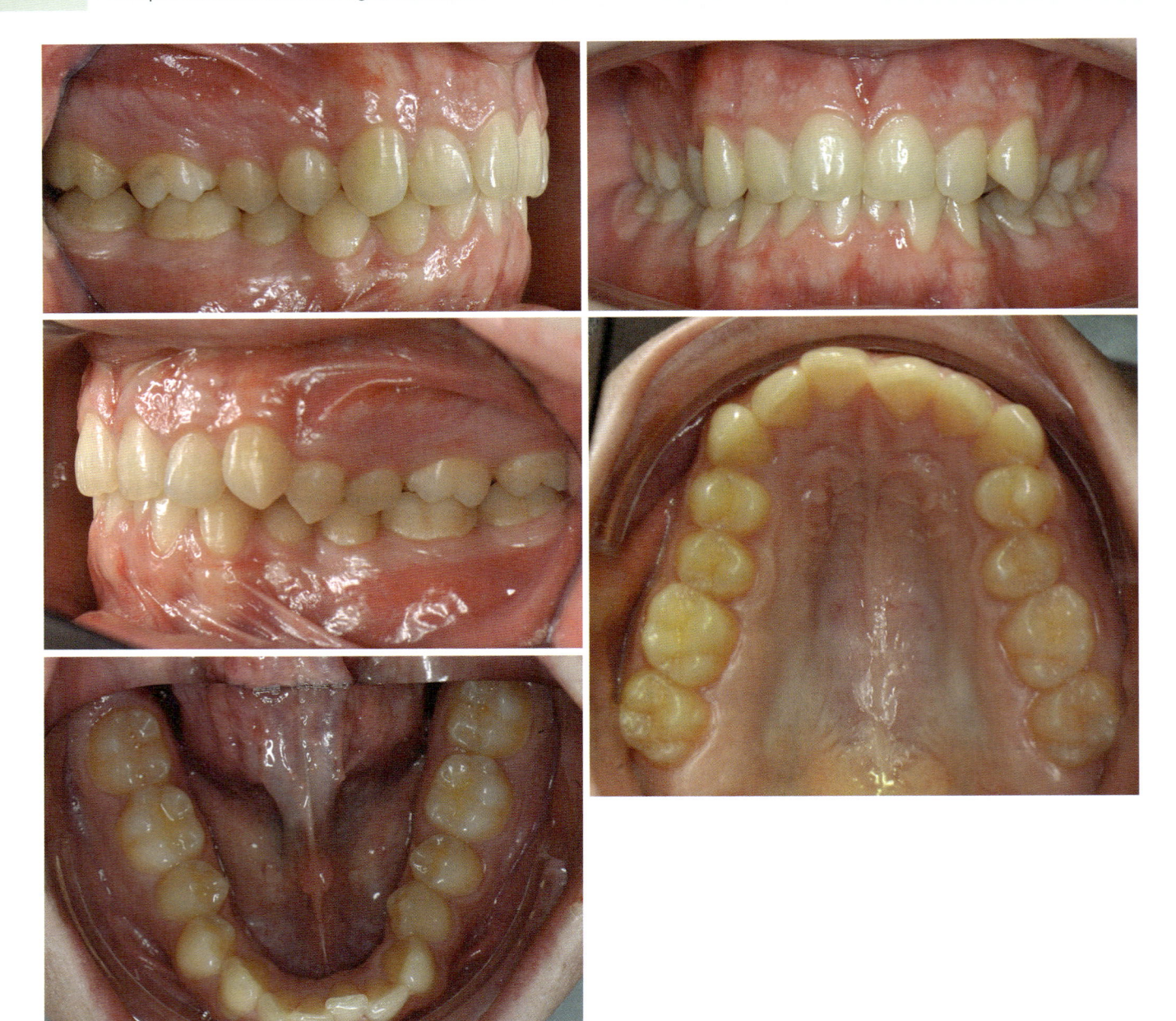

276　Principles and Biomechanics of Aligner Treatment

Fig. 20.1 Initial intraoral photographs of adult patient with class I malocclusion dentoalveolar contraction in both arches.

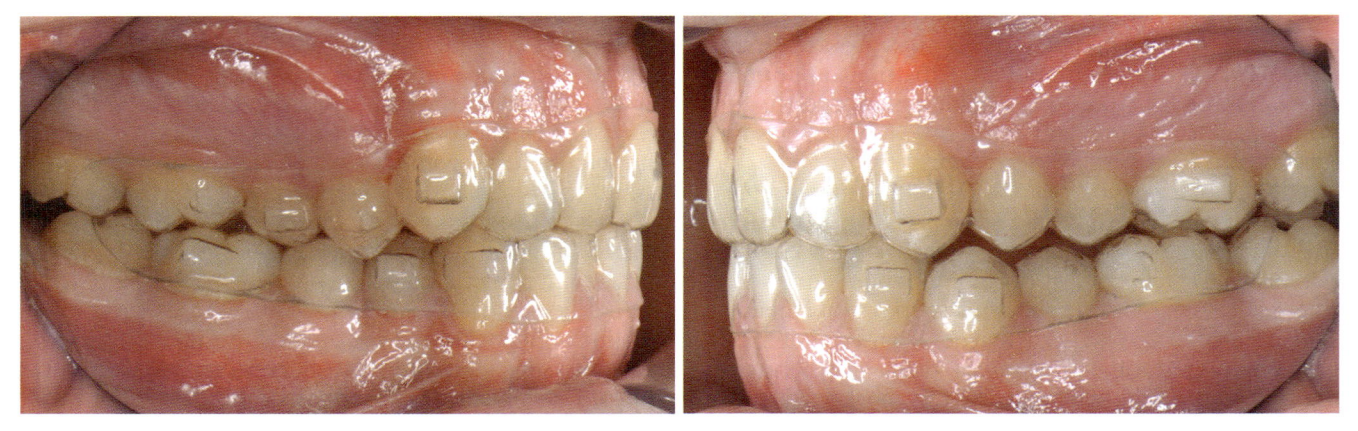

Fig. 20.2 Intraoral photographs during aligner therapy with composite buttons.

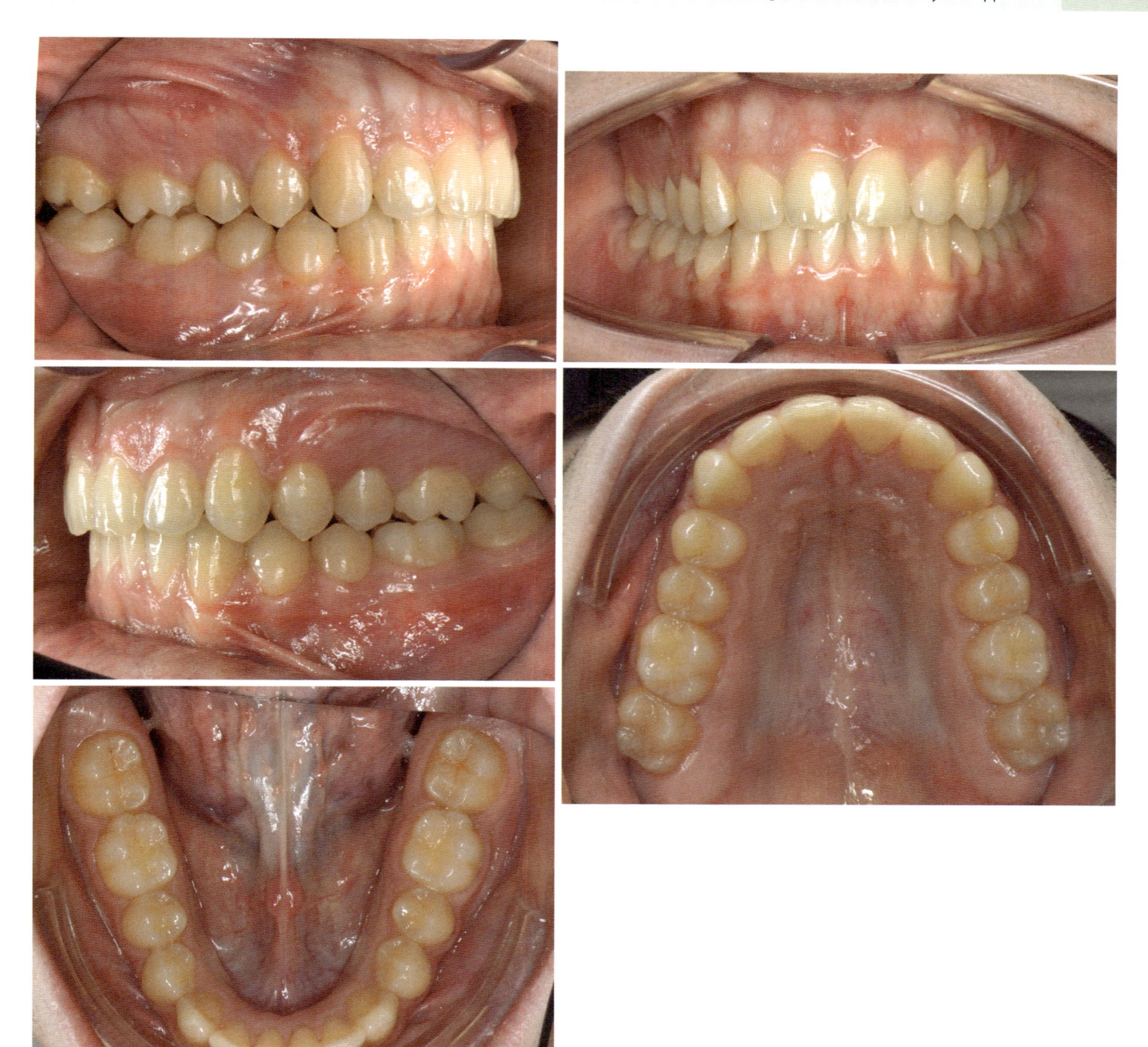

Fig. 20.3 Final intraoral photographs after 20-step aligner treatment.

permit correct eruption and improve the transverse and sagittal occlusal relationships. However, in such patients, aligners (Fig. 20.7) can be used as an efficacious tool for completing dental alignment and creating acceptable intercuspidation without decompensating the class III malocclusion (Fig. 20.8).

It is not only in children that such problems arise, however; in adult patients,[24] the predictability of transverse expansion via bodily movement of the premolars and molars is poor, and may be damaging in patients with thin periodontal tissues or gingival recession (Fig. 20.9). Hence in adults it is best to resolve issues of skeletal maxillary contraction via surgery or skeletal anchorage expanders (bone-bone rapid palatal expander) (Fig. 20.10). Only after the transverse deficit has been resolved should crowding be addressed, and in such cases the occlusion can be improved by means of aligners (Fig. 20.11), which can guide the extrusion of the teeth in a controlled fashion. This approach lessens the risk of premature contacts, unwanted vestibular movement, and worsening gingival recession (Fig. 20.12).

Canine and Premolar Rotation

It has been demonstrated that the mandibular canine is the most difficult tooth to control with aligners and that the

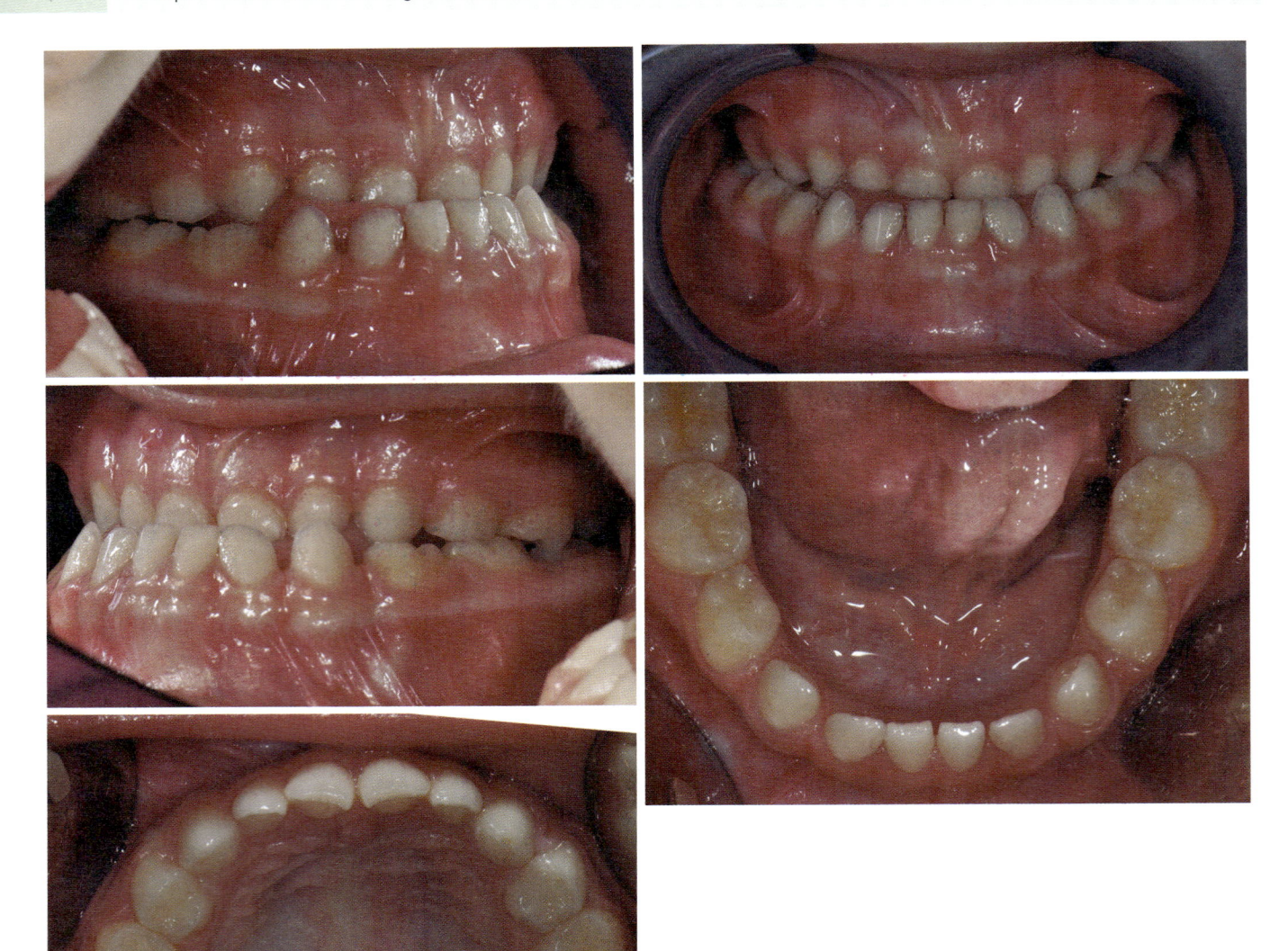

278 Principles and Biomechanics of Aligner Treatment

Fig. 20.4 Initial intraoral photographs of a young patient with skeletal and dental class III and narrow upper jaw.

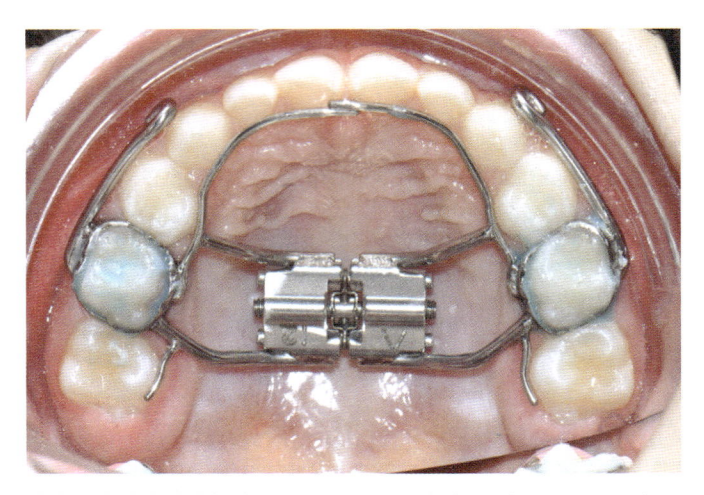

Fig. 20.5 Rapid palatal expansion with arms for Delaire mask on deciduous second molars.

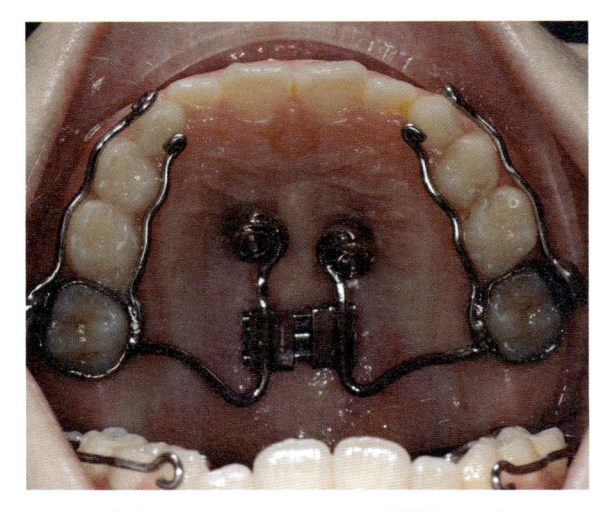

Fig. 20.6 Hybrid expander with dental and skeletal anchorage in upper jaw and arms for Delaire mask.

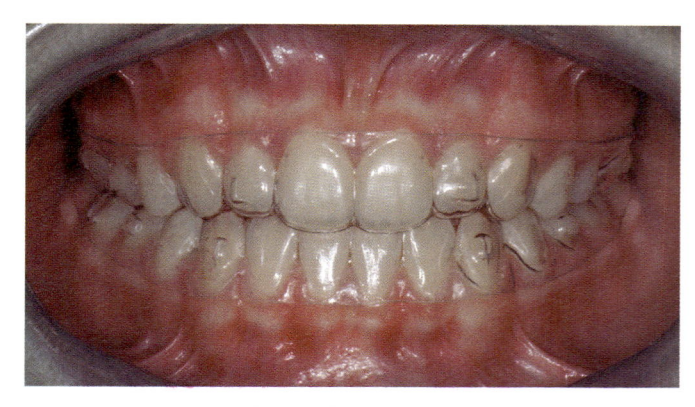

20 • Overcoming the Limitations of Aligner Orthodontics: A Hybrid Approach   **279**

Fig. 20.7 Intraoral photograph during aligner therapy.

amount of rotation actually achievable with the maxillary and mandibular canines is roughly a third of that predicted.[25] For premolars, the rotation accuracy of aligners has been reported within the range 23.2% to 41.8%.[26] The difficulty in derotating cylindrical teeth by means of aligners is likely due to the fact that they are unable to grip these teeth sufficiently to generate a force couple. This may be ascribable to poor aligner fitting and/or excessive stiffness of the appliance itself.

Numerous potential solutions to this problem have been proposed in recent years. For example, in a case of crowding with a severely rotated lower canine and upper incisor (Fig. 20.13), composite buttons were applied on the lingual side of the aligner (Fig. 20.14) to increase the grip, and derotation was planned in only 20 steps. The good elasticity[27] and fit (Fig. 20.15) of F22 aligners (Sweden & Martina, Due Carrare, Italy), in addition to careful stripping,

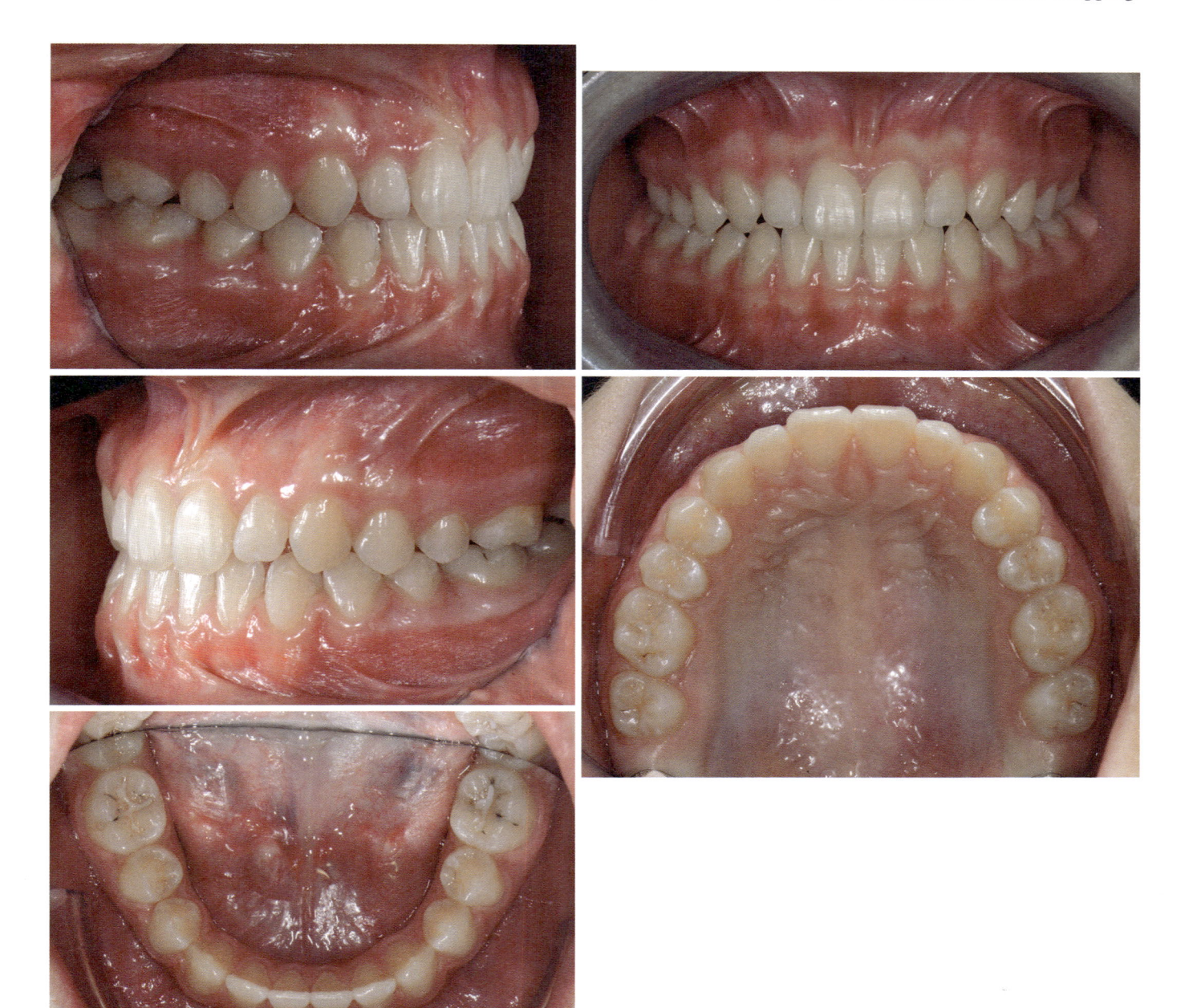

Fig. 20.8 Final intraoral photographs after 11-step aligner treatment.

280 Principles and Biomechanics of Aligner Treatment

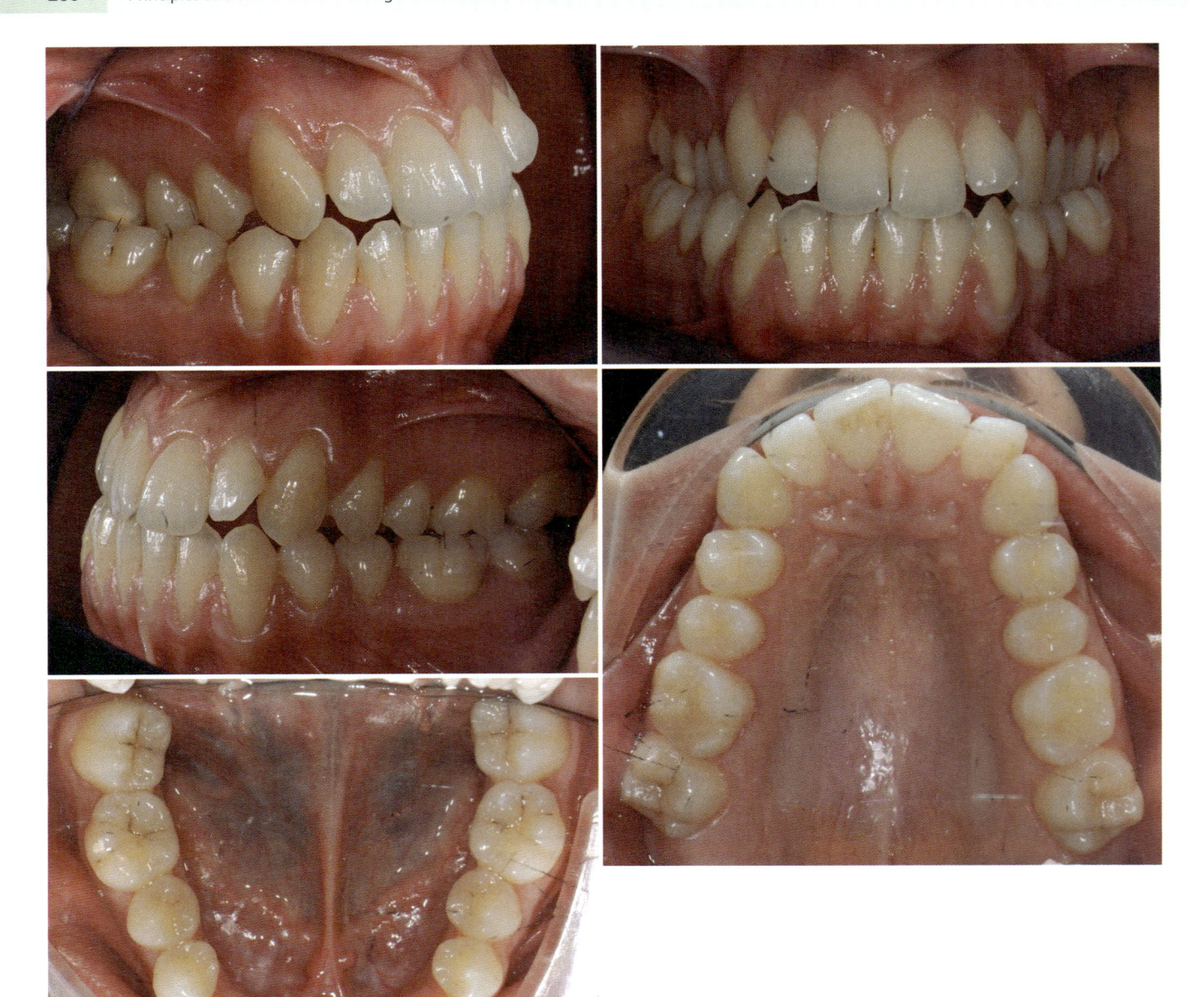

Fig. 20.9 Initial intraoral photographs of adult patient with skeletal contraction of upper jaw, class III tendency and gingival recession in both arches.

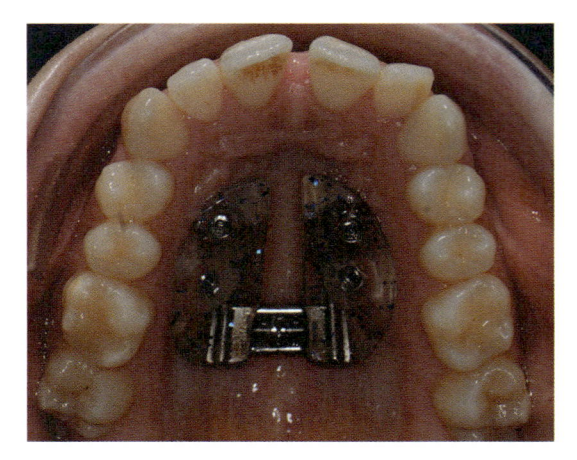

Fig. 20.10 Rapid palatal expansion with skeletal anchorage (MAPA method).

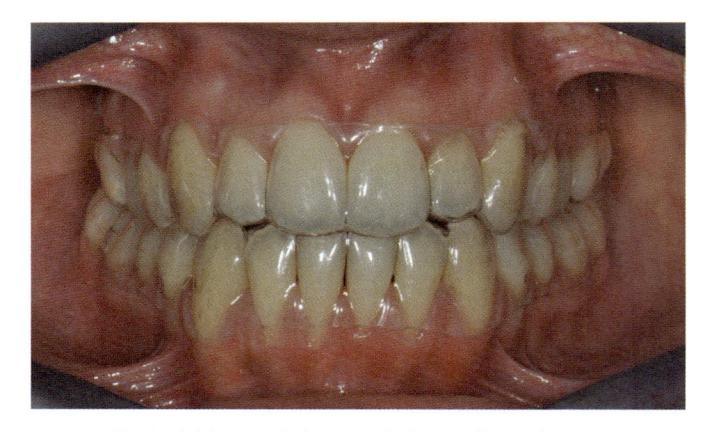

Fig. 20.11 Intraoral photograph during aligner therapy.

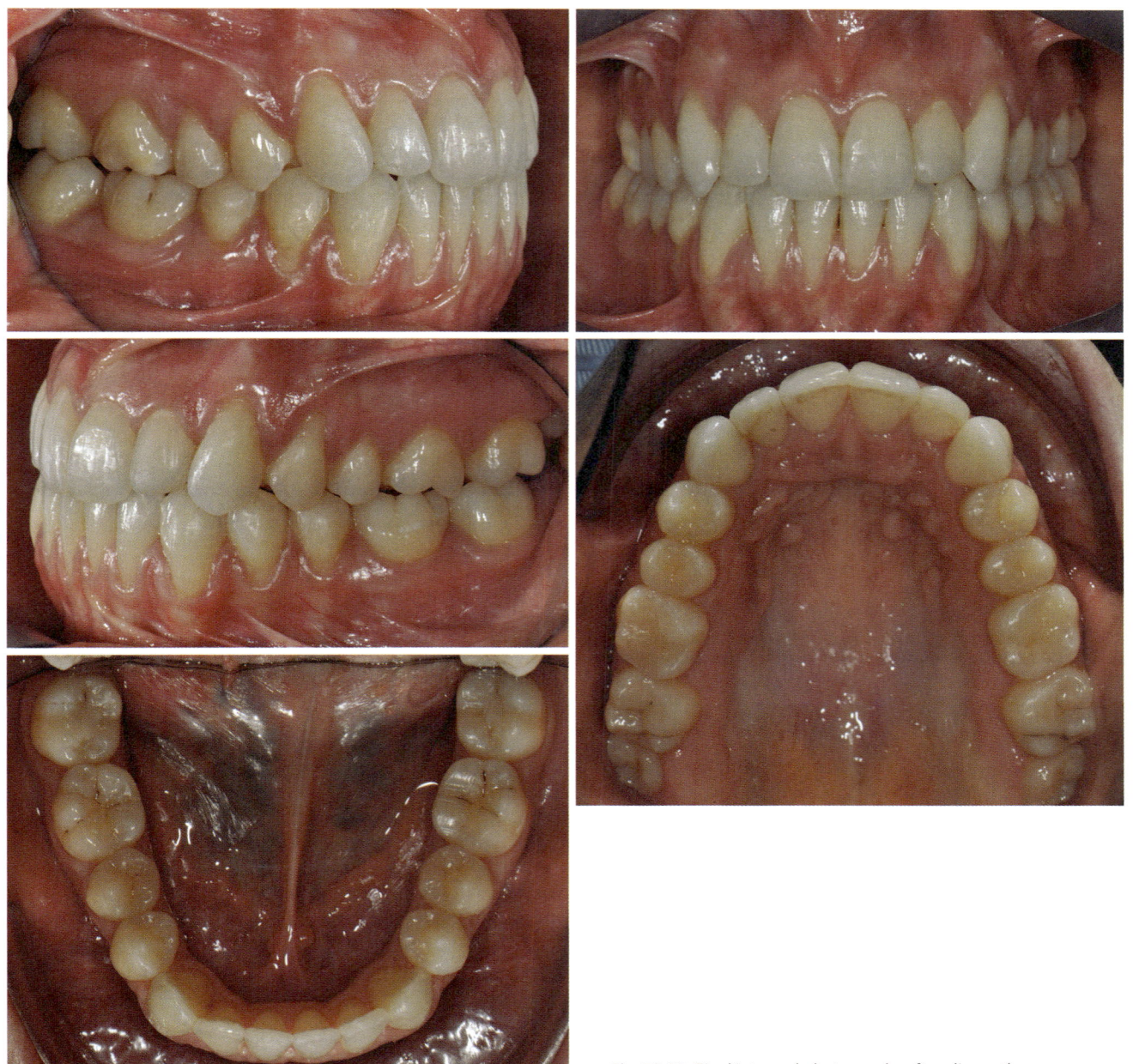

Fig. 20.12 Final intraoral photographs after aligner therapy.

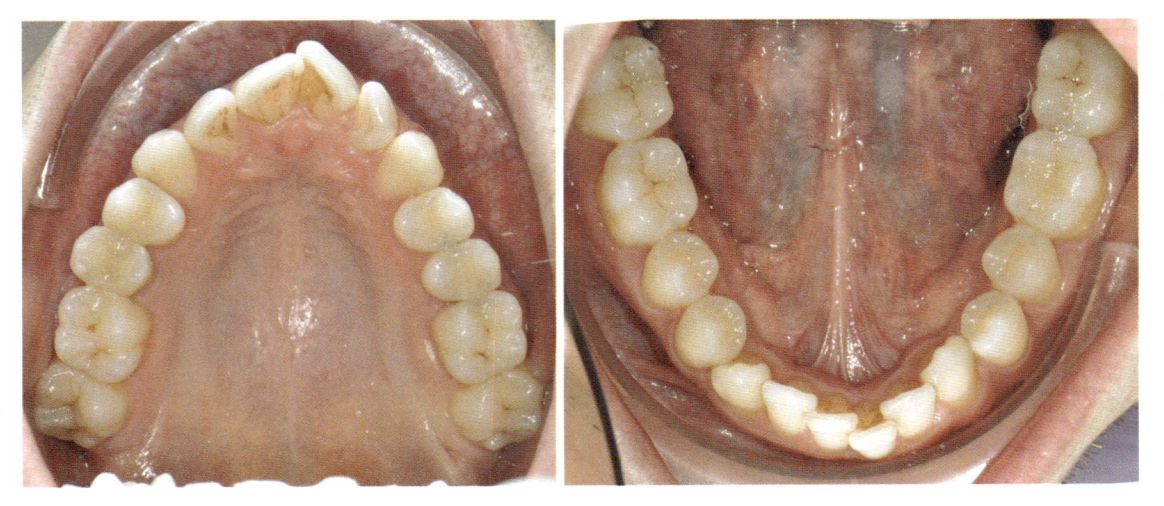

Fig. 20.13 Initial occlusal intraoral photographs of an adult patient with severe rotation of the upper incisors (A) and right lower canine (B).

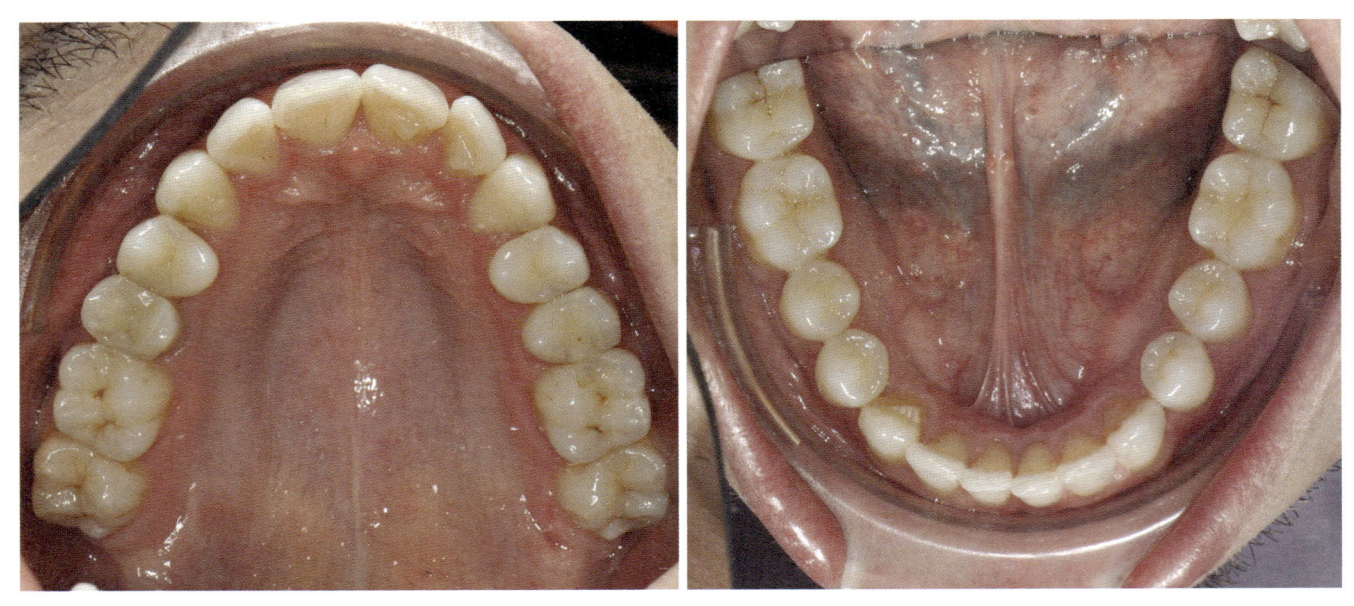

Fig. 20.14 Occlusal intraoral photographs during treatment with composite buttons on the lingual surfaces of teeth 1.3, 2.1, 2.2, and 4.3.

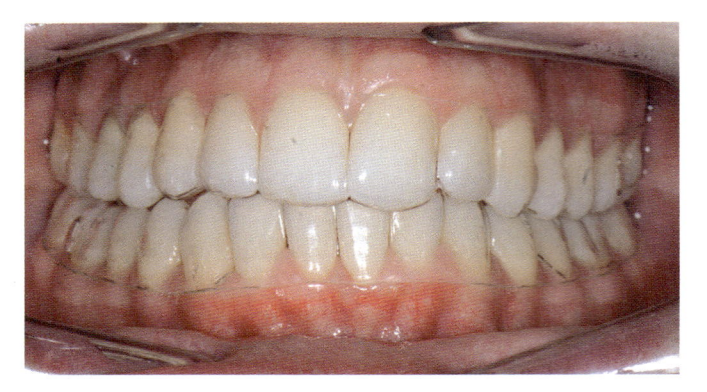

Fig. 20.15 Intraoral photograph during aligner therapy.

provided satisfactory alignment, without recourse to multiple refinements, within a limited timeframe (Fig. 20.16).

We have recently developed a new hybrid approach to increase the predictability of rotations, which is one of the major limitations of aligner treatment.[16-18] In cases of rotations of 20 degrees or above (Fig. 20.17), it is possible to include microtubes with a circular cross section in the setup to be positioned across the lingual surface of the rotated teeth (Fig. 20.18). The setup can be performed in such a way that the aligners cover these sections without actually touching them (Fig. 20.19). This enables the clear aligner to guide the movement of the teeth, eliminate unwanted movements, and increase patient comfort. By these means we achieved correct rotation in only 10 steps without any refinements or

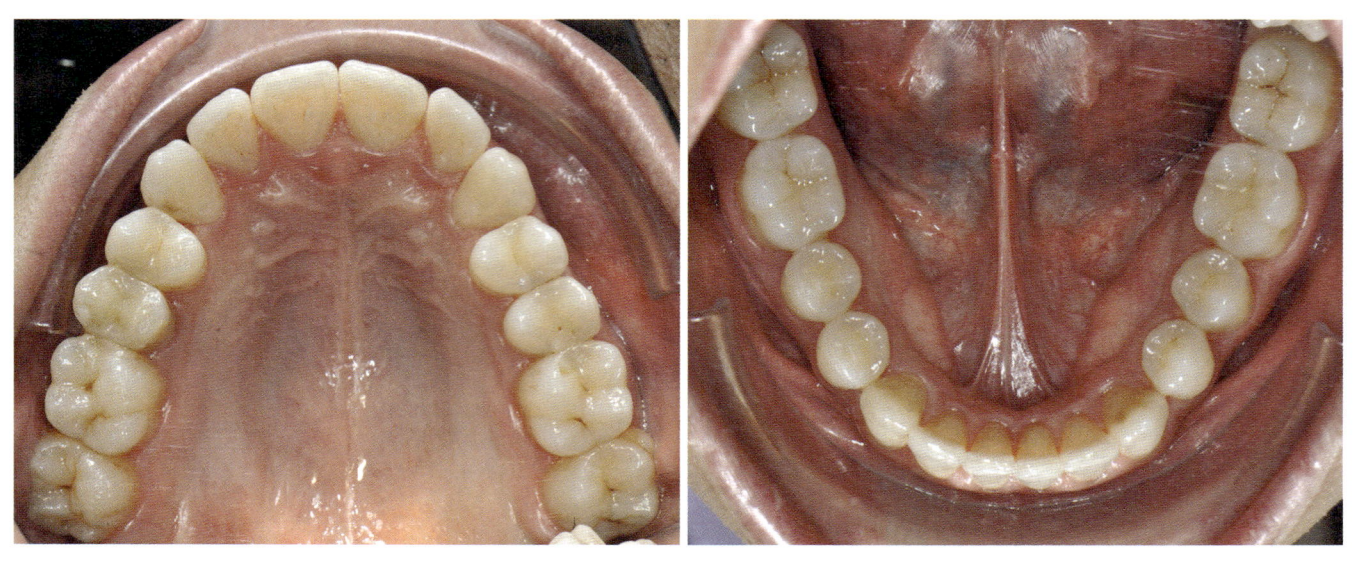

Fig. 20.16 Final intraoral photographs after 20-step aligner treatment.

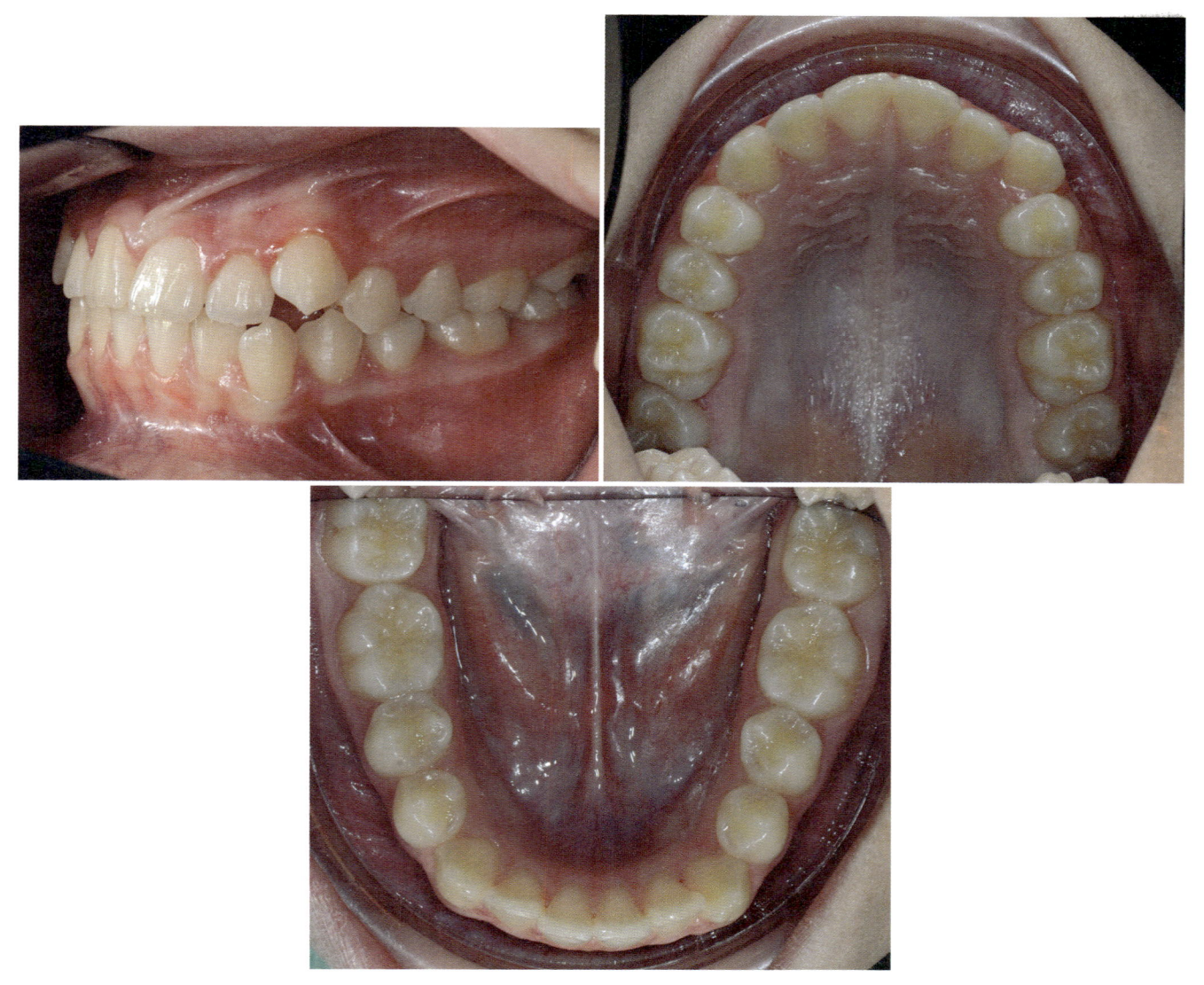

Fig. 20.17 Initial photographs of a young patient with rotation greater than 20 degrees of left upper canine and left second premolar.

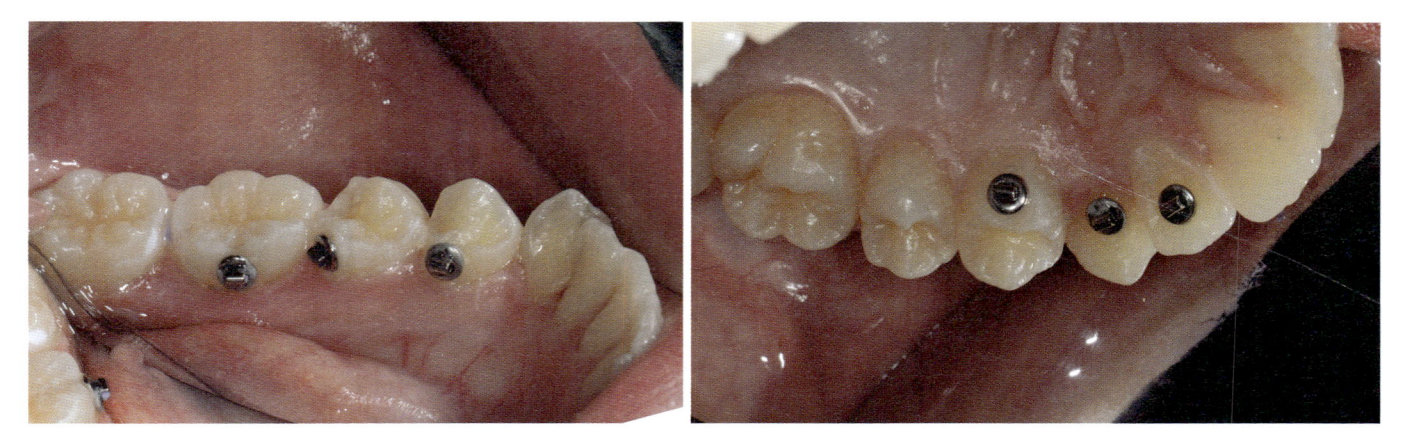

Fig. 20.18 Application of microtubes on rotated, mesial, and distal teeth.

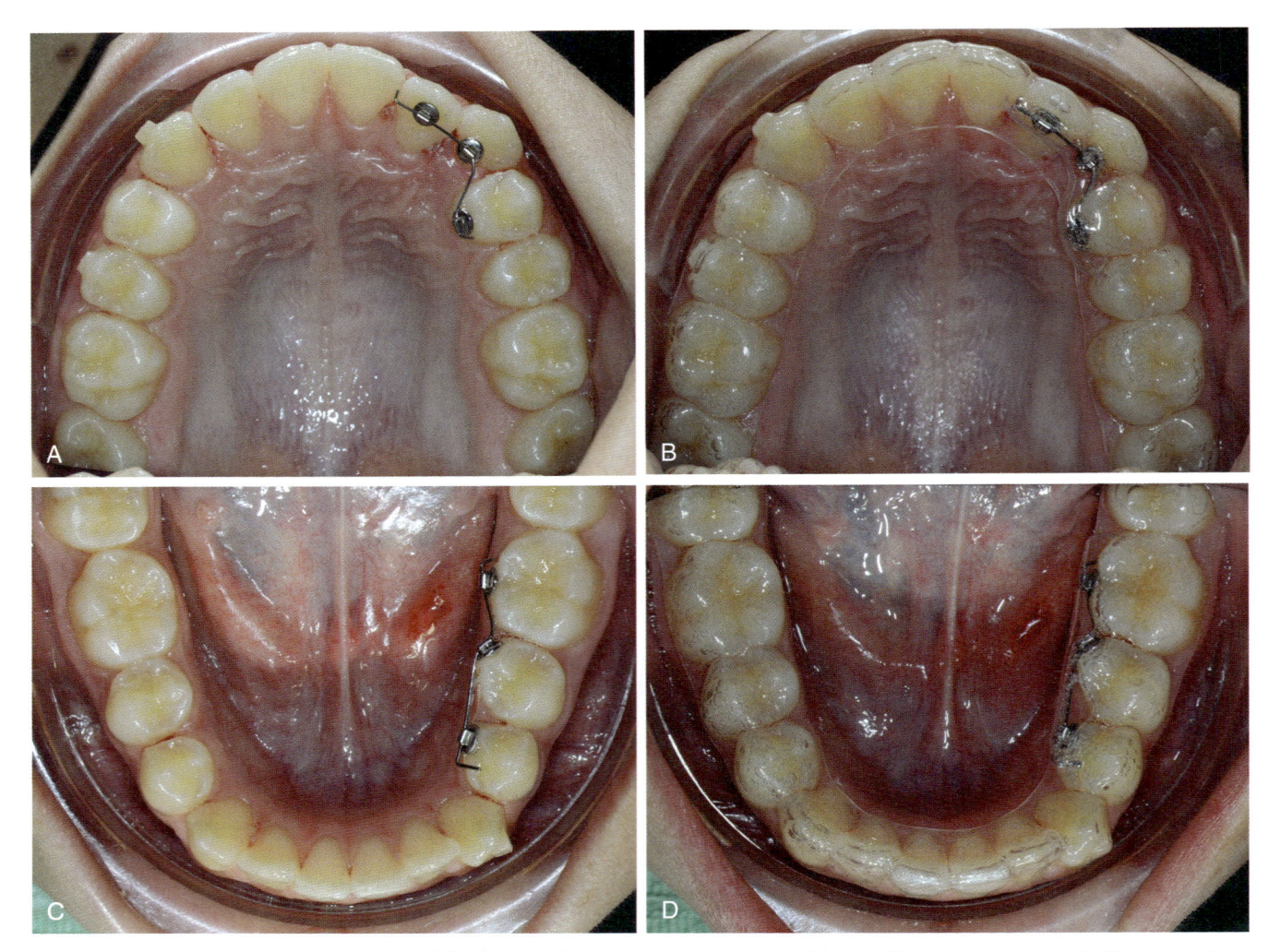

Fig. 20.19 Occlusal photographs. (A) Upper arch with thermal NiTi 0.013 sectional. (B) Upper arch with aligner covering thermal NiTi 0.013 sectional. (C) Lower arch with thermal NiTi 0.013 sectional. (D) Occlusal photograph of lower arch with aligner covering thermal NiTi 0.013 sectional.

composite buttons. In other words, this hybrid approach enabled us to improve both predictability and treatment time (Fig. 20.20).

Extrusion, Intrusion, and Overbite Control

According to Kravitz,[14] extrusion and intrusion are among the least predictable movements achievable with clear aligners; only 29.6% (extrusion) and 41.3% (intrusion) of the movements planned in the setup are achieved at the end of aligner treatment. Some authors have demonstrated that it is possible to achieve anterior bite closure using clear aligners,[14] but in the majority of cases this will involve uncontrolled lingual tipping of the upper and lower incisors, achieved via space creation through IPR and transverse maxillary expansion. The difficulty in achieving pure extrusion is likely due to the poor grip of the aligners on cylindrical teeth, which may be improved by the application of composite buttons. However, we have also had some success in overcoming this biomechanical limitation, resolving open bite using auxiliaries either before or during aligner therapy. We have found, for example, when open bite in growing patients is due to bad habits (thumb-sucking) and has already caused skeletal alterations (maxillary contraction) (Fig. 20.21), it is better to opt for an orthopedic approach (bite-block expander with grille) (Fig. 20.22) to normalize the upper jaw and allow correct eruption of the upper incisors (Fig. 20.23). Then, once these improvements have been achieved, aligners are the ideal solution for refining the occlusion (Fig. 20.24), guiding the erupting teeth into their proper positions within a limited timeframe and with minimal unwanted effects (Fig. 20.25).

At the opposite end of the spectrum, deep bite (Fig. 20.26) cannot generally be resolved by means of aligners alone, as intrusion of the upper and lower incisors is unpredictable, once again presumably due to poor grip on the anchoring teeth. Hence, in all cases in which it is indicated (class II, not excessive vestibular movement of the lower incisors), it may be very useful to employ class II elastics (Fig. 20.27). The effects of these devices that are commonly seen as undesirable (lower molar extrusion and vestibular movement of the lower incisors) enable rotation of the occlusal plane, appreciably aiding opening of the bite, and allow correction of the sagittal relationships (Fig. 20.28).

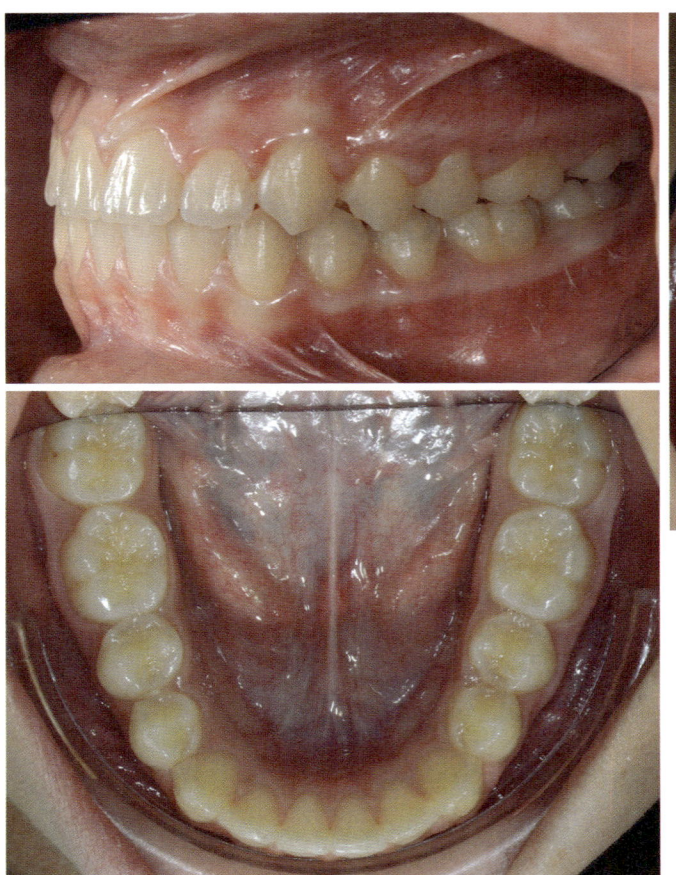

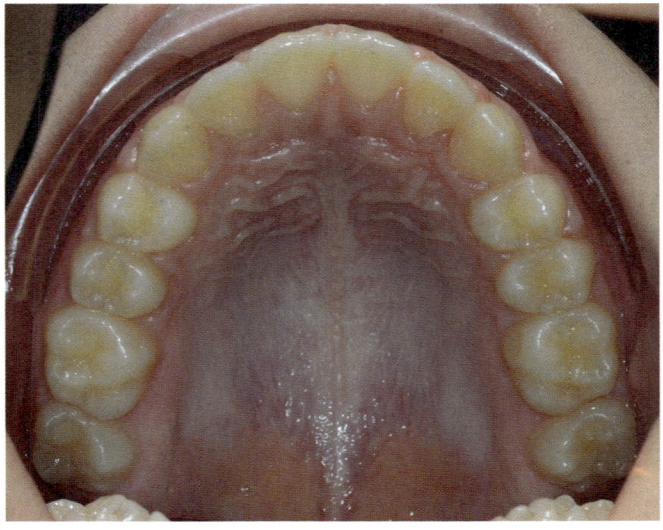

20 • Overcoming the Limitations of Aligner Orthodontics: A Hybrid Approach   285

Fig. 20.20 Final intraoral photographs after seven-step aligner treatment.

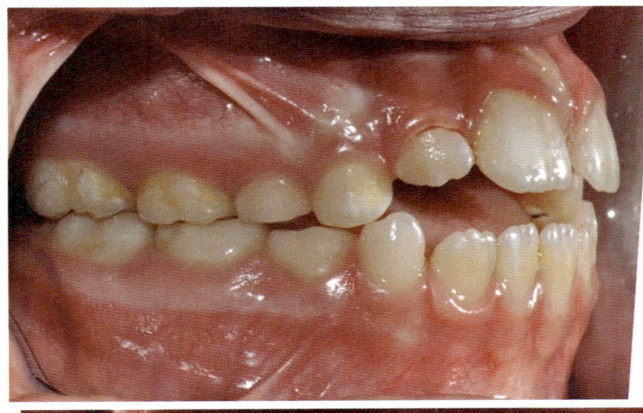

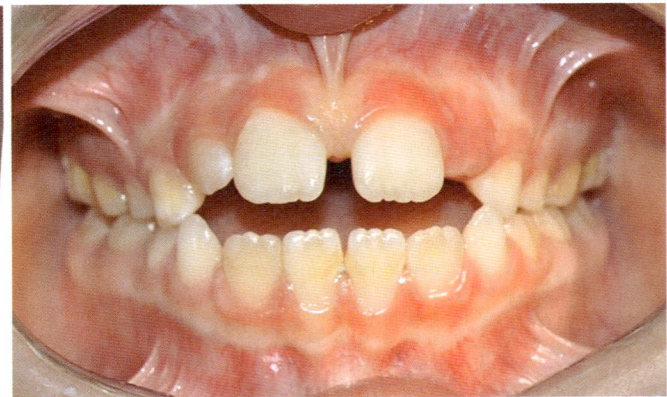

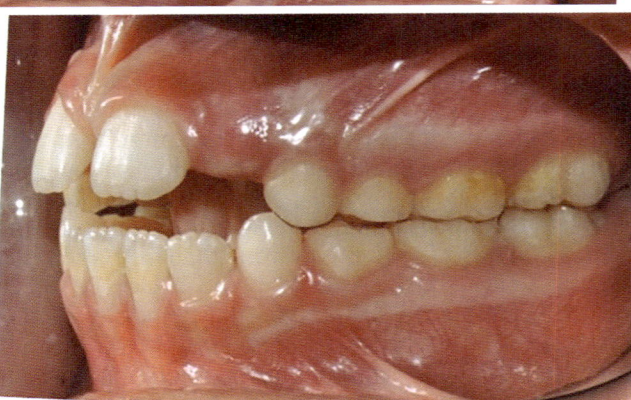

Fig. 20.21 Initial intraoral photographs of young patient with anterior open bite and maxillary contraction.

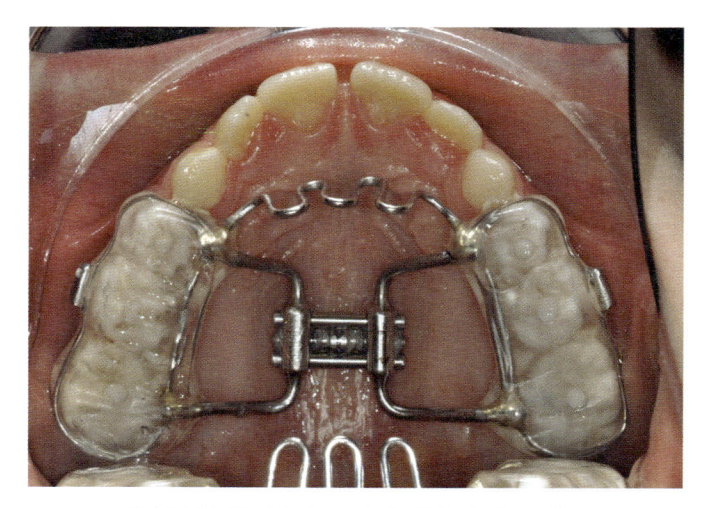

Fig. 20.22 Bite-block expander with anterior grille.

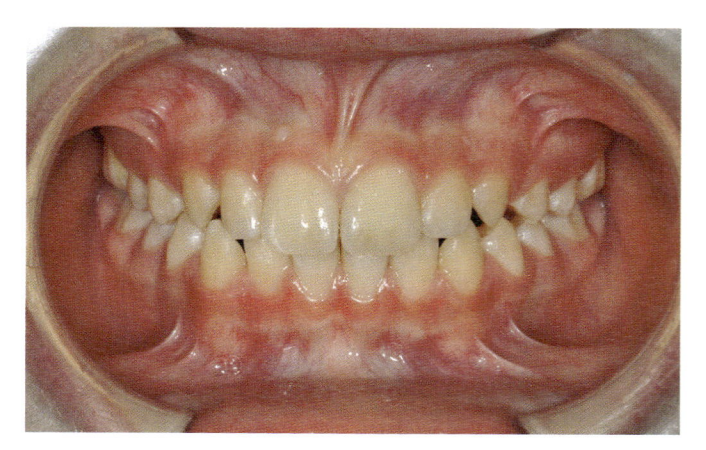

Fig. 20.23 Frontal intraoral photograph after the first stage of treatment with palatal expander and grille.

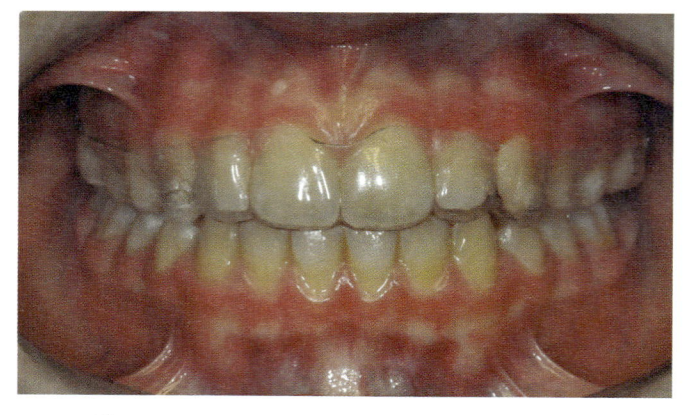

Fig. 20.24 Intraoral photograph during aligner therapy.

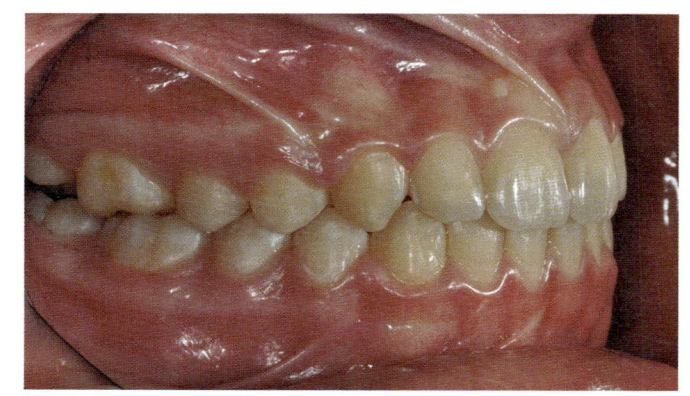

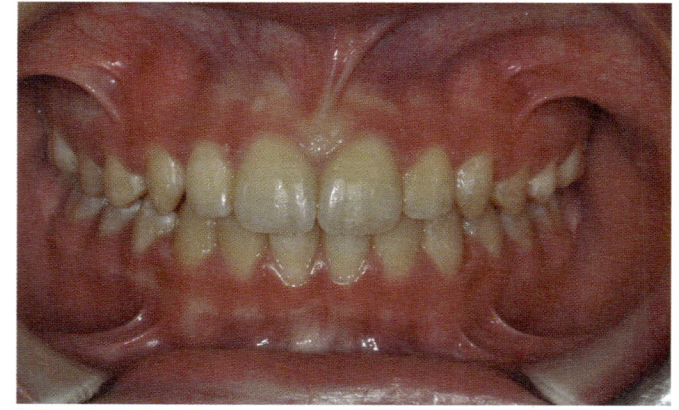

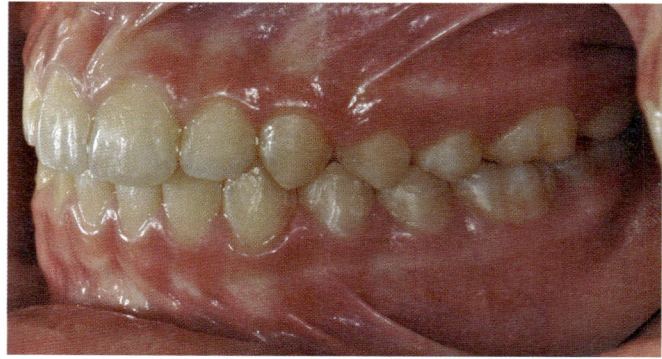

Fig. 20.25 Final intraoral photographs after 10-step aligner treatment.

Molar Distalization

It has been demonstrated that aligners are able to distalize the upper molars with a very high degree of efficacy (roughly 87%) when the extent of the planned movement is around 2.5 mm.[28] However, our clinical experience has shown that bodily molar distalization is not, in fact, achievable by means of aligners, as they provide only very limited root control. In 2015, Zhang[29] demonstrated, in a study of 32 patients who underwent cone-beam computed tomography (CBCT) before and after aligner treatment, that irrespective of the type of orthodontic movement planned, what was achieved were large crown movements but very small root movements. This made it clear that the aligners were acting to tilt the teeth rather than move them bodily.

With this in mind, in molar distalization cases[30] (Fig. 20.29), it is preferable to plan derotation around the palatal root, with distal inclination of the crown rather than bodily movement. Knowing that derotation of the upper molar is not sufficient to correct class II, and may cause anchorage loss, it is better to employ class II elastics (Fig. 20.30). The effect of these elastics is to mesially incline the teeth in the lower arch, preventing the upper canines and incisors from moving mesially (Fig. 20.31).

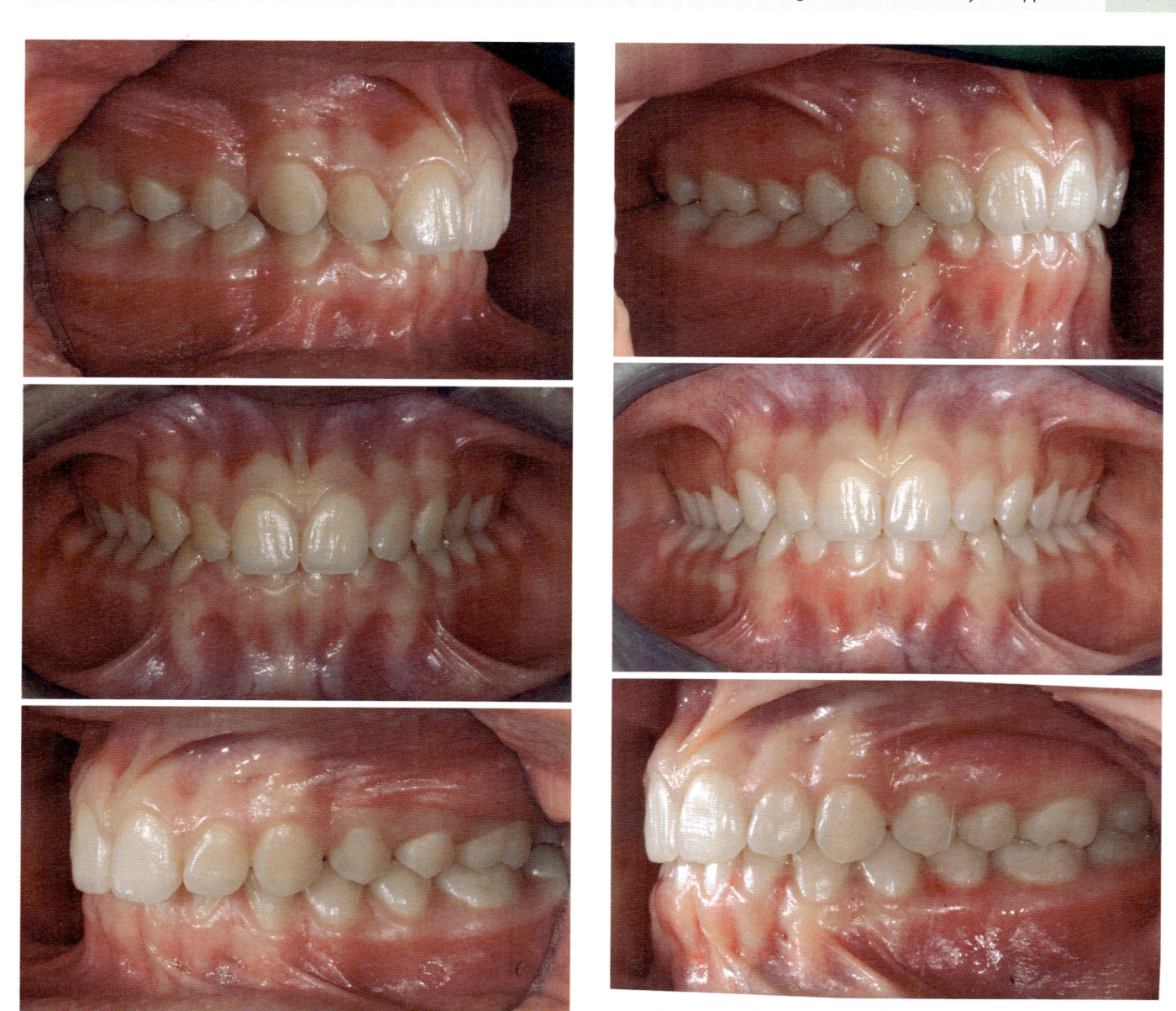

20 • Overcoming the Limitations of Aligner Orthodontics: A Hybrid Approach

Fig. 20.26 Initial intraoral photographs of a young patient with deep bite and class II.

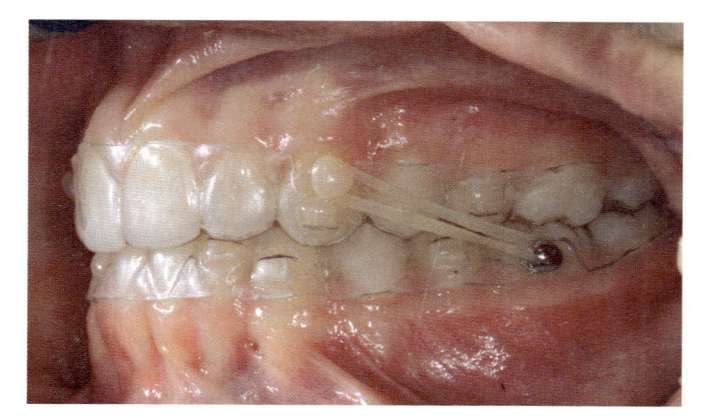

Fig. 20.27 Lateral intraoral photograph during aligner therapy combined with class II elastics.

Fig. 20.28 Final intraoral photographs after 14-step aligner treatment.

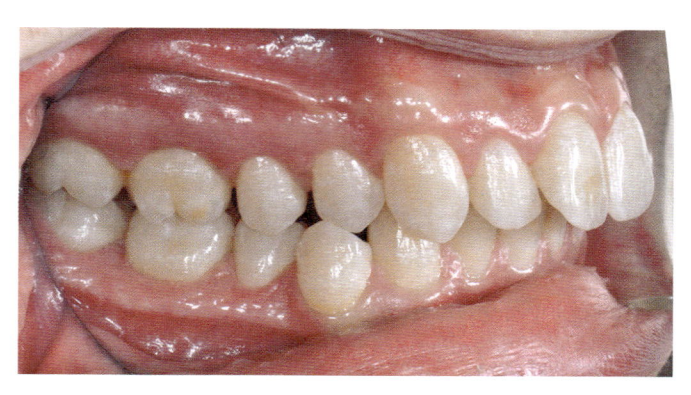

Fig. 20.29 Right initial intraoral photograph of a patient with class II subdivision and contraction of the upper jaw.

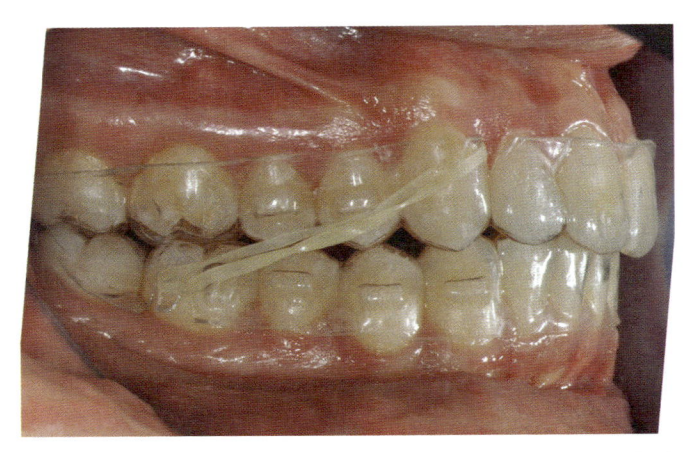

Fig. 20.30 Lateral intraoral photograph during aligner therapy combined with class II elastics.

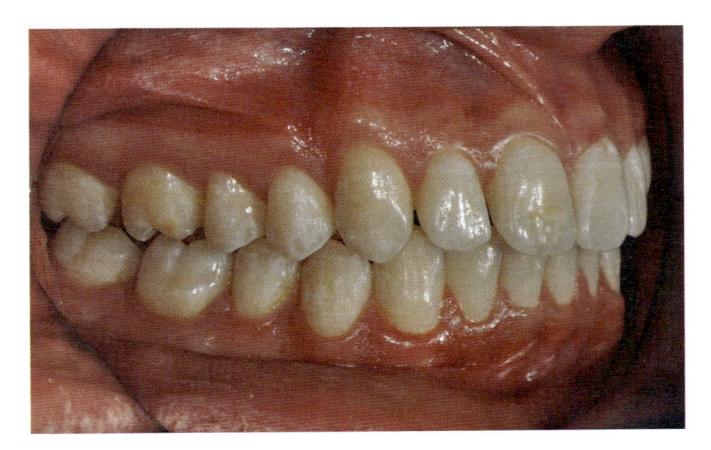

Fig. 20.31 Right lateral intraoral photograph lateral after aligner treatment.

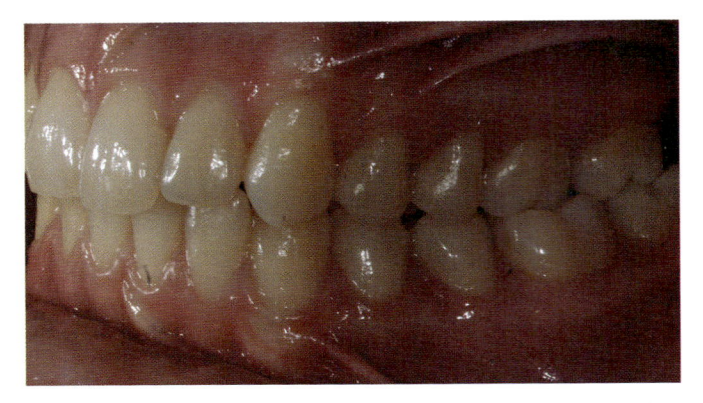

Fig. 20.32 Left initial intraoral photograph of a patient with class II subdivision and contraction of the upper jaw.

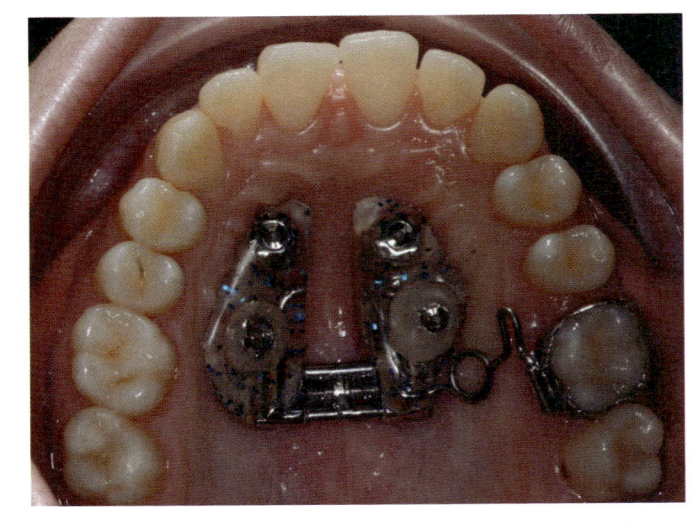

Fig. 20.33 Rapid palatal expansion and pendulum with skeletal anchorage (MAPA method).

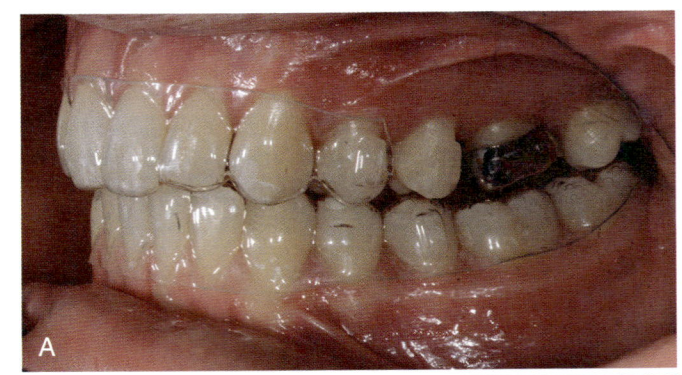

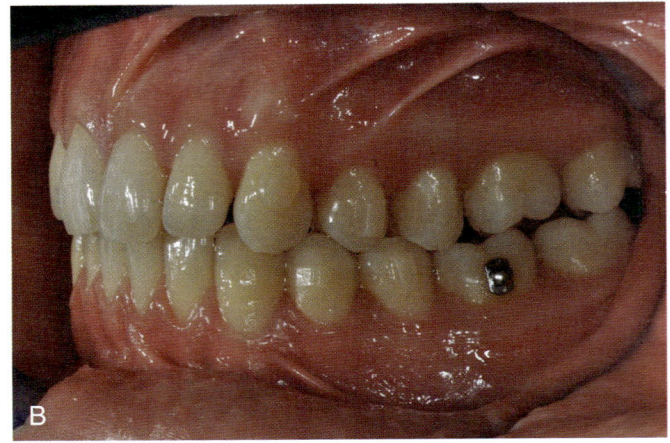

Fig. 20.34 Lateral intraoral photographs during aligner therapy (A) and combined with class II elastics (B).

That being said, there are cases in which the class II is so severe that molar distalization alone is not sufficient to resolve sagittal issues. In this patient (Fig. 20.32), for example, it would be unrealistic to expect to achieve 7-mm distalization via bodily movement with aligners. Hence we decided to expand the upper jaw using a rapid palatal expander anchored to four miniscrews, positioned using the MAPA method,[31-33] in combination with a monolateral pendulum (Fig. 20.33). This approach enabled us to resolve first the transversal issues and then the sagittal, quickly, unobtrusively, and without the need for patient compliance. Once class I had been achieved, a series of 14 aligners was planned to close the spaces in the upper arch and coordinate the arches (Fig. 20.34). In this case, the application of aligners in combination with class II elastics on the right

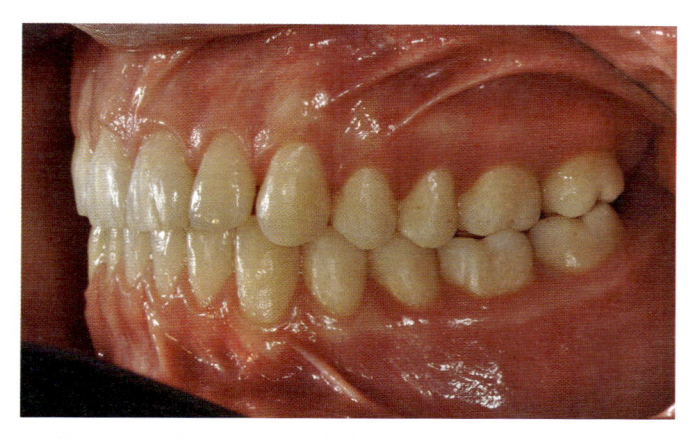

Fig. 20.35 Left lateral intraoral photograph after aligner therapy.

side (to promote distalization of the upper premolars and canines) enabled us to treat the malocclusion with satisfactory results over a short period of time (Fig. 20.35).

Conclusions

The scientific and clinical evidence now shows that aligners are able to resolve malocclusion in a growing number of cases. On the other hand, their limitations in terms of achieving transverse expansion via bodily movement has been amply documented. It also appears that they are unable to predictably derotate canines and premolars. What is more, limitations have been described for extrusion and intrusion movements and control of overbite and occlusal contacts. On the basis of these findings, and the knowledge that the solution to these problems cannot be an endless series of aligners, we propose a hybrid approach combining aligner therapy with different orthodontic devices to provide satisfactory and predictable clinical outcomes.

References

1. Kesling HD. The philosophy of tooth positioning appliance. *Am J Orthod.* 1945;31:297-304.
2. Ponitz RJ. Invisible retainers. *Am J Orthod.* 1971;59:266-272.
3. Sheridan JJ, LeDoux W, McMinn R. Essix retainers: fabrication and supervision for permanent retention. *J Clin Orthod.* 1993;27:37-45.
4. Bouchez R. *Clinical Success in Invisalign Orthodontic Treatment.* Paris: Quintessence International; 2010.
5. Sheridan JJ. The readers' corner 2: what percentage of your patients are being treated with Invisalign appliances? *J Clin Orthod.* 2004;38:544-545.
6. Joffe L. Invisalign: early experiences. *J Orthod.* 2003;30:348-352.
7. Baldwin DK, King G, Ramsay DS, et al. Activation time and material stiffness of sequential removable orthodontic appliances. Part 3: premolar extraction patients. *Am J Orthod Dentofacial Orthop.* 2008;133:837-845.
8. Kravitz ND, Kusnoto B, BeGole E, et al. How well does Invisalign work? A prospective clinical study evaluating the efficacy of tooth movement with Invisalign. *Am J Orthod Dentofacial Orthop.* 2009;135(1):27-35.
9. Womack WR. Four-premolar extraction treatment with Invisalign. *J Clin Orthod.* 2006;40(8):493-500.
10. Womack WR, Day RH. Surgical-orthodontic treatment using the Invisalign system. *J Clin Orthod.* 2008;42(4):237-245.
11. Kamatovic M. *A Retrospective Evaluation of the Effectiveness of the Invisalign Appliance Using the PAR and Irregularity Indices.* Toronto: University of Toronto (Canada); 2004.
12. Galan-Lopez L, Barcia-Gonzalez J, Plasencia E. A systematic review of the accuracy and efficiency of dental movements with Invisalign. *Korean J Orthod.* 2019;49:140-149.
13. Boyd RL. Increasing the predictability of quality results with Invisalign. *Proceedings of the Illinois Society of Orthodontists.* Oak Brook; 2005.
14. Kravitz ND, Kusnoto B, BeGole E, et al. How well does Invisalign work? A prospective clinical study evaluating the efficacy of tooth movement with Invisalign. *Am J Orthod Dentofacial Orthop.* 2009;135:27-35.
15. Lagravère MO, Flores-Mir C. The treatment effects of Invisalign orthodontic aligners: a systematic review. *J Am Dent Assoc.* 2005;136:1724-1729.
16. Rossini G, Parrini S, Castroflorio T, et al. Efficacy of clear aligners in controlling orthodontic tooth movement: a systematic review. *Angle Orthod.* 2015;85:881-889.
17. Rossini G, Parrini S, Castroflorio T, et al. Periodontal health during clear aligners treatment: a systematic review. *Eur J Orthod.* 2015;37:539-543.
18. Zheng M, Liu R, Ni Z, et al. Efficiency, effectiveness and treatment stability of clear aligners: a systematic review and meta-analysis. *Orthod Craniofac Res.* 2017;20:127-133.
19. Solano-Mendoza B, Sonnemberg B, Solano-Reina E, et al. How effective is the Invisalign system in expansion movement with Ex30' aligners? *Clin Oral Investig.* 2017;21(5):1475-1484.
20. Houle JP, Piedade L, Todescan Jr R, et al. The predictability of transverse changes with Invisalign. *Angle Orthod.* 2017;87(1):19-24.
21. Buschang PH, Ross M, Shaw SG, et al. Predicted and actual end-of-treatment occlusion produced with aligner therapy. *Angle Orthod.* 2015;85(5):723-727.
22. Lombardo L, Arreghini A, Ramina F, et al. Predictability of orthodontic movement with orthodontic aligners: a retrospective study. *Prog Orthod.* 2017;18(1):35.
23. Maino G, Turci Y, Arreghini A, et al. Skeletal and dentoalveolar effects of hybrid rapid palatal expansion and facemask treatment in growing skeletal class III patients. *Am J Orthod Dentofacial Orthop.* 2018;153:262-268.
24. Lombardo L, Carlucci A, Maino BG, et al. Class III malocclusion and bilateral cross-bite in an adult patient treated with miniscrew-assisted rapid palatal expander and aligners. *Angle Orthod.* 2018;88(5):649-664.
25. Kravitz ND, Kusnoto B, Agran B, et al. Influence of attachments and interproximal reduction on the accuracy of canine rotation with Invisalign. A prospective clinical study. *Angle Orthod.* 2008;78(4):682-687.
26. Simon M, Keilig L, Schwarze J, et al. Treatment outcome and efficacy of an aligner technique—regarding incisor torque, premolar derotation and molar distalization. *BMC Oral Health.* 2014;14:68.
27. Lombardo L, Arreghini A, Martines E, et al. Stress relaxation properties of four orthodontic aligner materials: a 24-hour in vitro study. *Angle Orthod.* 2017;87(1):11-18.
28. Guarneri MP, Oliverio T, Silvestre I, et al. Open bite treatment using clear aligners. *Angle Orthod.* 2013;83(5):913-919.
29. Zhang XJ, He L, Guo HM, et al. Integrated three-dimensional digital assessment of accuracy of anterior tooth movement using clear aligners. *Korean J Orthod.* 2015;45(6):275-281.
30. Lombardo L, Colonna A, Carlucci A, et al. Class II subdivision correction with clear aligners using intermaxillary elastics. *Prog Orthod.* 2018;19(1):32.
31. Maino G, Paoletto E, Lombardo L, et al. MAPA: a new high-precision 3D method of palatal miniscrew placement. *EJCO.* 2015;3(2):41-47.
32. Maino BG, Paoletto E, Lombardo III L, et al. A three-dimensional digital insertion guide for palatal miniscrew placement. *J Clin Orthod.* 2016;50(1):12-22.
33. Maino BG, Paoletto E, Lombardo L, et al. From planning to delivery of a bone-borne rapid maxillary expander in one visit. *J Clin Orthod.* 2017;51(4):198-207.

Index

Page numbers followed by "*f*" indicate figures and "*t*" indicate tables.

A

Afferent fibers, 253
Aging, of polymers, 30
Align appliance, 125–126, 125*f*, 126*f*
Aligner
  auxiliaries, 43–47
    attachments and pressure areas, 43–45, 44*f*
    interproximal reduction, 45–46
    intraoral elastics, 45
    temporary anchorage devices, 47
  discoloration, 36
  extrusion, 18–19, 18*f*, 19*f*
  plastics, 17
Aligner material properties
  clinical loading patterns, 40–41, 40*f*
  long-term loading, 37–40, 39*f*, 40*f*
  mechanical properties, 35
  optical changes, 36, 36*f*
  optical material changes, 35
  short-term mechanical loading
    multiple cycle, 37, 38*f*
    occlusal forces, 37
    single, 36–37, 37*f*
  water absorption, 35, 36*f*
Aligner orthodontics
  anchorage, 47
  application, 13
  attachments, 13
  basic attachment configurations
    anterior extrusion, 18–19, 18*f*, 19*f*
    first-order control, 19–21, 20*f*, 21*f*
    posterior intrusion, 19, 19*f*
    second-order control, 21–23, 21*f*, 22*f*, 23*f*, 24*f*
    third-order control, 24–26, 24*f*, 25*f*, 26*f*, 27*f*, 28*f*
    vertical control, 17
  biologic considerations, 48–49
  biomaterials, 13
  functions
    delivering predetermined force vectors, 17, 17*f*, 18*f*
    providing aligner retention, 16, 16*f*
    slipping avoid, 16, 17*f*
  geometry, 13, 15*f*
  hybrid approach
    canine and premolar rotation, 277–284, 281*f*, 282*f*, 283*f*, 284*f*, 285*f*
    extrusion, intrusion, and overbite control, 284, 285*f*, 286*f*, 287*f*
    molar distalization, 286–289, 287*f*, 288*f*, 289*f*
    transverse expansion, 275–277, 276*f*, 277*f*, 278*f*, 279*f*, 280*f*, 281*f*
  improvements, 13
  location, 14–15, 15*f*, 16*f*
  in prerestorative patients, 168–189
  sequentialization, 47
  size, 15
  translucent composites, 13
Aligner planning software, 191–194
Aligner "slipping," 16, 17*f*
Aligner-tooth mismatch, 13, 14*f*
American Dental Association Council on Scientific Affairs (CSA), 6
Anchorage management, 47

Anterior open bite
  biomechanics, for correction, 95
  diagnosis, 95
  treatment
    alternatives, 99, 104
    attachments, 96–97, 96*f*, 97*f*
    ClinCheck software design, 95–96
    objectives, 99, 100*t*, 104, 105*t*
    plan, 99, 104, 105*f*
    results, 100–102, 101*f*, 102*f*, 102*t*, 105, 106*f*, 107*f*, 108*f*, 108*t*
    sequence, 99–100, 100*f*, 105, 106*f*
Arch development, class I malocclusions treatment plan, 51

B

Beneslider, clinical procedure and rational of, 190–191, 191*f*
Bicuspids, with plastic aligners, 19
Biomaterials, for attachment fabrication, 13
Biomechanical conventional attachment, class I malocclusions treatment plan, 51, 52*f*
Bolton analysis, 53
Bracket-based biomechanics, 21
Buccal tipping, 25, 25*f*

C

Calcitonin gene-related peptide (CGRP), 252–253
Canine impaction
  adverse sequelae of, 149
  clinical case, 157–158, 158*f*, 159*f*, 162*f*, 163*f*, 164*f*, 165*f*, 166*f*
  early diagnosis and treatment, 149–153, 152*f*, 153*f*
  late diagnosis, 153–154, 154*t*
  pathologic condition, 149
  prevalence, 149
  treatment, 149–153, 152*f*, 153*f*
    planning, 154–157, 154*f*, 155*f*, 156*f*
Carriere Motion 3D Appliance (CMA), 137, 138
CAT. *See* Clear aligner therapy (CAT)
CBCT. *See* Cone-beam computed tomography (CBCT)
Cephalometric analysis, 83, 97, 99*f*
Cervical vertebral maturation (CVM), 121
Chemical aging, of polymers, 30, 32–33
Class II elastics, 190
Class II malocclusions, 123–126, 125*f*, 126*f*
  clinical protocol, 67–68
  elastic effect, 67
  extractions, 67
  hybrid approach in
    case report, 138–139, 139*f*, 140*f*, 141*f*, 142*f*, 143–146, 143*f*, 144*f*, 145*f*, 146*f*, 147*f*
    with distalizing device, 137–138
  mandibular advancement, 67
  maxillary distalization, 68–78, 68*f*, 70*f*, 72*f*, 73*f*, 74*f*, 75*f*, 76*f*, 77*f*, 78*f*, 80*f*
  maxillary molar distalization, 66–67
  maxillary molar rotation, 67
  orthognathic surgery, 67
  therapeutic options, 66

Class I malocclusions, 51
  dentoalveolar discrepancy, 52, 52*f*, 53*f*, 54*f*
  diagnosis, 51
  morphologic discrepancy, 58–60, 61*f*, 62*f*, 63*f*
  preprosthetic need, 60–62, 64*f*
  tooth size discrepancy, 53–56, 55*f*
  transverse discrepancy, 56–58, 56*f*, 57*f*, 58*f*, 59*f*
  treatment, 51–52
Clear aligner therapy (CAT), 137, 252
  case study, 240–244, 241*f*, 242*f*, 243–244*f*, 245*f*, 246*f*, 247*f*, 248*f*, 249*f*, 250*f*
  complex movements, 42
  fundamentals recap, 49
  with Invisalign, 235
  patient compliance, 49
  surgery first, 237–240
  theoretical and practical considerations, 43–48
    analysis of movements occurring, 43–48
    final position analysis, 43, 43*f*
  transitioning, 237, 238–239*f*, 238*f*, 239*f*, 240*f*
  with virtual setup software, 210
Clear aligner treatment (CAT)
  class II malocclusions, 66
  of crowding, 52
ClinCheck software, 68–69, 83
  design, 95–96
  tools, 52*f*
  treatment plan, 18*f*
Complementary force vectors, 17, 17*f*
Computer-assisted design/computer-assisted manufacturing (CAD/CAM), 1
Cone-beam computed tomography (CBCT), 1, 2*f*, 153
  advantages, 5
  ALADA, 5
  ALARA concept, 5
  benefits, 6–7, 6*f*, 7*f*, 8*f*, 9*f*, 10*f*
  cephalometrics, 5
  with conventional panoramic examinations, 6
  low-dose radiographic procedures, 5–6
  orthodontic diagnosis and treatment planning, 5
  orthognathic surgery, 7
  upper airway, 7
Conventional attachments, of aligner auxiliaries, 44, 44*f*
Conventional bracket techniques
  orthodontic tooth movement with, 13, 14*f*
  torque modification of, 24, 24*f*
Creep, 17, 33, 37
Curve of Spee, 109–110, 110*f*

D

Deep bite
  case report, 111–114, 111*f*, 112*f*, 113*f*, 114*f*, 115*f*, 116*f*, 117*f*, 118*f*, 119*f*, 120*f*
  correlation between, 109
  curve of Spee level, 109–110, 110*f*
  definition, 109
  treatment strategies, 109
  upper incisors level, 110–111

290

Index

Dental arches, 3
Dentoalveolar discrepancy, 52, 52f, 53f, 54f
Dentofacial orthopedics, 1
Differential scanning calorimetry (DSC), 32
Digital Imaging and Communications in Medicine (DICOM), 7
Digital imaging techniques, 11, 11f
Digital impressions, 3
Digital models, 1–5, 3f
Digital smile design (DSD), 169
Distalization, 67
Double conventional attachment, 54f
Duplex, 56

E

Elastic aligner deformation, 13, 14f
Elastic effect, of class II malocclusions, 67
Elastic wear, 67
Enamel, 3–5
Esthetic analysis, 169
Ethanol, 31–32
Evolution, 1
Extraction
 diagnosis, 83, 84f, 85f, 86f
 of posterior teeth, 95
 treatment
  plan, 83
  progress, 83–87, 87f, 88f, 89f, 90f
  results, 87–91, 91f, 92f, 93f

F

Fabrication process, 32
Facial three-dimensional scan, 2f
Fewer aligners, 67
Finite element analysis (FEA), 15, 20–21
Finite element method (FEM), 44–45
Free gingival graft (FGG), 205–207
Furcation defects, 207–208

G

Gingival crevicular fluid (GCF) biomarkers, 125
Glass transition temperature, 32
Glassy material, 31–32

H

Hand and wrist maturation (HWM), 121
Horseshoe-shaped geometry, 25–26
Hygroscopic expansion, 35

I

Incisor control, class I malocclusions treatment plan, 51
Insufficient force levels, 25–26, 26f, 27f, 28f
Interceptive orthodontics, 121
 case reports, 122–123, 123f, 124f, 124t
 maxillary expansion, 121–122, 122f
Intermaxillary elastics, 16
Interproximal contacts, 11
Interproximal enamel reduction (IPR), 45–46
Interproximal reduction, class I malocclusions treatment plan, 51–52
Intraoral scans (IOSs), 1–5, 3f
Invisalign aligners, 138–139
Invisalign system, 83

L

Labial fixed orthodontic appliances, 236–237, 236f

Labial impactions, 157
Laser scanning, 7–9
Leone appliance, 125, 125f
Loss of tracking, 17

M

Malocclusion, 1
Mandibular advancement, 126–132, 127f, 128f, 130f, 132f, 133f, 134f
 phase, 126
Mandibular fixation, 236–237
Maxillary distalization, 68–78, 68f, 70f, 72f, 73f, 74f, 75f, 76f, 77f, 78f, 80f
Maxillary expansion (ME), 121–122, 122f
Maxillary molar distalization, 66–67
Maxillary molar rotation, 67
Maxillary transverse deficiency, 6
Mesiodistal movements, 210
Mini-implants, 190
Molar distalization
 aligner orthodontics, in hybrid approach, 286–289, 287f, 288f, 289f
 upper
  in aligner treatment, 190
  clinical case, 191–200, 192f, 193t, 194f, 195f, 196f, 197f, 198f, 200f
  clinical considerations, 200
Molars, with plastic aligners, 19
Mucogingival junction (MGJ), 157

N

National Commission on Radiation Protection and Measurements, 5
Near infrared (NIR) technology, 3–5, 4–5f

O

Open-bite treatment
 alternatives, 99, 104
 attachments, 96–97, 96f, 97f
 ClinCheck software design, 95–96
 for correction, biomechanics, 95
 objectives, 99, 100t, 104, 105t
 plan, 99, 104, 105f
 results, 100–102, 101f, 102f, 102t, 105, 106f, 107f, 108f, 108t
 sequence, 99–100, 100f, 105, 106f
Optimized attachments, of aligner auxiliaries, 44, 44f
Optimized Root Control Attachments, 22
Orthodontic applications, in polymers, 30
Orthodontic pain
 biologic mechanisms of, 252–253
 in clear aligner therapy, 253–254
 clinical considerations, 255–256, 256t
 clinical correlates, 252–253
 importance of, 252
 psychological factors, 254–255
Orthodontics, 1
 advances in, 168
 aligner, 1
 diagnosis, 1, 2f
 digital evolution in, 1
 2D imaging modalities, 5–6
Orthodontic tooth movement (OTM), 42
 staging, 47–48
Orthodontic treatment. See Retention
Orthodontists, 42
Orthognathic surgery, 7, 67, 235
Orthopantomography (OPG), 116f, 120f, 149, 152f
OrthoPulse, 91–93
Overerupted molars, 179

P

Pain, 252
Palatal impactions, 157
Palatally displaced maxillary canine (PDC) teeth, 149
Panoramic x-ray, 147f
Pathologic tooth migration (PTM), 202
Pendulum K appliance, 138
Periodontal disease
 clinical case, 214–220, 215f, 216f, 217f, 218f, 219f, 221f, 222f, 223f, 224f, 225f, 226f, 227f, 228f, 229f, 230f, 231f
 diagnosis, 205–210
 malocclusions related to, 202, 203f
 optimal control, 210–214
  flowchart, 214
  mesiodistal movements, 210, 212f
  vertical movements, 213–214, 213f
  vestibulolingual movements, 213
 orthodontic movements, 210–214, 212f
 orthodontic treatment in, 202, 204f
 retention, 214
 treatment planning
  multidisciplinary team, 205
  orthodontic assessment, 208, 208t, 209f, 211f, 212f
  patient expectations, 205, 205f
  periodontal assessment, 205–208, 205t, 206f, 206t
Periodontal ligament (PDL) strain, 22, 22f
Periodontitis
 grades, 205t, 220t
 stages, 206t, 219t
PETG. See Polyethylene terephthalate glycol (PETG)
Physical aging, of polymers, 30, 32–33
Plastic foil, 210
Plastic materials, 42
Polyethylene terephthalate glycol (PETG), 31, 35
 material, chemical structure of, 31f
Polymers
 chemical aging, 30, 32–33
 definition, 30
 materials, 30
 mechanical stability, 30
 molecular structure, 30–32, 31f
 in orthodontic applications, 30
 physical aging, 30, 32–33
 thermal properties, 30–32
Polyurethane (PU), 31
 material, chemical structure of, 31f
Pre–mandibular advancement phase, 126
PU. See Polyurethane (PU)

R

Rapid maxillary expansion (RME), 121, 122
Retention
 appliances, 266, 266f, 267f, 268f, 269f
 in orthodontic treatment, 259–260
 protocol, 260–261f, 260–264, 262f, 263f, 264–265f, 265f, 270–272
 specifics, 266–270, 270f, 271f, 272f, 273f
Revolution, 1
Rotation control, class I malocclusions treatment plan, 51
Runner, 125, 125f

S

Sequentialization, 47
Severe dentofacial deformity, 235

Slow maxillary expansion (SME), 122
Soft tissue data extraction, 7–9
Space management
    in anterior region, 168–169
    case study, 169–170, 169f, 170f, 171f, 172f, 173f
    in posterior region, 170–174, 175f, 176f, 177f, 178f
Specific volume, 31
Splint-aided maxillary, 236–237
Stability, 259–260
Stereophotogrammetry, 7–9
Stress relaxation, 17, 37–39, 40f
Subepithelial connective tissue graft (SCTG), 205–207
Supercooled region, 31–32
Surgery first, with aligner therapy, 235–251

T

Tangential forces, 16, 17f
Teeth segmentation, 9
Temporary anchorage devices (TADs), 47, 95, 157
Temporomandibular disorders (TMDs)
    case study, 180–184, 180f, 181f, 182f, 183f, 184f, 185f, 186f, 187f, 188f
    diagnosis, 179–180
    management, 179
    treatment plan, 179–180

Temporomandibular joint (TMJ), 7
Tensile measurements, 37–39
Thermoplastic aligner materials, 40
Thermoplastic polymers, 31
Thermoplastic polyurethane (TPU), 35
Thodontics. *See* Aligner orthodontics
3D data integration, 11, 11f
3D facial reconstruction techniques, 7–9, 10f
3D imaging
    cone-beam computed tomography, 5–6
    benefits, 6–7, 6f, 7f, 8f, 9f, 10f
    3D data integration, 11, 11f
    3D facial reconstruction techniques, 7–9, 10f
    virtual setup, 9–11, 11f
TMDs. *See* Temporomandibular disorders (TMDs)
Tooth alignment
    after aligner sequence, 13, 14f
    and leveling, 11
Tooth displacement patterns, of posterior teeth, 22, 22f
Tooth size discrepancy, 53–56, 55f
Tooth-tooth-gingiva segmentation, 9
Torque modification, of anterior teeth, 24
Tracing superimposition, 116f
Transition phase, 126
Transverse deficiency
    correction of, 24
    maxillary, 6

Transverse discrepancy, 56–58, 56f, 57f, 58f, 59f
Tumor necrosis factor-α (TNF-α), 252–253

U

Upper molar distalization. *See also* Molar distalization
    in aligner treatment, 190
    clinical case, 191–200, 192f, 193t, 194f, 195f, 196f, 197f, 198f, 200f
    clinical considerations, 200
Uprighting moment, of posterior teeth, 22f

V

Vertical movements, 213–214
Vestibulolingual movements, 213
Viscoelasticity, 31–32
Viscoelastic material, mechanical behavior of, 37

W

Water absorption, of aligner material properties, 35, 36f
Width of keratinized gingiva (WKT), 208